Aortic Dissection and Acute Aortic Syndromes

Frank W. Sellke
Editor-in-Chief

Joseph S. Coselli • Thoralf M. Sundt
Joseph E. Bavaria • Neel R. Sodha
Editors

Aortic Dissection and Acute Aortic Syndromes

Springer

Editor-in-Chief
Frank W. Sellke
Rhode Island Hospital
Brown University
Providence, RI
USA

Editors
Joseph S. Coselli
Department of Surgery
Baylor College of Medicine
Houston
USA

Thoralf M. Sundt
Massachusetts General Hospital and
Harvard Medical School
Boston, Massachusetts
USA

Joseph E. Bavaria
Perelman Center for Advanced Medicine
University of Pennsylvania
Philadelphia, Pennsylvania
USA

Neel R. Sodha
Thoracic Cardiothoracic Surgery
Rhode Island Hospital and Alpert Medical
School of Brown University
Providence, RI,
USA

ISBN 978-3-030-66670-5 ISBN 978-3-030-66668-2 (eBook)
https://doi.org/10.1007/978-3-030-66668-2

This Springer imprint is published by the registered company Springer Nature Switzerland AG
The registered company address is: Gewerbestrasse 11, 6330 Cham, Switzerland

Contents

Part I
History, Presentation and Genetics of Acute Aortic Syndromes

Overview and History of Aortic Dissection and Other Acute Aortic Syndromes

Afshin Ehsan and Frank W. Sellke

Introduction

Acute aortic syndromes are complex and potentially life-threatening pathologies of the aorta that have only been successfully managed in the last 70 years. The spectrum of disease ranges from intra-mural hematomas and penetrating aortic ulcers to aortic dissections and ruptured aneurysms, with dissections being the most frequent of these aortic pathologies. The ability to diagnose and treat these conditions have required advances in imaging as well as open and endovascular surgical techniques. The historical evolution of our understanding of these conditions and subsequent management reflect the critical nature of acute aortic syndromes and the pioneering efforts of innovators determined to improve the outcomes of these complex patients.

History of Acute Aortic Syndromes

The earliest reports of aortic pathology were noted in the Ebers Papyrus, an Egyptian scroll named after the Egyptologist, George Ebers (1837–1898 CE), which dates back to 1550 BCE. The scrolls are believed to be copied from earlier texts and it's here that peripheral and abdominal aneurysms were first described [1]. The Greek physician, Galen de Pergamon (129-c. 200/c. 216 CE), described "localized pulsatile swellings" and a ruptured aneurysm: "when an aneurysm is wounded, the blood spouted out with so much violence that it can scarcely be arrested" [2]. A Greek surgeon and contemporary of Galen, Antyllos, further described aneurysms as being either false traumatic or true aneurysms. He also provided the earliest record of

A. Ehsan (✉) · F. W. Sellke
Warren Alpert Medical School of Brown University and Rhode Island Hospital, Providence, RI, USA
e-mail: aehsan@lifespan.org

J. S. Coselli et al. (eds.), *Aortic Dissection and Acute Aortic Syndromes*,
https://doi.org/10.1007/978-3-030-66668-2_1

performing surgery to treat small peripheral aneurysms by ligating them proximally and distally followed by opening of the sac and evacuation of the thrombus. He further opposed surgery for larger aneurysms given that he believed they were too dangerous to treat. His approach to managing peripheral aneurysms remained the treatment of choice until the end of the nineteenth century [3, 4]. The Flemish physician, Andreas Vesalius (1514–1564 CE) was the first to solely use human anatomic dissections for what served as the modern recording of human anatomy. He identified aneurysms of the thoracic and abdominal aorta and considered them untreatable [5, 6]. German physician, Daniel Sennert (1572–1637 CE) appears to be the first to report aortic dissections, describing them as a separation of the aortic wall layers" while Giovanni Battista Morgagni (1682–1771 CE) reported several cases whereby blood forced its way through the wall "coming out under the external coat of the artery" [7, 8].

In 1760 George II, King of England, (Fig. 1) died in Kensington palace "while straining on the toilet". The King had woken up at 6 am that morning and was following his morning routine when his "valet de chamber in waiting" heard a noise, after which he found the king lying on the floor, dead. The King's personal physician, Frank Nicholls (1699–1778 CE), was ordered to open and embalm the body, which provided him with the opportunity to carefully document the cause of death. His detailed account of the findings served as the first documentation of pericardial

Fig. 1 George II, King of England (1683–1760)

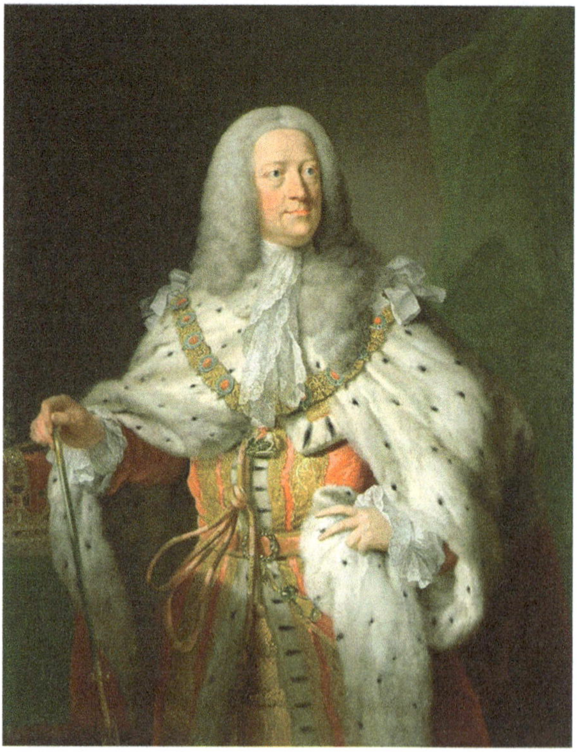

tamponade caused by an aortic dissection. He specifically noted "...the pericardium was found distended with a quantity of coagulated blood, nearly a pint...; the whole heart was so compressed as to prevent any blood contained in the veins from being forced into the auricles; therefore the ventricles were found absolutely void of blood...; and in the trunk of the aorta we found a transverse fissure on its inner side, about an inch and a half long, through which some blood had recently passed under its external coat and formed an elevated ecchymosis" [9, 10]. Interestingly, King George II was also Duke of Hannover. This is the same Hannover in Germany that has been the site of many advances in aortic surgery.

In 1802, Jean Pierre Maunoir proposed the term "aortic dissection", however in 1819, French surgeon René Théophile Laennec, the inventor of the stethoscope, was the first to use the term "dissecting aneurysm" [11, 12]. Since that time, this designation has created confusion regarding the nature of dissections and aneurysms and their distinct differences. In 1822, John Shekleton (1795–1824 CE) of Dublin was the first to report cases of chronic dissections, or what was described as "double barreled" aortas. His findings included a description of atheromatous changes on the lining of the aorta as well as the presence of a re-entry site into the original lumen [13]. In 1839, Viennese pathologist Carl von Rokitansky (1804–1878 CE) explained the difference between aortic dissection and spontaneous rupture [14]. In 1843 Thomas Peacock reported a case series of aortic dissections where he documented the importance of an intimal tear and hypothesized that the dissection was the result of a disruption of the "internal coats of the vessel". Through experimental models of aortic dissections, he also described the reentry of flow back into the original vessel considering it an "imperfect natural cure of the disease". He further described the difference in prognosis between dissections involving the ascending aorta versus those in the descending aorta [15, 16]. Other notable experts at that time offered an alternative theory to the concept of penetration of the aortic wall given that cases of dissection were identified that lacked a tear in the vessel. They believed that a primary cleavage of the media was the triggering event that led to dissection [17, 18]. At the end of the nineteenth century and into the early part of the twentieth century, several theories as to the pathophysiology of dissections existed. They varied from atheromatous ulcerations versus consequences of inflammation with "molecular changes of the elastic structures and subcellular events" along with stress from elevated blood pressure occurring in the wall of the aorta and lastly rupture of the vasa vasorum [19–21].

In 1934, Theodore Shennan published the largest series of aortic dissections at that time and proposed that degenerative changes in the media resulting in a loss of elasticity was an important factor leading to dissections. He also believed mechanical, inflammatory, and congenital factors could also be involved [22]. French pediatrician, Antoine Marfan, reported the first case of arachnodactyly in 1896 and studied the symptoms of the disease that would later bear his name but it was Helen Taussig and colleagues in 1943 that made the association between Marfan disease and aortic medianecrosis [23, 24]. That same year Lewis Etter reported the association between Marfan disease and aortic dissections [25]. In 1958, Albert E. Hirst published a report of over 500 aortic dissections that provided important detailed information about the etiology and pathogenesis of the disease along with valuable clinical insights. Also included in the report were the medical and surgical treatment strategies that had been employed up until that time [26].

Although less common than aortic dissection, intramural hematoma is another of the acute aortic syndromes. First described by Hans Eppinger Sr (1848–1916 CE) in 1887, it was Fredrich Krukenberg in 1920 that made the observation that a ruptured vaso vasorum can lead to a "dissection without intimal tear" [27, 28]. Penetrating aortic ulcer was first described as a clinical condition in 1986 by Anthony Stanson and colleagues and is also included in the scope of acute aortic syndromes [29].

Treatment of Acute Aortic Syndrome

Until surgical options became available, treatment of patients with aortic dissections centered largely around medical therapies. Mandatory bed rest was the mainstay of treatment in the eighteenth and nineteenth centuries and if patients were restless they received sedation along with morphine for pain. With the advent of antihypertensive medications, treating elevated blood pressures were felt to be of value by some, while others believed that the therapy itself encouraged dissections in patients with hypertension. In patients experiencing shock, the administration of whole blood plasma, intravenous fluids and vasoconstrictors were employed as these therapies became available [30–32]. Unfortunately, as can be expected, the success of these approaches was quite limited and reflected the need for more direct corrective therapies.

Throughout the nineteenth century, a variety of procedures were developed and used to address aortic aneurysms. Foreign bodies such as wires and needles were inserted into aneurysms along with the delivery of electrical currents with the idea of stimulating thrombus formation within the aneurysm sac. In doing so they would obliterate the artery thus stabilizing the aneurysm and preventing further growth or rupture [33–35]. The more sophisticated technique of endoaneurysmorrhaphy was introduced in the latter half of the century whereby surgeons would open the aneurysms with the intention of either obliterating the blood flow through the vessel from within versus reconstructing the vessel by creating a normal caliber lumen to maintain patency and excluding the aneurysm sac [36–38].

An alternative approach to addressing aneurysms and dissections were to wrap the involved vessels with either prosthetic or biologic materials in an attempt to stabilize the vessel and prevent rupture. The technique of wrapping cellophane around an aneurysm was introduced by Paul Harrison in 1943 whereby he wrapped two arteriovenous aneurysms of the subclavian artery resulting in their eventual elimination [39]. In 1948, James Edgar Paulin was the first to use cellophane to treat a dissection when he wrapped the material around a chronically dissected descending aorta [40]. Others reported the use of fascia lata, polyvinyl sponge, and dermal wrappings, all which were eventually abandoned due to poor results [41, 42]. After being diagnosed with an abdominal aortic aneurysm, Albert Einstein underwent cellophane wrapping of his aneurysm in 1948 but died 5 years later from subsequent rupture of the dilated vessel.

The first direct surgical treatment of an aortic dissection was performed by David Gurin and colleagues in 1935 to treat an ischemic leg caused by extension of the dissection into the right external iliac artery. Although the procedure was unsuccessful, Gurin attempted to reestablish blood flow into the leg by opening the vessel through the non-dissected segment and incising the intima into the dissected segment thus establishing a re-entry point for blood back into the true lumen [43]. In 1955, Robert S Shaw reported a similar strategy to improve blood flow back into the true lumen of a dissected thoracic and abdominal aorta. It was Shaw who coined the term "fenestration", and this remains the name of the procedure to date. Despite its improvement of flow into the true lumen, the procedure did not address the complexities associated with ascending and arch dissections and was soon recognized as a largely palliative procedure [44].

A critical step in the evolution of treating aortic pathology was the development of techniques that resected and subsequently replaced portions of the diseased vessel. The pioneering work of Nobel laureate Alexis Carrel along with Charles Guthrie led to the development of vascular anastomotic techniques and the use of homograft aortic substitutes [45]. Clarence Crafoord in 1944, was the first to resect a segment of the aorta and reestablish continuity with an end to end anastomosis to treat a coarctation and in 1948 Robert Gross was the first to replace a segment of the aorta using a homograft after resecting a coarctation [46, 47]. The direct repair of an aortic dissection was first performed by Michael DeBakey at Houston Methodist Hospital. In 1955 he reported a series of six cases whereby he repaired the descending thoracic aorta injured by dissection. In five of the procedures the aorta was transected and the false lumen was obliterated by sewing the true lumen circumferentially to the adventitia. Aortic continuity was then reestablished by either direct end to end anastomosis of the native aorta or placement of a homograft interposition (Fig. 2). The remaining case involved primary resection of a saccular aneurysm

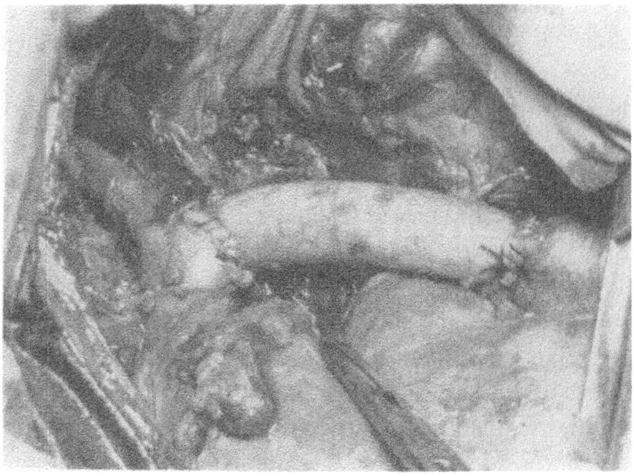

Fig. 2 Repair of descending thoracic dissection using homograft as demonstrated by DeBakey and colleagues in 1955. (Taken from: DeBakey ME, Cooley DA, Creech O. Surgical considerations of dissecting aneurysms of the aorta. Ann Surg. 1955;142:586–610)

distal to the left subclavian artery followed by primary closure of the resultant defect [48].

The success of treating thoracic aortic pathology using homografts initially generated great hope and enthusiasm for the definitive treatment of conditions that were until that time felt to be untouchable. However, the limited durability and availability of homografts as well as less than optimal long-term outcomes, soon tempered that enthusiasm. As a result, a more durable and readily available alternative to homografts was needed. The development of synthetic arterial grafts began with the work of Arthur Voorhees who proposed the use of a tube constructed from fabric. First using a silk handkerchief and subsequently a material called "vinyon-N", Voorhees reported the successful use of these prosthetic grafts in animal experiments in 1952 [49]. The first use of a synthetic graft to treat an aortic pathology was by Arthur Blakemore who used a graft made from vinyon-N to replace a ruptured abdominal aortic aneurysm in 1953 [50]. Charles Hufnagel reported the use of a Lucite tube containing his aortic assist valve to replace a large portion of descending thoracic aorta as a means of treating aortic insufficiency [51]. Although not intended to teat aortic pathology, this and the use of other synthetic grafts provided further proof of concept that the aorta can be replaced with a synthetic substitute. However, the poor physical adaptability, limited durability and inconsistent biocompatibility of vinyon-N and other materials such as Orlon and Teflon limited their wider acceptance and use. The polyester polymer Dacron, initially developed around 1939, was introduced to DeBakey in a department store when he was shopping for material to construct vascular grafts. Using his wife's sewing machine, he created grafts that he then trialed in animals beginning in 1954. He found Dacron to be easier to sew to then vinyon-N and more physically adaptable for use in arterial reconstruction. In collaboration with industry, he led the development of seamless knit Dacron grafts of various sizes that were either tube shaped or had bifurcating segments to accommodate a variety of anatomic needs. The grafts were also constructed with circumferential crimping to allow for greater flexibility to shape the grafts without kinking. After 2 years of animal testing, DeBakey and his colleagues began to use the new grafts in humans and in 1958 they reported their experience of over 800 cases using these grafts in patients with occlusive disease of the abdominal aorta as well as the iliac and femoral arteries [52–54]. Further advances with synthetic grafts addressed issues of porosity and improved suture handling to the point where they have become the mainstay of arterial reconstruction.

Advances in cardiopulmonary bypass allowed for more complex approaches to the management of aortic pathologies particularly those involving the ascending aorta and arch. Denton Cooley and DeBakey were the first to report the successful resection and reconstruction of an ascending aortic aneurysm using a homograft in 1956 [55]. The following year DeBakey and colleagues reported the first successful replacement of the aortic arch once again using a homograft [56]. The first report of successful treatment of an ascending aortic dissection was by William Muller in 1960. In this series of three patients with Marfan's syndrome and aortic aneurysms with aortic insufficiency, two were found to have dissections. As a result, the ascending aorta was resected and replaced with a Teflon graft. (Fig. 3) The aortic

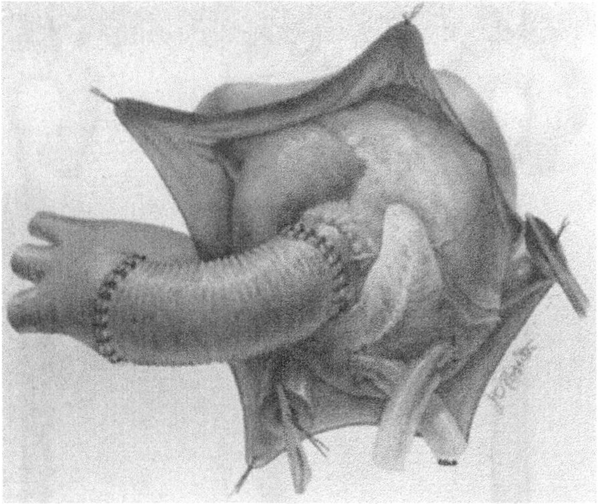

Fig. 3 Repair of ascending aortic dissection using a Teflon graft as demonstrated by Muller and colleagues in 1960. (Taken from: Muller WH Jr., Dammann JF Jr., Warren WD. Surgical Correction of Cardiovascular Deformities in Marfan's Syndrome. Ann Surg. 1960;152:506–516)

insufficiency was addressed using a bicuspidization technique that resulted in reducing the size of the dilated aortic annulus. The noncoronary sinus, leaflet and annulus were excised followed by primary closure of the defect resulting in a competent bicuspid aortic valve [57]. This report also served as the first to describe the management of an aortic dissection in Marfan's patients and addressed the treatment of aortic valve insufficiency that can result from dissections or dilation of the aortic root. Frank Spencer and colleagues also described repairing the aortic valve in patients with aortic dissections due to separation of the commissure from the aortic wall using commissural resuspension [58]. The first successful repair of an acute ascending aortic dissection performed emergently took place in 1962 once again by DeBakey and colleagues [59].

In an effort to simplify how aortic dissections were thought of and subsequently treated, DeBakey began publishing classification schemas as early as 1955. The schema he published in 1965, and then modified in 1982, serves as the classic DeBakey classification schema where he defined three types of aortic dissection. Type I was dissections originating in the ascending aorta and extending beyond the left subclavian to involve varying degrees of the descending thoracic and abdominal aorta. Type II dissections were those that originated and were isolated to the ascending aorta. And Type III dissections were those that originated in the descending thoracic aorta, sparing the ascending aorta and arch [60, 61]. In 1970 Pat Daily and his colleagues at Stanford reported their experience with treating acute aortic dissections and in doing so provided an alternative classification schema. They defined dissections that involved the ascending aorta, irregardless of distal extension, as Type A and dissections that spared the ascending aorta and arch as Type B (Fig. 4). The Stanford classification has become the more readily applied means of labeling dissections and with it has come the universal clinical understanding that Type A dissections are to be treated as a surgical emergency while uncomplicated Type B dissections are largely treated with medical therapy [62].

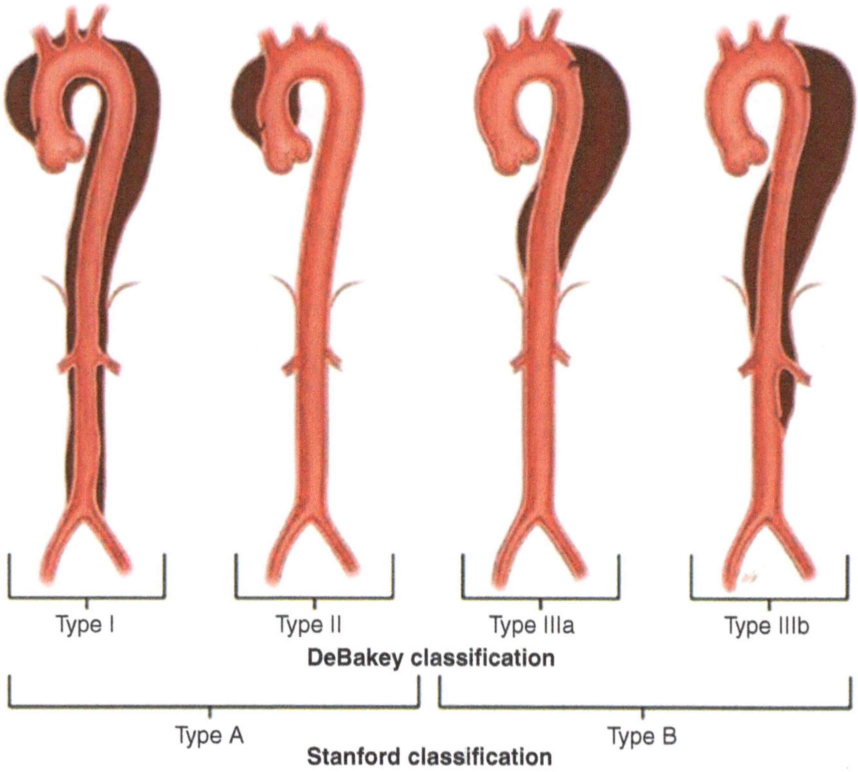

Fig. 4 Classification schemas for aortic dissection

The next phase in the advancement of treating aortic pathology was the development of procedures to address the aortic root. In 1962, Myron Wheat and colleagues reported the first replacement of the entire ascending aorta from the annulus to the innominate artery except for two small tongues of aortic wall containing the coronary ostia. The aorta was replaced with a woven Teflon graft and the aortic valve was replaced using a Starr-Edwards aortic prosthetic valve [63]. Hugh Bentall and Antony DeBono, in 1968, reported their technique for replacing the entire ascending aorta including the aortic root using a prosthetic valved conduit. The coronary ostia were anastomosed to corresponding openings on the graft while still in continuity with the native aortic tissue, given that the native aorta was then wrapped around the graft [64]. Kouchoukos and colleagues later described the resection of the pathologic aortic tissue and formation of coronary "buttons" that were anastomosed directly to the graft [65]. For patients with structurally normal aortic valves, valve sparing techniques were developed. Tyrone David introduced the technique of valve "reimplantation" in 1992 which entails implantating the native aortic valve inside a tube graft that is anchored to the aortic annulus and Magdi Yacoub, in 1993, reported the aortic remodeling technique which involves resecting the aorta to within 2–3 mm of the valve leaflets and commissures and anastomosing the graft to the cut edge of the aorta [66, 67]. These aortic root replacement procedures have been employed quite successfully in patients with dissections that leave the root either irreparably injured or with significant aneurysmal dilation [68, 69]. The choice of sparing the valve in the context of treating an acute dissection is dependent on the anatomy of the native valve and the degree to which the patient can withstand a potentially longer procedure, all the while being balanced against the expertise of the surgeon.

Other advances resulted in improved outcomes for patients with complex aortic pathology. Improved imaging modalities such as CT angiography, echocardiography, and MRI have made it possible to rapidly obtain detailed images in order to facilitate timely intervention. Deep hypothermic circulatory arrest and the use of cerebral perfusion techniques increased the safety of performing more complete arch procedures or procedures involving thoracoabdominal reconstructions [70–72]. The medical management of aortic dissections with a focus on reducing the "impulse" force of blood ejected from the left ventricle along with improved blood pressure control was introduced by Wheat and colleagues in 1965. This approach was the result of poor outcomes with the surgical management of aortic dissections and has since evolved into the practice of using pharmacologic therapy as the first line approach for uncomplicated Type B aortic dissections [73]. Endovascular treatment of arterial pathology began in the 1980s with the development of the first aortic stent grafts. The first clinical use was in 1985 when Nikolai Volodos placed a stent graft in the left common and external iliac artery of a patient to treat stenotic atherosclerotic disease manifesting signs of ischemia. Volodos and his colleagues were also the first to use a stent graft in the aorta to treat a post-traumatic pseudoaneurysm of the thoracic aorta [74]. Julio Palmaz developed the first balloon-expandable stent and in collaboration with Juan Parodi performed the first endovascular repair of an abdominal aortic aneurysm in 1990 [75]. The first use of an endovascular approach to treat a descending thoracic aneurysm was reported by Michael Dake and colleagues in 1994, and in 1999 two back-to-back reports detailed the use of this strategy towards treating Type B aortic dissections [76–78] (Fig. 5). In recent years, more sophisticated endovascular techniques have been developed in conjunction with more aggressive open surgical operations. The classic elephant trunk operation, first reported by Hans Borst and used to aggressively treat Type A aortic dissections, has been transformed to an endovascular frozen elephant trunk procedure [79, 80]. Lastly, the application of endovascular therapy has made its way to the ascending aorta as well, whereby direct treatment of high-risk patients with Type A aortic dissections have been reported, however, these have been limited to case series and single center experiences [81].

Treatment of the other acute aortic syndromes, and in particular intramural hematomas is somewhat controversial. Given that intramural hematomas have some similarities, but also some differences with acute aortic dissections, the management of this clinical entity has led to different schools of thought. In patients with involvement of the ascending aorta, some advocate surgical intervention based on a threshold of wall thickness, while others believe this presentation to be part of a spectrum of Type A dissections and should therefore be treated as such. Acute aortic

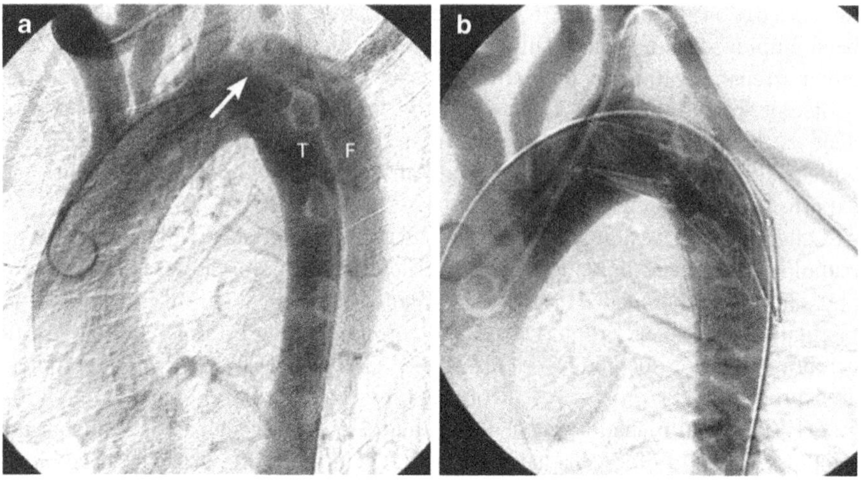

Fig. 5 Thoracic aortograms obtained before and immediately after stent–graft placement over the primary entry tear. (**a**) Before stent–graft deployment, there is flow of contrast medium from the true lumen (T) across the entry tear (arrow) into the false lumen (F). (**b**) After stent–graft placement, only the true lumen is evident. (Taken from: Dake MD, Kato N, Mitchell RS, Semba CP, Razavi MK, Shimono T, Hirano T, Takeda K, Yada I, Miller C. Endovascular stent-graft placement for the treatment of acute aortic dissection. N Engl J Med. 1999;340:1546–52

dissections, intramural hematomas and penetrating aortic ulcers can occur simultaneously or separately, but they share the characteristic of being potentially lethal and therefore needing sound clinical judgment for their treatment.

The purpose of this book is to gather the opinions of many of the world's experts in the treatment of acute aortic syndromes. It is meant to present a concise, practical approach to the diagnosis, treatment and surveillance of aortic disease. As with most difficult clinical conditions, opinions vary as to the best medical, surgical, and endovascular treatment. Importantly, it should be remembered that even though one author advocates one manner of treatment, there are many ways to manage acute aortic dissections and other acute aortic syndromes.

References

1. Ghalioungui P. The Ebers papyrus: a new English translation, commentaries and glossaries. Cairo: Academy of Scientific Research and Technology; 1987.
2. Galen J. Observations on aneurysms. London: Translated by John Eric Erichsen; 1986.
3. Daremberg C. Oevres d'Oribase. IV. Paris; 1867.
4. Sachs M. Die Methoden der Blutstillung in ihrer historischen Entwicklung. Hamostaseologie. 2000;20:83–9.
5. Vesalii A. De humani corporis fabrica libri septem. Padua; 1543.
6. Bonetus T. Sepulchretum anatomia practica ex cadaveribus morbo denatis. Book 3, Sect 2. Lugduni (Lyon); 1700. p. 290.

7. Sennertus Daniel. Opera. Op Omn Lib 5,1, Cap 42, p.306 Lugduni (Lyon); 1650.
8. Battista MG. De sedibus et causis morborum per anatomen indagates [the seats and causes of diseases investigated by anatomy; in five books, containing a great variety of dissections, with remarks]. Ep 26, Art 17 (Ep 48) F 50. Venice; 1761.
9. Nicholls L. Observations concerning the body of his late majesty. Philos Trans (Lond). 1761;52:265–74.
10. Leonard JC. Thomas Bevill peacock and the early history of dissecting aneurysm. Br Med J. 1979;2:260–2.
11. Maunoir JP. Mémoires Physiologiques et Practiques sur l'Aneurysme et la Ligature des Artères. Géneva; 1802.
12. Laennec RT. De l'Auscultations Médiate, ou Traité du Diagnostic des Maladies des Poumons et du Coeur. Paris: Fondé Principalemente sur ce Nouveau Moyen d'Esploration; 1819.
13. Shekleton J. Dublin Hosp. Rep. 1822;3:231.
14. Rokitansky VK. Über spontane Zerreissungen der Aorta. Schmidts Jahrbuch. 1839;24:30–3.
15. Peacock TB. Report on cases of dissecting aneurysms. Trans Path Soc Land. 1863;14:87.
16. Peacock TB. An account of some experiments illustrative of the mode of formation of the dissecting aneurysm. Monthly J Med Sci. 1843;3:871–8.
17. Whitman RG, Stein HB. A contribution to the pathogenesis of dissecting aneurysms: a case of dissecting Mesaortitis (babes and Mironescu), without dissecting aneurysm. J Med Res. 1924;44:579–92.
18. Babes V, Mironescu T. Über dissezierende Arteriitis und Aneurysma dissecans. Beitr Pathol Anat Allg Pathol. 1910;48:221.
19. Virchow R. Handbuch der speciellen Pathologie und Therapie. Erlangen; 1854.
20. Recklinghausen FD. Auserlesene pathologisch-anatomische Betrachtungen. Virchows Arch Pathol Anat Physiol. 1864;30:372–87.
21. Recklinghausen FD. Handbuch der allgemeinen Pathologie des Kreislaufs und der Ernährung. Stuttgart; 1883.
22. Shennan T. Dissecting aneurysm. In: medical research council special report, series no. 193. London: His Majesty's Stationary Office; 1934.
23. Marfan AB. Un cas de déformation congénitale des quatre members, plus prononcée aux extrémités, caracterisée par l' allongement des os avec un certain degréd' amincissement. Bull Mem Soc Med Hop Paris. 1896;13:220–6.
24. Baer RW, Taussig HB, Oppenheimer EH. Congenital aneurysmal dilation of the aorta associated with arachnodactyly. Bull John Hopk Hosp. 1943;72:309–32.
25. Etter LE, Glover LP. Arachnodactyly complicated by dislocated lens and death from rupture of dissected aneurysm of the aorta. J Am Med Assoc. 1943;123:88–9.
26. Hirst AE, Johns VJ, Kime SW. Dissecting aneurysms of the aorta: a review of 505 cases. Medicine. 1958;37:217–79.
27. Eppinger H. Pathogenesis, Histogenesis und Aetiologie der Aneurysmen, einschließlich des Aneurysma equi verminosum: Pathologisch-anatomische Studien. Berlin; 1887.
28. Krukenberg E. Beitrage zur Frage des Aneurysma dissecans. Beitr Pathol Anat Allg Pathol. 1920;67:329–51.
29. Stanson AW, Kazmier FJ, Hollier LH, et al. Penetrating atherosclerotic ulcers of the thoracic aorta: natural history and clinicopathologic correlations. Ann Vasc Surg. 1986;1:15–23.
30. Beaven DW, Murphy EA. Dissecting aneurysm during methonium therapy; report of nine cases treated or hypertension. Br M J. 1956;1:77–80.
31. MacCuish RK. Dissecting aortic aneurysm; varied clinical picture. Br M J. 1953;1:71–3.
32. Pyke DA. Dissecting aneurysm of aorta; recovery after treatment with hexamethonium. Lancet. 1953;2:1189–90.
33. Ciniselli L. Sugli aneurismi dell'aorta toracica finora trattati colla elettro-puntura. Ann Univ Med. 1870;214:292.
34. Weir RF, Page ED. Aneurysm of the ascending aorta treated by Macewen's needling method for inducing white thrombus. NY Med J. 1892;55:510–1.

35. Siddique K, Alvernia J, Fraser K, Lanzino G. Treatment of aneurysms with wires and electricity: a historical overview. J Neurosurg. 2003;99:1102–7.
36. Matas R. Traumatic aneurysm of the left brachial artery. Incision and partial excision of the sac-recovery. Med New NY. 1888;53:462–6.
37. Matas R. Personal experiences in vascular surgery: a statistical synopsis. Ann Surg. 1940;112:802–39.
38. Creech O. Endo-aneurysmorrhaphy and treatment of aortic aneurysm. Ann Surg. 1966;164:935–46.
39. Harrison P, Chandy J. A subclavian aneurysm cured by cellophane fibrosis. Ann Surg. 1943;118:478–81.
40. Paullin JE, James DF. Dissecting aneurysms of the aorta. Postgrad Med. 1948;4:291–9.
41. Warren WD, Beckwith J, Muller WH. Problems in the surgical management of acute dissecting aneurysms of the aorta. Ann Surg. 1956;144:530–48.
42. Kirschner M, Schubert A. Lehrbuch der Chirurgie. Allgemeine u. spezielle chirurgische Operationslehre. Berlin; 1927.
43. Gurin D, Bulmer JW, Derby R. Dissecting aneurysm of the aorta: diagnosis and operative relief of acute arterial obstruction due to this cause. NY J Med. 1935;35:1200–2.
44. Shaw RS. Acute dissecting aortic aneurysms: treatment by fenestration of the internal wall of the aneurysm. N Engl J Med. 1955;253:331–3.
45. Smith RB. Presedential address: the foundations of modern aortic surgery. J Vasc Surg. 1998;27:7–15.
46. Crafoord C, Nylin G. Congenital coarctation of the aorta and its surgical treatment. J Thorac Surg. 1945;14:347–61.
47. Gross RE, Hurwitt ES, Bill AH, Peirce EC. Preliminary observations on the use of human arterial grafts in the treatment of certain cardiovascular defects. N Engl J Med. 1948;239:578–9.
48. DeBakey ME, Cooley DA, Creech O. Surgical considerations of dissecting aneurysms of the aorta. Ann Surg. 1955;142:586–610.
49. Voorhees AB, Jaretzki A, Blakemore AH. The use of tubes constructed from Vinyon "N" cloth in bridging arterial defects. Ann Surg. 1952;135:332–6.
50. Levin SM. Breakthrough: Arthur Blakemore and Arthur Voorhees Jr. J Vasc Surg. 2012;55:1829–31.
51. Hufnagel CA, Harvey WP, Rabil PJ, McDermott TF. Surgical correction of aortic insufficiency. Surgery. 1954;35:673–83.
52. DeBakey ME, Jordon GL, Abbott JP, Halpert B, O'Neal RM. The fate of dacron vascular grafts. Arch Surg. 1964;89:757–82.
53. DeBakey ME, Cooley DA, Crawford ES, Morris GC Jr. Clinical applications of a new flexible knitted dacron arterial substitute. Am Surg. 1958;24:862–9.
54. DeBakey ME, Crawford ES, Cooley DA, Morris GC Jr. Surgical considerations of occlusive disease of the abdominal aorta and iliac and femoral arteries; analysis of 803 cases. Ann Surg. 1958;148:62–80.
55. Cooley DA, DeBakey ME. Resection of entire ascending aorta in fusiform aneurysm using cardiac bypass. J Am Med Assoc. 1956;162:1158–9.
56. DeBakey ME, Crawford ES, Cooley DA, Morris GC Jr. Successful resection of fusiform aneurysm of aortic arch with replacement by homograft. Surg Gynecol Obstet. 1957;105:657–64.
57. Muller WH Jr, Dammann JF Jr, Warren WD. Surgical correction of cardiovascular deformities in Marfan's syndrome. Ann Surg. 1960;152:506–16.
58. Spencer FC, Blake H. A report of the successful surgical treatment of aortic regurgitation from dissecting aortic aneurysm in a patient with the Marfan syndrome. J Thorac Cardiovasc Surg. 1962;44:238–45.
59. Morris GC, Henly WS, DeBakey ME. Correction of acute dissecting aneurysm of aorta with valvular insufficiency. J Am Med Assoc. 1963;184:185–6.
60. DeBakey ME, Henly WS, Cooley DA, Morris GC, Crawford ES, Beall AC. Surgical management of dissecting aneurysms of the aorta. J Thorac Cardiovasc Surg. 1965;49:130–49.

61. DeBakey ME, McCollum CH, Crawfrom ES, Morris GC Jr, Howell J, Noon GP, Lawrie G. Dissection and dissecting aneurysms of the aorta: twenty-year follow-up of five hundred twenty-seven patients treated surgically. Surgery. 1982;92:1118–34.
62. Daily PO, Trueblood HW, Stinson EB, Wuerflein RD, Shumway NE. Management of acute aortic dissections. Ann Thor Surg. 1970;10:237–47.
63. Wheat MW Jr, Wilson JR, Bartley TD. Successful replacement of the entire ascending aorta and aortic valve. J Am Med Assoc. 1962;188:717–9.
64. Bentall H, DeBono A. A technique for complete replacement of the ascending aorta. Thorax. 1968;23:338–9.
65. Kouchoukos NT, Wareing TH, Murphy SF, Perrillo JB. Sixteen-year experience with aortic root replacement. Results of 172 operations. Ann Surg. 1991;214:308–18.
66. David TE, Feindel CM. An aortic valve-sparing operation for patients with aortic incompetence and aneurysm of the ascending aorta. J Thorac Cardiovasc Surg. 1992;103:617–21.
67. Sarsam MA, Yacoub M. Remodeling of the aortic valve annulus. J Thorac Cardiovasc Surg. 1993;105:435–8.
68. Irimie V, Atieh A, Kucinoski G, Jankulovski A, Zacher M, Urbanski PP. Long-term outcomes after valve-sparing anatomical aortic root reconstruction in acute dissection involving the root. J Thorac Cardiovasc Surg. 2019 Apr 25 [Online ahead of print].
69. Rosenblum JM, Leshnower BG, Moon RC, Lasanajak Y, Binongo J, McPherson L, Chen EP. Durability and safety of David V valve-sparing root replacement in acute type A aortic dissection. J Thorac Cardiovasc Surg. 2019;157:14–23.
70. Griepp RB, Stinson EB, Hollingsworth JF, Buehler D. Prosthetic replacement of the aortic arch. J Thorac Cardiovasc Surg. 1975;70:1051–63.
71. Kouchoukos NT, Wareing TH, Izumoto H, Klausing W, Abboud N. Elective hypothermic cardiopulmonary bypass and circulatory arrest for spinal cord protection during operations on the thoracoabdominal aorta. J Thorac Cardiovasc Surg. 1990;99:659–64.
72. Stamou SC, Rausch LA, Kouchoukos NT, Lobdell KW, Khabbaz K, Murphy E, Hagberg RC. Comparison between antegrade and retrograde cerebral perfusion or profound hypothermia as brain protection strategies during repair of type A aortic dissection. Ann Cardiothorac Surg. 2016;5:328–35.
73. Wheat MW Jr, Palmer RF, Bartley TD, Seelman RC. Treatment of dissecting aneurysms of the aorta without surgery. J Thorac Cardiovasc Surg. 1965;50:364–73.
74. Volodos NL. Historical perspective: the first steps in endovascular aortic repair: how it all began. J Endovasc Ther. 2013;20:S3–23.
75. Parodi JC, Palmaz JC, Barone H. Transfemoral intraluminal graft implantation for abdominal aortic aneurysms. Ann Vasc Surg. 1991;5:491–9.
76. Dake MD, Miller DC, Semba CP, Mitchell RS, Walker PJ, Liddell RP. Transluminal placement of endovascular stent-grafts for the treatment of descending thoracic aortic aneurysms. N Engl J Med. 1994;331:1729–34.
77. Nienaber CA, Fattori R, Lund G, Dieckmann C, Wolf W, von Kodolitsch Y, Nicolas V, Pierangeli A. Nonsurgical reconstruction of thoracic aortic dissection by stent-graft placement. N Engl J Med. 1999;340:1539–45.
78. Dake MD, Kato N, Mitchell RS, Semba CP, Razavi MK, Shimono T, Hirano T, Takeda K, Yada I, Miller C. Endovascular stent-graft placement for the treatment of acute aortic dissection. N Engl J Med. 1999;340:1546–52.
79. Borst HG, Walterbusch G, Schaps D. Extensive aortic replacement using the "elephant trunk" prosthesis. Thorac Cardiovasc Surg. 1983;31:37–40.
80. Karck M, Chavan A, Hagl C, Friedich H, Galanski M, Haverich A. The frozen elephant trunk technique: a new treatment for thoracic aortic aneurysms. J Thorac Cardiovasc Surg. 2003;125:1550–3.
81. Vallabhajosyula P, Gottret J-P, Bavaria J, Desai ND, Szeto WY. Endovascular repair of the ascending aorta in patients at high risk for open repair. J Thorac Cardiovasc Surg. 2015;149:S144–50.

Aortic Anatomy and the Pathophysiology of Acute Aortic Syndromes

Lauren V. Huckaby and Thomas G. Gleason

Introduction

Fascination with the pathogenesis of acute aortic dissection dates back to the death of King George II in 1760 who, after collapsing suddenly, was found at autopsy to have a "transverse fissure on the inner side of the ascending aorta 3.75 cm long, through which blood had recently passed in its external coat to form a raised ecchymosis" [1]. This was one of the first reports of aortic dissection and underscores key themes of acute aortic disease that remain true today. Though much progress has been made in the diagnosis, management, and prevention of aortic catastrophe, knowledge gaps remain in the understanding of the pathophysiology of thoracic aortic disease and in the identification of those patients most at risk for acute aortic events.

The foundations for optimal management of patients with thoracic aortic disease lie in the appreciation of the anatomy and pathophysiology of the thoracic aorta. Furthermore, recognition of the distinct etiologies and presentations of acute aortic syndromes is also a key component of management decisions. Consider, for instance, the case of an acute aortic dissection in a 20-year-old with Marfan syndrome compared to that of a 70-year-old with a degenerative thoracic aortic aneurysm. The underlying etiology will inform intra-operative decision-making and post-operative care and may be responsible for widely varying outcomes in these two patients. Technology has also driven a renewed focus on the anatomy and pathophysiology of aortic disease. Advances in radiologic imaging have increasingly been able to delineate subtle findings, such as intramural hematoma or

L. V. Huckaby
Department of Surgery, University of Pittsburgh, Pittsburgh, PA, USA

T. G. Gleason (✉)
Division of Cardiac Surgery, Department of Surgery, University of Maryland School of Medicine, Baltimore, MD, USA
e-mail: tgleason@som.umaryland.edu

J. S. Coselli et al. (eds.), *Aortic Dissection and Acute Aortic Syndromes*,
https://doi.org/10.1007/978-3-030-66668-2_2

penetrating atherosclerotic ulcer, which demand further investigation to accurately incorporate these findings into what is already known about the prognosis and natural history of thoracic aortic disease. Adoption of new operative techniques, including endovascular approaches, should also be accompanied by thorough consideration of the characteristics of the native aorta. This chapter reviews the embryology, anatomy, histology and pathophysiology of the normal and diseased thoracic aorta (Fig. 1).

Embryology

The third week of gestation marks the onset of development of the aorta and great vessels. By the eighth week, coordinated regression and persistence of the embryologic branches has resulted in the formation of an aortic arch more closely resembling that seen in the adult (Fig. 2). The thoracic aorta and its branches begin as two aortae, the dorsal and ventral, which are connected by six paired branchial arch arteries. These arches form in a craniocaudal manner. By the end of the fourth week, only the third, fourth and six arches are still present. The first and second arches have regressed, and the fifth arch never fully forms. By the fifth week, the internal carotid arteries form from the third arch. The dorsal aorta between the third and fourth aortic arches begins to atrophy, and this is complete by the end of the sixth week. The seventh cervical intersegmental arteries, which arise from the dorsal aorta, enlarge to contribute to the bilateral subclavian arteries. Additionally, by the end of the sixth week, the pulmonary arteries are formed from the ventral portion of the sixth aortic arch. While the right-sided dorsal portion of the sixth arch ultimately atrophies, the left dorsal sixth arch gives rise to the ductus arteriosus.

At this point, asymmetric development is responsible for the most common aortic configuration, with the aorta taking a leftward course. The aortic arch and proximal descending aorta develop from the left fourth aortic arch and left dorsal aorta, the right dorsal aorta having atrophied. The right subclavian artery develops from the right fourth aortic arch, a portion of the remaining right dorsal aorta and the intersegmental artery. The innominate artery on the right and the left common carotid artery form from the ventral aorta. The left subclavian artery arises from a left intersegmental artery. At the end of the eighth week, the primitive aorta resembles that seen in the adult.

Neural crest cells migrate to the primitive aortic arches to contribute to branching patterns and ultimately give rise to medial smooth muscle cells. Neuroectoderm has a significant contribution in aortopulmonary septation, driving differentiation of the aortic root and pulmonary trunk. The most proximal aspect of the aorta appears to have a greater influence from neural crest cells compared to the arch and descending aorta, although the exact role of neural crest in aortic development has yet to be fully elucidated. The origin of the coronary arteries is not firmly established but they likely arise from the epicardium of the heart and later connect with the aorta. The aortic valve itself is primarily derived from mesodermal cells.

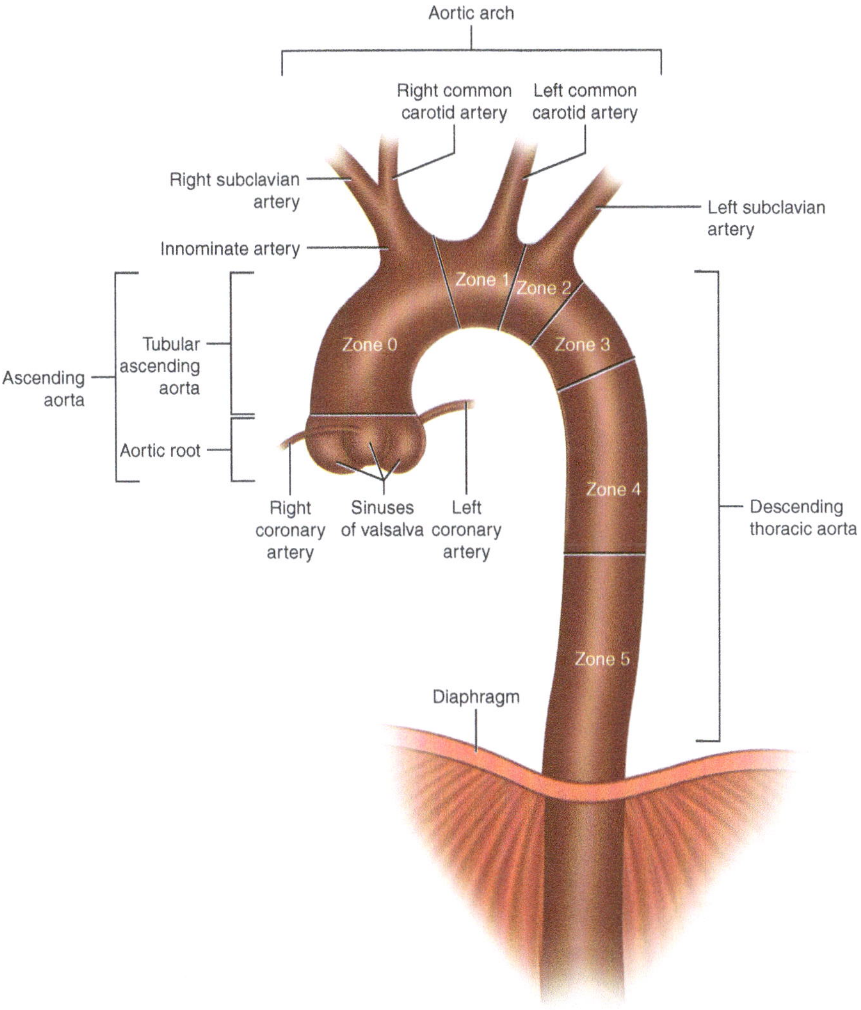

Fig. 1 Thoracic aorta. The thoracic aorta, from the aortic valve to the diaphragmatic hiatus, is divided into the ascending aorta (including the aortic root and tubular ascending aorta), aortic arch and descending aorta. The aortic root includes the aortic valve, aortic annulus, sinuses of Valsalva and the origins of the right and left coronary arteries

Regions of the Thoracic Aorta

The thoracic aorta can be subdivided into three regions: the ascending aorta, the aortic arch, and the descending thoracic aorta, and these have more recently been subdivided into six zones (Fig. 1). Aberrations in course and branching patterns may occur as a result of altered embryological development. The most common

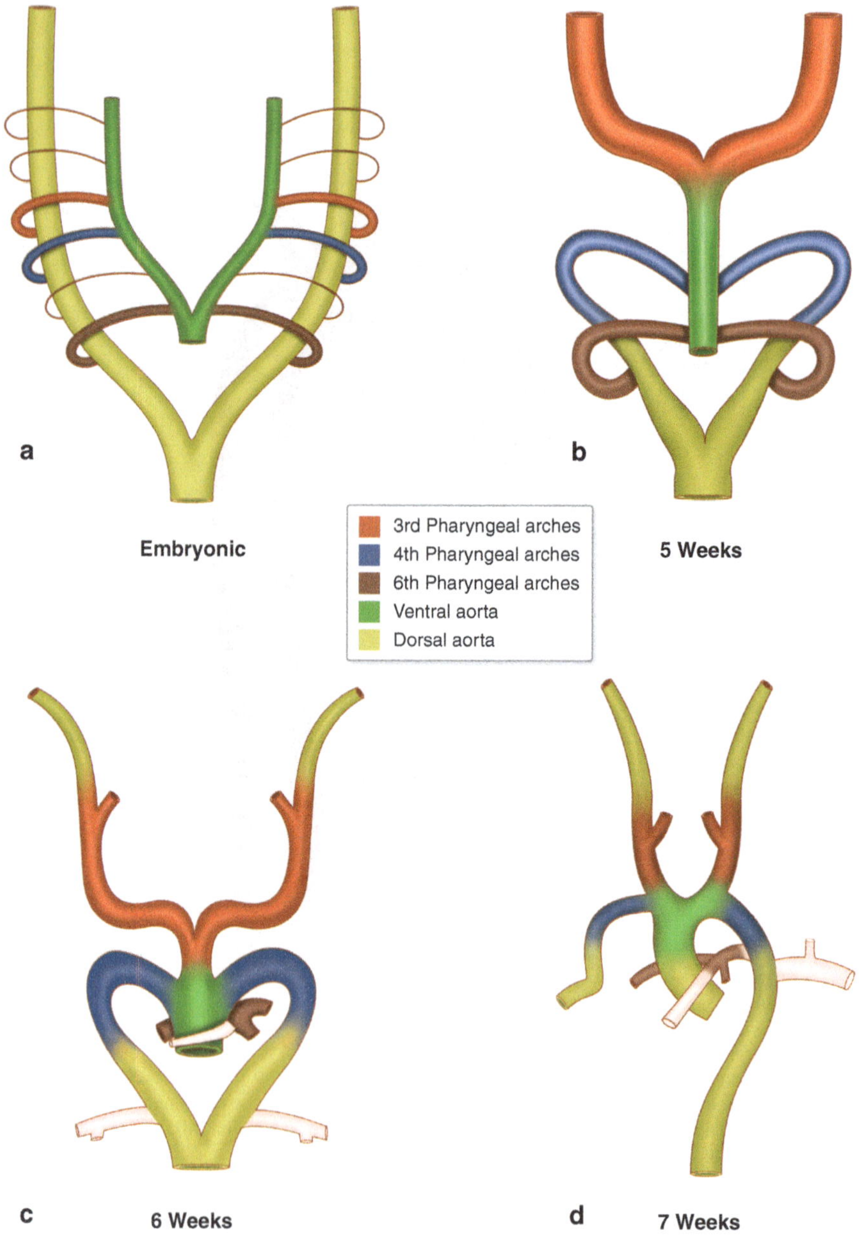

Fig. 2 Embryology of the thoracic aorta. The thoracic aorta is derived from the dorsal and ventral aortae and the paired pharyngeal vascular arches. Coordinated regression and persistence of the arches determines the course of the aortic arch and the configuration of the branches

configurations will be described first, and further attention will be directed to these anomalies in the next section.

Aortic Root and Ascending Aorta

The ascending aorta is composed of the aortic root and the tubular ascending aorta. The aortic root is the most proximal component and begins at the aortic annulus, a fibrous ring that supports the aortic valve and marks the transition from the left ventricle. From there, the aorta balloons slightly outward to form the three sinuses of Valsalva. The origins of the right and left coronary arteries are present at these sinuses and the aortic cusps and sinuses are named accordingly: right, left and non-coronary. The sinotubular junction delineates the transition between the aortic root and the beginning of the tubular ascending aorta. At this point, the aorta assumes a mostly uniform caliber and begins a superior path towards the arch. The aortic diameter is positively correlated with age. Variations in imaging modalities and in the level of aortic measurements in relation to other structures can influence reported values of normal aortic diameter. With these caveats, a study of 1442 subjects undergoing computed tomography angiography (CTA) showed that the ascending aorta at the level of the mid-pulmonary artery measures approximately 3.1 cm in females and is larger at approximately 3.4 cm in males [2]. In the retrosternal position, the remnant of the thymus overlies the aorta. The right atrial appendage lies anteromedial to the proximal ascending aorta with the pulmonary trunk coursing posterolaterally. Immediately to the right of the ascending aorta lies the superior vena cava (SVC). The transition from the ascending aorta to the arch also marks the superior extent of the pericardium.

Aortic Arch

The aortic arch commences at the origin of the innominate (brachiocephalic) artery which arises from the superior aspect of the aorta (Fig. 3a). This trunk is situated slightly anterior to the other arch vessels and takes a right and posterior course where it branches into the right subclavian and right common carotid arteries. The aortic arch curves posteriorly and to the left with its superior convexity reaching the level of the mid-manubrium. The subsequent great vessel branches from the arch are the left common carotid and left subclavian arteries, each arising successively posterior to the takeoff of the innominate artery. The left brachiocephalic vein courses anteriorly to all three head vessels at their most proximal aspects. The arch is intimately related to multiple mediastinal structures. It passes immediately anterior to the trachea (Fig. 3b). The left phrenic nerve runs anteriorly at the distal portion of the arch, and the right phrenic nerve lies lateral to the SVC. The right vagus nerve passes anterior to the right subclavian artery, giving

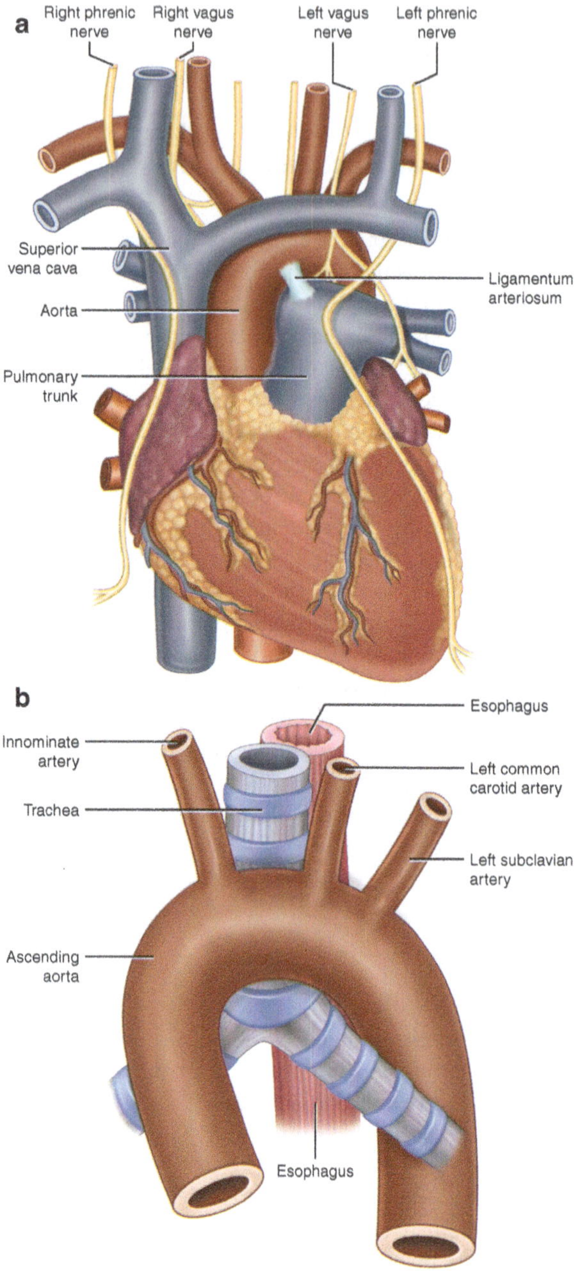

Fig. 3 Thoracic aorta and surrounding structures. (**a**) shows the aortic root and tubular ascending aorta. (**b**) shows the arch and proximal descending aorta. Note the proximity of the thoracic aorta to the pulmonary arteries, superior vena cava, vagus and phrenic nerves, trachea and esophagus. The vertebral column (not shown) lies directly posterior and to the right of the descending thoracic aorta

off its recurrent branch and then descending posterior to the right pulmonary hilum. The left vagus nerve passes anterior to the arch just at or medial to the take-off of the left subclavian artery and gives off the left recurrent laryngeal branch which continues inferiorly along the concave border of the arch just lateral to the ligamentum arteriosum, the fibrous remnant of the fetal ductus arteriosus and then ascends in the tracheoesophageal groove. The left pulmonary artery lies in close contact to the lesser curve of the arch. The aortic arch ends at approximately the T4-T5 vertebral level.

Descending Thoracic Aorta

The descending thoracic aorta begins after the origin of the left subclavian artery at vertebral level T4. This section runs immediately to the left of the vertebral bodies early in its course and gradually assumes a more medial position so that it lies almost at midline as it passes through the diaphragm. The descending aorta gives rise to pericardial, bronchial, esophageal, mediastinal, intercostal, and superior phrenic artery branches. The esophageal artery branches provide blood supply to the mid-esophagus. The posterior intercostal artery branches consist of nine paired vessels running along the undersurface of the lower nine intercostal spaces. The artery of Adamkiewicz originates from the 9th through 12th intercostal arteries and feeds the anterior spinal artery. In cases of descending thoracic aorta and thoracoabdominal aorta repair, reimplantation of intercostal vessels may be necessary to ensure adequate spinal perfusion via this artery. The descending aorta enters the diaphragm at the aortic hiatus at T12. The mid-descending thoracic aorta diameter is slightly smaller than the normal ascending aorta and measures approximately 2.70 cm in men and 2.46 cm in women [3].

Congenital Anomalies of the Thoracic Aorta

Left Aortic Arch with Aberrant Branching

In the majority of the population, the aortic arch takes a leftward course and descends to the left of the thoracic spine (Fig. 4a). With this configuration, up to 30% of the population display a bovine arch in which the left common carotid arises from the innominate artery (Fig. 4b). The aortic arch may also have four branches, as is the case with an aberrant right subclavian artery. With this, the right subclavian originates on the arch distal to the left subclavian, often from a dilated portion termed a diverticulum of Kommerell (Fig. 4c). It then runs posterior to the esophagus. The etiology of this configuration is an early regression of the right fourth pharyngeal arch in combination with persistence of the eighth segment of the dorsal aorta. The majority of individuals are asymptomatic, however dilatation of the aberrant

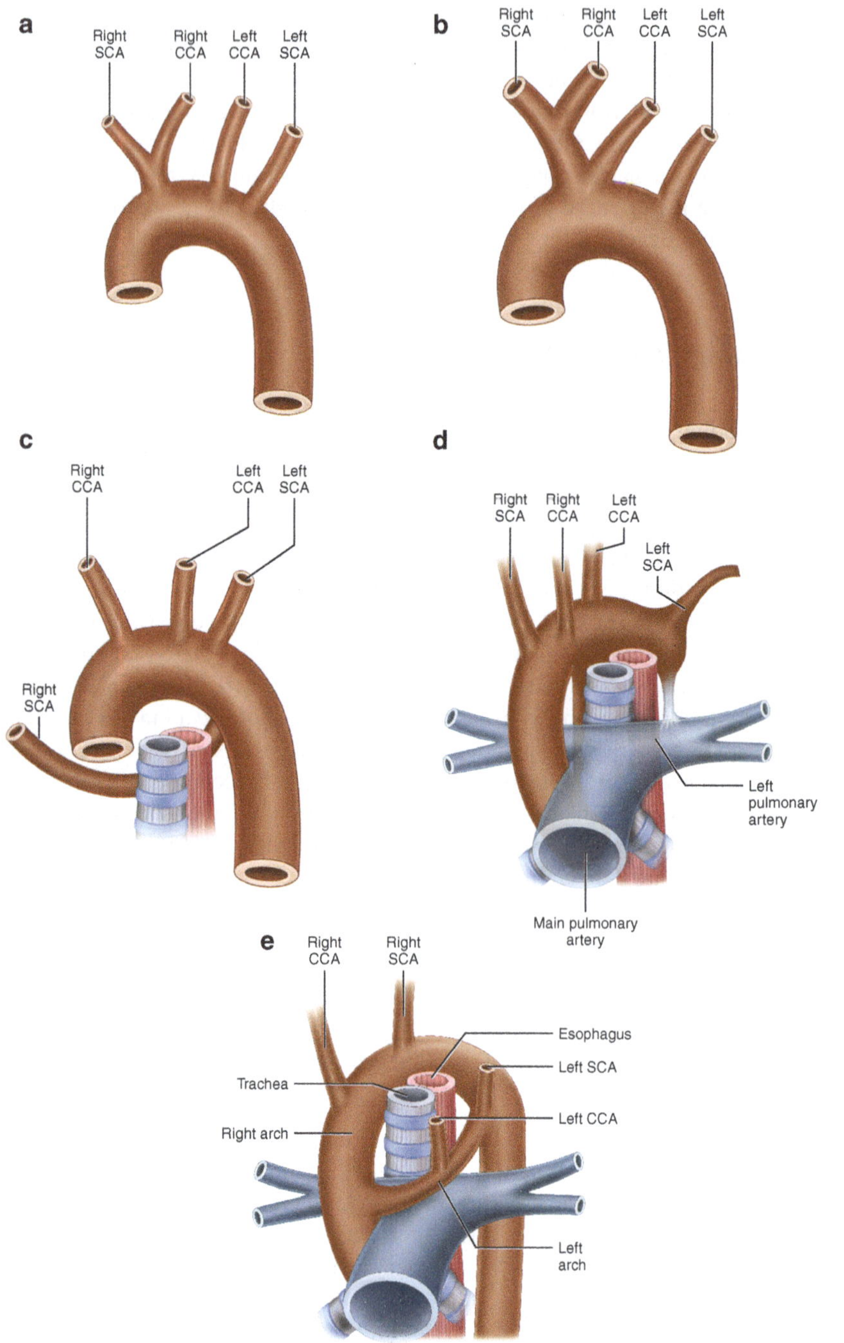

Fig. 4 Congenital variants of the aortic arch and branches. The most common aortic configuration (**a**) consists of a left-sided aorta which may display aberrant branching such as a bovine arch (**b**) or an aberrant right subclavian artery (**c**). A right-sided aortic arch (**d**) results from persistence of the right fourth pharyngeal arch whereas a double aortic arch (**e**) occurs as a result of persistence of both the right and left fourth pharyngeal arches. Common carotid artery (CCA), subclavian artery (SCA)

subclavian may compress the esophagus resulting in dysphagia lusoria. The left vertebral artery may also originate from the arch independent of the left subclavian artery in 3–4% of people [4].

Right Aortic Arch

A right-sided aortic arch is marked by an arch that crosses anterior to the right pulmonary bronchus (Fig. 4d). This occurs in less than 1% of the population. The anomaly is due to persistence of the right fourth pharyngeal arch in combination with regression of the left fourth pharyngeal arch and of the eighth dorsal aortic segment. The descending aorta usually runs to the right of the spine but may course on the left side. Vascular rings may result from incomplete regression and may cause compressive symptoms.

Double Aortic Arch

Persistence of both the right and left fourth pharyngeal arches in addition to the dorsal aorta results in a double aortic arch (Fig. 4e). Each arch serves as the origin for the ipsilateral carotid and subclavian arteries. The arches themselves may either be patent or atretic. The right arch typically extends more superiorly and posteriorly and is larger than the left. As this represents a true vascular ring, compressive symptoms may develop from obstruction of the trachea and/or esophagus.

Aortic Coarctation

Aortic coarctation is found more frequently than many of the aforementioned arch anomalies, accounting for approximately 5% of congenital heart disease diagnoses. Focal hyperplasia of the aortic media results in narrowing near the location of the fetal ductus arteriosus. Coarctation is associated with bicuspid aortic valve, Turner syndrome and ventricular septal defect. More severe lesions often present in infancy, however, development of collateral vessels may render this partial obstruction asymptomatic until incidentally detected in adulthood. In rare cases, coarctation may occur more distally in the descending thoracic aorta.

Histology of the Aortic Wall

Appreciation of the microscopic structure of the thoracic aortic wall helps to contextualize the thoracic aortic pathologies and the natural history of relevant disease processes that will be described in the following sections. Like other arterial

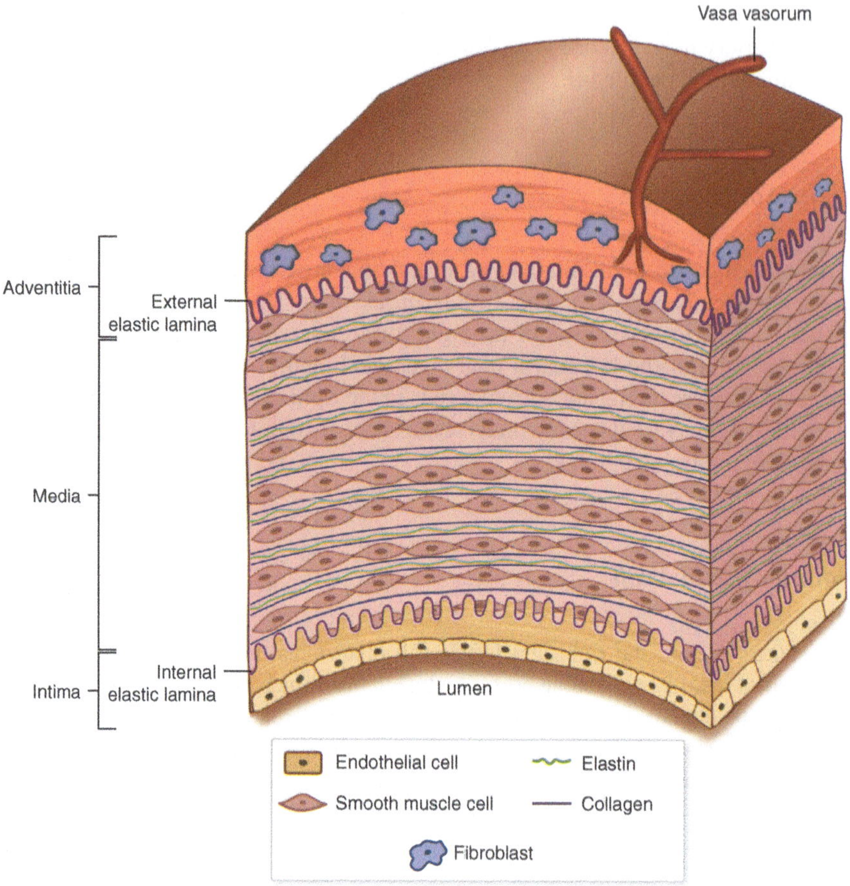

Fig. 5 Composition of the aortic wall. The outermost layer, the adventitia, consists of a collagen-based strength layer and provides blood supply to the aortic wall through the vasa vasorum. The aortic media is comprised of smooth muscle cells (SMCs) with structural extracellular matrix (ECM) components and the external elastic lamina. The intima is composed of an endothelial monolayer, connective tissue and the internal elastic lamina

structures, the aortic wall consists of three layers which, from the lumen moving outwards, are termed the intima, media and adventitia (Fig. 5).

The innermost layer, the intima, can be further subdivided into the single cell layered endothelium and subendothelial connective tissue. Endothelial cells mediate signaling between the lumen and the deeper layers of the aortic wall. For example, endothelial cells, in response to mechanical and biochemical signals, may influence the function of aortic smooth muscle cells in the medial layer. The intimal layer receives its blood supply via diffusion from the aortic lumen, which is also the source of oxygen and nutrients for the innermost portions of the medial layer. The internal elastic lamina, a fenestrated sheet of elastic fibers, separates the intimal layer from the media.

The medial layer has been a focus of investigation since Austrian pathologist Jakob Erdheim first described "medionecrosis aortae idiopathica" in 1929 [5]. While the exact pathogenesis of medial changes leading to aortic aneurysm or dissection have been debated since that time, there is no doubt that the thoracic aortic media plays a key role in both normal physiology as well as in pathophysiologic states. The media is the thickest of the three layers. Aortic smooth muscle cells (SMCs) constitute the main cell type and function to maintain the structural integrity of the aortic wall. Particularly important for aortic aneurysm pathophysiology, they are responsible for regulation of the extracellular matrix (ECM), consisting mainly of the fibrillar proteins collagen and elastin. Intact collagen fibers and elastin fibers, organized into elastic lamellae, confer strength and resist hemodynamic forces; fragmentation of these fibers is seen in diseased aortas, similar to that historically described as cystic medial necrosis. Fibrillin-1 is an essential component of the ECM, critical to organized elastin deposition, and mutations of this gene are responsible for the Marfan syndrome. The outermost portion of the media is delineated by the external elastic lamina.

The adventitia is the outermost layer of the aorta and contains the vasa vasorum, or blood vessels of the blood vessel. The vasa vasorum supplies the adventitia and outer portions of the media which do not receive sufficient blood supply via diffusion from the aortic lumen. In this layer, fibroblasts are the main contributing cell and are responsible for production of collagen fibers, mainly type I and type III, which constitute a majority of the volume of the adventitia. A layer of periadventitial fat often surrounds the three-layered vessel wall and may itself secrete paracrine factors which regulate aortic function, though investigation into its role is ongoing.

Thoracic Aortic Aneurysm

Dilatation of the aortic wall may be associated with heritable aortopathies, but more commonly is degenerative in nature and is therefore associated with aging. While often clinically silent and frequently diagnosed incidentally, thoracic aortic aneurysm (TAA) connotes an associated risk of aortic catastrophe, i.e. aorta dissection and/or rupture. Characteristics common to TAA of all etiologies include focal or global aortic wall integrity loss manifesting as saccular or fusiform aortic enlargement.

Aside from the heritable causes of TAA which are discussed in subsequent sections, risk factors for TAA include hypertension, smoking, age, and sex. Medial degeneration is the predominant histologic feature and may be driven by local cellular perturbations or result from the failure of the aortic wall to appropriately adapt and respond to physiologic hemodynamic forces (Fig. 6a–b). A systematic review of TAA growth identified larger diameter and distal aneurysmal disease as risk factors for accelerated aortic growth with an average growth rate of 0.2–4.2 mm/year [6].

Histologic features in descending thoracic aortic aneurysms often demonstrate the coexistence of atherosclerotic disease, which is not thought to be a driving factor in the pathogenesis of TAA in the ascending aorta. Extent of thoracoabdominal aneurysms follows the Crawford classification (with Safi modification): type 1 includes aneurysms originating distal to the left subclavian and terminating proximal to the renal vessels, type 2 extends the zone covered by type 1 to the aortoiliac bifurcation, type 3 involves aneurysms originating in the distal descending aorta

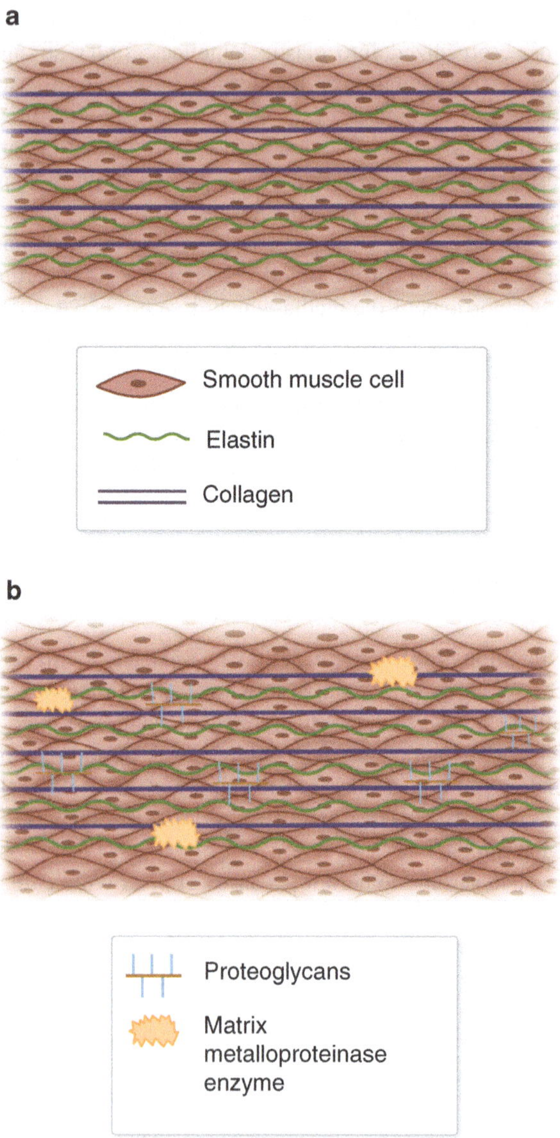

Fig. 6 Histology of the diseased aortic wall. Graphic depictions of normal (**a**) and aneurysmal (**b**) histology of the aortic wall are shown. Thoracic aortic aneurysm has historically been characterized by medial degeneration, consisting of the classic findings of smooth muscle cell (SMC) apoptosis, proteoglycan accumulation and extracellular matrix degradation

that extend to the aortic bifurcation, type 4 involves only the abdominal aorta with aneurysm originating at or around the mesenteric arteries extending to the aortic bifurcation, and type 5 aneurysms involve the distal descending aorta from around the sixth thoracic vertebrae to the mesenteric arteries [7].

Penetrating Atherosclerotic Ulcer and Intramural Hematoma

Improvements in radiologic technology, particularly computed tomography (CT), have expanded the spectrum of aortic pathologies that must be risk-stratified and appropriately managed. Penetrating atherosclerotic ulcer (PAU) is one such finding that was previously only detected histologically (Fig. 7a). PAU begins as an atheromatous plaque and progresses to ulceration of the intima with disruption of the internal elastic lamina and may lead to hematoma formation within the media. It

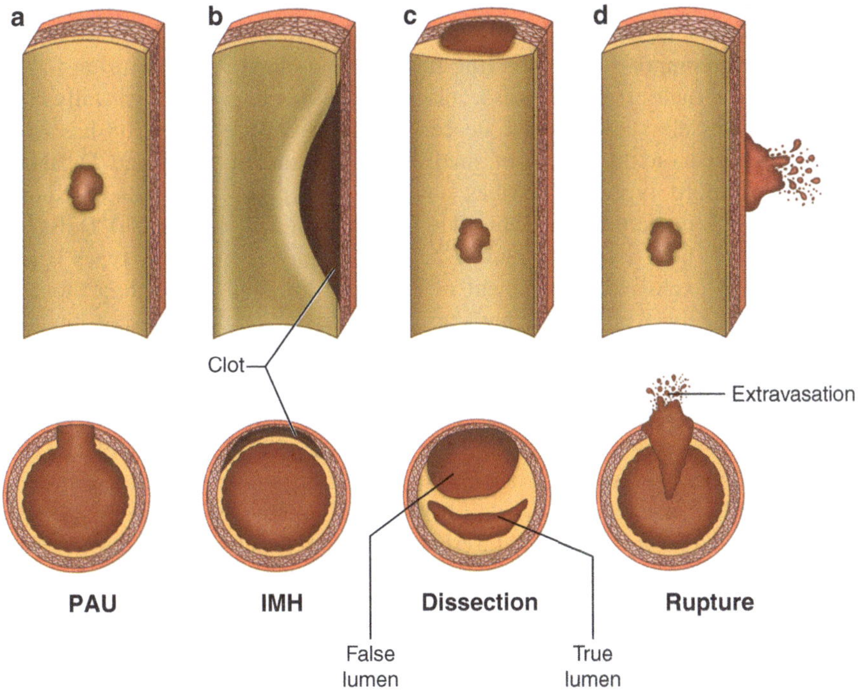

Fig. 7 Spectrum of acute aortic processes. Penetrating atherosclerotic ulcer (PAU), intramural hematoma (IMH) and acute aortic dissection (AAD) constitute radiologic and gross findings of acute aortic syndromes. PAU (**a**) represents ulceration of an atherosclerotic plaque into the medial layer. IMH (**b**) results from hemorrhage within the medial layer in the absence of intimal disruption. Aortic dissection (**c**) occurs when an intimal tear permits blood flow through a false lumen within the medial layer. Rupture of the aortic wall (**d**) may also occur these entities

may progress to intramural hematoma (IMH) formation, aortic dissection/rupture, or result in pseudoaneurysm formation. The majority of PAUs are located in the descending thoracic aorta [8].

In contrast, IMH can result from rupture of the vasa vasorum within the media creating focal accumulation of blood in the wall in the absence of a direct communication to the lumen (Fig. 7b). IMH may be present with concurrent PAU and may progress to frank aortic dissection in 28–47% of cases [8]. Spontaneous resolution of IMH has also been reported. IMH location is also important with those found in in the ascending aorta necessitating urgent operative intervention due to a higher risk of dissection or rupture.

Aortic Dissection and Rupture

Aortic catastrophic, thoracic aortic dissection and/or rupture constitute the sequelae of terminal structural failure of the aortic wall (Fig. 7d). Aortic dissection is defined by local intimal disruption permitting blood flow through a false lumen within the medial layer. Longitudinal propagation through this false lumen and resulting compression of the true lumen may compromise perfusion to the arch vessels at their origins and dissection can continue to propagate distally both along arch vessels and down the descending aorta. Aortic dissection has been classified based on the extent of involvement by the Stanford and DeBakey schema. Stanford type A describes any involvement of the ascending aorta whereas type B is exclusively localized to the descending aorta (Fig. 8a). DeBakey type I involves both ascending and descending thoracic aorta while types II and IIIA describe exclusive involvement of the ascending and descending thoracic aorta, respectively; type IIIB is characterized by dissection in the descending and abdominal aorta (Fig. 8b).

Approximately 67% of all acute aortic dissections are type A, with two-thirds of dissection patients being male; the average age of presentation is 63 years [9]. Presence of hypertension as well as pre-existing aortic dilatation are significant risk factors for dissection. Although aortic diameter may correlate to some extent with intrinsic wall weakening, a majority of patients who experience aortic dissection have diameters below the surgical threshold of 5.5 cm for elective aneurysm repair [10]. Quantification of focal mechanical stresses on the aortic wall may improve understanding of individualized risk, particularly in those patients with smaller aortic diameters [11, 12].

Aortic rupture results from full thickness failure of the aortic wall and may be preceded by PAU, IMH or dissection, indicating a sequence of failure of the adventitia to contain the blood after the initial pathologic insult. True incidence is unknown due to the propensity for sudden death. Contained rupture into the pericardium may result in tamponade while free rupture into a pleural cavity often leads to rapid, lethal exsanguination.

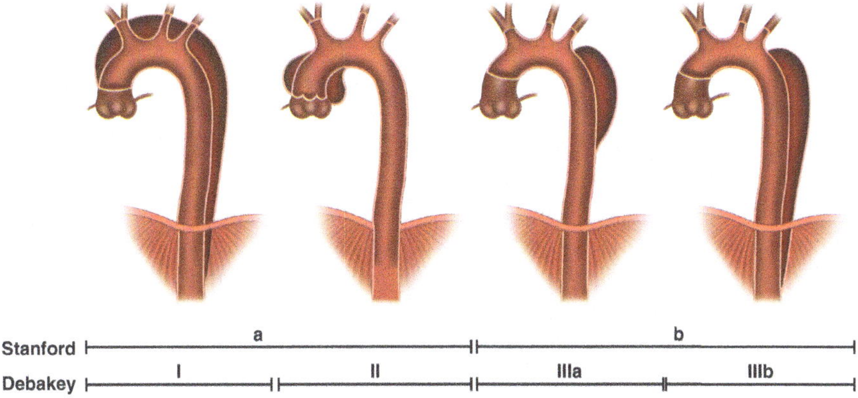

Fig. 8 Dissection classification. Aortic dissection involving the ascending and/or descending thoracic aorta is classified using the Stanford (**a**) or DeBakey (**b**) schema which each delineate areas of involvement

Special Cases

Iatrogenic

Iatrogenic aortic injury has been associated with both open and percutaneous interventions. Spinal hardware, commonly vertebral pedicle screws, may encroach upon the descending aorta causing dissection in an acute or delayed fashion. Resulting injury ranges from acute or delayed perforation, which may occur years later, or pseudoaneurysm formation [13, 14]. The natural history of screws abutting but not penetrating the aorta is unknown, however, the high mortality rates of vascular complications of spinal procedures suggest consideration of screw removal [15].

Despite quick recognition and appropriate management, iatrogenic type A dissection associated with open heart surgery carries a high mortality rate of 40% [16]. A retrospective review by Ahn et al. found an incidence of 0.29% among cardiac surgery cases with the aortic tear related to the cannulation site in 9 of 10 cases [16]. Of those patients with available pre-operative CT imaging, ascending aortic size ranged from 31 to 55 mm, however, the low sample size precluded analysis of risk factors for injury resulting in dissection.

In addition to open surgery, interventional procedures harbor a low but notable risk of aortic injury. Aortic dissection following percutaneous coronary intervention is rare, with an incidence of 0.06% in one series, but is often detected immediately and thus associated with relatively low mortality [17]. Retrograde type A dissection may occur secondary to endovascular stenting of the descending aorta. In one report, retrograde dissection occurred in 1.9% of patients undergoing TEVAR [18]. All cases were associated with placement of the proximal extent of the graft in the ascending aorta or arch and incidence was increased among those with an aortic diameter of greater than or equal to 4.0 cm [18].

Blunt Trauma

Traumatic aortic rupture may occur with blunt chest trauma and is most commonly seen with sudden deceleration, such as motor vehicle accidents. Insult to the aortic wall is most commonly localized to the aortic isthmus near the ligamentum arteriosum, which may serve as a rigid point of fixation allowing a shearing effect on the surrounding aorta. Alternatively, clinical data supports the so-called "osseous pinch" theory whereby the aorta is directly sheared between bony structures of the anterior thoracic (manubrium, first ribs and clavicular heads) and the posterior vertebral column [19, 20]. While approximately two-thirds of injuries occur at the isthmus, the ascending and more distal descending thoracic aorta can also be at risk. Rupture is thought to occur in a stepwise fashion with the traumatic insult first generating a tear in the intimal/medial layers which progresses to full thickness rupture, thus providing a potential window of opportunity for intervention [21]. Although the true incidence is unknown, in one study 35% of trauma victims undergoing autopsy showed evidence of traumatic thoracic aortic injury, of whom 80% died at the scene [22]. Given the spectrum of aortic injury severity, radiologic imaging may reveal injuries less prone to rupture, such as isolated intimal disruptions or small pseudoaneurysms, yet risk stratification for such findings in the context of trauma has not been fully defined.

Pregnancy

Pregnancy may predispose individuals to highly morbid vascular phenomena, such as the risk of splenic artery rupture, hemorrhagic stroke, and aortic pathologies. Both hormonal fluctuation and hemodynamic changes have been proposed as potential risk factors. Pregnancy-associated aortic catastrophe in Marfan syndrome (MFS), the most common heritable aortopathy, has received the most attention. A retrospective review of 98 women with MFS revealed increased aortic growth rate during pregnancy with an overall increased risk of dissection and elective repair on long-term follow-up compared to nulliparous MFS women [23]. In this cohort, no women experienced aortic events during pregnancy. However, those MFS patients with pre-existing risk factors for aortic dissection, such as aortic diameter greater than 40 mm, appear to be at a heightened risk for experiencing an aortic event during pregnancy [24]. Among the general population, aortic dissection and rupture remains elevated during pregnancy, as demonstrated by a study of over six million pregnant and postpartum women [25]. Nevertheless, the occurrence is rare though caution must be exercised in those with known aortopathy.

Cocaine Use

Use of cocaine has been linked to acute coronary syndrome and arrhythmia and has anecdotally been associated with acute aortic dissection in a younger population than that seen with degenerative TAA and dissection. In a retrospective review of patients who experienced dissection comparing those who did and did not use cocaine, dissection location and extent did not appear to differ [26]. These patients presented at an average of 12.8 h after substance ingestion [26]. Cocaine functions as a sympathomimetic, raising intracellular calcium and leading to transient tachycardia and hypertension. Given the temporality between substance ingestion and symptomatic presentation, it is plausible that acute changes in blood pressure may incite intimal tear and subsequent dissection. The relative contribution of repetitive cocaine usage on aortic wall pathology has not yet been investigated.

Bicuspid Aortic Valve Aortopathy

The most common congenital heart defect, affecting 1–2% of the population, is a bicuspid aortic valve (BAV). While characterized by its valvular morphology, BAV is strongly associated with an ascending aortopathy with a majority of BAV patients having a larger diameter ascending aorta compared to age- and sex-matched controls with many (up to 84%) developing aneurysmal features [27, 28]. Two hypotheses have been proposed to relate concomitant valve disease and aneurysm: one posits that dilatation results from an intrinsic aortic wall defect, possibly related to similar embryologic origins as the valve tissue, and the other implicates altered blood flow through the bicuspid valve with eccentric jets creating focal strain on the ascending aortic wall. To date, no singular genetic mutation has been ascribed to the presence of BAV, although its heritability is understood [29, 30]. Various mechanisms for BAV aortopathy have been proposed including: multifactorial genetic contributions, defective cellular response to oxidative stress, alterations in extracellular matrix remodeling, and modified epigenetic control [31–34]. By 30 years of age, over half of BAV patients demonstrate aortic dilatation and the prevalence increases to 88% for those over 60 [35]. The relative risk of aortic dissection in patients with TAA associated with BAV, in comparison with those with TAA and a normal aortic valve, is similar [36], although this topic of relative risk has been controversial. Further studies will be necessary to identify BAV-specific risk factors for aortic dissection and thereby direct decisions for elective aortic replacement.

Inherited Aortopathies

Marfan Syndrome

First described in 1896 by Antoine Marfan, the Marfan syndrome (MFS) is the most common known genetically-triggered aortopathy and is marked by early and extensive TAA and aortic dissection. Phenotypic manifestations include ectopia lentis, tall stature, and arachnodactyly. Pathogenesis is linked to a mutation in the ECM structural protein fibrillin-1, which regulates transforming growth factor (TGF)-β signaling. A spectrum of disease is seen that appears to relate to the specific mutations seen involving fibrillin-1 giving rise to some but not all MFS features in some patients, so-called Marfan forme fruste. Aortic disease, the primary cause of early death among MFS patients, is characterized by a root phenotype, with enlargement of the sinuses of Valsalva, and occurs in 15–44% of patients [37]. Involvement of the root has been attributed to alterations in elastin content with resultant tissue weakening under physiologic hemodynamic forces [38]. Aortic disease, however, is not limited to the root. Examination of long-term outcomes in MFS patients by Kari et al. revealed that 68% of dissections were DeBakey type I, which paralleled their findings of high rates of reintervention for descending aortic disease [39]. Histologically, features of cystic medial degeneration are seen although this is not pathognomonic.

EDS

Multiple subtypes constitute Ehlers-Danlos syndrome (EDS), however, type IV, the vascular subtype, is most commonly associated with thoracic aortic disease. Characterized by a defect in the *COL3A1* gene encoding type III procollagen, the EDS type IV phenotype consists of predisposition to bowel, uterine and arterial rupture in addition to characteristic facial features and thinned skin with visible vessels. Inheritance is autosomal dominant. Patients with EDS experience early death at a mean age of 50 years with the majority of these being attributable to arterial rupture [40, 41]. Widespread medium and large vessel involvement is typical in EDS with a complication involving the aorta leading to death in 68% of cases [40]. Animal models of *COL3A1* haploinsufficiency demonstrate aortic dissection in the absence of aneurysm and with associated decreases in medial collagen content [42]. Owing to the high risk of sudden death and the rarity of the EDS, there is a lack of knowledge about the natural history of thoracic aortic disease and of the histologic findings in those who undergo resection. Nevertheless, these clinical manifestations highlight the importance of collagen type III in maintaining extracellular matrix function in the aorta.

LDS

Loeys-Dietz syndrome (LDS) is an autosomal dominant connective tissue disorder first described in 2005 that results from a genetic mutation in TGF-β or its receptor [43]. Fibrillin-1, which is mutated in MFS, binds TGF-β thus regulating downstream signaling including TGF-β receptor-mediated pathways. Similar histologic findings to MFS, including elastic fiber fragmentation and proteoglycan accumulation, are present in LDS patients [44]. Phenotypic manifestations include cardiovascular, craniofacial, cognitive and skeletal abnormalities [43]. LDS is marked by arterial tortuosity with accompanying predisposition to dissection and rupture. Cases of thoracic aortic dissection have been reported in infancy [45]. The rarity of this condition limits thorough epidemiologic studies, however the burden of aortic dilatation among this population is significant with cases of dissection and fatality due to aortic or vascular disease accounting for premature death. Guidelines for management of thoracic aortic disease reflect the aggressiveness of this heritable aortopathy: recommendations include early and frequent screening, beginning at 6 months of age, and a lower threshold for consideration of aortic repair [46].

Familial Thoracic Aortic Aneurysm and Dissection (FTAAD)

Familial Thoracic Aortic Aneurysm and Dissection (FTAAD) defines a subset of patients with isolated aortic disease characterized by more rapid aortic growth and earlier presentation. Analysis of over 100 patients with a familial pattern of TAA but without MFS revealed a predominantly autosomal dominant inheritance with a male predilection [47]. Mutations in *TGFB2*, which encodes TGF-β2 may represent the genetic driving factor for a subset of these patients [48]. This etiology underscores the importance of considering family medical history in the prognostication of all patients with thoracic aortic disease.

Turner Syndrome

Turner syndrome (TS) is characterized by complete or partial absence of one of the sex chromosomes in females, resulting in short stature and premature ovarian failure. TS also harbors a 100-fold increased risk of aortic dissection compared to the general population [49]. Associated findings of hypertension, BAV, aortic coarctation, and treatment with growth hormone all contribute to the increased risk. Approximately 25% of patients with Turner syndrome have BAV. In the absence of the aforementioned risk factors, TS is independently associated with aortic dilatation in the aortic root and ascending aorta [50]. Aortic dissection presents at median age of 35 years and most commonly involves the ascending aorta [51]. The mechanism of aortic degeneration in TS is unknown however histologic analyses have described both cystic medial necrosis and an altered ratio of collagen subtypes [51]. The range of aortic anomalies in the presence of the monosomy of TS suggests a genetic origin, though no specific defect has been identified.

References

1. Leonard JC. Thomas Bevill Peacock and the early history of dissecting aneurysm. Br Med J. 1979;2:260–2.
2. Mao SS, et al. Normal thoracic aorta diameter on cardiac computed tomography in healthy asymptomatic adults. Impact of age and gender. Acad Radiol. 2008. https://doi.org/10.1016/j.acra.2008.02.001
3. McComb BL, et al. Normative reference values of thoracic aortic diameter in American College of Radiology Imaging Network (ACRIN 6654) arm of National Lung Screening Trial. Clin Imaging. 2016;40:936–43.
4. Popieluszko P, Henry M, Sanna B, Hsieh C. A systematic review and meta-analysis of variations in branching patterns of the adult aortic arch. J Vasc Surg. 2018;68:298–306.
5. J E. Medionecrosis aortae idiopathiea cystica. Virchows Arch Pathol Anat Physiol Klin Med. 1930;276(1):187–229.
6. Oladokun D, et al. Systematic review of the growth rates and influencing factors in thoracic aortic aneurysms. Eur J Vasc Endovasc Surg. 2016;51:674–81.
7. Safi HJ. Thoracoabdominal aortic aneurysm repair: how I do it. Cardiovasc Surg. 1999;7:597–606.
8. Eggebrecht H, Plicht B, Kahlert P, Erbel R. Intramural hematoma and penetrating ulcers: indications to endovascular treatment. Eur J Vasc Endovasc Surg. 2009;38:659–65.
9. Hagan PG, et al. The international registry of acute aortic dissection (IRAD) new insights into an old disease. JAMA. 2000;283:897–903.
10. Pape LA, et al. Aortic diameter ≥5.5 cm is not a good predictor of type A aortic dissection: observations from the international registry of acute aortic dissection (IRAD). Circulation. 2007;116:1120–7.
11. Emerel L, et al. Pre-dissection-derived geometric and distensibility indices reveal increased peak longitudinal stress and stiffness in patients sustaining acute type a aortic dissection: implications for predicting dissection. J Thorac Cardiovasc Surg. 2018;15232:1–10.
12. Nathan DP, et al. Pathogenesis of acute aortic dissection: a finite element stress analysis. Ann Thorac Surg. 2011;91:458–63.
13. Lavigne F, Mascard E, Laurian C, Dubousset J, Wicart P. Delayed-iatrogenic injury of the thoracic aorta by an anterior spinal instrumentation. Eur Spine J. 2009;18(Suppl 2):265–8.
14. Kakkos SK, Shepard AD. Delayed presentation of aortic injury by pedicle screws: report of two cases and review of the literature. J Vasc Surg. 2008;47:1074–82.
15. Sandhu HK, Charlton-Ouw KM, Azizzadeh A, Estrera AL, Safi HJ. Spinal screw penetration of the aorta. J Vasc Surg. 2013;57:1668–70.
16. Hwang HY, Jeong DS, Kim K-H, Kim K-B, Ahn H. Iatrogenic type A aortic dissection during cardiac surgery. Interact Cardiovasc Thorac Surg. 2010;10:896–9.
17. Nóñez-Gil IJ, et al. Incidence, management, and immediate- and long-term outcomes after iatrogenic aortic dissection during diagnostic or interventional coronary procedures. Circulation. 2015;131:2114–9.
18. Williams JB, et al. Retrograde ascending aortic dissection as an early complication of thoracic endovascular aortic repair. J Vasc Surg. 2012;55:1255–62.
19. Cohen A, Crass J, Thomas H, Fisher R, Jacobs D. CT evidence for the 'osseous pinch' mechanism of traumatic aortic injury. Am Roentgen Ray Soc. 1992;159:271–4.
20. Javadpour H, O'Toole JJ, McEniff JN, Luke DA, Young VK. Traumatic aortic transection: evidence for the osseous pinch mechanism. Ann Thorac Surg. 2002;73:951–3.
21. Neschis DG, Scalea TM, Flinn WR, Griffith BP. Blunt aortic injury. N Engl J Med. 2008;359:1708–16.
22. Teixeira PGR, et al. Blunt thoracic aortic injuries: an autopsy study. J Trauma Inj Infect Crit Care. 2011;70:197–202.

23. Donnelly RT, Pinto NM, Kocolas I, Yetman AT. The immediate and long-term impact of pregnancy on aortic growth rate and mortality in women with Marfan syndrome. J Am Coll Cardiol. 2012;60:224–9.
24. Lind J, Wallenburg HC. The Marfan syndrome and pregnancy: a retrospective study in a Dutch population. Eur J Obs Gynecol Reprod Biol. 2001;98:28–35.
25. Kamel H, Roman MJ, Pitcher A, Devereux RB. Pregnancy and the risk of aortic dissection or rupture: a cohort-crossover analysis. Circulation. 2016. https://doi.org/10.1161/CIRCULATIONAHA.116.021594
26. Daniel JC, et al. Acute aortic dissection associated with use of cocaine. J Vasc Surg. 2007;46:427–33.
27. Verma S, Siu SC. Aortic dilatation in patients with bicuspid aortic valve. N Engl J Med. 2014;370:1920–9.
28. Keane MG, et al. Bicuspid aortic valves are associated with aortic dilatation out of proportion to coexistent valvular lesions. Circulation. 2000;102:III35–9.
29. Ward C. Clinical significance of the bicuspid aortic valve. Heart. 2000;83:81–5.
30. Cripe L, Andelfinger G, Martin LJ, Shooner K, Benson DW. Bicuspid aortic valve is heritable. J Am Coll Cardiol. 2004;44:138–43.
31. Prakash SK, et al. A roadmap to investigate the genetic basis of bicuspid aortic valve and its complications: insights from the international BAVCon (bicuspid aortic valve consortium). J Am Coll Cardiol. 2014. https://doi.org/10.1016/j.jacc.2014.04.073
32. Phillippi JA, et al. Basal and oxidative stress-induced expression of metallothionein is decreased in ascending aortic aneurysms of bicuspid aortic valve patients. Circulation. 2009. https://doi.org/10.1161/CIRCULATIONAHA.108.770776
33. Phillippi JA, et al. Bicuspid aortic valve Morphotype correlates with regional antioxidant gene expression profiles in the proximal ascending aorta. Ann Thorac Surg. 2016;104:79–87.
34. Ikonomidis JS, et al. Expression of matrix metalloproteinases and endogenous inhibitors within ascending aortic aneurysms of patients with bicuspid or tricuspid aortic valves. J Thorac Cardiovasc Surg.2007. https://doi.org/10.1016/j.jtcvs.2006.10.083
35. Della Corte A, et al. Predictors of ascending aortic dilatation with bicuspid aortic valve: a wide spectrum of disease expression. Eur J Cardio-thoracic Surg. 2007. https://doi.org/10.1016/j.ejcts.2006.12.006
36. Kim JB, et al. Risk of aortic dissection in the moderately dilated ascending aorta. J Am Coll Cardiol. 2016;68:1209–19.
37. Milewicz DM, Dietz HC, Miller DC. Treatment of aortic disease in patients with Marfan syndrome. Circulation. 2005;111:150–7.
38. Cãadas V, Vilacosta I, Bruna I, Fuster V. Marfan syndrome. Part 1: pathophysiology and diagnosis. Nat Rev Cardiol. 2010;7:256–65.
39. Rylski B, et al. Type A aortic dissection in marfan syndrome: extent of initial surgery determines long-term outcome. Circulation. 2014;129:1381–6.
40. Pepin MG, et al. Survival is affected by mutation type and molecular mechanism in vascular Ehlers-Danlos syndrome (EDS type IV). Genet Med. 2014;16:881–8.
41. Pepin M, Schwarze U, Superti-Furga A, Byers PH. Clinical and genetic features of the Ehlers-Danlos syndrome type IV, the vascular type. N Engl J Med. 2000;342:673–80.
42. Smith LB, et al. Haploinsufficiency of the murine Col3a1 locus causes aortic dissection: a novel model of the vascular type of EhlersDanlos syndrome. Cardiovasc Res. 2011;90:182–90.
43. Loeys BL, et al. A syndrome of altered cardiovascular, craniofacial, neurocognitive and skeletal development caused by mutations in TGFBR1 or TGFBR2. Nat Genet. 2005;37:275–81.
44. Lindsay ME, et al. Loss-of-function mutations in TGFB2 cause a syndromic presentation of thoracic aortic aneurysm. Nat Genet. 2012;44:922–7.
45. Williams JA, et al. Early surgical experience with Loeys-Dietz: a new syndrome of aggressive thoracic aortic aneurysm disease. Ann Thorac Surg. 2007;83
46. Hiratzka LF, et al. 2010 ACCF/AHA/AATS/ACR/ASA/SCA/SCAI/SIR/STS/SVM guidelines for the diagnosis and management of patients with thoracic aortic disease: a report of

the American College of Cardiology Foundation/American Heart Association Task Force on Practice Guidelines, A. Circulation. 2010;121:e266–369.
47. Albornoz G, et al. Familial thoracic aortic aneurysms and dissections-incidence, modes of inheritance, and phenotypic patterns. Ann Thorac Surg. 2006;82:1400–5.
48. Boileau C, et al. TGFB2 mutations cause familial thoracic aortic aneurysms and dissections associated with mild systemic features of Marfan syndrome. Nat Genet. 2012;44:916–21.
49. Mortensen KH, Erlandsen M, Andersen NH, Gravholt CH. Prediction of aortic dilation in turner syndrome – enhancing the use of serial cardiovascular magnetic resonance. J Cardiovasc Magn Reson. 2013;15:1–11.
50. Lopez L, et al. Turner syndrome is an independent risk factor for aortic dilation in the Young. Pediatrics. 2008;121:e1622–7.
51. Gravholt CH, et al. Clinical and epidemiological description of aortic dissection in Turner's syndrome. Cardiol Young. 2006;16:430–6.

Histopathology of Acute Aortic Syndromes

David Ranney and Ryan P. Plichta

Normal Anatomy and Histology

The aorta is the largest arterial vessel in the human body, providing a conduit for blood flow from the heart to the iliac artery bifurcation. The wall of the aorta is composed of three distinct layers: the intima, media, and adventitia [1] (Fig. 1).

The innermost layer, the intima, is in direct contact with the circulating blood volume via a layer of squamous epithelial cells known as the endothelium [2]. The endothelium participates in hemostasis, coagulation, and is semi-permeable to the blood and blood components. Beneath the endothelium is a layer of subendothelial tissue comprised of collagen, elastic fibers, and smooth muscle cells. The middle layer of the aorta, the media, consists mostly of smooth muscle and elastic fibers. As the thickest layer of the aortic wall, it provides both the tensile strength necessary to withstand repetitive impulses from cardiac ejection as well as the elastic recoil required to maintain diastolic pressure and continuous blood flow [3]. Elastic fibers are more prevalent in the proximal aorta compared to the distal aorta, and thus offer more compliance to accommodate undampened left ventricular ejection. The outermost layer of the aortic wall, the adventitia, is a layer of collagenous connective tissue that contains lymphatics, nerve fibers, and in the thoracic aorta, the vaso vasorum, a small arterial network that provides blood flow to the outer portion of the aortic wall. The inner portion is nourished by diffusion from the aortic lumen [1].

D. Ranney · R. P. Plichta (✉)
Duke University, Durham, NC, USA
e-mail: ryan.plichta@duke.edu

J. S. Coselli et al. (eds.), *Aortic Dissection and Acute Aortic Syndromes*,
https://doi.org/10.1007/978-3-030-66668-2_3

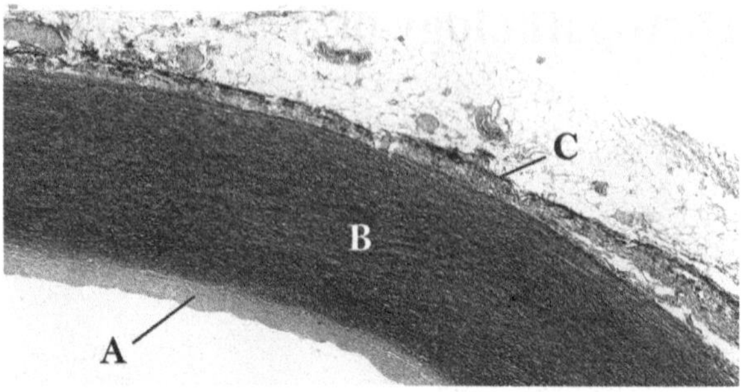

Fig. 1 Cross section of the aorta demonstrating the (**a**) intima, (**b**) media, and (**c**) adventitia. *Duke University School of Medicine*

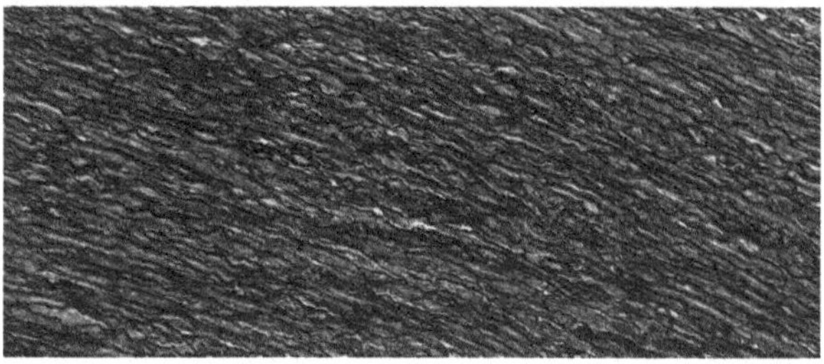

Fig. 2 Aortic media stained for elastin. *Duke University School of Medicine*

Predisposing Histopathology

The aorta is a dynamic organ that is vulnerable to several processes known to precede clinical disease. With increasing age, the native aorta experiences degeneration and fragmentation of elastic fibers, which reduces the compliance of the vessel and hence its ability to withstand repetitive impulses [4, 5] (Fig. 2).

Additional histologic changes take place with aging that contribute to elongation of the aorta and eventual tortuosity [3]. Aging also leads to increasing aortic diameters, particularly in the ascending aorta, though this is not considered to be aneurysmal until its diameter exceeds dilation by at least 50% of normal. Rates of increase in diameter vary according to the segment of the aorta, with a rate of change of 0.07 to 0.2 cm/year for the ascending aorta and arch [6]. The effects of aging on the aorta are exacerbated by hypertension and atherosclerosis, which are frequent comorbidities in the same patient population. Smoking and COPD are additional risk factors that accelerate these degenerative processes.

Atherosclerosis is a distinct process that is commonly observed in settings such as coronary, carotid, and peripheral vascular disease. This same process also contributes to the development of aortic disease. The endothelial damage incurred by circulating lipoproteins, inflammation, and deposition of debris and smooth muscle cells leads to degradation of the aortic wall that can be seen on a histologic level. This atherosclerotic weakening then follows a similar mechanism by which either aneurysmal development occurs, or intimal injury followed by AAS. Atherosclerotic changes tend to predominate in the descending thoracic and abdominal aorta, as compared to the ascending aorta, where degradation of elastic tissue is more frequently encountered [3].

A separate common pathway for aortic disease is characterized histologically by both elastic fragmentation and loss of smooth muscle cells in the aortic media. These components are replaced by ground substance forming cyst-like structures, a process referred to as *cystic medial degeneration* (CMD) (previously *cystic medial necrosis*). CMD is observed in the aging aorta as well as conditions such as Marfan's syndrome and Ehlers-Danlos syndrome [4, 7]. It is frequently seen in the setting of aortic aneurysm and dissection, thus it is recognized as a predisposing factor for AAS.

Acute Aortic Syndromes

Aortic Dissection

Aortic dissection is a highly morbid and lethal condition with an incidence of 2000 patients per year in the U.S. alone [3]. This disease process is characterized by a tear in the aortic intima that communicates with a channel forming within the aortic media (Fig. 3).

This channel, referred to as the "false lumen" has the tendency to propagate in either the antegrade or retrograde direction, as it is pressurized by the blood flow within the aorta. The torn intima produces a flap that compresses the "true lumen" and, along with an expanding false lumen, can lead to various malperfusion syndromes or aortic valve insufficiency depending on the location and extent of the injury. Some of these malperfusion syndromes have lethal consequences, such as bowel or cerebral ischemia, and high rates of morbidity with carotid or spinal cord ischemia. Furthermore, the false lumen is bounded only by adventitia and a thin, outer remnant of aortic media. As a result, sustained pressurization can lead to rupture, or subsequent aneurysmal degeneration if not repaired during the acute phase, as is often the case with uncomplicated aortic dissections of the descending and abdominal aorta [4, 8].

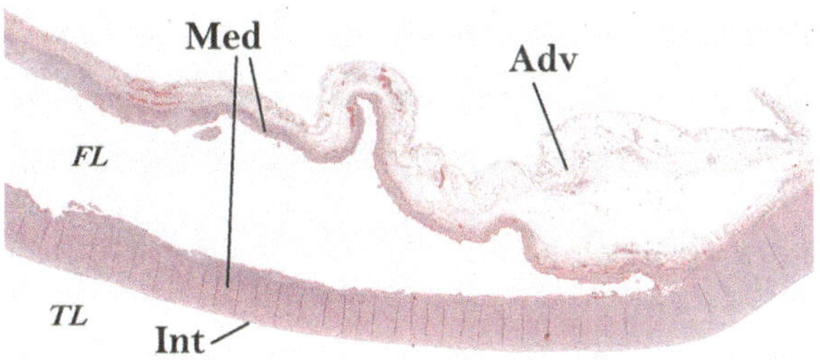

Fig. 3 Aortic dissection, as characterized by separation of layers within the media, and associated intimal flap. *Intima (Int), media (Med), adventitia (Adv), true lumen (TL), false lumen (FL). University of Michigan Medical School*

While it is commonly accepted that an intimal tear is an inciting event for aortic dissection, there are several conditions which facilitate its occurrence. With regard to the quality of the aortic tissue, connective tissue disorders (CTD), CMD, and atherosclerosis are all risk factors for dissection. With regard to hemodynamics; hypertension, states of hypervolemia, and catecholamine release are risk factors for AAS. Intimal damage, trauma, and iatrogenic injury are also prerequisites for dissection [3].

Intramural Hematoma

Intramural hematoma (IMH) is a variant of aortic dissection, and, like dissection, is characterized by hemorrhage/thrombus formation within the aortic media with variable distances of propagation. Unlike dissection, however, the overlying intima remains intact. IMH is hypothesized to occur as a result of rupture of the vaso vasorum [3, 4]. Untreated, pressure necrosis or injury of the overlying intima can occur, leading to communication with the aortic lumen, a condition indistinguishable from aortic dissection. As such, IMH is managed as an AAS (Fig. 4).

Penetrating Atherosclerotic Ulcer (PAU)

In the setting of atherosclerotic disease, intimal damage can result in a small tear with contained extravasation into the aortic media. Known as a penetrating atherosclerotic ulcer (PAU), these lesions are at risk for propagation and thus evolving into an IMH or dissection. PAUs arise in different locations and geometries, and management is determined accordingly.

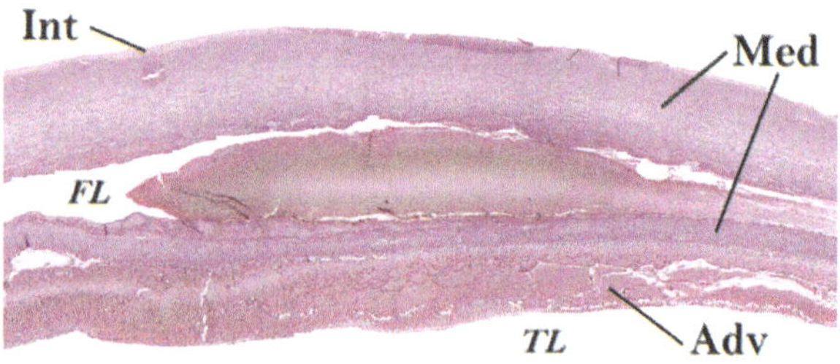

Fig. 4 Intramural hematoma. *Intima (Int), media (Med), adventitia (Adv), true lumen (TL), false lumen (FL). Duke University School of Medicine*

Special Populations

Connective Tissue Disorders

CTDs exist in many forms and subtypes and are a significant risk factor for aneurysm and dissection. Marfan Syndrome (MFS) is an autosomal dominant CTD, though sporadic forms are also encountered. This disorder is characterized by derangements in the gene encoding fibrillin-1, a structural protein found in the aortic wall that is necessary for functional elastic structure. As such, aneurysmal disease is present in up to 80% of MFS patients, necessitating surgical intervention in the majority [3]. The aortic root is more typically involved in MFS compared to other aneurysmal etiologies. As aortic diameter increases, so does the risk for rupture and dissection. Loeys-Deitz Syndrome (LDS) is another autosomal dominant CTD characterized by a mutation in transforming growth factor beta (TGF-B), also leading to medial elastic fiber fragmentation and aortic root aneurysms. Compared to MFS, patients with LDS tend to develop complications of aneurysm and dissection at younger ages, and typically at smaller aortic diameters [9]. Ehler-Danlos syndrome is another CTD characterized by defective type III collagen production. The result is a thin, friable aortic wall, particularly in the arch and descending thoracic aorta, predisposing to aneurysm and dissection. Ehler-Danlos also affects large and small arteries throughout the body, leading to rupture at various locations.

Bicuspid Aortic Valve Syndrome

Approximately 1–2% of the general population have a bicuspid aortic valve [3]. Associated with this finding is dilation of the proximal aorta that predisposes to aneurysm and dissection. While this syndrome is not fully understood, there are both sporadic and familial patterns observed, as well as additional associations with other conditions such as Turner's syndrome and coarctation of the aorta. Abnormal neural crest cell migration has also been suggested as a mechanism for BAV development, given its role in outflow tract septation and semilunar valve modeling [10]. The BAVS phenotype appears to be an endpoint for several genetic, structural, and hemodynamic mechanisms, or combinations thereof [11]. Histologically, the aortic wall in BAVS is characterized by elastic fragmentation, loss of smooth muscle, and increased levels of matrix metallic proteinases. These proteinases, though necessary for normal extracellular matrix maintenance, can lead to elastic destruction when overproduced, resulting in histologic findings that precede aneurysm and dissection.

Familial Thoracic Aortic Disease

It is estimated that 20% of patients with thoracic aortic aneurysms have a first degree relative with an aortic aneurysm, and similar associations among patients with aortic dissection has been observed [3]. This demonstrates the presence of underlying genetic predispositions for aortic disease, beyond those that exist among patients with CTD. Although patterns of inheritance are quite variable, there are certain gene mutations that have been linked to aortic aneurysm and dissection, such as TGFBR1, TGFBR2, MYH11, and SMAD3. The histologic manifestations of these mutations result in similar phenotypes of disease, leading to often earlier surgical intervention in an effort to prevent AAS.

Conclusion

Acute aortic syndromes remain a challenging clinical entity that carries significant morbidity and mortality. Improved understanding of the genetic, histologic, and pathology mechanisms behind these syndromes will lead to better patient specific management and novel clinical therapies.

References

1. Ovalle WK, Nahirney PC. Netter's essential histology. 2nd ed. Philadelphia, PA: Elsevier/Saunders; 2013.
2. Hossler FE. Ultrastructure atlas of human tissues. Wiley-Blackwell: Hoboken, NJ; 2014.
3. Cohn LH, Adams DH. Cardiac surgery in the adult. 5th ed. New York: McGraw-Hill Education; 2018.
4. Buja LM, Butany J. Cardiovascular pathology. 4th ed. Amsterdam: Elsevier/Academic; 2016.
5. Bode-Jänisch S, Schmidt A, Günther D, Stuhrmann M, Fieguth A. Aortic dissecting aneurysms—histopathological findings. Forensic Sci Int. 2012;214(1–3):13–7.
6. Patel HJ, Deeb GM. Ascending and arch aorta: pathology, natural history, and treatment. Circulation. 2008;118(2):188–95.
7. Halushka MK, Angelini A, Bartoloni G, Basso C, Batoroeva L, Bruneval P, et al. Consensus statement on surgical pathology of the aorta from the Society for Cardiovascular Pathology and the Association For European Cardiovascular Pathology: II. Noninflammatory degenerative diseases – nomenclature and diagnostic criteria. Cardiovasc Pathol. 2016;25(3):247–57.
8. Tsai TT, Nienaber CA, Eagle KA. Acute aortic syndromes. Circulation. 2005;112(24):3802–13.
9. Zanotti G, Vricella L, Cameron D. Thoracic aortic aneurysm syndrome in children. Semin Thorac Cardiovasc Surg Pediatr Card Surg Annu. 2008:11–21.
10. Phillips HM, Mahendran P, Singh E, Anderson RH, Chaudhry B, Henderson DJ. Neural crest cells are required for correct positioning of the developing outflow cushions and pattern the arterial valve leaflets. Cardiovasc Res. 2013;99(3):452–60.
11. Hiratzka LF, Creager MA, Isselbacher EM, Svensson LG, Nishimura RA, Bonow RO, et al. Surgery for aortic dilatation in patients with bicuspid aortic valves: a statement of clarification from the American College of Cardiology/American Heart Association Task Force on Clinical Practice Guidelines. J Thorac Cardiovasc Surg. 2016;151(4):959–66.

Genetically-Triggered Aortic Dissections

Melissa L. Russo and Jia Jennifer Ding

Introduction

Aortic aneurysm and aortic dissection are life-threatening events that can greatly influence a person's life. Greater than 20% of all thoracic aortic aneurysms have been attributed to a genetic etiology [1]. The estimation of the genetic contributions to aortic dissection may actually be an underestimate secondary to silent thoracic aneurysms being undiagnosed and an under-utilization of genetic testing in the clinical arena [2]. Therefore, it is imperative for the cardiologist and cardiovascular surgeon to have an understanding of the genetic conditions associated with an increased risk for aortic dissection.

The genetic conditions with a predisposition for aortic aneurysm and dissection can be classified into syndromic conditions versus non-syndromic alterations in gene expression that predispose to aortic aneurysm and dissection (Table 1). The syndromic conditions are typically autosomal dominant and have characteristic features on history and physical exam that identify these individuals. The syndromic conditions include Marfan syndrome, Loeys-Dietz syndrome, vascular Ehlers-Danlos syndrome, Turner syndrome and bicuspid aortic valve aortopathy. In contrast, non-syndromic genetic conditions do not have any identifying systemic features. Modern genomic sequencing technology has identified pathogenic variants in genes important for functioning of vascular smooth muscle cells. The non-syndromic genetic conditions have familial aggregation. The non-syndromic genetic

M. L. Russo (✉)
Maternal-Fetal Medicine and Clinical Genetics, Women and Infants Hospital, Warren Alpert Medical School of Brown University, Providence, RI, USA
e-mail: MLRusso@Wihri.org

J. J. Ding
PGY4 Resident Educational Chief, Obstetrics and Gynecology Residency, Women and Infants Hospital, Warren Alpert Medical School of Brown University, Providence, RI, USA

J. S. Coselli et al. (eds.), *Aortic Dissection and Acute Aortic Syndromes*,
https://doi.org/10.1007/978-3-030-66668-2_4

Table 1 Genetic conditions with predisposition for aortic aneurysm and dissection

Genetic condition	Gene affected	Clinical features
Marfan syndrome	FBN1	• Aortic root dilation • Ectopia lentis • Skeletal features
Loeys-Dietz syndrome	TGFBR1 TGFBR2 SMAD3 TGFB2 TGFB3 SMAD2	• Aortic and arterial aneurysms • Arterial tortuosiy • Craniofacial features-hypertelorism, bifid uvula/cleft, craniosynostosis • Cutaneous features-translucent skin
Vascular Ehlers Danlos syndrome (type IV)	COL3A1	• Arterial, intestinal or uterine rupture • Thin, translucent skin • Easy bruising • Characteristic facial appearance-pinched nose, thin lips, prominent eyes
Turner syndrome	Karyotype XO	• Aortic dilation at root/ascending • Short stature • Premature ovarian failure
Bicuspid Aortic Valve Aortopathy	NOTCH1[a]	None unless with underlying syndrome
Familial thoracic aortic aneurysm	ACTA2 MYH11 MYLK PRKG1 LOX	None

[a]Association only in some cases

conditions with increased risk for aortic dissection include pathogenic variants in *ACTA2*, *MYH11*, *MYLK*, *PRKG1* and *LOX* [3].

This chapter will outline the major features and method of diagnosis for genetic conditions with a predisposition for aortic dissection. In addition, this chapter will highlight national and international recommendations on imaging surveillance, pharmacotherapy, prophylactic surgical guidelines and surgery recommendations in regards to these conditions.

General Guidelines with Genetic Conditions with Predisposition for Aortic Dissection

Over the few decades, there have been tremendous medical advancements for some of genetically-triggered aortic dissections conditions with prophylactic aortic surgery, revised methods for diagnosis with clinical criteria and genetic testing, and medical treatment.

The diameter of the enlarged aortic root is an important risk factor for future aortic dissection in the setting of monogenetic disorders where increased wall tension in the presence of weakened connective tissues causes the aorta to enlarge slowly before dissection occurs. A majority of aortic aneurysms in these conditions arise at the aortic root or ascending aorta. The key points of optimal care include early diagnosis, close surveillance of aneurysms, eliminating modifiable risk factors and appropriate medical and surgical treatment.

Diagnosis

- Early diagnosis is critical in order for individuals to have proper surveillance and treatment to slow aortic root growth and mitigate risk for aortic dissection.
- A clinical diagnosis is made after a thorough history and detailed physical exam focused on signs of connective tissue condition.
- Detailed three generation family history is recommended as some of these conditions have reduced penetrance and variable expressivity. It is important to ask about family history of thoracic aortic aneurysm/dissection, aneurysms in any location, or sudden cardiac death before age 45 [5].
- Syndromic conditions have clinical criteria that will be reviewed in the individual sections and genetic testing is recommended to confirm diagnosis in most cases.

Screening

- Once a diagnosis is made, serial imaging is recommended to assess the aortic root with transthoracic echocardiograms and assessment of the entire vascular tree is also recommended.
- Frequency of imaging surveillance will be reviewed in individual sections but generally is performed on a yearly basis.
- Screening other first relatives in a family is also recommended as a majority of these conditions are autosomal dominant in inheritance.

Management

- Pharmacotherapy of beta-blockers, angiotensin receptor blockers or a combination of the two medications is recommended to slow aortic root growth. However their role in prevention of aneurysm is equivocal in some of the previous studies.
- Mitigation of risk with smoking cessation, treatment of dyslipidemia and hypertension is a part of the treatment plan to prevent aortic dissection.
- Recommendations for prophylactic aortic root repair in genetic conditions based on aortic root threshold measurements have been put forth by national and inter-

national societies (Table 2). Prophylactic surgery has been the main driving force that has increased life expectancy in some of these conditions.
- Individuals with these conditions are advised to avoid high-stress isometric exercises, contact sports and competitive sports. However, there are no evidence-based guidelines for exercise in this population. Animal models have shown that some exercise is beneficial to prevent aortic root growth [6].
- Pregnancy is higher risk period for aortic dissection secondary to hemodynamic and hormonal changes of the physiological state of pregnancy. Therefore, it is important for providers to have a discussion about a person's reproductive plans and ensure they understand the risks. It is also advisable to involve maternal-fetal medicine specialists in these discussions.
- For management of type A dissections in genetic conditions, open thoracic surgery with resection of the affected part of the aorta and replacement with synthetic Darcon vascular prosthesis is performed. If required, reimplantation of the coronary arteries can also be performed at this time. Secondary to these surgeries being performed earlier in life aortic root replacement sparing the aortic valve is preferred if possible.
- With type B dissections that require surgical intervention, thoracic endovascular aortic repair (TEVAR) is traditional approach in the general population. However, in individuals with weakened connective tissues, this approach may be problematic and is not generally recommended except for emergent cases. Open surgery for repair of type B dissections is preferred for this population currently.

Table 2 Recommended indications for prophylactic aortic surgery in genetic conditions

Genetic syndrome	Indications for surgery (maximal aortic root diameter)
Marfan syndrome	• >50 mm—No risk factors • >45 mm—growth rate > 3 mm/year, desire for pregnancy, severe valve regurgitation
Loeys-Dietz syndrome	• >42 mm
Vascular Ehlers-Danlos syndrome	• Role of prophylactic surgery has not been established • Surgery reserved for life-threatening complications • May be considered for large aneurysm/rapid growth
Bicuspid Aortic Valve Aortopathy	• >55 mm—No risk factors • >50 mm- growth rate > 3 mm/year, systemic hypertension, desire for pregnancy
Turner syndrome	• ASI[a] > 27 mm/m^2
Familial Thoracic Aneurysms	• No specific recommendations due to heterogeneity and lack of data on natural history-management individualized with attention to family history

[a]ASI is Max aortic diameter/body surface area [17, 18]

Marfan Syndrome

Marfan syndrome is an autosomal dominant condition with *FBN1* as the causative gene that encodes an extracellular matrix protein, fibrillin-1. There have been over 1800 different mutations identified in *FBN1* that cause Marfan syndrome. This genetic condition is highly penetrant and with variable expression between individuals and additionally there is variability in family members with the same pathogenic mutation. Marfan syndrome affects 1 in 5000 individuals and is implicated as the cause in 3–5% of all aortic dissections [7, 8]. It mainly affects the cardiovascular, ocular and musculoskeletal systems. The primary cause of death in persons with Marfan syndrome is progressive aortic root dilatation that leads to subsequent aortic dissection. Advancements mainly in surgical management of aortic aneurysms coupled with medical management have improved survival. The average life expectancy historically was 45 years however now is 70 years, closer to the general population's life expectancy [9, 10].

Fibrillin-1 is large extracellular matrix protein encoded by *FBN1* and fibrillin-1 microfibrils maintain connective tissue structural integrity. The original hypothesis was that pathogenic variants in *FBN1* led to structural weakness of the aortic wall, however this was not the full story. In addition to its structural role, fibrillin-1 is an essential player regulating cell signaling by sequestering transforming growth factor-beta (TGFβ) in the extracellular matrix. The loss of fibrillin-1 leads to increased bioavailable TGFβ and activation of both canonical SMAD-dependent and non-canonical SMAD-independent TGFβ signaling pathways, which lead to aneurysmal dilation (Fig. 1) [11]. Increased TGFβ signaling has been shown in aneurysmal tissue from aortas in individuals with Marfan syndrome [12].

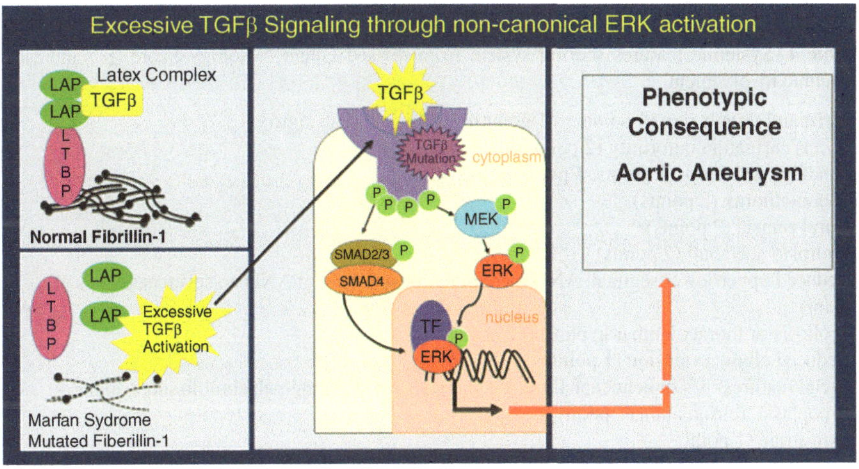

Fig. 1 Mechanism of aortic aneurysm in Marfan syndrome

Diagnosis

- The Ghent nosology is a set of clinical criteria used to diagnose Marfan syndrome [13]. This was revised in 2010 to put more weight on the cardiovascular manifestations (Tables 3 and 4). With this nosology ectopia lentis and aortic root aneurysm are cardinal features and family history is taken into account.
- An *FBN1* mutation is not necessary, nor sufficient for diagnosis, however is incorporated into the clinical criteria.

Screening and Surveillance

- In the condition Marfan syndrome, 75% of cases are familial and 25% are sporadic, de novo mutations [4].

Table 3 Revised Ghent criteria for diagnosis of Marfan syndrome

In the absence of family history:
1. Ao ($Z \geq 2$) and Ectopia lentis
2. Ao ($Z \geq 2$) and *FBN1* pathogenic variant
3. Ao ($Z \geq 2$) and systemic score (≥7 points)
4. Ectopia lentis and *FBN1* with known Ao
In the presence of family history:
5. Ectopia lentis and family history of Marfan syndrome
6. Systemic score of (≥7 points) and family history of Marfan syndrome
7. Ao ($Z \geq 2$ above 20 years old and Ao $Z \geq 3$ below 20 years old) and family history of Marfan syndrome

Loeys et al. 2010

Table 4 Systemic features scoring system from revised Ghent Nosology Score ≥ 7 indicates systemic involvement

Wrist and thumb sign (3 points vs 1 point for wrist or thumb sign)
Pectus carinatum deformity (2 points)
Hindfoot deformity (2 points, 1 point for pes planus)
Pneumothorax (2 points)
Dural ectasia (2 points)
Protrusio acetabuli (2 points)
Reduced upper/lower segment AND increased arm span/height AND no severe scoliosis (1 point)
Scoliosis or thoracolumbar kyphosis (1 point)
Reduced elbow extension (1 point)
Facial features- 3/5 dolichocephaly, enopthalmos, downslanting palpebral fissures, malar hypoplasia, retrognathia (1 point)
Skin striae (1 point)
Myopia >3 diopters (1 point)
Mitral valve prolapse (1 point)

- Since a majority of cases are familial, with a new diagnosis for an individual, it is important to additionally screen first and second degree family members for this condition if they have any clinical signs genetic testing can be sent.
- Aortic root aneurysms should be followed with serial imaging. Annual imaging of the root and ascending aorta is recommended along with clinical visit with specialist on a yearly basis.

Management

- The goal of beta-blockers and angiotensin-receptor blockers is to slow the growth of aneurysmal expansion. Beta-blockers have been shown to decrease the rate of aortic root growth however a meta-analysis has refuted the effect of this medication [14–16].
- Prophylactic aortic root surgery is recommended at >5 cm and lower diameter for additional risk factors of rapid growth, fam history of dissection, desired pregnancy, severe aortic or mitral regurgitation (Table 2) [17, 18].

Loeys-Dietz Syndrome

Loeys-Dietz syndrome (LDS) is an autosomal dominant condition with variable expression. There can be variability among family members with the same gene mutation and there is wide clinical spectrum of disease [19]. The genes associated with Loeys-Dietz syndrome encode receptors, ligands and downstream signals in the TGFβ signaling pathway. Pathogenic variation in these genes lead to dysregulation and increased signaling in the TGFβ pathway.

When this condition was first described, Loeys-Dietz syndrome was classified into two types with pathogenic genetic changes in the receptors *TGFBR1* and *TGFBR2*. These individuals had manifestations of disease in the cardiovascular, craniofacial, neurocognitive and skeletal systems with features of arterial aneurysms, congenital heart disease, craniosynostosis, cleft palate, and mental retardation. The tissues from these persons showed perturbation of TGFβ signaling [20]. One of the largest series of individuals with *TGFBR1* and *TGFBR2* mutations showed 80% survive until 60 years of age. In this cohort, 23% of individuals with *TGFBR1* and *TGFBR2* mutations had aortic dissections and of these cases 18% had prophylactic aortic surgery prior to rupture. Extra-aortic features in this population were hypertelorism (29%), cervical arterial tortuosity (53%), widened scars (27%). Aortic root diameter at dissection was smaller <4.5 cm and congenital heart defects (bicuspid aortic valve, atrial septal defect, patent ductus arteriosus) were also more common in *TGFBR2* patients. The rate of aortic dissection in this cohort was 1.7% [21].

There are now six different sub-types of Loeys-Dietz syndrome (LDS I-VI) that have been described with pathogenic variants in six different genes (Table 5) [22, 23]. Individuals with LDS type I (*TGFBR1*) have prominent craniofacial features including cleft palate, craniosynostosis, micrognathia and bifid or broad uvula [24]. Type II LDS has pathogenic variants in *TGFBR2* and these individuals have less prominent craniofacial features, easy bruising, atrophic scars, thin translucent skin and visceral rupture events, similar to vascular Ehlers-Danlos syndrome. Type III LDS, also known as aneurysm-osteoarthritis syndrome, with pathogenic variants in *SMAD3* typically have early onset joint abnormalities, arterial tortuosity, aneurysm and aortic dissections. LDS types IV, V and VI are less common and typically have milder phenotypic features and less severe clinical course [22].

Diagnosis

- There are no formal criteria for clinical diagnosis, however MacCarrick et al. has suggested revised nosology of arterial aneurysm or dissection in combination with pathogenic variant in one of the Loeys-Dietz genes or family member with known diagnosis of Loeys-Dietz syndrome is sufficient for diagnosis [25]. This nosology reduces the emphasis on dysmorphic features and focuses on cardiovascular manifestations in conjunction with genetic information.
- Data has suggested that those with more prominent craniofacial features have more severe disease with cardiovascular complications at younger ages than those with less prominent facial features [24]. Similar observations about specific features being associated with worse cardiovascular outcomes were noted in another cohort with hypertelorism, translucent skin and arterial tortuosity being associated with higher odds ratio of prophylactic surgical aortic repair and aortic dissection [21].
- Another cardinal feature that should prompt consideration of Loeys-Dietz as a diagnosis is tortuous cerebrovascular vessels especially those of the head and neck seen on imaging [26].
- One third of individuals with Loeys-Dietz syndrome have skeletal features including joint contractures, talipes equinovarus (clubbed foot), camptodactyly, pectus deformity, arachnodactyly, joint hypermobility or scoliosis [19].

Table 5 Different types of Loeys-Dietz syndrome

Type	Gene mutation
Type I	TGFBR1
Type II	TGFBR2
Type III	SMAD3
Type IV	TGFB2
Type V	TGFB3
Type VI	SMAD2

Screening and Surveillance

- With a new diagnosis of Loeys-Dietz, 25% of cases are familial thus first degree family members should also be screened for aneurysms and potential diagnosis of Loeys-Dietz syndrome [27].
- Baseline imaging of the aortic root and entire vascular tree is recommended as 50% of individuals with have aneurysm distant from aortic root [23, 27]. The size of the aortic root can be monitored with transthoracic echocardiograms however the rest of the vascular tree is examined with CT or MRA. This cardiovascular surveillance is preliminarily every 6 months and once determined to be stable, imaging surveillance is recommended at 1–2 year intervals. MRA scans are used alternatively to CT scans to avoid long-term exposure to radiation [25].
- Individuals with Loeys-Dietz may have cervical spine abnormalities including cervical spine subluxation, instability, scoliosis or kyphosis. In order to assess the cervical spine, flexion/extension X-rays are recommended, especially prior to any planned procedure or surgery [28, 29].

Management

- Pharmacotherapy with beta-blockers or angiotensin-receptor blockers is recommended to avoid hypertension and also decrease shear forces on blood vessels [21, 25].
- Patients should be given exercise recommendations that include avoidance of contact and competitive sports, intense isometric exercise and exercise to the point of exhaustion [21, 25].
- The decision to proceed with prophylactic aortic surgery is based on the absolute dimension of the aortic root, rate of progression, valve function, severity of non-cardiac features, family history of dissection [25]. There are specific guidelines set forth by national and international organizations about guidelines for prophylactic surgery (Table 2) [17, 18].
- Vascular surgery is generally well tolerated by individuals with Loeys-Dietz syndrome. One study stated survival after vascular surgery of 94% [30]. Another study showed fatal complications during vascular surgery or immediately after surgery were 1.7–4.8% in types I and II LDS [24].
- With aortic surgery, there is a long-term risk for need for a subsequent operation and this risk is higher if the original procedure was performed for a type A dissection and not prophylactic aortic surgery [31, 32].
- With type B dissections that require surgery, open repair is generally preferred in these patients over endovascular repair. Thoracic endovascular repair of aortic root (TEVAR) is relatively contraindicated secondary to progressive aortic dilatation and dissection at the landing zones of these devices. Nevertheless, TEVAR can be considered in an emergency situation as a bridge to later open surgical repair [25, 27, 31, 32].

Vascular Ehlers-Danlos Syndrome

Vascular Ehlers-Danlos syndrome (vEDS) is an autosomal dominant condition with features of thin, translucent skin, easy bruising and risk for rupture of arteries and hollow organs such as bowel, spleen or uterus. vEDS has been classified as type IV Ehlers-Danlos syndrome and there are currently 13 sub-types with vEDS subtype comprising 5–10% of the total Ehlers-Danlos population [33]. The prevalence of this condition is 1 in 10,000 to 25,000 [33]. Pathogenic variants in type III procollagen (*COL3A1*) affect the amount and/or properties of normal type III collagen. This results in a loss of tensile strength of arteries, vascular fragility and affects walls strength of hollow organs.

With vEDS, the type III collagen produced is either defective from substitutions of glycine residues, exon skip or splice site mutations or, there is less type III collagen produced with null/haploinsufficiency mutations. Substitution of glycine residues in Gly-X-Y repeats of a triple helical domain disturbs the type III collagen folding process, weakening the collagen, and these alterations account for a majority of identified pathogenic variants in COL3A1. There are also variants in splice acceptor or donor site which lead to exon skipping or frameshift mutations and results in defective type III collagen. Complications are rare in childhood with vEDS however about one fourth of individuals have their first major adverse event by age 29 and greater than 80% have had a major adverse event by age 40. The median survival is 51 years old and most deaths result from arterial rupture [34–36]. Bowel rupture ultimately affects 20–30% of individuals but rarely leads to death. There is a milder form of vEDS in individuals with null mutations where a premature stop codon leads to nonsense-mediated decay and there is half of the normal type III collagen. These nonsense mutations result in a milder phenotype and individuals have a longer life span with the age of first vascular event delayed about 15 years and complications are limited to vascular events [37, 38]. In this group, the median survival is 51 years and in those taken to surgery 70% survive.

Diagnosis

- Traditionally, diagnosis has been based on clinical signs, non-invasive imaging of vascular system and identification of pathogenic variants in type III collagen (*COL3A1*) [33].
- The phenotypical features of vEDS include thin skin with visible veins, easy bruising, thin pinched nose, thin lips, prominent ears, hollow cheeks and tight facial skin [34].
- There has been revised nosology [39] suggested that clinical diagnosis should be considered with two of the following features:
  - Thin, translucent skin
  - Arterial, intestinal or uterine rupture

  - Easy bruising
  - Characteristic facial appearance

- In the absence of family history, the diagnosis of vEDS is not often considered until after a major event of arterial or hollow organ rupture.
- Confirmatory genetic testing is performed on cultured dermal fibroblasts to examine type III collagen mRNA or genetic testing for *COL3A1* pathogenic variants.
- With vEDS, it has been suggested that genetic testing to confirm diagnosis is essential as clinical criteria alone are inadequate to establish diagnosis. The clinical features of vEDS overlap with other types of Ehlers-Danlos syndrome and other connective tissue conditions. In addition, the correct diagnosis of vEDS and the type of mutation of *COL3A1* has serious implications on prognosis, lifelong surveillance, and medical/surgical management decisions [40].

Screening and Surveillance

- Individuals with vEDS have aneurysms, dissections, rupture, pseudoaneurysms, thrombosis or carotid cavernous malformations [40]. The most severe complications arise from arterial rupture or rupture of hollow organs. Unfortunately, there are no biomarkers or imaging criteria to accurately predict these events.
- Currently imaging surveillance and prophylactic surgery guidelines are less well established in this population with surgery typically being reserved for life-threatening vascular complications. This lack of guidance has led to programs and institutions varying in their approach to surveillance that ranges from no regular evaluations to arterial imaging on a yearly basis. Byers and colleagues have recommended if possible annual assessment of vascular system with ultrasound, CTA or MRA [36].
- Fifty percent of those with COL3A1 pathogenic variants have a de novo mutation and the other half have an affected family member with vEDS [36]. Therefore, it is important when a new diagnosis in made in a family to screen first degree family members examining clinical features, imaging findings and genetic testing.

Management

- The major goal of pharmacotherapy is to maintain lower blood pressure and decrease arterial wall tension in an attempt to minimize the likelihood of arterial dissection. The medical therapy that is currently given as treatment includes beta-blockers, angiotensin receptor blockers or combination therapy.

- There was a trial of the mixed β1antagonist and β2 agonist, celiprolol, that suggested treatment with this drug extended time to vascular events compared to those not treated with this medication. The conclusion from this study are weakened by the fact that a third of participants did not have *COL3A1* mutations and there was a failure to ensure those in the comparison group were equivalent in disease severity to those in the treatment group [41]. Thus, there is not yet evidence based guidance for medical treatment in vEDS.
- Some of the arterial events in smaller arteries are self-limiting and do not require surgical intervention. Typically the location of the arterial rupture determines the method of treatment. Surgery is typically reserved for life-threatening vascular complications
- Surgical morbidity has been historically described as high as 40%, attributed to tissue fragility, poor wound healing, excess bleeding, fistula formation, and adhesions [38]. However, more recent, larger studies in this population have shown improved surgical outcomes with cautionary measures in regards to tissue handling and open repair of aneurysms/dissection is well tolerated [40].
- Similar to other connective tissue recommendations, the use of TEVAR is generally not advised as this carries a significant risk of erosion at the fixation zones secondary to fragility of the aortic wall and concern for retrograde aortic dissection [40].

Turner Syndrome

Turner syndrome is a sex chromosome disorder caused by partial or complete monosomy of the X chromosome in a female. It accounts for 1/2500 live female births. Women with Turner syndrome have a 100-fold increased risk for aortic dissection compared to the general population and this adverse cardiovascular outcome typically occurs in the third or fourth decade of life [42].

Individuals with Turner syndrome have an imbalance in TIMP and MMPs due to hemizygosity of TIMP1. This imbalance is further exacerbated by TIMP3 risk alleles. As a result, loss of inhibition of MMP 2 and 9 proteolytically degrade extracellular matrix of the aortic wall. This degradation releases more active TGFβ which is normally sequestered by extracellular matrix proteins. As TGFβ activity increases, there is more fibrosis and inflammation and increased MMP activity which leads to aortic aneurysm [43, 44].

Diagnosis

- Clinical features of short stature, early onset ovarian failure, metabolic and hormonal aberrations, aortic disease and congenital heart abnormalities suggest this diagnosis [45].

- Karyotype confirms the partial or complete monosomy X.
- Congenital heart abnormalities occur in up to 50% of individuals, mainly affecting the left side of the heart including bicuspid aortic valve, coarctation of the aorta, and thoracic aortic aneurysm.

Surveillance

- Because of the high prevalence of congenital and acquired cardiovascular disease in Turner syndrome, noninvasive cardiac imaging using echocardiogram, cardiac magnetic resonance and computed tomography is recommended for diagnosis, management and risk assessment [46].
- Unlike other connective tissue conditions, the predictors of aortic dissection risk have not been extensively studied.
- The ascending aortic diameter divided by body surface area is the aortic size index (ASI); the ASI has been used to assess risk for aortic dissection in the Turner syndrome population [47]. The ASI >2.3 and presence of congenital heart disease have been used to stratify individuals into higher versus lower risk groups for aortic dissection and defines the frequency of surveillance with imaging.
- It is important to note that women with Turner syndrome can have aortic dissection at smaller ascending aortic diameters than those with other genetic aortopathies.

Management

- In contrast to other aortopathy conditions, the aortic size index (ASI), which takes into account stature and body surface area, is utilized to decide when someone should have prophylactic aortic surgery. However, there is not complete consensus on what this threshold should be for prophylactic surgery [46].
- Women with Turner syndrome are at increased risk to develop hypertension and should be treated medically if this develops. Treatment for aortic dilatation includes beta-blocker, angiotensin receptor blocker or combination of both.
- Women should be counseled that pregnancy may be a higher risk time for aortic dissection. In addition, contraception counseling should be given to reproductive age women.
- Similar to other genetic-aortopathy conditions, avoidance of intense weight training and competitive, contact sports are not recommended if there is aortic root dilation [46].

Bicuspid Aortic Valve Aortopathy

Bicuspid aortic valve (BAV) is one of the most common heart defects affecting approximately 1–2% of the U.S. population with male:female ratio of 2:1 [48]. Of those with a bicuspid aortic valve, 40–60% of these individuals have aortic root or ascending aorta dilatation [8, 49]. There is a six- to ninefold increases risk for aortic complications such as dissection and rupture with bicuspid aortic valve aortopathy compared to the general population [49]. There have been efforts to classify BAV based on location of aortic dilation versus morphological classification to define distinct patterns however to date no uniform classification exists [50].

Bicuspid aortic valve aortopathy is autosomal dominant however it has decreased penetrance and variable expressivity [51]. Despite knowledge of this being a heritable condition, the genetic pathogenic variants that results in BAV aortopathy have not been identified in a majority of cases however there are some genes including *NOTCH1* that have been associated with predisposition for aortopathy [52, 53].

Diagnosis

- BAV aortopathy is a clinical diagnosis from transthoracic echocardiogram and vascular imaging studies of CT and MRA

Screening and Surveillance

- As mentioned earlier, this is a heritable condition but with reduced penetrance with this condition being present in 9% of first degree relatives [51].
- There are many risk factors that are taken into account along with aortic root and ascending aorta size and frequency and approach to surveillance has not been streamlined amongst providers. An individualized plan for surveillance based on aorta dimensions and other risk factors.

Management

- Persons with BAV aortopathy are treated with beta-blockers to normalize blood pressure and decrease wall stress.
- There are national and international guidelines for surgical decision making about prophylactic aortic surgery with BAV aortopathy based on aortic root size measurements. Prophylactic surgery is to be considered with aortic root measurements >5.5 cm or >5 cm with other risk factors present (Table 2) [54].

- However, in clinical practice these decisions may be more complex than consideration of the aortic root size [50]. In a survey of 100 surgeons, there were differences in surgical approaches and decisions based on attitude of surgeon about the disease and genetic versus hemodynamic etiology beliefs [55]. In addition, the threshold sizes suggested for prophylactic surgery are not based on conclusive data but instead expert opinion. Some authors suggest considerations of BSA, gender, age, lifelong growth of aortic root diameter and should be taken into account with aortic root measurements [50].

Familial Thoracic Aortic Aneurysms

This is a group of conditions with heritable thoracic aortic aneurysms however there are no systemic signs of disease. A majority of these pathogenic variants are autosomal dominant with reduced penetrance and variable expressivity. A majority of altered genes are responsible for the contractile apparatus of smooth muscle cells including pathogenic variants in the genes: *ACTA2*, *MYH11*, *MYLK*, and *PRKG1*. The *ACTA2* mutations account for 10–15% of familial thoracic aneurysms. *MYH11* encodes myosin heavy chain 11 and accounts for 2% of familial thoracic aneurysms. These individuals have ascending thoracic aneurysms and there is an association with patent ductus arteriosus. *MYLK* encodes myosin light chain kinase and can lead to acute aortic dissection without preceding aneurysm. PRGKG1 encodes type I cGMP-dependent protein kinase that is responsible for smooth muscle relaxation. Pathogenic variants in this gene are associated with coronary aneurysms and aortic dissections at younger ages. These are very rare conditions and currently there are no formal recommendations for surveillance as aortic root dilation does not predict these events and no formal recommendations in management.

Other Genetic Syndromes Associated with Aortic Dissection

There are some other syndromes or genetic conditions associated with aortic aneurysm and dissection that should be mentioned. Arterial tortuosity syndrome is a rare autosomal recessive condition with loss of function mutations in *SLC2A10* which encodes facilitative glucose transporter GLUT10 for glucose homeostasis. This syndrome is characterized by arterial tortuosity, stenosis of medium and large sized arteries and a propensity for aneurysm formation and dissection. They can have Marfanoid skeletal features or craniofacial features. Some of these individuals have poor prognosis with mortality as high as 40% in first 5 years of life or less severe phenotype [56]. Autosomal dominant polycystic kidney disease and Noonan syndrome have also been associated with higher risk for aortic dissection compared to the general population.

References

1. Albornoz G, Coady MA, Roberts M, Davies RR, Tranquilli M. Familial thoracic aortic aneurysms and dissections—incidence, modes of inheritance, and phenotypic patterns. Ann Thorac Surg. 2006;82(4):1400–5.
2. Elefteriades JA, Farkas EA. Thoracic aortic aneurysm clinically pertinent controversies and uncertainties. JACC. 2010;55(9):841–57.
3. Renard M, Francis C, Ghosh R, Scott AF, Witmer PD, et al. Clinical validity of genes for heritable thoracic aortic aneurysm and dissection. JACC. 2018;72(6):605–15.
4. Verstraeten A, Alaerts M, Van Laer L, Loeys B. Marfan syndrome and related disorders: 25 years of gene discovery. Hum Mutation. 2016;37:524–31.
5. Verhagen JM, Kempers M, Cozijnsen L, Bouma BJ, Duijnhouwer AL, et al. Expert consensus recommendations on the cardiogenetic care for patients with thoracic aortic disease and their first-degree relatives. Int J Cardiol. 2018;258:243–8.
6. Mas-Stachurska A, Siegert AM, Batlle M, Del Blanco DG, Meirelles T, et al. Cardiovascular benefits of moderate exercise training in Marfan syndrome: insights from an animal model. J Am Heart Assoc. 2017;6(9):e006438.
7. Pape LA, Awais M, Woznick EM, Suzuki T, Trimarchi S et al. Presentation, diagnosis, and outcomes of acute aortic dissection: 17-Year trends from the international registry of acute aortic dissection. JACC. 2015;66(4):350–8.
8. Paterick TE, Humphries JA, Ammar KA, Jan MF, Loberg R, et al. Aortopathies: etiologies, genetics, differential diagnosis, prognosis and management. Am J Med. 2013;126(8):670–8.
9. Silverman DI, Burton KJ, Gray J, Bosner MS, Kouchoukos NT. Life expectancy in Marfan syndrome. 1995;75(2):157–60.
10. Finkbohner R, Johnston D, Crawford ES, Coselli J, Milewicz D. Aortas/pulmonary arteries: Marfan syndrome: long-term survival and complications after aortic aneurysm repair. Clin Investig Rep. 1995;91(3):728–33.
11. Habashi JP, Judge DP, Holm TM, Cohn RD, Loeys BL, Cooper TK, et al. Losartan, an AT1 antagonist, prevents aortic aneurysm in a mouse model of Marfan syndrome. Science. 2006;312(5770):117–21.
12. Neptune ER, Frischmeyer PA, Arking DA, Myers L, Bunton TE. Dysregulation of TGF-beta activation contributes to pathogenesis in Marfan syndrome. Nat Genetics. 2003;33(3):407–11.
13. Loeys BL, Dietz HC, Braverman AC, Callewaert BL, De Backer J, et al. The revised Ghent nosology for the Marfan syndrome. J Med Genetics. 2010;47:476–85.
14. Shores J, Berger KR, Murphy EA, Pyretiz RE. Progression of aortic dilatation and the benefit of long-term beta-adrenergic blockade in Marfan's syndrome. NEJM. 1994;330:1335–41.
15. Ladouceur M, Fermaniam C, Lupoglazoff JM, et al. Effect of beta-blockade no ascending aortic dilatation in children with Marfan syndrome. Am J Cardiol. 2007;99:406–9.
16. Gersony DR, McClaughin MA, Jin Z, Gersony WM. The effect of beta-blocker therapy on clinical outcome in patient's with Marfan syndrome: a meta-analysis. Int J Cardiol. 2007;114:303–8.
17. Hiratzka LF, Bakris GL, Beckman JA, et al. 2010 ACCF/AHA/AATS/ACR/ASA/SCA/SCAI/SIR/STS/SVM Guidelines for the diagnosis and management of patients with thoracic aortic disease. A Report of the American College of Cardiology Foundation/American Heart Association Task Force on Practice Guidelines, American Association of Thoracic Surgery, American College of Radiology, American Stroke Association, Society of Cardiovascular Anesthesiologists, Society of Cardiovascular Angiography and Interventions, Society of Interventional Radiology, Society of Thoracic Surgeons and Society of Vascular Medicine. J Am Coll Cardiol. 2010;55:e27–129.
18. Erbel R, Aboyans V, Boileau C, Bossone E, Bartolomeo RD, et al. ESC guidelines on the diagnosis and treatment of aortic diseases: document covering acute and chronic aortic diseases of the thoracic and abdominal aorta of the adult. The task force for the diagnosis

and treatment of aortic diseases of the European Society of Cardiology (ESC). Eur Heart J. 2014;2014:2873–926.
19. Attias D, Sthenuer C, Roy C, Collod-Beroud G, Detaint D, et al. Comparison of clinical presentations and outcomes between patients with TGFBR2 and FBN1 mutations in Marfan syndrome and related disorders. Circulation. 2009;120:2541–9.
20. Loeys BL, Chen J, Neptune ER, Judge DP, Podowski M, et al. A syndrome of altered cardiovascular, craniofacial, neurocognitive and skeletal development caused by mutations in TGFBR1 or TGFBR2. Nat Genetics. 2005;37(3):275–81.
21. Jondeau G, Ropers J, Regalado E, Braverman A, Evangelista A, et al. International registry of patients carrying TGFBR1 or TGRBR2 mutations, results of MAC (Montalcino Aortic Consortium). Circ Cardiovasc Genetics. 2016;9:548–58.
22. Meester JAN, Verstraeten A, Schepers D, Alaerts M, Van Laer L, et al. Differences in manifestations of Marfan syndrome, Ehlers-Danlos syndrome and Loeys-Dietz syndrome. Ann Cardiothorac Surg. 2017;6(6):582–94.
23. Loeys BL, Dietz HC. Loeys-Dietz syndrome. Gene Reviews [Internet]. Seattle (WA) Updated March 2018.
24. Loeys BL, Schwarze U, Holm T, Cakkewaert BL, Thomas GH, et al. Aneurysm syndromes caused by mutations in the TGF-beta receptor. N Engl J Med. 2006;355(8):788–98.
25. MacCarrick G, Black J, Bowdin S, El-Hamamsy I, Frischmeyere-Guerrerio P, et al. Loeys-Dietez syndrome: a primer for diagnosis and management. Genet Med. 2014;16(8):576–87.
26. Tran-Fadulu V, Pannu H, Kim DH, Vick GW, Lonsford CM, et al. Analysis of multigenerational families with thoracic aortic aneurysms and dissections due to TGFBR1 or TGFBR2 mutations. J Med Genetics. 2009;46:607–13.
27. Van Hemelrijk C, Renard M, Loeys B. The Loeys-Dietz syndrome: an update for the clinician. Curr Opin Cardiol. 2010;25:546–51.
28. Erkula G, Sponseller PD, Paulsen LC, Oswald GL, Loeys B, et al. Musculoskeletal findings of Loeys-Dietz syndrome. J Bone Joint Surg Am. 2010;92:1876–83.
29. Sousa SB, Lambot-Juhan K, Rio M, et al. Expanding the skeletal phenotype of Loeys-Dietz syndrome. Am J Med Genetics. 2011;155A:1178–83.
30. Krohg-Sorensen K, Lingaas PS, Lundblad R, Seem E, Paus B, et al. Cardiovascular surgery in Loeys-Dietz syndrome types 1-4. Eur J Cardiothorac Surg. 2017;52:1125–31.
31. Aftab M, Cikach F, Zhu Y, Idrees JI, Rigelsky CM, et al. Loeys-Dietz syndrome: intermediate-term outcomes of medically and surgically managed patients. J Thorac Cardiovasc Surg. 2019;157(2):439–50.
32. Williams JA, Loeys BL, Nwakanma LU, et al. Early surgical experience with Loeys-Dietz: a new syndrome of aggressive thoracic aortic aneurysm disease. Ann Thor Surg. 2007;83:S757–63.
33. Germain DP. Ehlers-Danlos syndrome type IV. Orphanet J Rare Dis. 2007;2:32.
34. Pepin M, Schwarze U, Superti-Furga A, Byers PH. Clinical and genetic features of Ehlers-Danlos syndrome type IV, the vascular type. N Engl J Med. 2000;342(10):673–80.
35. Frank M, Albuisson J, Ranque B, Golmard L, Mazzella JM, et al. The type of variants at the COL3A1 gene associates with phenotype and severity of vascular Ehlers-Danlos syndrome. Eur J Hum Genet. 2015;23:1657–64.
36. Byers PH, Belmont J, Black J, De Backer J, Frank M, et al. Diagnosis, natural history, and management in vascular Ehlers-Danlos syndrome. AJMG. 2017;175C:40–7.
37. Leistritz DF, Pepin MG, Schwarze U, Byers PH. COL3A1 haploinsufficiency results in a variety of Ehlers-Danlos syndrome type IV with delayed onset of complications and longer life expectancy. Genet Med. 2011;13(8):717–22.
38. Pepin MG, Schwarze U, Rice KM, Liu M, Leistritz D, Byers PH. Survival is affected by mutation type and molecular mechanism in vascular Elhers-Danlos syndrome (EDS type IV). Genet Med. 2014;16(12):881–8.
39. Beighton P, De Paepe A, Steinmann B, Tsipouras P, Wenstrup RJ. Ehlers-Danlos syndromes: revised nosology, Villefranche, 1997. Ehlers-Danlos National Foundation (USA) and Ehlers-Danlos support group (UK). Am J Med Genet. 1998;77(1):31–7.

40. Shalhub S, Byers PH, Hicks KL, Coleman DM, Davis FM, et al. A multi-institutional experience in vascular Ehlers-Danlos syndrome diagnosis. J Vasc Surg. 2020;71(1):149–57.
41. Ong KT, Perdu J, DeBacker J, Bozec E, Colligan P, et al. Effect of celiprolol on prevention of cardiovascular events in vascular Ehlers-Danlos syndrome: a prospective randomized, open, blinded-endpoints trial. Lancet. 2010;376:1476–84.
42. Matura LA, Ho VB, Rosing DR, Bondy CA. Aortic dilatation and dissection in Turner syndrome. Circulation. 2007;116(15):1663–70.
43. Corbitt H, Gutierrez J, Silberbach M, Maslen C. The genetic basis of Turner syndrome aortopathy. AmJ Genet C Semin Med Genet. 2019;181(1):117–25.
44. Corbitt H, Morris SA, Gravholt CH, Mortensen KH, Tippner-Hedges R, et al. TIMP3 and TIMP1 are risk genes for bicuspid aortic valve and aortopathy in turner syndrome. PLoS Genet. 2018;14(10):e1007692.
45. Turtle EJ, Sule AA, Bath LE, Denvir M, Gebbie A, et al. Assessing and addressing cardiovascular risk in adults with Turner syndrome. Clin Endocrinol. 2013;78(5):639–45.
46. Silberbach M, Roos-Hesselink JW, Andersen NH, Braverman AC, Brown N, et al. Cardiovascular health in Turner syndrome: a scientific statement from the American Heart Association. Circ Genomics Precis Med. 2018;11(10):e000048.
47. Corbitt H, Maslen C, Prakash S, Morris SA, Silberbach M. Allometric considerations when assessing aortic aneurysms in Turner syndrome: implications for activity recommendations and medical decision-making. AJMG. 2018;176:277–82.
48. Ward C. Clinical significance of bicuspid aortic valve. Heart. 2000;83:81–5.
49. Michelena HI, Khanna AD, Mahoney D, Margaryan E, Topilsky Y, et al. Incidence of aortic complications in patients with bicuspid aortic valves. JAMA. 2011;306:1104–12.
50. Stock S, Mohammed SA, Sievers HH. Bicuspid aortic valve related aortopathy. Gen Thorac Cardiovasc Surg. 2019;67:93–101.
51. Cripe L, Andelfinger G, Martin LJ, Shooner K, Benson W. Bicuspid aortic valve is heritable. JACC. 2004;44(1):138–43.
52. Mohamed SA, Aherrahrou Z, Liptau H, Erasmi AW, Hagemann C, et al. Novel missense mutations (p.T596M and p.P1797H) in NOTCH1 in patients with bicuspid aortic valve. Biochem Biophys Res Commun. 2006;345:1460–5.
53. McKellar SH, Tester DJ, Yagubyan M, Majumdar R, Ackerman MJ, et al. Novel NOTCH1 mutations in patients with bicuspid aortic valve disease and thoracic aneurysms. J Thorac Cardiovasc Surg. 2007;134:290–6.
54. Hiratzka LF, Creager MA, Isselbacher EM, Svensson LG. AHA/ACC Guidelines for the Management of Patients with Valvular Heart Disease Representative Members. Surgery for aortic dilatation in patients with bicuspid aortic valves: a statement of clarification from the American College of Cardiology/American Heart Association Task Force on Clinical Practice Guidelines. J Thoracic Cardiovasc Surg. 2016;151:959–66.
55. Verma S, Yanagawa B, Kalra S, Ruel M, Peterson MD, et al. Knowledge, attitudes and practice patterns in surgical management of bicuspid aortopathy: a survey of 100 cardiac surgeons. J Thoracic Cardiovasc Surgery. 2013;146:1033–4.
56. Morris SA. Arterial tortuosity in genetic arteriopathies. Curr Opinion Cardiology. 2015;30(6):587–93.

Presentation of Acute Aortic Syndromes

Santi Trimarchi, Hector W. L. de Beaufort, and Theodorus M. J. van Bakel

History

The majority of patients with acute aortic syndromes, especially those affecting the distal thoracic aorta, have a history of hypertension. Other conditions in the patient's history that should increase the suspicion of an acute aortic syndrome are known thoracic aneurysm, pregnancy, repaired or unrepaired coarctation of the aorta, and aortic valve abnormalities. Moreover, connective tissue disorders and genetic defects (Marfan, Ehlers-Danlos, Noonan, and Turner syndrome) predispose to aneurysm and dissection.

Signs and Symptoms

The most common presenting symptom of acute aortic syndromes is pain, regardless of whether the eventual diagnosis is aortic dissection, intramural hematoma, or symptomatic penetrating aortic ulcer. It is reported by 95.5% of acute dissection patients, and is usually described as severe or as the worst pain ever experienced, with a sudden onset (Table 1) [1]. The abrupt onset and unremitting nature of the pain may help to distinguish from myocardial infarction, in which the pain tends to be more crescendo in nature. The quality of the pain is most commonly described as

S. Trimarchi (✉)
Fondazione IRCCS Ca' Granda Ospedale Maggiore Policlinico Milano, Milan, Italy

Department of Clinical Sciences and Community Health, University of Milan, Milan, Italy
e-mail: santi.trimarchi@unimi.it

H. W. L. de Beaufort · T. M. J. van Bakel
Thoracic aortic research program, University of Milan, Milan, Italy

J. S. Coselli et al. (eds.), *Aortic Dissection and Acute Aortic Syndromes*,
https://doi.org/10.1007/978-3-030-66668-2_5

Table 1 Pain in aortic dissection, percentage of patients who report characteristic (adapted from Hagan et al. [1])

	Type A dissection (%)	Type B dissection (%)
Any pain	95.5	93.8
Abrupt onset	84.8	85.4
Chest pain	72.7	78.9
Back pain	53.2	46.6
Abdominal pain	29.6	21.6
Severe or worst ever pain	90.6	90.1
Sharp pain	64.4	62.0
Tearing or ripping pain	50.6	49.4
Radiating	28.3	27.2
Migrating	16.6	14.9

sharp, or as a tearing or ripping sensation [1]. Intensive physical activity or involving rapid movement, such as lifting weights, chopping wood with an axe, and playing sports are sometimes mentioned as provoking factors [2].

The pain is reported in the chest, anterior and/or posterior, and in abdomen. A proximal dissection more typically starts as anterior chest pain that progresses down the back or even into the thighs, and a distal dissection as back pain that migrates down into the abdomen. However, these findings are not specific, as there is a substantial overlap in reported location of the pain. Another characteristic is radiating or migratory pain (Fig. 1) that should heighten suspicion of dissection, although this is reported in just 16.6% of patients [1]. Abdominal pain can be a symptom of mesenteric malperfusion, which may also cause watery or bloody defecation. It is present in about 3.7% of type A dissection and 7% of type B dissection patients [3]. Increased lactate levels can help to confirm the diagnosis but take longer to develop, so in many cases, the decision to intervene will be based on high clinical suspicion. Abdominal pain may also be associated with renal ischemia, which is reported preoperatively in 18% of the patients, while leg pain points to peripheral malperfusion involving the iliac and femoral arteries, reported in 9.7% of cases [3].

A small minority of dissection patients, particularly those with Marfan syndrome or who are on steroid medication [2], as well as those with previous cardiac surgery [4], may present without pain. In these patients, syncope or focal neurologic deficits ("giving way or collapse of the legs") are the main presenting symptoms [4].

Overall, syncope is reported by up to 10% of patients [1]. In slightly over half of patients, it indicates the presence of cardiac tamponade or extension of the dissection into the brachiocephalic vessels and stroke [5]. In the other half, the syncope may be related to other pathophysiologic mechanisms, including vasovagal reactions. However, in contrast to myocardial ischemia, nausea or vomiting are less frequent in aortic dissection [2]. If the dissection leads to obstruction of a coronary artery, symptoms of myocardial ischemia are present. When dyspnea is present, this is usually caused by acute severe aortic valve insufficiency.

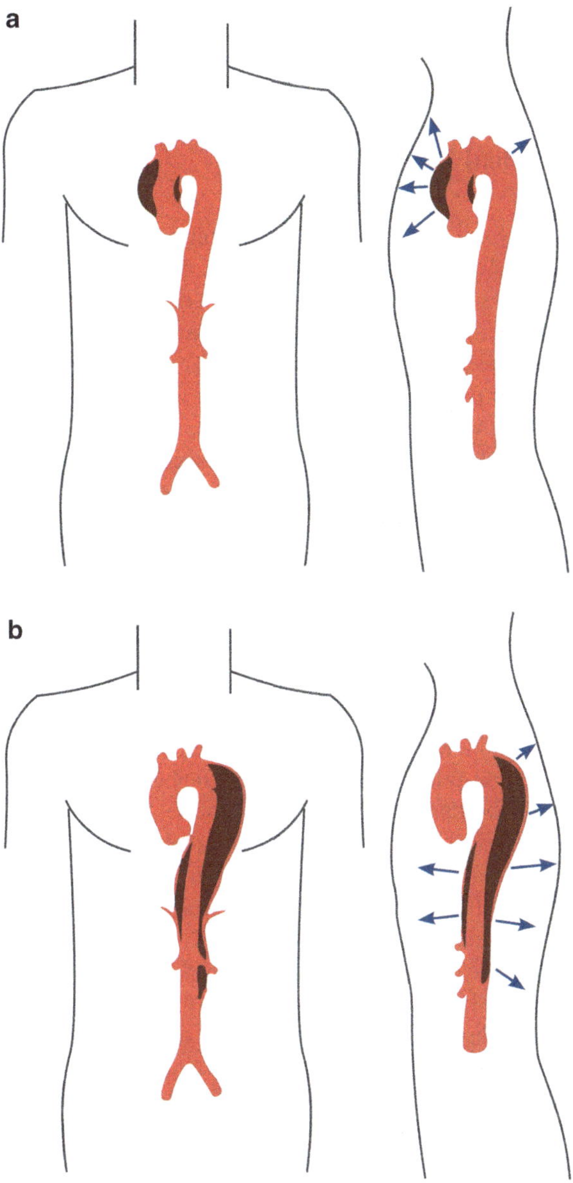

Fig. 1 Radiating pain in (**a**) Stanford type A aortic dissection (**b**) Stanford type B aortic dissection

Neurologic symptoms are related either to branch vessel obstruction, which may be expressed as stroke or reduced consciousness when the carotid artery is involved, and as acute paraplegia when the blood supply to the spinal cord is obstructed. The latter is more common in distal dissection, but is still rare. Even rarer neurologic symptoms are caused by a mass effect of the enlarging aorta, and include Horner syndrome, from compression of the superior cervical sympathetic ganglion, and hoarseness, from compression of the left recurrent laryngeal nerve.

Physical Exam

On physical examination, the patient may give a restless, agitated or apprehensive impression, and appear shocked, cold, clammy, with the sensation of imminent death. Tachycardia is almost always noted [2]. The rest of the findings on physical examination depend on the location and extent of the dissection. While a history of hypertension is present in about 80% of patients, only 35.7% of type A dissection patients present with hypertension, while 24.6% are hypotensive, which can be caused by aortic valve insufficiency, cardiac tamponade, or less commonly, coronary occlusion as a result of the dissection [1]. Moreover, if the dissection leads to malperfusion of the brachiocephalic vessels, brachial cuff pressures may be falsely depressed. Hypotension is rarely present in type B dissection, and is usually a sign of aortic rupture with hemothorax or hemoperitoneum.

On auscultation, a new onset diastolic decrescendo murmur points to the presence of aortic valve insufficiency. This is noted in 31.6% of dissections, most of which are ascending dissections [1]. Prolapse of the cusp due to a single commissure being dissected affects leaflet coaptation, which in some cases returns when the dissection spreads further proximally into the annulus. Aortic insufficiency can also be due to a tear in the aortic root with prolapse of the entire valve. The murmur of dissection-related aortic valve insufficiency is most commonly heard along the right sternal border (in contrast to pre-existent aortic valve insufficiency, which is most commonly heard along the left sternal border). Auscultation might also reveal a pericardial rub or distant heart sounds, indicative of cardiac tamponade. Findings of pleural effusion, especially on auscultation of the left hemithorax, point to distal aortic rupture.

Obstruction of branch vessels by the dissection flap can lead to weak or absent peripheral pulses, which is noted in 15.1% of patients [1]. These pulse deficits of the carotid, brachial or femoral arteries are associated with upper or lower extremity and brain malperfusion, and are associated with an increased risk of mortality [6]. Leg ischemia is a marker of extensive dissection and may be accompanied by compromise of other vascular territories. On the other hand, it is well known that pulse deficits change in nature as the dissection expands distally and produces re-entries. Spontaneous return of pulses is noted in up to a third of patients with lower extremity malperfusion [7]. Moreover, pulse deficits are a quite specific finding and can thus lead to a swifter diagnosis of dissection. This could explain why pulse deficits do not always lead to higher mortality.

The electrocardiogram is generally normal or shows nonspecific changes, which is an important way to differentiate the cause of chest pain from myocardial ischemia. However, in proximal dissections extending into the coronary ostia, S-T segment and T-wave changes may be observed. Heart block can result from extension of the hematoma into the aortic root, interatrial septum, and atrioventricular node.

Laboratory tests are usually normal, or have non-specific changes. Mild anemia and mild leukocytosis are not uncommon. In cases of hemothorax, important anemia can be detected. Bilirubin and lactic acid dehydrogenase levels may be increased due to hemolization of blood trapped within the false lumen. In cases of malperfusion syndrome, metabolic acidosis may be present, and renal malperfusion can lead to oliguria/anuria and microscopic hematuria. D-dimer is generally highly increased in acute dissection, so dissection can be reliably ruled out with D-dimer levels below a cut-off of 500 ng/ml [8].

Differences in Presentation of Intramural Hematoma and Penetrating Aortic Ulcer

There are few, if any, differences in presentation between intramural hematoma and aortic dissection [9], although patients with any kind of intramural hematoma appear less likely to present with pulse deficits [10, 11]. Other differences with aortic dissection are that those with type A intramural hematoma are less likely to present with aortic regurgitation, and those with type B intramural hematoma are more likely to present with chest pain [10, 11]. Penetrating aortic ulcer (PAU) is still included in the acute aortic syndromes, although the typical PAU patient is elderly with hypertension, and generally does not present with symptoms, being diagnosed occasionally after CT scan. In these patients, pain can be present in those with impending PAU rupture, sudden diameter increase, or frank rupture. Due to the focal nature of the lesion, the thoracic pain, which is characteristic of all acute aortic syndromes, is usually not accompanied by signs of aortic valve insufficiency, pulse deficits, or neurologic deficits [12].

References

1. Hagan PG, Nienaber CA, Isselbacher EM, Bruckman D, Karavite DJ, Russman PL, et al. The international registry of acute aortic dissection (IRAD): new insights into an old disease. JAMA. 2000;283(7):897–903.
2. Svensson LG, Crawford ES. Aortic dissection and aortic aneurysm surgery: clinical observations, experimental investigations, and statistical analyses. Part II. Curr Probl Surg. 1992;29(12):913–1057.
3. Evangelista A, Isselbacher EM, Bossone E, Gleason TG, Eusanio MD, Sechtem U, et al. Insights from the international registry of acute aortic dissection: a 20-year experience of collaborative clinical research. Circulation. 2018;137(17):1846–60.
4. Imamura H, Sekiguchi Y, Iwashita T, Dohgomori H, Mochizuki K, Aizawa K, et al. Painless acute aortic dissection. Diagnostic, prognostic and clinical implications. Circ J. 2011;75(1):59–66.

5. Nallamothu BK, Mehta RH, Saint S, Llovet A, Bossone E, Cooper JV, et al. Syncope in acute aortic dissection: diagnostic, prognostic, and clinical implications. Am J Med. 2002;113(6):468–71.
6. Bossone E, Rampoldi V, Nienaber CA, Trimarchi S, Ballotta A, Cooper JV, et al. Usefulness of pulse deficit to predict in-hospital complications and mortality in patients with acute type A aortic dissection. Am J Cardiol. 2002;89(7):851–5.
7. Cambria RP, Brewster DC, Gertler J, Moncure AC, Gusberg R, Tilson MD, et al. Vascular complications associated with spontaneous aortic dissection. J Vasc Surg. 1988;7(2):199–209.
8. Suzuki T, Distante A, Zizza A, Trimarchi S, Villani M, Salerno Uriarte JA, et al. Diagnosis of acute aortic dissection by D-dimer: the international registry of acute aortic dissection substudy on biomarkers (IRAD-bio) experience. Circulation. 2009;119(20):2702–7.
9. Falconi M, Oberti P, Krauss J, Domenech A, Cesareo V, Bracco D, et al. Different clinical features of aortic intramural hematoma versus dissection involving the descending thoracic aorta. Echocardiography. 2005;22(8):629–35.
10. Harris KM, Braverman AC, Eagle KA, Woznicki EM, Pyeritz RE, Myrmel T, et al. Acute aortic intramural hematoma: an analysis from the international registry of acute aortic dissection. Circulation. 2012;126(11 Suppl 1):S91–6.
11. Tolenaar JL, Harris KM, Upchurch GR Jr, Evangelista A, Moll FL, di Eusanio M, et al. The differences and similarities between intramural hematoma of the descending aorta and acute type B dissection. J Vasc Surg. 2013;58(6):1498–504.
12. Coady MA, Rizzo JA, Hammond GL, Pierce JG, Kopf GS, Elefteriades JA. Penetrating ulcer of the thoracic aorta: what is it? How do we recognize it? How do we manage it? J Vasc Surg. 1998;27(6):1006–15. discussion 15-6

Classification Systems of Acute Aortic Syndromes

Arminder S. Jassar, Rizwan Q. Attia, and Eric M. Isselbacher

Introduction

Acute aortic syndromes (AAS) characterize closely related life-threatening clinical conditions that include aortic dissection, intramural hematoma, and penetrating aortic ulcer. The suggested etiology of these conditions is pathologically different [1]. Although numerous classification systems have been proposed, rather than exhaustively list them all, the objective of this chapter is to highlight the most commonly used and most recently described classifications that would be of greatest utility for those caring for patients with AAS.

Anatomic Classification Systems

Stanford and DeBakey Classifications

The most commonly used classification system for AAS are the DeBakey and the Stanford systems [2, 3] (Fig. 1). For these, the ascending aorta refers to the part of the aorta proximal to the brachiocephalic artery, the aortic arch extends from the brachiocephalic artery to the distal ostium of the left subclavian artery, and the descending aorta from left subclavian artery to the iliac bifurcation. Stanford type A dissection involves the ascending aorta and type B the descending aorta distal to the left subclavian artery (without involvement of the ascending aorta). DeBakey type I dissection involves the ascending aorta, the aortic arch and the descending aorta; DeBakey type II is limited to the ascending aorta only. DeBakey type III involves

A. S. Jassar · R. Q. Attia · E. M. Isselbacher (✉)
Thoracic Aortic Center, Massachusetts General Hospital, Boston, MA, USA
e-mail: eisselbacher@mgh.harvard.edu

J. S. Coselli et al. (eds.), *Aortic Dissection and Acute Aortic Syndromes*,
https://doi.org/10.1007/978-3-030-66668-2_6

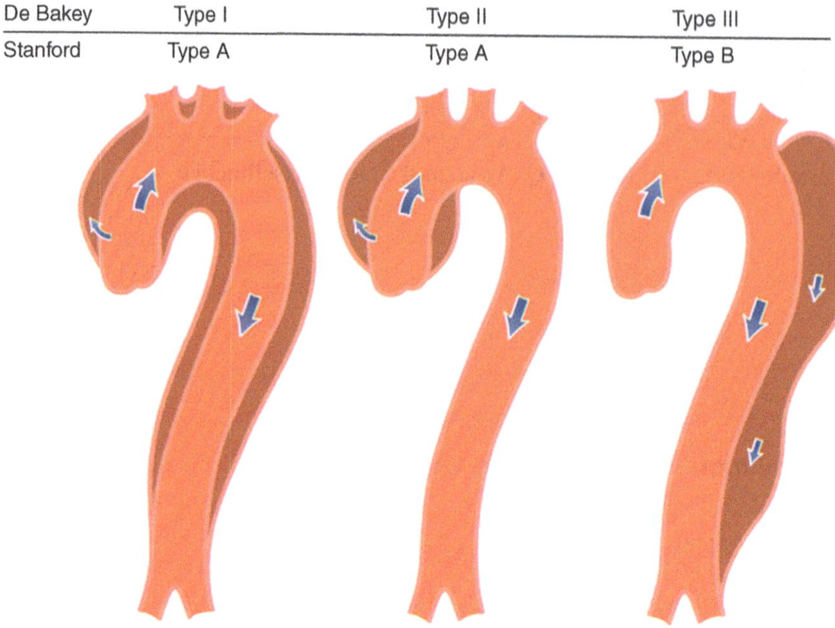

Fig. 1 Traditional classification of aortic dissection. Schematic drawing of aortic dissection subdivided into DeBakey types I, II, III and Stanford A and B. DeBakey type III may be further differentiated into subtypes IIIa (limited to the thoracic aorta) and IIIb (extending into the abdominal aorta). (Figure courtesy of 2014 ESC guidelines on the diagnosis and treatment of aortic diseases [4])

the descending aorta, distal to the subclavian artery. DeBakey type III is further divided into IIIa (limited to the thoracic aorta) and IIIb (extending into the abdominal aorta).

These two classification systems have stood the test of time and are the most widely used classification methodologies. The simplicity of the Stanford classification system has made it the most commonly used system by the non-surgical specialties, including those frequently making the initial diagnosis, i.e., radiologists and emergency medicine physicians. It has the advantage of stratifying treatment strategy based on the type A or B designation, with type A dissection patients treated with emergency aortic replacement, while patients with type B dissection are generally managed medically with aggressive blood pressure control unless there is end-organ malperfusion, risk of aortic rupture, uncontrolled hypertension, or uncontrolled symptoms, in which case intervention can be considered.

Data from the International Registry of Acute Aortic Dissection (IRAD) suggest that the patients with type A dissection who were treated with surgery have a mortality of 15–23%, whereas those treated medically have a mortality of 56–58% [4, 5]. In most instances, the patients treated medically are those who are thought to carry a high risk of death prior to the operation and hence not offered surgery. Longer term survival in surgically managed patients is 97% to 90% at 1 and 3 years, respectively. The medically managed type A patients who survive the initial hospitalization have survival rates of 88% and 68% at 1 and 3 years [5, 6]. Mortality for type B aortic dissection is 7–10% for patients managed medically, 7–32% for patients treated with open surgery, and 1.5–8% for patients treated with endovascular techniques [7, 8]. Longer term survival at 1–3 years is approximately 77% in the medical, 85% in the surgical, and 77–98% in the endovascular cohorts [4, 7, 9].

Dissections of the Aortic Arch: "Non-A, Non-B"

One important limitation of the Stanford and DeBakey classification systems is the lack of a clear and consistent designation for aortic dissections that involve the aortic arch and the descending aorta but spare the ascending aorta. This has prompted some authors to coin the term "non-A non-B" dissection [10]. This entity can be further differentiated into the descending-entry type or the arch-entry type, based on the location of the intimal tear [11]. There is still debate regarding the optimal management of the non-A non-B dissections. In a series of 101 patients in the IRAD registry who had retrograde extension of a descending aortic dissection into the aortic arch, early mortality rate was 9%, 18%, and 13%, for patients treated medically, with open surgical repair, or with endovascular therapies, respectively ($P = 0.51$) [12, 13]. A favorable early mortality rate was observed in patients with retrograde extension limited to the arch at 9% vs. into the ascending aorta at 19%, $P = 0.14$.

In their series of 43 patients with non-A non-B dissection patients, Rylski et al. found that emergency open or endovascular aortic repair was necessary due to malperfusion or aortic rupture in 29% of the 21 patients with an entry site in the descending aorta and 36% of the 22 patients with an entry in the aortic arch, with an in-hospital mortality of 1/6 and 3/8, respectively, of those undergoing aortic repair [11]. Moreover, at 2 weeks following the dissection, aortic repair was required (due to new organ malperfusion, rapid aortic growth, aortic rupture, or persistent pain) in 43% of descending-entry and 36% of arch-entry patients. Indeed, by the end of the 4.4 mean years of follow-up, 88% of patients had undergone aortic intervention.

SVS/STS Classification

Recently, the Society for Vascular Surgery (SVS) and the Society of Thoracic Surgeons (STS) published reporting standards for acute type B dissection and proposed a new anatomic classification system for thoracic aortic dissection. This novel SVS/STS classification is based on the proximal and distal extent of the dissection flap at various zones in the aorta (Fig. 2). This is akin to the well accepted classification of the aortic arch into zones as proposed by Ishimaru [15]. According to this schema, the distinction between type A and type B is determined by the location of

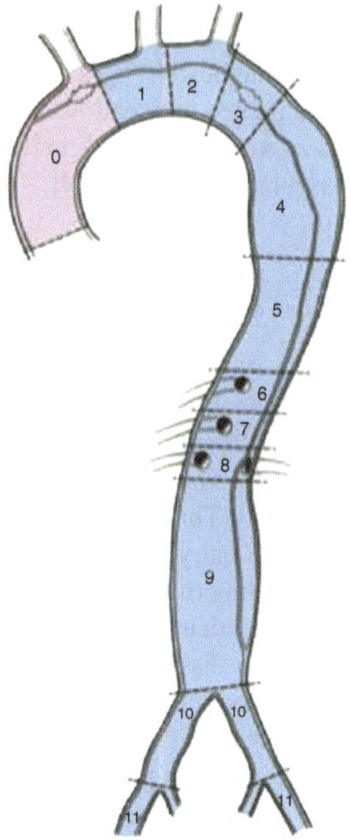

Type	Proximal Extent	Distal Extent
A_D Entry tear: **Zone 0**	0 1 2 3	0 1 2 3
B_{PD} Entry tear: **≥Zone 1**	4 5 6 7 8	4 5 6 7 8
I_D Unidentified entry tear involving **Zone 0**	9 10 11 12	9 10 11 12

Fig. 2 Society for Vascular Surgery/Society of Thoracic Surgeons Aortic Dissection Classification System. (Courtesy SVS/ STS standards reporting committee [14])

the primary entry tear. Any dissection with an entry tear in zone 0 is classified as type A. In addition, a subscript is added to denote the most distal zone to which the dissection extends (A_D). For example, a dissection with an entry tear in the ascending aorta that extends to the infrarenal aorta would be termed A_9. Conversely, any dissection with an entry tear in Zone I or beyond is defined as a type B dissection, and the proximal and distal extents are denoted by a respective pair of subscripts ($B_{P,D}$). For example, a dissection with its intimal tear just distal to the left subclavian artery and extending to the infrarenal aorta would be designated $B_{3,9}$. When considering the proximal and distal extent of a given dissection, any aortic segment that has true and false lumens, a thrombosed false lumen, or intramural hematoma (IMH) are to be included. This classification system designates dissections as indeterminate (rather than type A or B) when the location of the entry tear cannot be determined on diagnostic imaging; and, as with type B dissection, the letter I is followed by a pair of subscripts denoting the proximal and distal extent of the dissection ($I_{P,D}$). The SVS and STS also recommend that patients with IMH and penetrating atherosclerotic ulcers (PAU) also have the extent of their aortic pathology described in a similar manner, namely $IMH_{P,D}$ or $PAU_{P,D}$. Finally, the classification scheme suggests that after a type A dissection repair, any residual distal dissection should be designated as such and include similar subscripts, e.g., residual $B_{P,D}$ (Fig. 2).

While the SVS/STS classification system enables clinicians to accurately define the extent of a dissection, the authors acknowledge that this system is not indented to replace the Stanford or DeBakey classifications, which are both simpler and familiar to the broad medical and surgical community. Indeed, so ingrained is the clinical distinction between the Stanford type A and B dissections, if a patient presents to an emergency with a dissection that involves the ascending aorta but whose entry site is in zone 3, a radiology report that were to classify it as a type B rather than type A dissection could lead to confusion, at the least, and potential mismanagement, at the worst.

Another limitation of the SVS/STS classification system is that although it takes onto account the location of the entry tear in distinguishing type A from type B dissections, it oddly ignores the location of the entry tear in subtyping type B dissections. Indeed, the location of the entry tear is a key determinant of the feasibility of endovascular repair of type B dissections. These limitations suggest that there is ample opportunity to further refine this classification system before it is promoted for routine clinical use.

Chronicity-Based Classification of Aortic Dissection

Historically, acute dissection has been considered to be "acute" when a patient presents 14 days or fewer from symptom onset and "chronic" when presenting more than 14 days from symptom onset. This distinction has been derived from the seminal work of Hirst et al. in the 1950s [16], who observed that mortality in untreated patients with both type A and B dissection significantly declined after 14 days. The estimates of mortality were 21% at 24 h, 49% in the first 4 days, and 74% at 14 days from symptom onset [16]. After 14 days, although mortality continued to rise, the curve flattened significantly during the 2–6-week time frame. Nevertheless, by 3 years the mortality had risen to 95%, indicating that aortic dissection remained lethal well after entering the "chronic" phase. Since this temporal classification system predated the current advances in diagnostic imaging and medical, endovascular, and surgical treatment of aortic dissection, several modifications have been proposed more recently.

IRAD Classification: Hyperacute, Acute, Subacute and Chronic

In a study of over 1800 patients in the IRAD database, Booher et al. [17] examined time-related survival in patients presenting with acute aortic dissection. The survival estimates were stratified by dissection type (Stanford A vs. B) and treatment strategy (medical vs. surgical vs. endovascular). The authors noted that survival continues to decrease significantly for up to 30 days after presentation for both type A and B dissection and across treatment strategies. Based on the inflection points noted in survival (Fig. 3a–c), the time from symptom onset was divided into four

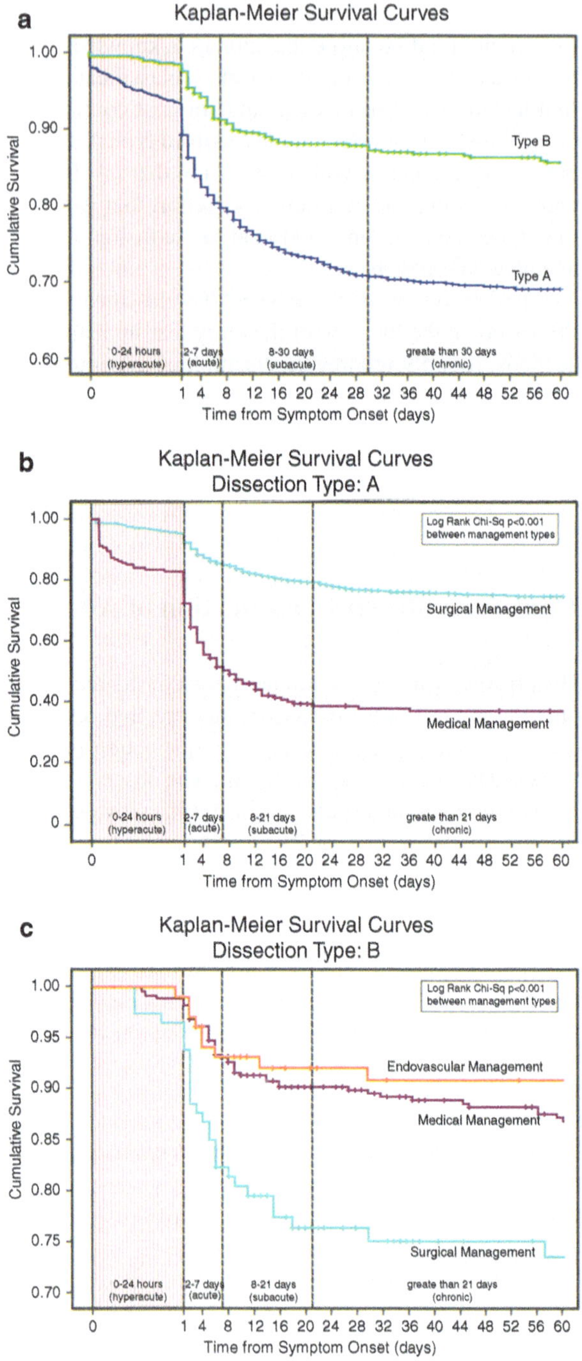

Fig. 3 Kaplan-Meier survival curves for type A and type B dissection. (Booher et al. [17], used with permission)

periods and defined as: hyperacute (0–24 h), acute (2–7 days), subacute (8–30 days), and chronic (>30 days). Importantly, for both type A and B dissection, whether managed medically or with intervention, survival progressively declined during the subacute period.

SVS/STS Classification

The SVS/STS recently proposed a modified classification for aortic dissection based on chronicity. They identify four distinct time periods, as did the IRAD group, but define the four as follows: hyperacute (<24 h); acute (1–14 days); subacute (15–90 days); and chronic (>90 days) (Table 1). Given the increasing role of endovascular therapies in the treatment of type B dissection, a key consideration in designing this classification was the behavior of the dissection flap over time. In the acute phase, the dissection flap tends to be thin and mobile but, as time passes, the dissection flap becomes thicker and less mobile. A rigid flap is much less likely to re-approximate to the aortic wall after TEVAR, thereby reducing the odds of false lumen thrombosis and positive aortic remodeling. In a study of patients undergoing TEVAR for aortic dissection, there was no significant difference in thoracic aortic remodeling between those treated at <14 days and those treated between 15 and 90 days. Thus, the European Society of Cardiology guidelines on the diagnosis and treatment of aortic disease also define the subacute phase of aortic dissection as 15–90 days [4, 18].

Classification Systems Based on Malperfusion and Other Complications at Presentation

The patient's clinical presentation is also an important consideration in classification of patients with acute aortic dissection, as malperfusion is a major determinant of the outcome. Indeed, the presence of malperfusion syndromes increases mortality rates several-fold, with an in-hospital mortality as high as 63% in patients with type A dissection complicated by mesenteric malperfusion [19]. As 30-day mortality following surgical repair of type A dissection remains relatively steady at ~20%

Table 1 Society for Vascular Surgery/Society of Thoracic Surgeons (SVS/STS) Chronicity Classification of Aortic Dissection [14]

Chronicity	Time from onset of symptoms
Hyperacute	<24 h
Acute	1–14 days
Subacute	15–90 days
Chronic	>90 days

[7], there has been increasing attention on the prompt diagnosis and treatment of malperfusion to improve outcomes in these patients.

In recent years, advances in endovascular and hybrid (e.g., frozen elephant trunk) therapies have provided new approaches to address the complications of acute dissection [8, 20, 21]. Resolution of malperfusion may require restoration of flow using endovascular techniques such as intimal fenestration, targeted endografting to seal entry tears, and opening branch vessels central aortic reconstruction [22]. Several classification systems have been proposed that consider the patient's clinical condition and organ system malperfusion at initial presentation.

Penn Classification

This classification system proposed by the group at the University of Pennsylvania is based upon the Stanford system of type A and type B dissection, but further classifies these according to the following: The "absence" of ischemic symptoms (class A), "branch" vessel malperfusion resulting in end-organ ischemia (class B), "circulatory" collapse that produces generalized ischemia (class C), or both regional ischemia from branch vessel malperfusion and generalized ischemia from circulatory collapse (class B and C), as summarized in Tables 2 and 3).

The mortality for acute type A dissection per the Penn classification is reported to be 3–6% for class A, 25–27% for class B, 15–17% for class C, and 40% for class B and C [23]. The mortality for acute type B dissection per the Penn classification is reported to be 6% for class A, 30% for class B, and 33% and B and C (no patients had class C) [25].

TEM Classification

A novel classification system, modeled after the TNM staging system that is widely used for cancer, has recently been proposed for aortic dissection. This classification extends the Stanford classification to include "Type," "Entry" location, and

Table 2 University of Pennsylvania integrated classification of acute Stanford Type A dissection [23]

Penn class	Clinical presentation
Class A	Absent (no) ischemia
Class B	Branch vessel malperfusion (presenting as stroke, paraplegia, mesenteric ischemia, and/or an ischemic limb)
Class C	Circulatory collapse (due to cardiac tamponade, acute aortic regurgitation, coronary artery dissection, or free aortic rupture)
Class B and C	Both branch vessel malperfusion and circulatory collapse

Table 3 University of Pennsylvania integrated classification of acute Stanford Type B dissection [24]

Penn class	Clinical presentation
Class A (uncomplicated)	Absent branch vessel malperfusion or circulatory compromise Type I: High risk for future aortic complications (false lumen diameter > 21 mm, patent or partially thrombosed false lumen, ulcer-like projections, aortic diameter > 40 mm, and intimal tear size and location—proximal, on concavity of the aortic arch) Type II: Low risk for future aortic complications
Class B (complicated)	Branch vessel malperfusion with visceral, renal, lower limb, spinal hypoperfusion based on clinical or laboratory data
Class C (complicated)	Circulatory compromise Type I: Aortic rupture with hemorrhage outside the aortic wall with/without cardiac arrest, shock and hemothorax Type II: Threatened aortic rupture with heralded refractory pain and or hypertension
Class BC (complicated)	Branch vessel malperfusion combined with circulatory compromise

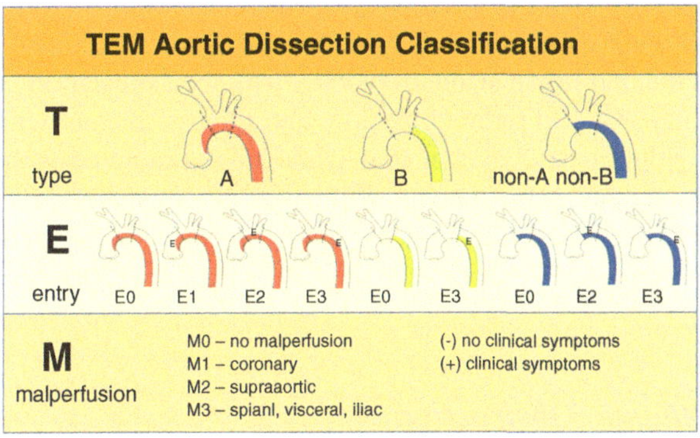

Fig. 4 TEM aortic dissection classification based on dissection type, the site of entry tear, and the presence or absence of malperfusion. (Courtesy Sievers et al. [26], used with permission)

"Malperfusion" in a system known by the acronym TEM [26]. Notably, for the dissection type (T), the authors also added non-A non-B dissection to the traditional Stanford types A and B. The location of the primary entry tear (E) is designated as 1, if the tear is in the ascending aorta; 2, in the arch; 3, in the descending aorta; and 0, if the primary entry tear is not visible (i.e., E0, E1, E2, E3). Malperfusion, based on the vessels radiographically affected, is denoted by the letter M and designated as 1, for coronary arteries; 2, for supra-aortic vessels; 3, for visceral/renal and/or a lower extremity; and 0, if malperfusion is absent (i.e., M0, M1, M2, M3). A plus sign (+) is added if there is clinical evidence of malperfusion (abdominal pain, ileus, bloody diarrhea, anuria, chemical renal failure, or clinical symptoms of limb ischemia) and minus (−) if malperfusion is present only as an imaging finding (Fig. 4).

The rationale for this classification is to help better plan treatment strategies, inform patients of their prognosis, and evaluate treatment results. The authors report in-hospital mortality rates of 16%, 5%, and 8% in patients with type A, type B, and non-A non-B dissection, respectively (P = 0.01); 22%, 14%, 40%, and 0% in patients with type A E0, E1, E2, and E3, respectively (P = 0.023); and 10% and 23% in patients with type A M0 and M3, respectively (P = 0.13). The main limitations of this system are that primary entry tears are not always detectable on CTA. The proximal and the distal extent of the dissection is not well defined in this system. Additionally, this classification has not been validated in larger cohort of clinical cases.

Classification of the Mechanism of Branch Vessel Malperfusion

Mortality for patients with aortic dissection and branch vessel malperfusion remains high. This has led to increasing use of TEVAR for acute type B dissections with malperfusion. In the cases of type A dissection, immediate central aortic repair remains the traditional standard of care, with the expectation that the closure of proximal entry tear and redirecting flow into the true lumen will resolve distal malperfusion. Studies have shown that while this strategy may be effective in majority of the patients, some patients will have ongoing malperfusion after surgical repair [27]. This is dependent on the morphology of the dissection flap in the branch vessel.

Static vs. Dynamic Obstruction

The group from the University of Michigan have described "static" and "dynamic" pathophysiology of the dissection flap involving the visceral branch vessels (Fig. 5) [28]. Dynamic obstruction is said to occur when the true lumen is compressed due to false lumen pressurization, which results in the occlusion of the branch vessel orifice by the dissection flap. Static malperfusion occurs due to the extension of the intimal flap into branch vessels, with subsequent thrombosis of the false lumen and occlusion of the true lumen (Fig. 5). In many cases, a combination of both static and dynamic components may be present. While central aortic repair may relieve dynamic obstruction, once end organ damage has occurred or static occlusion of the branch vessel due to thrombosis of the false lumen is present, malperfusion is not reliably resolved by proximal aortic repair alone.

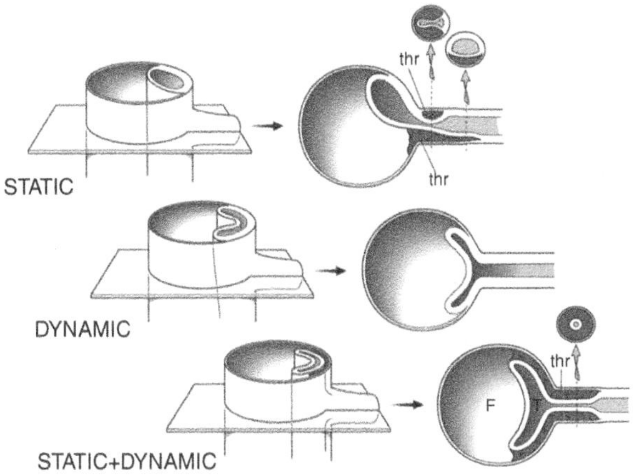

Fig. 5 Static vs. dynamic compression as mechanism of branch vessel occlusion (Courtesy of Kamman et al. [28], used with permission)

Classification of Branch Artery Perfusion by Nagamine et al.

Nagamine and colleagues have proposed a more detailed classification system for branch artery perfusion pattern that emphasizes physiologic and perfusion characteristics over anatomic and morphological criteria [29]. According to their classification, the perfusion patterns can be categorized into three classes:

- Class I, dissection involving but not extending into the branch artery
- Class II, dissection extending into the branch artery
- Class III, dissection causing branch artery ostial avulsion

Each class is further categorized based on branch perfusion pattern and the presence or absence of branch blood flow obstruction due to compression by the dissection flap, or false lumen thrombosis (Fig. 6). After central aortic repair, the resulting perfusion patterns were compared to the pre-repair blood flow and categorized into four possible results: (1) improvement compared to baseline; (2) no change in low-risk patterns (3) no improvement or worsening in high-risk patterns, and (4) postoperative presence of Class II-a or III-a pattern (low-risk), as detailed in Fig. 7 [29]. High risk subtypes that are less likely to improve after central aortic repair alone were identified (Figs. 6 and 7). The authors recommend that for arch vessel malperfusion, preoperative high-risk perfusion patterns such as Classes I-b, I-c and II-b-2 should be treated with immediate central surgical repair. For abdominal vessels, preoperative high-risk perfusion patterns such as Classes I-b, I-c, II-b-2, and III-b should be treated with central surgical repair, if there are no signs of visceral malperfusion. If signs of visceral malperfusion are evident, Classes I-b and I-c should be treated with immediate central surgical repair, with evaluation for additional endovascular repair. Classes II-b-2 and III-b should be treated with endovascular intervention prior to aortic repair. The abdominal branch Class III-c pattern is best

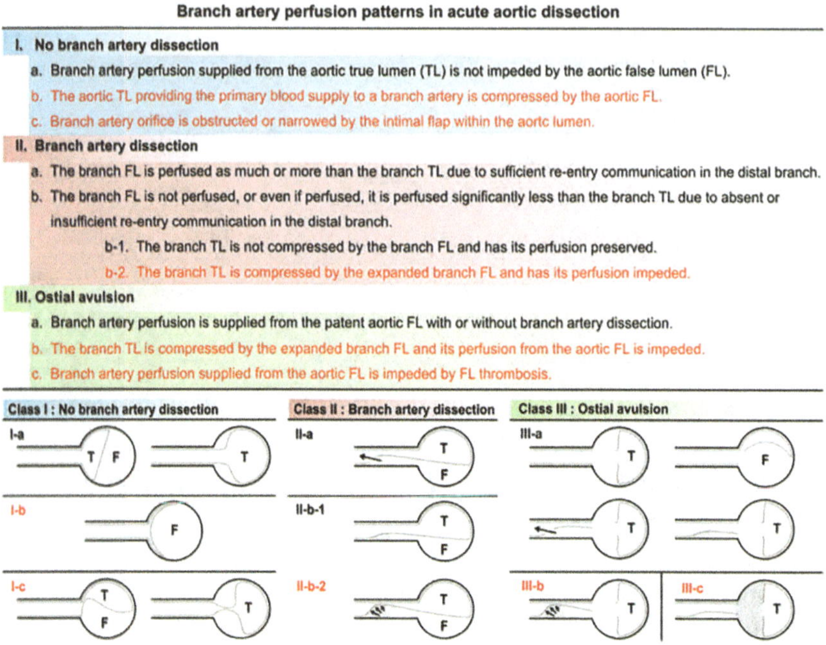

Fig. 6 Branch artery perfusion patterns in acute aortic dissection. Class I: blue-shaded background, Class II: red-shaded background, Class III: green-shaded background. Red lettering: high risk of developing end-organ malperfusion. T: true lumen, F: false lumen. (Adapted from Nagamine et al. [29], used with permission)

treated with simultaneous central repair and peripheral bypass, given that endovascular intervention may not be feasible or effective.

Similar to the Michigan classification of static vs. dynamic obstruction, patients in the Nagamine classification who had direct branch vessel involvement by the dissection were at a higher risk of having persistent malperfusion after aortic repair. While the classification system by Nagamine et al. is more comprehensive than the Michigan system, and includes classification of the supra-aortic vessels in addition to the visceral vessels, it is cumbersome to remember. Both classification systems can be applied to each branch vessel individually and provide the care providers with an "index of suspicion" when caring for these often critically ill patients.

DISSECT Classification

The DISSECT classification system is a mnemonic-based approach for evaluating aortic dissection that includes several of the characteristics that have been described above. The mnemonic "DISSECT" refers to: **D**uration, **I**ntimal tear, **S**ize of aorta,

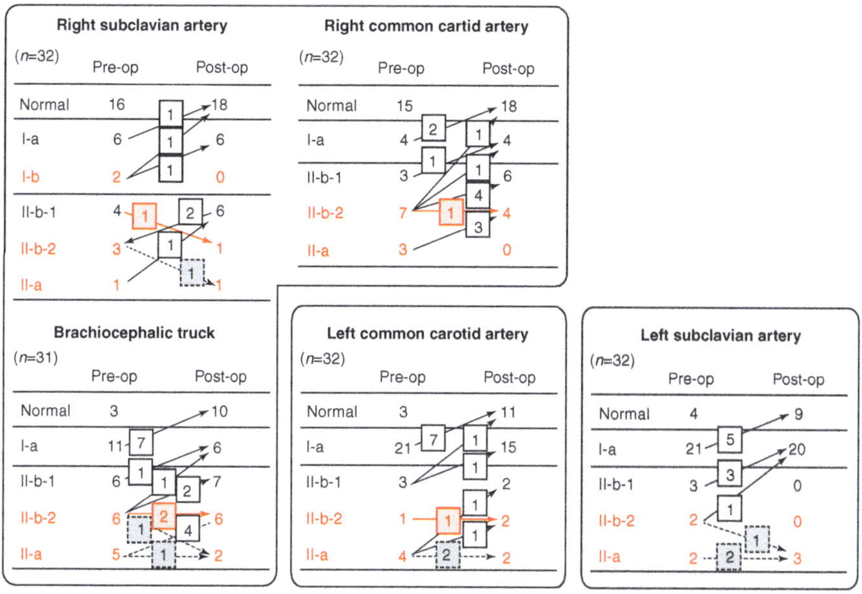

Fig. 7 Changes between pre- and postoperative perfusion patterns in cervical branches in 32 cases. White box and grey arrow: improvement; grey box and dotted arrow: settled into Class II-a or III-a; red box and red arrow: no improvement in high-risk perfusion patterns, such as Classes I-b, I-c and II-b-2, or worsening. Red lettering: high-risk perfusion patterns developing end-organ malperfusion (Class II-b-2 or I-b). Orange lettering: perfusion patterns, in which distal perfusion was supplied through the patent branch false lumen (Class II-a). One case of aberrant subclavian artery syndrome was included in the 32 cases and, therefore, the total number of brachiocephalic trunks was 31. (From Nagamine et al. [29], used with permission)

Segmental extent of involvement, Clinical complications, and Thrombosis of the false lumen, as detailed in Table 4 [30].

The DISSECT system is comprehensive and allows evaluation of any patient with aortic dissection, highlighting the factors relevant to formulating a treatment plan [30]. The primary entry tear determines the intervention for the patient. Tear location in the aortic arch and the abdominal aorta are addressed. The extent of the aorta involved by the dissection is defined, which might affect the presentation, treatment and prognosis. This remains true when patients are followed up after aortic dissection repair or when they are managed conservatively. The patency of false lumen, which influences late complications and is a risk factor for chronic aneurysmal degeneration of the dissection, is considered in this system. Following surgical repair for type A dissection, persistent flow in the distal false lumen predicts both late death and the need for subsequent treatment for the dissected descending aorta [31]. This has also been demonstrated in type B dissection, in which partial false lumen thrombosis is associated with increased mortality [32]. Less of a typical classification system, this system is more of a tool to facilitate the methodical evaluation of patients with aortic dissection.

Table 4 The DISSECT classification system [30]

DISSECT Classification	Subcategories
D = Duration	Acute = <2 weeks from onset Subacute = 2 weeks to 3 months Chronic = after 3 months
I = Intimal tear (primary) location within the aorta	A = Ascending aorta Ar = Arch D = Descending aorta Ab = Abdominal aorta U = Unknown
S = Size	Maximum transaortic diameter based on center line analysis (true lumen) in mm at any level within dissected segment of the aorta
SE = Segmental Extent of aortic involvement from proximal to distal boundary	A = Ascending aorta exclusively Ar = Aortic arch exclusively D = Descending exclusively Ab = Abdomen exclusively AAr = Ascending to arch AD = Ascending to descending AAb = Ascending to abdomen AI = Ascending to iliac ArD = Arch to descending ArAb = Arch to abdomen Arl = Arch to iliac DAb = Descending to abdomen DI = Descending to iliac
C = Complications related to dissection	C = Complicated • Aortic valve involvement • Cardiac tamponade • Rupture • Branch vessel malperfusion—symptomatic branch vessel involvement as defined as anatomic and clinical manifestations of branch vessel compromise. This can be static or dynamic disruption to flow leading to stroke, paraplegia, coronary, mesenteric, renal and/or peripheral limb ischemia) • Progression of aortic involvement with proximal or distal extension of dissection • Uncontrollable hypertension or clinical symptoms, or rapid false lumen expansion due to pressurization and aortic diameter of >10 mm within 2 weeks of presentation UC = Uncomplicated dissection
T = Thrombosis of aortic false lumen (evaluation of patency within the dissected aortic segments as assessed by CT, MRI or echocardiography)	**P** = Patent aortic false lumen as evident by flow or contrast into the false lumen of the entire dissected vessel **CT** = Complete thrombosis of the aortic false lumen with no flow or contrast into the vessel segments **A** = Ascending aorta **Ar** = Arch **D** = Descending **Ab** = Abdominal **PT** = Partial thrombosis of the aortic false lumen with segments of false lumen having flow with incomplete thrombosis

Conclusion

In this chapter we have summarized various systems of categorization of aortic dissection. Some are simple (DeBakey, Stanford), whereas others are complex but more comprehensive (SVS/STS, TEM, DISSECT). Each system has its own merits and limitations. While the simplicity of the earlier systems makes them universally adoptable, the greater anatomic detail in the newer systems facilitates targeted evaluation of patient eligibility for evolving treatment strategies and simplifies the universal reporting of results. It is likely that, as our understanding of aortic dissection pathology continues to expand, additional factors that impact patient outcomes are recognized, and newer treatment modalities are developed, these classification systems will be further refined.

References

1. Pape LA, et al. Aortic diameter >or = 5.5 cm is not a good predictor of type A aortic dissection: observations from the International Registry of Acute Aortic Dissection (IRAD). Circulation. 2007;116:1120–7.
2. Daily PO, Trueblood HW, Stinson EB, Wuerflein RD, Shumway NE. Management of acute aortic dissections. Ann Thorac Surg. 1970;10:237–47.
3. DeBakey ME, et al. Surgical considerations in the treatment of aneurysms of the thoraco-abdominal aorta. Ann Surg. 1965;162:650–62.
4. Reul GJ, et al. Dissecting aneurysm of the descending aorta: improved surgical results in 91 patients. Arch Surg. 1975;110:632–40.
5. Erbel R, et al. ESC guidelines on the diagnosis and treatment of aortic diseases. Eur Heart J. 2014;35:2873–926.
6. Rampoldi V, et al. Simple risk models to predict surgical mortality in acute type A aortic dissection: the International Registry of Acute Aortic Dissection score. Ann Thorac Surg. 2007;83:55–61.
7. Pape LA, et al. Presentation, diagnosis, and outcomes of acute aortic dissection: 17-year trends from the International Registry of Acute Aortic Dissection. J Am Coll Cardiol. 2015;66:350–8.
8. Nienaber CA, et al. Endovascular repair of type B aortic dissection: long-term results of the randomized investigation of stent grafts in aortic dissection trial. Circ Cardiovasc Inter. 2013;6:407–16.
9. Olsson C, et al. Mortality and reoperations in survivors operated on for acute type A aortic dissection and implications for catheter-based or hybrid interventions. J Vasc Surg. 2013;58:333–339.e1.
10. von Segesser LK, et al. Dissection of the descending thoracic aorta extending into the ascending aorta. A therapeutic challenge. J Thorac Cardiovasc Surg. 1994;108:755–61.
11. Rylski B, et al. Acute non-A non-B aortic dissection: incidence, treatment and outcome. Eur J Cardiothorac Surg. 2017;52:1111–7.
12. Nauta FJH, et al. Early outcomes of acute retrograde dissection from the International Registry of Acute Aortic Dissection. Semin Thorac Cardiovasc Surg. 2017;29:150–9.
13. Nauta FJH, et al. Impact of retrograde arch extension in acute type B aortic dissection on management and outcomes. Ann Thorac Surg. 2016;102:2036–43.
14. Lombardi JV, et al. Society for Vascular Surgery (SVS) and Society of Thoracic Surgeons (STS) reporting standards for type B aortic dissections. Ann Thorac Surg. 2020;109:959–81.
15. Ishimaru S. Endografting of the aortic arch. J Endovasc Ther. 2004;11(Suppl 2):II62–71.

16. Hirst AE, et al. Dissecting aneurysm of the aorta: a review of 505 cases. Medicine (Baltimore). 1958;37:217–79.
17. Booher AM, et al. The IRAD classification system for characterizing survival after aortic dissection. Am J Med. 2013;126:730.e19–24.
18. Lombardi JV, et al. Aortic remodeling after endovascular treatment of complicated type B aortic dissection with the use of a composite device design. J Vasc Surg. 2014;59:1544–54.
19. Di Eusanio M, et al. Clinical presentation, management, and short-term outcome of patients with type A acute dissection complicated by mesenteric malperfusion: observations from the International Registry of Acute Aortic Dissection. J Thorac Cardiovasc Surg. 2013;145:385–390.e1.
20. Axtell A, et al. Total arch replacement and frozen elephant trunk for acute complicated type B dissection. Ann Thorac Surg. 2020;110(3):e213–6. https://doi.org/10.1016/j.athoracsur.2019.12.077.
21. Vallabhajosyula P, et al. Central repair with antegrade TEVAR for malperfusion syndromes in acute Debakey I aortic dissection. Ann Thorac Surg. 2017;103:748–55.
22. Leshnower BG, et al. The 'thoracic endovascular aortic repair-first' strategy for acute type A dissection with mesenteric malperfusion: initial results compared with conventional algorithms. J Thorac Cardiovasc Surg. 2019;158:1516–24.
23. Augoustides JGT, et al. Classification of acute type A dissection: focus on clinical presentation and extent. Eur J Cardiothorac Surg. 2011;39:519–22.
24. Augoustides JGT, Szeto WY, Woo EY, et al. The complications of uncomplicated acute type-B dissection: the introduction of the Penn classification. J Cardiothorac Vasc Anesth. 2012;26:1139–44. PMID 22920842.
25. Tien M, et al. The Penn classification predicts hospital mortality in acute Stanford type A and type B aortic dissections. J Cardiothorac Vasc Anesth. 2020;34:867–73.
26. Sievers HH, et al. Aortic dissection rethought: a new classification system adding clarity and allowing prediction of in-hospital mortality. Inter Cardiovacs Thorac Surg. 2019;3:451–7.
27. Grimm JC, et al. Differential outcomes of type A dissection with malperfusion according to affected organ system. Ann Cardiothorac Surg. 2016;5:202–8.
28. Kamman AV, et al. Visceral malperfusion in aortic dissection: the Michigan experience. Semin Thorac Cardiovasc Surg. 2017;29:173–8.
29. Nagamine H, et al. A new classification system for branch artery perfusion patterns in acute aortic dissection for examining the effects of central aortic repair. Eur J Cardiothorac Surg. 2013;44:146–53.
30. Dake MD, et al. DISSECT: a new mnemonic-based approach to the categorization of aortic dissection. Eur J Vasc Endovasc Surg. 2013;46:175–90.
31. Fattouch K, et al. Long-term results after repair of type a acute aortic dissection according to false lumen patency. Ann Thorac Surg. 2009;88:1244–50.
32. Tsai TT, et al. Partial thrombosis of the false lumen in patients with acute type B aortic dissection. N Engl J Med. 2007;357:349–59.

Medical Conditions Predisposing to Aortic Dissection and Preventive Strategies

Eduardo Bossone, Valentina Russo, Andrea Salzano, and Kim Eagle

Introduction

Acute aortic dissection (AAD)—characterized by the presence of an intimal flap separating the true and false lumen—represents a life-treating medical condition affecting the aorta wall interesting predominantly media aorta layer (Fig. 1) [1–3]. Most frequently it affects men (~65%), in the sixth decade of life (mean age 63 years) [4].

Overall incidence ranges from approximately 2.6 and 3.5 cases per 100,000 person-years (6000–10,000 cases annually in the USA) [5, 6].

It is commonly classified by the Stanford system into two anatomic categories regardless of the site of origin: type A involving the ascending aorta, and type B not involving the ascending aorta (Figs. 2, 3 and 4) [1–3, 7–9]. If the elapsed time from symptoms onset to presentation is considered, three domains are identified: acute (<14 days), subacute (15–90 days), and chronic dissection (>90 days) [2, 3]. As etiology concerns, AAD may be caused by a wide spectrum of congenital or acquired diseases, either acute or chronic variably leading to increased aortic wall stress and/or aortic media abnormalities (Table 1) [1–3].

E. Bossone (✉)
Division of Cardiac Rehabilitation - Echo Lab, Department of Internal Medicine, A. Cardarelli Hospital, Naples, Italy
e-mail: eduardo.bossone@aocardarelli.it

V. Russo
Department of Advanced Biomedical Sciences, Federico II University of Naples, Naples, Italy

A. Salzano
IRCCS SDN, Naples, Italy

K. Eagle
University of Michigan Frankel Cardiovascular Center, Ann Arbor, MI, USA
e-mail: keagle@med.umich.edu

J. S. Coselli et al. (eds.), *Aortic Dissection and Acute Aortic Syndromes*,
https://doi.org/10.1007/978-3-030-66668-2_7

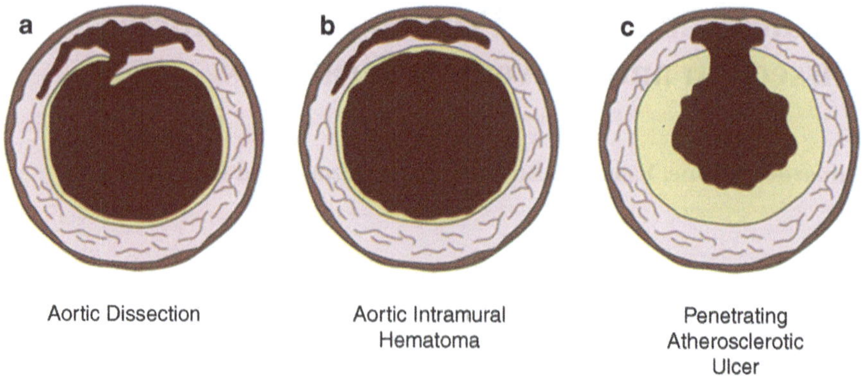

Fig. 1 Acute Aortic Syndromes. (**a**) Classic aortic dissection. (**b**) Aortic intramural hematoma. (**c**) Penetrating atherosclerotic aortic ulcer. Reprinted, with permission, from Braverman AC and Schermerhorn M. Diseases of the aorta. *In*: Braunwald's Heart Disease: A Textbook of Cardiovascular Medicine. 11th ed. Philadelphia, PA: Elsevier Inc.; 2018, p1295–1337 [1]. *Definitions [2]: Acute aortic syndromes (AAS):* Life-threatening medical conditions characterized by breakdown of the intima and media. They include classic acute aortic dissection (AAD), aortic intramural hematoma (IMH) and penetrating aortic ulcer (PAU). *Classic Aortic Dissection (AAD):* disruption of the media layer of the aorta with bleeding within and along the wall of the aorta resulting in separation of the layers of the aorta. *Intramural Hematoma (IMH):* hematoma develops in the media of the aortic wall in the absence of a false lumen and intimal tear. *Penetrating Atherosclerotic Ulcer (PAU):* ulceration of an aortic atherosclerotic plaque penetrating through the internal elastic lamina into the media

Herein we discuss the conditions predisposing to AAD along with preventive strategies at individual and population levels.

Conditions Associated with Increased Aortic Wall Stress

Systemic Hypertension

History of systemic hypertension (mostly poorly controlled) is by far the most common AAD risk factor (observed in about 75–80% of cases), more frequent in type B AAD than in type A AAD (81% versus 74%) [1–4]. Interestingly it represents per se along with increasing age a predictor of AAD independent of aortic diameter size [10]. Thus, blood pressure should be tightly controlled (optimal blood pressure <120/80 mm Hg) in order to limit organ structural and/or functional damages (i.e. the heart, aorta, brain, retina, kidney) [11].

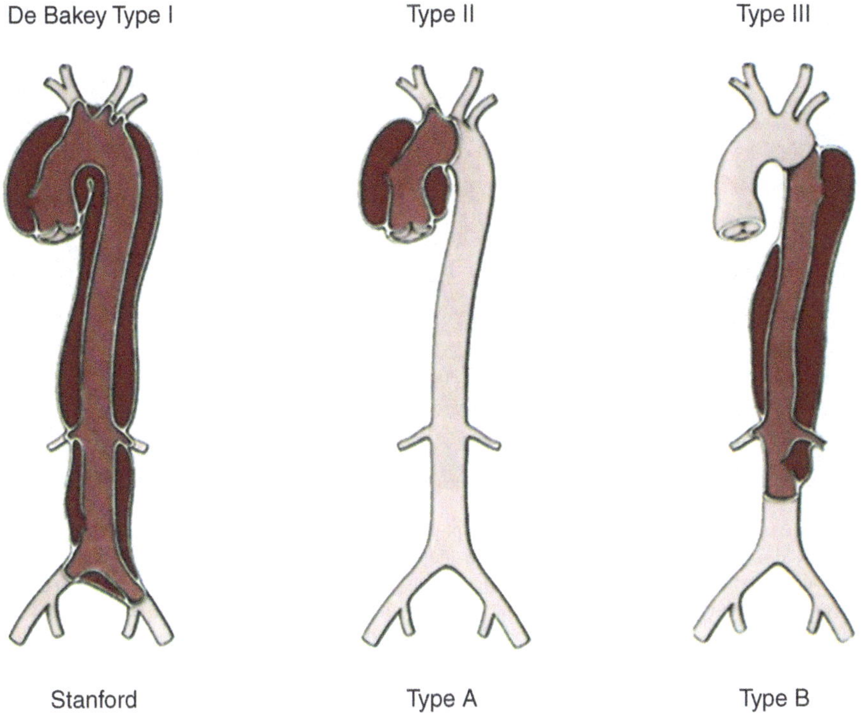

Fig. 2 De Bakey and Stanford Classification of Aortic Dissection. The DeBakey classification system categorizes dissections on the basis of the origin of the intimal tear and the extent of the dissection [7, 8]. Type I Dissection tear in the ascending aorta propagating distally to include at least the aortic arch and typically the descending aorta. Type II: Dissection tear only in the ascending aorta. Type III: Dissection tear in the descending aorta propagating most often distally. The Stanford classification system divides dissections into 2 categories, those that involve the ascending aorta and those that do not. Type A: All dissections involving the ascending aorta irrespective of the site of tear. Type B: All dissections that do not involve the ascending aorta; note that involvement of the aortic arch without involvement of the ascending aorta in the Stanford classification is labelled as Type B. Reprinted, with permission, from Hiratzka LF, et al. 2010 ACCF/AHA/AATS/ACR/ASA/SCA/SCAI/SIR/STS/SVM guidelines for the diagnosis and management of patients with thoracic aortic disease: a report of the American College of Cardiology Foundation/American Heart Association Task Force on Practice Guidelines, American Association for Thoracic Surgery, American College of Radiology, American Stroke Association, Society of Cardiovascular Anesthesiologists, Society for Cardiovascular Angiography and Interventions, Society of Interventional Radiology, Society of Thoracic Surgeons, and Society for Vascular Medicine. J Am Coll Cardiol 2010;55:e27–129 [3]

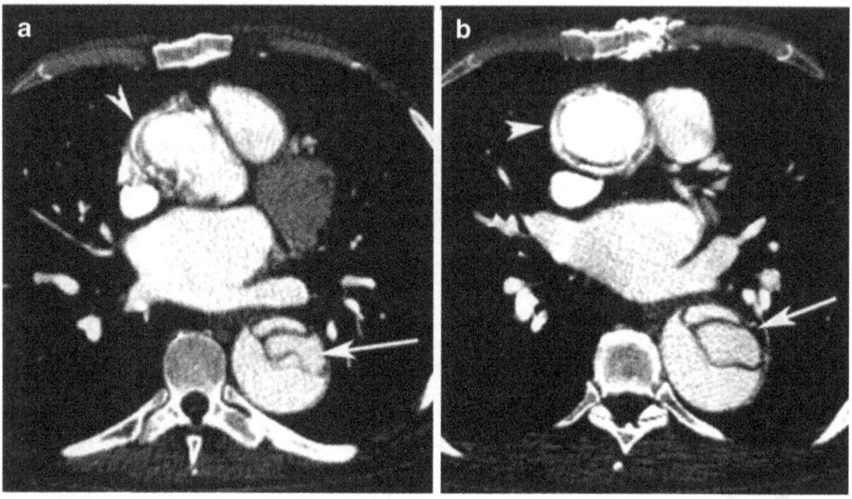

Fig. 3 Axial postcontrast computed tomography (CT) in a patient with type A acute aortic dissection (AAD). Axial postcontrast CT images (**a** and **b**) showing irregularity of the aortic wall with an intimal flap between the true and false aortic lumens. There is compression of the true lumen of the ascending aorta (white arrowheads, **a** and **b**) and of the descending aorta (white arrows, **a** and **b**) by expanding false lumen. (*Courtesy of* the Department of General and Emergency Radiology, A. Cardarelli Hospital, Naples, Italy). Reprinted, with permission, from Bossone E, et al. Acute Aortic Syndromes: Diagnostic and Therapeutic Pathways. Heart Fail Clin. 2020;16(3):305–315 [9]

Pheochromocytoma

Pheochromocytoma (rare usually benign tumor arising from the chromaffin cells of the adrenal medulla) may cause sudden uncontrolled substantial increase in arterial blood pressure (elevated catecholamines secretion) and in turn AAD or aortic aneurysms rupture [1]. In literature, there are few cases reporting on pheochromocytoma revealed by an AAD and *viceversa* [12, 13].

Cocaine and/or Other Stimulant Use

Several reports have documented the occurrence (~2.5% of type B AAD, ~ 1.4% of type A AAD) of AAD in cocaine—using subjects [14, 15]. It may be linked to the direct effects of cocaine on cardiovascular system as the increase in sympathetic output and catecholamines. The typical cocaine using AAD patient is usually young black male with a history of tobacco use and systemic hypertension. In addition to the standard therapeutic interventions it should be underlined the necessity to call for specific addiction counseling [14, 15].

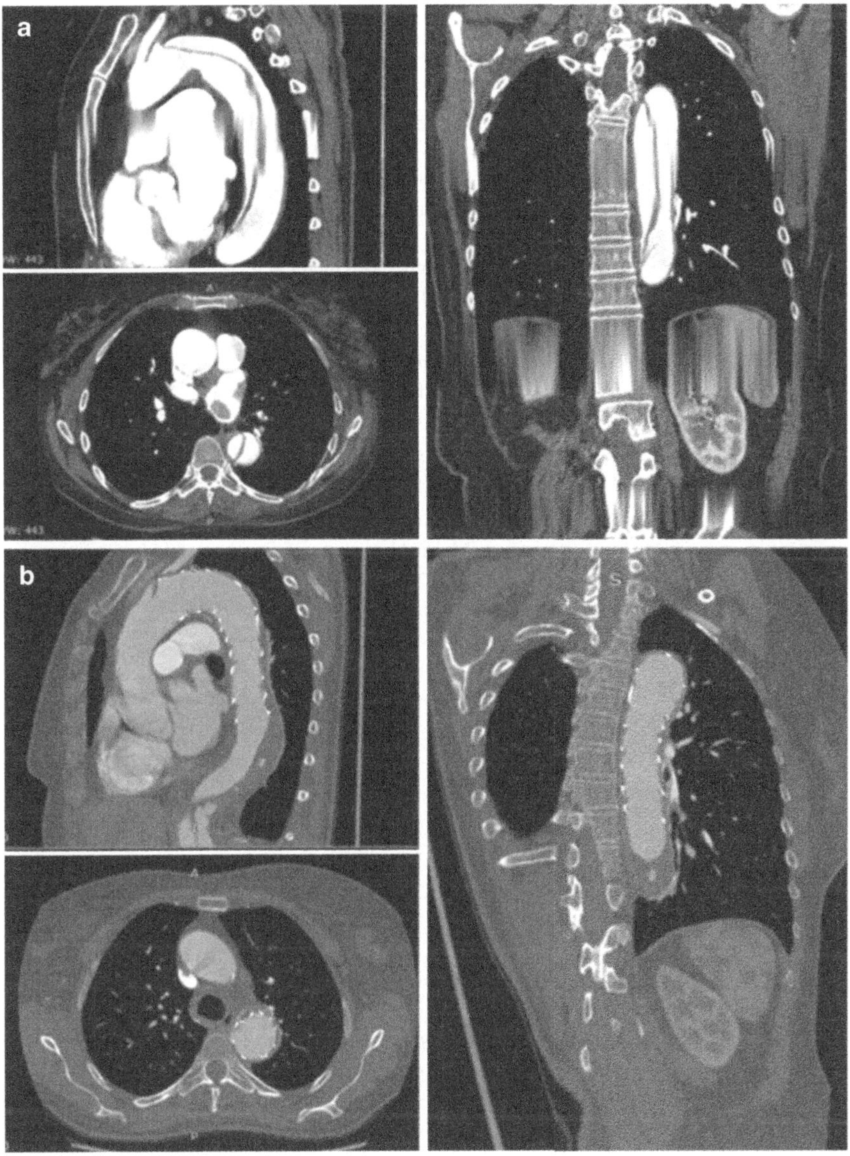

Fig. 4 Contrast-enhanced computed tomography (CT) scan with multiplanar reconstruction of type B acute aortic dissection (AAD) complicated by malperfusion before (**a**) and after thoracic endovascular aortic repair (**b**). (*Courtesy of* the Cardiac Surgery Department, Federico II Medical School University, Naples, Italy). Reprinted, with permission, from Bossone E, et al. Acute Aortic Syndromes: Diagnostic and Therapeutic Pathways. Heart Fail Clin. 2020;16(3):305–315 [9]

Table 1 Risk factors for development of aortic aneurysms and aortic dissections

1. Conditions associated with increased aortic wall stress	1.1 Hypertension, particularly if uncontrolled
	1.2 Pheochromocytoma
	1.3 Cocaine or other stimulant use
	1.4 Weight lifting or other Valsalva maneuvers
	1.5 Coarctation of the aorta
	1.6 Traumatic aortic injuries (partial or complete transection of the aorta)
	1.6.1 High-speed motor vehicle accident
	1.6.2 Falling from a great height
2. Conditions associated with aortic media abnormalities	2.1 Genetic
	2.1.1 Syndromic
	2.1.1.1 Marfan syndrome
	2.1.1.2 Loeys-Diez syndrome
	2.1.1.3 Ehlers-Danlos syndrome, vascular form
	2.1.1.4 Turner syndrome
	2.1.1.5 Arterial tortuosity syndrome
	2.1.1.6 Aneurysms-osteoarthritis syndrome
	2.1.1.7 Others
	2.1.2 Non syndromic familial thoracic aortic aneurysm and dissection syndrome
	2.1.2.1 Known gene mutations
	2.1.2.2 Known gene mutations
	2.1.2.2.1 Fibrillin
	2.1.2.2.2 Tumor growth factor-beta receptor
	2.1.2.2.3 SMAD3
	2.1.2.2.4 MYH11
	2.1.2.2.5 ACTA2
	2.1.2.2.6 MYLK
	2.1.2.2.7 PRKG1
	2.1.3 Bicuspid aortic valve (including prior aortic valve replacement)
	2.2 Non genetic
	2.2.1 Inflammatory vasculitis
	2.2.1.1 Takayasu arteritis
	2.2.1.2 Giant cell arteritis
	2.2.1.3 Behçet arteritis
	2.3 Other
	2.3.1 Atherosclerosis
	2.3.2 Pregnancy
	2.3.3 Polycystic kidney disease
	2.3.4 Chronic corticosteroid or immunosuppression agent administration
	2.3.5 Fluoroquinolones exposure
	2.3.6 Infection involving the aortic wall (from bacteremia or adjacent infection extension)

Table 1 (continued)

3. Iatrogenic	Cardiac surgery, coronary angiography and/or intervention, other

ACTA2 smooth muscle alpha-actin 2, *MYH11* smooth muscle cell–specific myosin heavy chain 11, *MYLK* myosin light chain kinase, *PRKG1* protein kinase cGMP-dependent 1, *SMAD3* mothers against decapentaplegic homolog 3

Modified from Hiratzka LF, et al. 2010 ACCF/AHA/AATS/ACR/ASA/SCA/SCAI/SIR/STS/SVM guidelines for the diagnosis and management of patients with thoracic aortic disease: a report of the American College of Cardiology Foundation/American Heart Association Task Force on Practice Guidelines, American Association for Thoracic Surgery, American College of Radiology, American Stroke Association, Society of Cardiovascular Anesthesiologists, Society for Cardiovascular Angiography and Interventions, Society of Interventional Radiology, Society of Thoracic Surgeons, and Society for Vascular Medicine. J Am Coll Cardiol 2010;55:e27–129 [2].

Weight Lifting and/or Other Valsalva Maneuver

Sudden increase in systemic arterial blood pressure associated with weight lifting and/or Valsalva manoeuvres may trigger AAD or aortic aneurysms rupture [3]. Indeed, the substantial sudden elevation in intrathoracic and systolic blood pressure (it may reach very high value) put a great stress on the aortic wall increasing dramatically the risk of AAD. In this regard individuals with known aortic aneurysm should avoid isometric physical activities (i.e. weight lifting, carrying heavy objects, pushing, etc.). Furthermore it is advised athletes engaging in heavy strength training should undergo routine echo—cardiovascular screening [16].

Coarctation of the Aorta

Coarctation of the aorta is a complex disease (prevalence of isolated forms is 3 per 10,000 lives births with a 2:1 ratio in males versus females) occurring as a discrete stenosis or a long hypoplastic aortic segment, typically located at the area of ductus arteriosus [1–3]. It is characterised by upper body systolic hypertension and lower body hypotension, with a difference >20 mm Hg. If not treated, about 80% of patients die for its complication, with at least 25% of these for AAD or rupture [1–3].

Traumatic Aortic Injuries

Traumatic aortic injurie (TAI)—partial or complete transection of the aorta—is an emergency and life-threatening condition causing death in the majority of cases (80%) [1–3]. It is usually associated with high-speed motor vehicle crashes (20% of road accident victims have evidence of ruptured aorta on autopsy), or falling from a great height [2, 3]. The aortic isthmus being the less mobile aortic segment represents the most frequent TAI anatomic site (90% of cases, Fig. 5) [1–3, 9]. Due to no

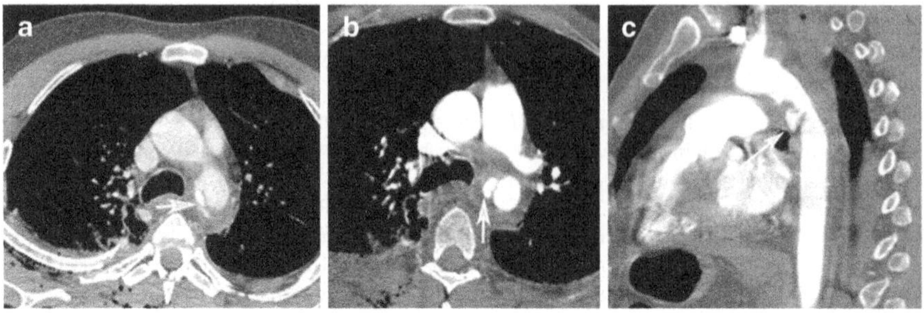

Fig. 5 Postcontrast computed tomography (CT) of aortic traumatic injury. (**a**) Axial postcontrast CT image showing a posttraumatic aortic dissection at the level of the aortic isthmus. An intimal flap is present with aortic contour irregularity and extravasation of contrast medium (white arrow) associated with a mediastinal hematoma. (**b**) Axial postcontrast CT image showing a posttraumatic aortic pseudoaneurysm at the level of the aortic isthmus (white arrow) associated with a mediastinal hematoma. (**c**) Oblique sagittal postcontrast CT reconstruction showing a posttraumatic aortic pseudoaneurysm at the level of the aortic isthmus with contrast agent outpouching extending beyond the aortic wall (white arrow). (*Courtesy of* the Department of General and Emergency Radiology, A. Cardarelli Hospital, Naples, Italy). Reprinted, with permission, from Bossone E, et al. Acute Aortic Syndromes: Diagnostic and Therapeutic Pathways. Heart Fail Clin. 2020;16(3):305–315 [9]

specific symptoms and signs (often covert by the co-existent thoracic or abdominal injuries) an high clinical suspicion is needed by the treating team in order to prompt an imaging test [2, 3]. In this regard computed tomography (CT) angiography (high accuracy, widely available, rapid and non invasive assessment of all aorta along with the skeletal system and all internal organs) is considered to be diagnostic technique of choice [transoesophageal echocardiography (TEE) second choice taking into account polytrauma patients contraindications] [2, 3]. Urgent endovascular (thoracic endovascular aortic repair/ endovascular aortic repair) rather than surgical repair is recommended if the anatomy is favorable and local expertise available [2, 3].

Conditions Associated with Aortic Media Abnormalities

Conditions associated with aortic media abnormalities can be categorized in genetic and non-genetic.

Genetic Conditions

Genetic conditions can be categorized in syndromic (Marfan syndrome, Loeys-Diez syndrome, Ehlers- Danlos syndrome, Turner syndrome) and non-syndromic. Furthermore a non-syndromic familial aortic aneurism and dissection syndrome has been described. Aortic diseases associated with the presence of a bicuspid aortic valve (BAV) should also be considered [1–3].

Syndromic Conditions

Marfan Syndrome

Marfan syndrome (MFS) (prevalence 15/100,000; incidence 25/100,000; male:female = 1:1) is the most frequent heritable (autosomal dominant) disorder of the connective tissue [1–3, 17]. It results from the mutation of the FBN1 gene encoding for fibrillin-1, a glycoprotein in the extracellular matrix [1–3]. Moreover, a second locus for MFS has been identified to be caused by mutations in the transforming growth factor-beta type II receptor (TGFBR2) [3]. The diagnosis of MFS relies on a set of clinical criteria (the Ghent nosology) along with DNA for sequencing. MFS patients may present cardiovascular, skin and skeletal, ocular, pulmonary, and dura mater abnormalities [1–3]. Among cardiovascular manifestations, MFS highly predisposes to thoracic aortic aneurysm/dissection with all patients having evidence of aortic disease at some point [2, 3]. It is mostly observed a dilatation of the aortic root or the ascending aorta or type A AAD [2, 3]. A subset of patients may also present with type B AAD, rarely with abdominal aortic aneurism making mandatory a clinical-imaging surveillance program [2, 3]. Current guidelines recommend a 2D transthoracic echocardiography (TTE) color doppler at the time of MFS first diagnosis and 6 months after, in order to estimate the rate of aorta enlargement [3]. In the case of a stable aortic dimensions, annual imaging is recommended [3]. Conversely if there is a significant growth from baseline or if the maximal aortic diameter is 4.5 cm, more frequent imaging should be considered [3].

Loeys-Dietz Syndrome

Loeys-Dietz syndrome (reported in 52 families) is an autosomal dominant very aggressive syndrome (mean age of death of 26 years) resulting from mutations in the transforming growth factor receptor type 1 or type 2 (TGFBR1/2) [1–3, 17]. Diagnosis is based on DNA testing and a clinical triad characterized by arterial tortuosity (most commonly observed in the head and neck vessels) and aneurysms (98% at the level of aortic root) throughout the arterial tree, hypertelorism and bifid uvula [1–3].

Notably, acute aortic dissection may occur at younger ages and smaller sizes as compare to MFS [18–20]. A comprehensive aortic imaging [TTE + CT or magnetic resonance imaging (MRI)] at initial diagnosis and 6 months thereafter is recommended [2, 3].

Ehlers- Danlos Syndrome, Vascular Form or Type IV

Type IV of Ehlers- Danlos syndrome, or vascular form, is a rare autosomal dominant disorder (prevalence 1/100,000; incidence 1/10,000–25,000) caused by the mutation of the COL3A1 gene, coding for type III procollagen [1–3, 17]. Diagnosis is based on clinical signs and DNA testing [1–3]. The clinical features consisted of easy bruising, thin/premature skin aging with visible veins and characteristic facial appearance (pinched and thin nose, thin lips, prominent ears, hollow cheeks, and tightness of skin over the face) [1–3]. Patients have also a significantly increased risk of rupture of visceral organs (usually not fatal) or blood vessels (high mortality) [1–3]. In particular, there is a tendency in alterations of the large and medium arteries with involvement of the aorta and arterial tree [1–3]. Notably, arteries may dissect without previous dilatation [1–3].

Turner Syndrome

Turner syndrome (prevalence 5.5/100,000; incidence 1/2000–2500) is characterised by the partial or complete monosomy of the X chromosome (karyotype 45X0) [1–3, 17]. Diagnosis is based on clinical findings and cytogenetic analyses [1–3]. The incidence of AAD in Turner syndrome is higher than in general population [21], occurring in the third-forth decade of age, with a very high mortality (about 50%); however, it is lower if compared to MFS or Loeys-Dietz syndrome [2, 3].

Arterial Tortuosity Syndrome

This rare autosomal recessive syndrome (prevalence <1/100,000; incidence unknown) is caused by mutations in the SLC2A10 gene, encoding for the facilitative glucose transporter GLUT-10 [1–3, 17]. Firstly reported in families from Italy, Morocco, and the Middle East, it is characterized by tortuosity, elongation, stenosis, and aneurysms of the large and middle-sized arteries [2]. Patients also show altered facial features (elongated face, blepharophimosis and down-slanting palpebral fissures, a beaked nose, a highly arched palate and micrognathia) and signs of skin (soft, hyperextensible skin) and skeleton (arachnodactyly, chest deformity, joint laxity, and contractures) and connective tissue disorders [2]. The prognosis of this syndrome, initially reported as very poor with mortality rate up to 40% before 5 years of life, seems to be less severe than estimated [2].

Aneurysms-Osteoarthritis Syndrome

This autosomal dominant syndrome (prevalence <1/100,000; incidence unknown) is caused by a mutation of SMAD3 gene, which encodes for an intracellular effector of the TGF-beta signalling [1–3, 17]. It is characterised by tortuosity, aneurysms, and dissection of all the arteries [2]. Patients may present also mild craniofacial-, skin-, and skeletal features [2]. Aneurysm-osteoarthritis syndrome represents at least 2% of all the syndromic familial thoracic acute aortic dissections [2].

Other Syndromic Conditions

Aortic root dilatation has been described in patients with other forms of Ehlers-Danlos syndrome, but the progression to AAD is rare. Furthermore aortic root enlargement (without progression to dissection) may be present in congenital contractural arachnodactyly or Beals syndrome (mutation in FBN2). Similarly to Noonan syndrome and Alagille syndrome, patients with autosomal dominant polycystic kidney disease have vascular complications including AAD [3].

Non Syndromic Familial Thoracic Aneurysm and Dissection Conditions [22]

Non syndromic familial thoracic aneurysm and dissection conditions can be categorized in those without and with known gene mutation. One on five of those without known genetic mutation shows a familial aggregation, with a first degree relative affected. These patients have an autosomal dominant transmission, with a great clinical variability and a decreased penetrance.

On the other hand when a mutation is recognised the followings are the most important genes identified: MYH11: encoding a myosin heavy chain produced in smooth muscle cell (SMC), is associated also with patent ductus arteriosus; ACTA2: encoding the SMC-specific alpha actin, is associated also with coronary artery disease, stroke and Moyamoya disease; MYLK: encoding myosin light chain kinase. Patients with this mutation usually experience AAD without aortic enlargement; TGFB2: encoding TGF-beta Type 2, has some features overlapping MFS; PRKG1: encoding PKGI, a type I cGMP-dependent protein kinase that controls SMC relaxation. Patients present aortic aneurysm and acute ADs at relatively young ages [1, 2].

Bicuspid Aortic Valve

Bicuspid aortic valve (BAV) is the most common congenital cardiac defect (prevalence at birth of 1–2%; the male:female ratio ranges from 2:1 to 4:1) [1–3]. It has been associated with Notch1 gene mutations, with a high rate of familial clustering, resulting in an autosomal dominant inheritance with reduced penetrance [2, 3]. BAV in the majority of cases (70%) is the result of a fusion between left coronary cusp (LCC)—with right coronary cusp (RCC) [2]. Patients with BAV may have a higher risk of develop an aortic dilatations [2]. In particular, LCC-RCC fusion is associated with dilatation in both ascending and aortic root [2]. Notably the prevalence of BAV in patients with AAD is only slightly higher than in the general population [2]. Among 3393 patients with AAD enrolled in the IRAD registry, 113 (3.3%) had BAV of which 82.3% type A AAD and 17.7% type B AAD [23].

Non Genetic Conditions

Inflammatory Vasculitis

Takayasu Arteritis

Takayasu arteritis is an idiopathic vasculitis, characterised by a T-cell-mediated panarteritis, involving the aorta and its branches [1–3]. With an overall rate of 2.6 per million of inhabitants, the most common onset of the disease is in the third decade, with a more prominence in the female sex [1–3]. Firstly described in Japan, it has been demonstrated to affect all ethnic groups, even if with an Asian overrepresentation, with two specific disease distribution (Japanese and India), which differ for vessels involved. Indeed, thoracic aorta and great vessels are prevalently involved in Japanese distribution, whereas abdominal aorta and renal arteries are typical in Indian one [3]. Clinically it may be distinguished an acute phase (characterised by systemic symptoms) and a chronic phase (with vascular symptoms, such as upper extremity claudication, dizziness, vision loss, stroke, carotid artery pain) [3]. Malignant hypertension suggests involvement of the renal arteries [3]. Different cohort studies have reported different localisation of the aneurysm formation (in about 30% of the population) [3]. Also stenosis of the aorta are very common (in about 53% of patients) [3]. In this regard it is important to obtain an imaging assessment of the entire aorta (TTE + CT or MRI). Positron Emission Tomography (PET)/CT or MRI is useful to visualise active disease [3].

Giant Cell Arteritis

Giant cell arteritis, also known as temporal arteritis, affects the aorta and its secondary and tertiary branches in about 20–25% of the patients (Fig. 6) [1–3, 24]. Typically, giant cell arteritis affects patients over 50 years, with a trend in older population (around 80 years) [3]. When the aorta is involved, dilatations of the aortic root and of the ascending aorta are the typical features, with a risk of aneurysms rupture or AD [25]. Epidemiological studies suggest a genetical predisposition, with a higher incidence for patients with northern Europe ancestry (e.g. higher in Scandinavian than in Southern Europe) [3]. However, when compared to Takayasu arteritis, aortic involvement is less common [3].

Behçet Arteritis

One third of the patients affected with Behçet disease (characterised by the classic triad of oral ulcerations, recurrent genital ulceration, uveitis or retinal vasculitis or skin lesions) have a vascular involvement [3]. Any vessels can be affected, and aneurysms formation may occur in multiple and different sites over follow-up [3]. Even if not common, aortic aneurysm rupture can be a fatal event [3].

Other

Atherosclerosis

Atherosclerosis along with systemic hypertension and advance age is considered to be a major determinant of the AAD pathophysiologic process [1–3]. Lipid accumulation in the aortic intima-media layer may lead to aortic plaque formation and in turn weaken the underlying media [1–3]. Thus it remains "*conditio sine qua no*" to adopt preventive measures targeting cardiovascular risk factors [1–3].

Pregnancy

Due to substantial hemodynamic changes and related increase in wall stress, AAD may rarely occur during pregnancy mostly in the last three months and in the peripartum period [3]. In this regard, among 6,566,826 pregnancies in 4,933,697

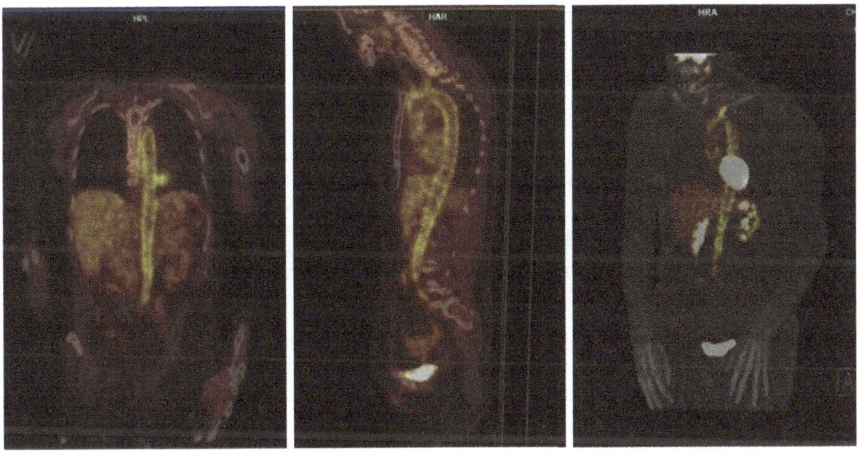

Fig. 6 ^{18}F-FDG positron emission tomography (PET) scan of a woman with giant cell arteritis. The PET scan reveals aortitis affecting the whole aorta. Reprinted, with permission, from Bossone E, et al. Aortitis. Vascul Pharmacol. 2016;80:1–10 [24].

women, only 36 cases of AAD or rupture have been identified [26]. Thus it is advised all pregnant women with known aortic root or ascending aortic dilatation should undergo monthly (or bimonthly) clinical -imaging (two dimensional echocardiography doppler exam) surveillance [3]. If clinically indicated, MRI (without contrast agents) has to be preferred to CT in order to avoid exposing both the mother and fetus to ionizing radiation [3].

Polycystic Kidney Disease

Autosomal dominant polycystic kidney disease may present AAD as a complication, although AAD is less common than cerebral aneurysms in these patients [3]. However, to date there is no enough evidence to recommend a focused screening in this population [3].

Chronic Corticosteroid or Immunosuppression Agent Administrations

Chronic corticosteroid or immunosuppression agents represent risk factors for infective aortitis (in particular, tuberculosis and fungal infections). In addition, oral steroid usage per se have been associated with abdominal aortic aneurysm expansion and aortic dissection [27].

Fluoroquinolones Exposure

Fluoroquinolones (one of the most commonly prescribed class of antibiotics) treatment seems to increase the risk of aortic aneurysm and dissection. For this reason, clinicians should consider alternative class of antibiotics in patients with connective tissue disorder or pre-existing aortic aneurysm [28].

Infections Involving the Aortic Wall

Several microorganisms have been associated with aortic aneurysms namely *Staphylococcus aureus*, Salmonella species, *Escherichia coli*, Streptococcus species, Neisseria species, and gram negative bacilli [1]. Tertiary syphilis (caused by Treponema pallidum) may involve the cardiovascular systems including ascending aorta aneurysms, coronary arterial stenosis and aortic valvulitis with mitral regurgitation in ~40%, ~30% and ~29% of cases respectively. However it should be point out that over the last decades the prevalence of tertiary syphilis is dramatically decreasing due to early stage antibiotic treatment [1]. Fungal (e.g. Candida or Aspergillus) are more frequent in the setting of impaired immunity (such as patients affected with human immunodeficiency virus, or under immunosuppressive therapy) [2, 24, 29, 30].

Iatrogenic

Iatrogenic AAD may occur (although rarely) during cardiac catheterization, coronary artery bypass graft surgery (CABG), or other invasive vascular procedures [4, 31]. The Registry on Aortic Iatrogenic Dissection (RAID) reported only 74 cases (0.07%) of ascending AAD (66.9 ± 10.8 years, 67.6% male) among 108,083 consecutive cardiac catheterizations (62% diagnostic and 38% therapeutic procedures) [31]. Interestingly they had favourable in hospital (only 2 deaths due to cardiogenic shock) and long term outcome (no deaths and/or major dissection-related complications) with conservative approach (36 underwent only medical treatment, 35 angioplasty with stenting, and 3 cardiac surgery) [31].

Preventive Strategies

Despite diagnostic and therapeutic exponential progress, the aortic diseases burden remains still high [32]. Thus, there is an increasing need to promote at individual and population levels healthy lifestyles including no exposure to tobacco in any form, low saturated fat diet, regular vigorous physical activity (30–60 min most days) optimal LDL-C and blood pressure levels, HbA1c <7%. Population screening programs should also be design and implement in relation to systemic hypertension and abdominal aneurysm [2, 7, 33]. In addition the usefulness of screening patients at risk of MFS (positive family history and/or the presence of characteristic clinical physical features) is well recognized [2, 3]. On the other hand the value of screening first-degree relatives of BAV patients remains debatable (no data support the cost-effectiveness of a screening programme) [2].

Population Screening Programs

Systemic Hypertension

Systemic hypertension is frequently an asymptomatic condition (silent killer) warrants population screening programmes or opportunistic blood pressure measurements in all adults (18 years or older). In fact a substantial number (>50%) of screened subjects are unaware to have hypertension. An optimal office blood pressure is defined as systolic <120 mmHg and diastolic <80 mmHg [11, 33].

Abdominal Aortic Aneurysm

Current evidence supports cost effectiveness abdominal ultrasound (A-US) population screening for abdominal aortic aneurysm (AAA) in all men >65 years of age [2]. It may be considered in women >65 years of age with history of current/past smoking and in first-degree siblings of a patient with AAA [2]. In the absence of structured screening programs it is suggested among above high risk cohorts to perform during TTE an A-US "opportunistic glimpse" for AAAs [2].

AAD: Long Term Follow Up

AAD is a lifelong disease affecting the entire aorta (holistic approach). Thus, patients with AAD need close clinical and imaging follow-up regardless of the initial therapeutic strategy [2, 3]. MRI (in addition to TTE/A-AUS) should be considered the first imaging technique choice (CT second choice) being radiation free [2, 3]. Medical treatment "cornerstone" includes an optimal blood pressure and heart rate control (blood pressure <120/80 mmHg, heart rate <60 bpm (first line: beta-blockers) as well as HDL-C <1.4 mmol/L (<55 mg/dL), or a reduction of at least 50% if the baseline (first line: statins) [11, 34]. Furthermore the patient should avoid isometric exercise while may perform mild to moderate aerobic exercise (walking, slow jogging, and recreational cycling) (Table 2) [7, 33, 35–38].

Table 2 Acute aortic dissection: long-term follow-up

Ten-year survival rate from 30% to 60%
Late complications
Progressive aortic insufficiency.
Progressive diameter increase, aneurysm formation, and rupture.
Recurrent dissection or progression of dissection.
Leakages/haemorrhage at surgical anastomoses/stent-grafted sites.
Malperfusion.
Patients at particularly high risk
Those with Marfan syndrome—very high risk of recurrent dissection or aneurysm formation with rupture.
Those with a patent false lumen—increased incidence of late complications and death.
Medical treatment
A. Optimal blood pressure (<120/80 mmHg) and heart rate (<60 b.p.m.) control.
First line: beta-blockers.
Second line: ACE-inhibitors or ARBs.
Third line: calcium channel blockers (long-acting dihydropyridine).
B. Lipid-lowering therapy: target <1.4 mmol/L (<55 mg/dL), or a reduction of at least 50% if the baseline. First line: statins. Second line: statins + ezetimibe. Third line: statins + ezetimibe + PCSK9 inhibitors.

Table 2 (continued)

Imaging surveillance
TTE + A-US + CT or MRI of chest and abdomen before discharge and at 1, 3, 6, and 12 months and annually thereafter[a]
Patient education and lifestyle goals
Adherence to medical treatment.
Genetic counselling.
Smoking cessation and risk factor modification for atherosclerotic disease.
Avoid cocaine or other stimulating drugs such as methamphetamine, strenuous physical activities (isometric exercise, pushing, or straining that would require a Valsalva manoeuvre), and contact sports (e.g. competitive football, ice hockey, or soccer, etc.).
Mild aerobic exercise and daily activities are not restricted. Common sense approach to sexual activity, avoiding straining or maximal exertion.

ACE angiotensin-converting enzyme, *ARBs* angiotensin II receptor blockers, *b.p.m.* beats per minute, *CT* computed tomography, *LDL* low-density lipoprotein, *MRI* magnetic resonance imaging, *PCSK9* proprotein convertase subtilisin/kexin type 9, *TTE* transthoracic echocardiography, *A-US* Abdominal ultrasound

Modified from Bossone E, LaBounty TM, Eagle KA. Acute aortic syndromes: diagnosis and management, an update. Eur Heart J. 2018;39(9):739–749d [7].

[a]Similar surveillance strategy for intramural haematoma and penetrating aortic ulcer is recommended [2]

Acknowledgments We are grateful to Dr. Brigida Ranieri and to Chiara Sepe for data management and technical support.

References

1. Braverman AC, Schermerhorn M. Diseases of the aorta. In: Braunwald's heart disease: a textbook of cardiovascular medicine. 11th ed. Philadelphia, PA: Elsevier; 2018. p. 1295–337.
2. Erbel R, Aboyans V, Boileau C, Bossone E, Bartolomeo RD, Eggebrecht H, et al. 2014 ESC Guidelines on the diagnosis and treatment of aortic diseases: document covering acute and chronic aortic diseases of the thoracic and abdominal aorta of the adult. The Task Force for the Diagnosis and Treatment of Aortic Diseases of the European Society of Cardiology (ESC). Eur Heart J. 2014;35:2873–926. https://doi.org/10.1093/eurheartj/ehu281.
3. Hiratzka LF, Bakris GL, Beckman JA, Bersin RM, Carr VF, Casey DE, et al. 2010 ACCF/AHA/AATS/ACR/ASA/SCA/SCAI/SIR/STS/SVM Guidelines for the diagnosis and management of patients with thoracic aortic disease. A Report of the American College of Cardiology Foundation/American Heart Association Task Force on Practice Guidelines, American Association for Thoracic Surgery, American College of Radiology, American Stroke Association, Society of Cardiovascular Anesthesiologists, Society for Cardiovascular Angiography and Interventions, Society of Interventional Radiology, Society of Thoracic Surgeons, and Society for Vascular Medicine. J Am Coll Cardiol. 2010;55:e27–e129. https://doi.org/10.1016/j.jacc.2010.02.015.
4. Evangelista A, Isselbacher EM, Bossone E, Gleason TG, Eusanio MD, Sechtem U, et al. Insights from the international registry of acute aortic dissection: a 20-year experience of collaborative clinical research. Circulation. 2018;137:1846–60. https://doi.org/10.1161/CIRCULATIONAHA.117.031264.

5. Mészáros I, Mórocz J, Szlávi J, et al. Epidemiology and clinicopathology of aortic dissection. Chest. 2000;117:1271–8. https://doi.org/10.1378/chest.117.5.1271.
6. Clouse WD, Hallett JW Jr, Schaff HV, et al. Acute aortic dissection: population-based incidence compared with degenerative aortic aneurysm rupture. Mayo Clin Proc. 2004;79:176–80. https://doi.org/10.4065/79.2.176.
7. Bossone E, LaBounty TM, Eagle KA. Acute aortic syndromes: diagnosis and management, an update. Eur Heart J. 2018;39:739–749d. https://doi.org/10.1093/eurheartj/ehx319.
8. Nienaber CA, Clough RE. Management of acute aortic dissection. Lancet. 2015;385:800–11. https://doi.org/10.1016/S0140-6736(14)61005-9.
9. Bossone E, Ranieri B, Romano L, et al. Acute aortic syndromes: diagnostic and therapeutic pathways. Heart Fail Clin. 2020;16:305–15. https://doi.org/10.1016/j.hfc.2020.03.002.
10. Pape LA, Tsai TT, Isselbacher EM, Oh JK, O'gara PT, Evangelista A, et al. Aortic diameter >or = 5.5 cm is not a good predictor of type A aortic dissection: observations from the International Registry of Acute Aortic Dissection (IRAD). Circulation. 2007;116:1120–7. https://doi.org/10.1161/CIRCULATIONAHA.107.702720.
11. Williams B, Mancia G, Spiering W, Agabiti Rosei E, Azizi M, Burnier M, et al. 2018 ESC/ESH Guidelines for the management of arterial hypertension [published correction appears in Eur Heart J. 2019 Feb 1;40:475]. Eur Heart J. 2018;39:3021–104. https://doi.org/10.1093/eurheartj/ehy339.
12. Runyan B, Hanak CR, Mahendiran S, Allamaneni S, Vester S. Type A aortic dissection complicated by pheochromocytoma. Ann Thorac Surg. 2019;107:e13–4. https://doi.org/10.1016/j.athoracsur.2018.05.084.
13. Lenders JW, Duh QY, Eisenhofer G, Gimenez-Roqueplo AP, Grebe SK, Murad MH, et al. Pheochromocytoma and paraganglioma: an endocrine society clinical practice guideline. J Clin Endocrinol Metab. 2014;99:1915–42. https://doi.org/10.1210/jc.2014-1498.
14. Eagle KA, Isselbacher EM, De Sanctis RW, International Registry for Aortic Dissection (IRAD) Investigators. Cocaine-related aortic dissection in perspective. Circulation. 2002;105:1529–30. https://doi.org/10.1161/01.cir.105.13.1529.
15. Dean JH, Woznicki EM, O'Gara P, Montgomery DG, Trimarchi S, Myrmel T, et al. Cocaine-related aortic dissection: lessons from the International Registry of Acute Aortic Dissection. Am J Med. 2014;127:878–85. https://doi.org/10.1016/j.amjmed.2014.05.005.
16. Hatzaras I, Tranquilli M, Coady M, Barrett PM, Bible J, Elefteriades JA. Weight lifting and aortic dissection: more evidence for a connection. Cardiology. 2007;107:103–6. https://doi.org/10.1159/000094530.
17. January 2020 - n°1 by Orphanet: an online database of rare diseases and 890 orphan drugs. Copyright, INSERM 1997. Available at http://www.orpha.net
18. Aftab M, Cikach FS, Zhu Y, Idrees JJ, Rigelsky CM, Kalahasti V, et al. Loeys-Dietz syndrome: Intermediate-term outcomes of medically and surgically managed patients. J Thorac Cardiovasc Surg. 2019;157:439–50.e5. https://doi.org/10.1016/j.jtcvs.2018.03.172.
19. Loughborough WW, Minhas KS, Rodrigues JCL, et al. Cardiovascular manifestations and complications of Loeys-Dietz syndrome: CT and MR imaging findings. Radiographics. 2018;38:275–86. https://doi.org/10.1148/rg.2018170120.
20. Williams JA, Hanna JM, Shah AA, et al. Adult surgical experience with Loeys-Dietz syndrome. Ann Thorac Surg. 2015;99:1275–81. https://doi.org/10.1016/j.athoracsur.2014.11.021.
21. Thunström S, Krantz E, Thunström E, Hanson C, Bryman I, Landin-Wilhelmsen K. Incidence of aortic dissection in turner syndrome. Circulation. 2019;139:2802–4. https://doi.org/10.1161/CIRCULATIONAHA.119.040552.
22. D'Souza RS, Slavov D, Graw S, Jirikowic J, Todd E, Rogers RK, et al. Clinical and genetic characterization of adult patients presenting with non-syndromic vascular aneurysms and dissections. Int Angiol. 2017;36:417–27. https://doi.org/10.23736/S0392-9590.17.03757-9.
23. Di Eusanio M, Pape L, Braverman AC, et al. Characteristics of acute aortic dissection in patients with bicuspid 781 aortic valve: insights from the IRAD registry [abstract]. Circulation. 2013;128:A15913.

24. Bossone E, Pluchinotta FR, Andreas M, et al. Aortitis. Vasc Pharmacol. 2016;80:1–10. https://doi.org/10.1016/j.vph.2015.11.084.
25. Yoshimoto R, Tanaka K, Kawahata T, Takatori S, Takatori K, Eguchi K, et al. Unusual manifestations of giant cell arteritis and granulomatosis with polyangiitis. Immunol Med. 2019;42:94–8. https://doi.org/10.1080/25785826.2019.1657377.
26. Kamel H, Roman MJ, Pitcher A, Devereux RB. Pregnancy and the risk of aortic dissection or rupture: a cohort-crossover analysis. Circulation. 2016;134:527–33. https://doi.org/10.1161/CIRCULATIONAHA.116.021594.
27. Tajima Y, Goto H, Ohara M, Hashimoto M, Akamatsu D, Shimizu T, et al. Oral steroid use and abdominal aortic aneurysm expansion - positive association. Circ J. 2017;81:1774–82. https://doi.org/10.1253/circj.CJ-16-0902.
28. Lee CC, Lee MG, Hsieh R, Porta L, Lee W-C, Lee SH, Chang S-S. Oral fluoroquinolone and the risk of aortic dissection. J Am Coll Cardiol. 2018;72:1369–78. https://doi.org/10.1016/j.jacc.2018.06.067.
29. Hartlage GR, Palios J, Barron BJ, et al. Multimodality imaging of aortitis. JACC Cardiovasc Imaging. 2014;7:605–19. https://doi.org/10.1016/j.jcmg.2014.04.002.
30. Meel R, Gonçalves R. Human immunodeficiency virus associated large artery disease. In Aortic aneurysm and aortic dissection [Working Title]. IntechOpen (2019). doi:https://doi.org/10.5772/intechopen.85956.
31. Núñez-Gil IJ, Bautista D, Cerrato E, Salinas P, Varbella F, Omedè P, et al. Incidence, management, and immediate- and long-term outcomes after iatrogenic aortic dissection during diagnostic or interventional coronary procedures. Circulation. 2015;131:2114–9. https://doi.org/10.1161/CIRCULATIONAHA.115.015334.
32. Sampson UK, Norman PE, Fowkes FG, et al. Global and regional burden of aortic dissection and aneurysms: mortality trends in 21 world regions, 1990 to 2010. Glob Heart. 2014;9:171–180.e10. https://doi.org/10.1016/j.gheart.2013.12.010.
33. Piepoli MF, Hoes AW, Agewall S, Albus C, Brotons C, Catapano AL, et al. 2016 European Guidelines on cardiovascular disease prevention in clinical practice: The Sixth Joint Task Force of the European Society of Cardiology and Other Societies on Cardiovascular Disease Prevention in Clinical Practice (constituted by representatives of 10 societies and by invited experts) Developed with the special contribution of the European Association for Cardiovascular Prevention & Rehabilitation (EACPR). Eur Heart J. 2016;37:2315–81. https://doi.org/10.1093/eurheartj/ehw106.
34. Mach F, Baigent C, Catapano AL, et al. 2019 ESC/EAS Guidelines for the management of dyslipidaemias: lipid modification to reduce cardiovascular risk. Eur Heart J. 2020;41:111–88. https://doi.org/10.1093/eurheartj/ehz455.
35. Chaddha A, Kline-Rogers E, Woznicki EM, Brook R, Housholder-Hughes S, Braverman AC, et al. Cardiology patient page. Activity recommendations for postaortic dissection patients. Circulation. 2014;130:e140–2. https://doi.org/10.1161/CIRCULATIONAHA.113.005819.
36. Chaddha A, Kline-Rogers E, Braverman AC, et al. Survivors of aortic dissection: activity, mental health, and sexual function. Clin Cardiol. 2015;38:652–9. https://doi.org/10.1002/clc.22418.
37. Chaddha A, Eagle KA, Braverman AC, et al. Exercise and physical activity for the post-aortic dissection patient: the clinician's conundrum. Clin Cardiol. 2015;38:647–51. https://doi.org/10.1002/clc.22481.
38. Chaddha A, Erickson S, Kline-Rogers E, et al. Medication adherence patterns in aortic dissection survivors. Indian J Med Res. 2018;147:183–8. https://doi.org/10.4103/ijmr.IJMR_1198_15.

What Do the Guidelines Say for the Treatment of Acute Aortic Syndromes?

Jordan P. Bloom, Navyatha Mohan, and Thoralf M. Sundt

Guidelines in General

Before delving deeply into the guidelines that exist regarding acute aortic syndromes, a few general concepts about guidelines are in order. First, it is important to clarify our terminology. Clinical practice guidelines are commonly defined as "systematically developed statements to assist practitioner and patient decisions about appropriate healthcare for specific clinical circumstances" [1]. Typically, the standards of evidence and the formality of the process for constructing guidelines is more rigorous than that for "consensus documents" or "expert opinion" pieces. Still, there can be considerable confusion generated around these terms, motivated in no small measure by the high citation rates such publications achieve, benefiting both editors and authors. Hybrid terms such as "consensus guidelines" have even been proffered [2].

The drive to produce guidelines is understandable. Clinical practice guidelines exist as tools to provide evidence-based decision support for busy clinicians in the face of an ever-accelerating volume literature on almost any subject. In the current era, with a proliferation of cardiovascular techniques, technologies and pharmacologies, it is impossible for an individual to keep truly up-to-date on all aspects of cardiovascular care. The deluge of information, good and bad, and the focus on evidence-based care has generated such an appetite for guidelines that we now find ourselves with the second-order problem of being inundated with guidelines themselves. A current PubMed search of the word guidelines results in close to 15,000 published manuscripts.

J. P. Bloom · N. Mohan · T. M. Sundt (✉)
Division of Cardiac Surgery, Corrigan Minehan Heart Center, Massachusetts General Hospital, Harvard Medical School, Boston, MA, USA
e-mail: TSUNDT@mgh.harvard.edu

J. S. Coselli et al. (eds.), *Aortic Dissection and Acute Aortic Syndromes*,
https://doi.org/10.1007/978-3-030-66668-2_8

Not infrequently, multiple guidelines on the same topic will be produced by medical and surgical subspecialty groups with disturbingly frequent disagreements and discrepancies. Moreover, the language used and the process employed in creating these guidelines, including issues as fundamental as the specific level of evidence acceptable is not standardized and the processes used to develop them varies significantly from one society to another. With numerous organizations of multinational origin and multidisciplinary composition writing about complex topics each from its own perspective, both inconsistencies in specific recommendations and glaring gaps are inevitable [3]. Shaneyfelt et al. conducted a structured review of 279 guidelines focused on the process whereby they were constructed. They concluded that guidelines published in the peer-reviewed medical literature do not adhere well to established methodological standards. They went on to say that the greatest improvement is needed in the identification, evaluation and synthesis of the scientific evidence [4].

In response to this chaos, guidelines for guidelines have been established. The Institute of Medicine (Clinical Practice Guidelines We Can Trust. Report Brief 2011) has published standards [5]. They state specifically that practice guidelines must be based on a systematic review of the evidence, be developed by a multidisciplinary panel of experts, consider important patient subgroups, be based on a transparent process that minimizes biases and conflicts of interest, explain clearly alternative care options and be revised as appropriate. In particular, there is a focus on the composition of the writing group and management of conflicts of interest. As adopted by the American College of Cardiology, this includes a requirement that the chairperson and at least 51% of the members have no relationships with industry. Attention to the importance of including methodologists is also increasing.

One of the major problems guideline writing groups face is the paucity of "high quality" evidence. Accordingly, an explicit system of grading evidence is employed by the American Heart Association and American College of Cardiology Task Force on Clinical Practice Guidelines. The classification of recommendations and level of evidence is shown in Table 1. The class represents the strength of recommendation and ranges from Class I (strong) to Class III (harm), with many recommendations being IIa ("it is reasonable to consider") and IIb ("may be considered"). The level of evidence is based not on the strength of opinion of the authors, but on the quality of evidence ranging from level A (multiple high quality randomized clinical trials) to level C-EO (consensus based on expert opinion). In this way, there is transparency about the evidence base for the recommendation. It should be apparent that there should be few Class I recommendations based on Level C evidence.

A final note should be made regarding the application of guideline recommendations to individual patients in the clinical setting. Since the data on which the recommendations are based are, of necessity, derived from application of statistical methodologies to populations of patients, the statistical probabilities are informative for the population as a whole but not directly for individuals [3]. The guidelines cannot account for all of the comorbidities and risk factors of the individual patient.

Table 1 Definitions of classification of recommendations and level of evidence

Classification of recommendation	
Class I	Conditions for which there is evidence and/or general agreement that a given treatment is useful or effective
Class II	Conditions for which there is conflicting evidence and/or a divergence of opinion about the usefulness/efficacy of a procedure or treatment IIa: Weight of evidence is in favor of usefulness/efficacy IIb: Usefulness/efficacy is less well established by evidence/opinion
Class III	Conditions for which there is evidence and/or general agreement that the procedure treatment is not useful/effective, and in some cases may be harmful
Level of evidence	
LOE A	Data derived from multiple randomixed clinical trials
LOE B	Data derived from a single randomized trial or non-randomized studies
LOE C	Consensus opinion of experts

Accordingly, guideline recommendations can only be considered a foundation upon which a patient specific recommendation can be made. They are the beginning of the conversation, not the end.

Societal Guidelines

Acute aortic syndromes consist of three related conditions with similar clinical characteristics and include aortic dissection, intramural hematoma and penetrating aortic ulcer. Current societal guidelines pertaining to these entities include the 2010 US ACCF/AHA/AATS/ACR/ASA/SCA/SCAI/SIR/STS/SVM [6], the 2011 Japanese Circulation Society (JCS) [7], the 2014 European Society of Cardiology (ESC) [8] and the 2016 Canadian CCS/CSCS/CSVS guidelines [9]. All of these guidelines define Acute AD as occurring within 14 days.

The ACCF/AHA, JCS and ESC guidelines are categorized by the Class of Recommendation (COR) and Level of Evidence (LOE) (Table 1). While COR reflects the magnitude of benefit over risk and corresponds to the strength of the recommendation, the LOE denotes the confidence in or certainty of the evidence supporting the recommendation based on quality of pertinent research findings. Therefore, COR and LOE are assessed independently. When a recommendation is designated as LOE C, that does not imply that the recommendation itself is weak. In some cases, clinical benefit is self-evident and the intervention is unlikely to undergo randomized study [10].

The guidelines from the Canadian panel were developed using Grading of Recommendations Assessment, Development and Evaluation (GRADE) methodology, with "Values and Preferences" to provide context to the recommendations [11].

Acute Type A Aortic Dissection (AAD), Intramural Hematoma (IMH) and Penetrating Aortic Ulcer (PAU)

The most widely utilized classification scheme for acute aortic dissection (AAD) is the Stanford classification system in which any aortic dissection involving the ascending aorta is an AAD [12, 13]. The alternative DeBakey scheme subdivides those AAD involving the ascending and descending aorta as Type I and a dissection involving only the ascending aorta as Type II [12, 13].

The recommendations for initial management of AAD are fairly uniform across society guidelines (Table 2). All societies advocate for therapeutic reduction in wall stress to limit the extension of the dissection and reduce the risk of developing end-organ damage and rupture. Both the US and European guidelines specifically recommend titrating intravenous beta-blockers as first-line agents (Class I LOE C)

Table 2 Summary table of guidelines for the management of acute aortic syndromes from the discussed international societies

Recommendations		ACCF/ AHA 2010	JCS 2011	ESC 2014	CCS 2016
Any thoracic aortic dissection regardless of anatomic location	Urgent surgical consultation recommended	Class I, LOE C	No specific recommendation	Class I, LOE C	No specific recommendation
Type A acute dissection	Initial management with medical therapy including pain relief and blood pressure control is recommended	Class I, LOE C (vasodilator therapy should not be initiated prior to rate control: Class III, LOE C)	No specific recommendation	Class I, LOE C	No specific recommendation
	Definitive management with urgent surgery recommended	Class I, LOE B	Class I, LOE C	Class I, LOE C	Strong Recommendation, Low-Quality Evidence[a]
	With organ malperfusion—a hybrid approach[b] should be considered	Class I, LOE C[c]	Class IIa, LOE C	Class IIa, LOE B	
Type A IMH, PAU	Urgent treatment recommended is	Surgery Class IIa, LOE C	Medical, Class I, LOE C	Surgery Class I, LOE C	

(continued)

Table 2 (continued)

Recommendations		ACCF/ AHA 2010	JCS 2011	ESC 2014	CCS 2016
Uncomplicated type B aortic dissection	Medical therapy is always recommended	Class I, LOE B	Class I, LOE C	Class I, LOE C	Strong Recommendation, Medium Quality Evidence
	Consider TEVAR	n/a	Class IIb, LOE C Surgery: Class III, LOE C	Class IIa, LOE B	First-line Strong Recommendation, Medium Quality Evidence
Complicated type B aortic dissection	TEVAR is recommended	n/a	Class I, LOE C	Class I, LOE C	n/a
	Surgery is recommended	n/a	Class I, LOE C[d]	Class IIb, LOE C	n/a
Uncomplicated type B IMH, PAU	Initial approach is medical treatment	n/a	n/a	Class I, LOE C	n/a
	Repetitive imaging (MRI/ CT) is indicated	n/a	n/a	Class I, LOE C	n/a
Complicated type B IMH/ PAU	TEVAR should be considered	n/a	n/a	Class IIa, LOE C	n/a
	Surgery may be considered	n/a	n/a	Class IIb, LOE C	n/a

[a]Extended distal arch repair, if presenting with primary intimal tear or significant aneurysmal disease

[b]Hybrid approach—Ascending aorta and/or arch replacement associated with any percutaneous aortic or branch artery procedure

[c]For patients with ascending thoracic aortic dissection, all of the aneurysmal aorta and the proximal extent of the dissection should be resected. A partially dissected aortic root may be repaired with aortic valve resuspension. Extensive dissection of the aortic root should be treated with aortic root replacement with a composite graft or with a valve sparing root replacement. If a Debakey Type II dissection is present, the entire dissected aorta should be replaced

[d]With severe complications directly related to aortic dissection where surgery is expected to achieve improvement or stop progression

and non-dihydropyridine calcium channel-blocking agents as second line (Class I, LOE C) to a heart rate of 60 beats per minute or less. Both societies suggest adding additional agents such as other vasodilators or angiotensin-converting enzyme inhibitors if necessary, to reduce systolic blood pressure less than 120 mm Hg (Class I, LOE C). Both societies warn that beta blockers should be used cautiously in the setting of acute aortic regurgitation because they will block the compensatory tachycardia (Class I, LOE C).

The recommendations for definitive management of AAD are also similar across the society guidelines. The US guidelines recommend urgent surgical consultation for all patients diagnosed with thoracic aortic dissection regardless of the anatomic location (ascending versus descending) as soon as the diagnosis is made or highly suspected (Class I, LOE C). All three societies recommend emergency surgical intervention for acute thoracic aortic dissection involving the ascending aorta because of the high risk of associated life-threatening complications such as rupture (Class I, LOE B). The Canadian guidelines specifically recommend replacement of the ascending aorta during systemic circulatory arrest with an open distal anastomosis to be used routinely for repair of acute type A dissections (Strong Recommendation, Low-Quality Evidence). They go on to recommend that an extended distal arch repair technique be considered for patients who present with acute type A dissection and one of the following:

(a) Primary intimal entry tear in the arch or descending aorta
(b) Significant aneurysmal disease of the arch (Strong Recommendation, Low-Quality Evidence).

According to the US guidelines, in patients with ascending thoracic aortic dissection all of the aneurysmal aorta and the proximal extent of the dissection should be resected. A partially dissected aortic root may be repaired with aortic valve resuspension. Extensive dissection of the aortic root should be treated with aortic root replacement with a composite graft or with a valve sparing root replacement. If a DeBakey Type II dissection is present, the entire dissected aorta should be replaced. (Class I, LOE C).

There are certain scenarios where non-operative management of AAD is recommended. The JCS guidelines suggest medical treatment to be started under certain conditions for type A dissection without complications or persistent pain where the false lumen of the ascending aorta is thrombosed (Class IIa, LOE C). The European guidelines suggest that a 'wait-and-watch' strategy (optimal blood pressure and pain control with serial imaging) may be an option to be considered on an individual patient basis, particularly in the case of substantial surgery risk (advanced age and severe co-morbidities), smaller aortic dimensions (<50 mm), and decreased IMH thickness (<11 mm) (Class I, LOE C).

Type A Intramural Hematoma and Penetrating Aortic Ulcers

ACC and ESC recognize IMH as separate but related conditions, however JCS does not use the term IMH, and instead considers it to be a non-communicating aortic dissection and apply those treatment guidelines to IMH.

The ACC and ESC guidelines conclude that the guidelines for treatment of Type A IMH and PAU correspond to the treatment guidelines described for Type A AAD. Therefore, emergency surgery is indicated in complicated cases of with pericardial effusion, periaortic hematoma, or large aneurysms and urgent surgery (<24 h after diagnosis) is required in most Type A IMHs (Class I, LOE C). It is worth noting that PAUs are less frequently located in the aortic arch and involvement of the ascending aorta is rare. Surgical intervention is recommended in case of Type A PAU (Class IIa, LOE C).

Acute Type B Aortic Dissection (AAD), Intramural Hematoma (IMH) and Penetrating Aortic Ulcer (PAU)

Aortic dissection isolated to the descending aorta is classified as Type B according to the Stanford system, or Type III according to the Debakey system [14]. Ascending aortic dissections are almost twice as common as descending dissections. Aortic IMHs more commonly involve the descending aorta [15]. Most penetrating ulcers are also located in the descending thoracic aorta (85–95%) [16]. This section will discuss management and treatment guidelines for Type B dissections, intramural hematomas and penetrating aortic ulcers.

Initial Management

As with Type A dissections, the ACCF guidelines recommend that Type B aortic dissections are also initially managed medically with the goal of decreasing aortic wall stress and controlling pain (Class I, LOE B). While the ACCF guidelines do not offer detailed recommendations for management of TBAD, the ESC and JCS offer more detailed guidelines regarding endovascular and surgical repair. An urgent surgical consult is recommended as soon as the diagnosis is made or suspected (Class I, LOE C).

Contrary to Type A AD, surgical intervention is typically reserved for patients with dissection associated complications—including end-organ malperfusion, recurrent and refractory pain or refractory hypertension, rapid expansion of the false lumen found during imaging surveillance, or dissection expansion and impending rupture (Class II, LOE C). Broadly, the recommendations for treatment overlap across the guidelines with minor differences in the level of evidence.

Uncomplicated Type B AD

Medical therapy is unequivocally recommended for all uncomplicated TBAD (Class I, LOE B by ACC, Class I, LOE C by JSC and ESC, Strong Recommendation, Medium Quality Evidence by CCS).

There remains some controversy with regard to the beneficial role of early Thoracic endovascular aortic repair (TEVAR) in uncomplicated TBAD compared to medical therapy alone (Class IIa, LOE B by ESC and Class II, LOE C by JCS). The CCS suggests that TEVAR may be considered for patients with uncomplicated disease to improve aorta-specific endpoints (Weak Recommendation, Low Quality

Evidence). Two trials have been conducted to assess the benefit of elective TEVAR in uncomplicated TBAD.

The INSTEAD trial randomized 140 patients with sub-acute (>14 days) type B AD. Two year follow up indicated that TEVAR is effective in aortic remodeling (91.3 vs. 19.4% with medical therapy, $P < 0.001$), however, no survival benefit was observed [17]. The INSTEAD-XL trial included extended follow up of the INSTEAD trial, and showed that aorta related mortality (6.9 vs. 19.3%, respectively; $P = 0.04$) and disease progression (27.0 vs. 46.1%, respectively; $P = 0.04$) were lower after 5 years in TEVAR patients compared to those receiving medical therapy. As with the initial trial, no difference was found in overall mortality [18].

The ADSORB trial compared medical therapy alone vs. medical therapy + TEVAR in acute complicated TBAD and showed that TEVAR conferred benefits in terms of aortic remodeling and lower rates of incomplete false lumen thrombosis. This trial was underpowered to draw conclusions regarding survival benefit [19]. Further studies are required to determine predictors of complications in patients presenting with uncomplicated TBAD.

Complicated Type B AD

Based on IRAD data, a significant one-third of patients with acute TBAD present with complications such as malperfusion or hemodynamic instability. ESC and JCS recommend TEVAR for complicated Type B AD (Class I, LOE C). The CCS also recommends that endovascular repair be first-line therapy for these patients (Strong Recommendation, Medium Quality Evidence). TEVAR helps to close the primary entry tear and perforation sites in the descending aorta, redirecting blood flow into the true lumen. This leads to improved distal perfusion by decompression. It also helps resolve malperfusion of visceral or peripheral arteries and promotes thrombosis of the false lumen, which is the initiation for aortic remodeling and stabilization.

There are no RCTs comparing TEVAR with open surgery in patients with acute complicated TBAD. In a propensity analysis from IRAD, open surgical repair was associated with an independent increased risk of in-hospital mortality (OR: 3.41, 95% CI, 1.00–11.67, $P = 0.05$) [14]. In-hospital complications occurred in 20% of patients subjected to endovascular techniques, and in 40% after open surgical repair. In-hospital mortality was significantly higher after open surgery (33.9%) than after endovascular treatment (10.6%, $P = 0.002$) [15]. Additionally, in the IRAD series, endovascular treatment seems to offer better short term outcomes in terms of mortality and associated complications compared to open repair [16].

Results from the single arm, STABLE trial suggests that TEVAR therapy is associated with increased true lumen size, and favorable clinical and anatomic results [20]. Subsequently, 1 year follow up from STABLE II demonstrated that

TEVAR + medical therapy is associated with favorable clinical and anatomical outcomes for rupture and malperfusion in acute complicated TBAD [21]. TEVAR might therefore offer better outcomes compared with open surgical approaches in complicated cases.

Indications for open surgery in acute complicated TBAD include—lower extremity artery disease, severe tortuosity of iliac arteries, sharp angulation of the aortic arch, and the absence of a proximal landing zone for the stent graft (Class IIb, LOE C).

The aim of open surgical repair is to replace the descending aorta with a Dacron prosthesis and redirect the flow into the true lumen of the downstream aorta by closing the false lumen at the distal anastomotic site, thereby improving perfusion and TL decompression, which may resolve malperfusion [22].

Although the results of open surgical repair have improved over the last decades, they still have an in-hospital mortality rate of about 25–50%. Predictors of poor prognosis include patient age > 70, hypotension/shock, severe visceral malperfusion and spinal cord ischemia preoperatively. In addition, extensive co-morbidity, such as end stage malignant disease and severe chronic obstructive pulmonary disease are considered contraindications for surgical aortic repair.

Type B Intramural Hematoma and Penetrating Aortic Ulcers

As with TBAD, the initial approach to Type B IMH and PAU is medical treatment (Class I, LOE C). The recommendations for endovascular therapy (Class IIa, LOE C) and surgery (Class IIb, LOE C) are similar to those for Type B ADs as well. The subgroup of patients with aortic dilation or ulcer-like projection (ULP) should be followed up closely and treated more aggressively if symptoms persist or reappear, or if progressive aortic dilation is observed [23] (Class I, LOE C). For patients presenting with expansion of the IMH despite medical therapy, or disruption of intimal tear on CT with contrast enhancement in the acute phase, the recommended intervention is TEVAR rather than surgery.

The most common location of PAU is the middle and lower descending thoracic aorta. The aim of treatment for PAU is to prevent propagation of the ulcerative process, leading to IMH, pseudoaneurysm or aortic rupture and progression to acute AD. Studies have suggested that indications for intervention include refractory or recurrent symptoms, penetration of the lesion through the aortic wall, expansion of aortic diameter and PAU diameter > 20 mm and depth > 10 mm [24, 25]. While unrelenting pain and rupture are clear indications for repair, the other indications are not as absolute [26].

As for IMH, there are no RCTs directly comparing TEVAR vs. open surgery in patients with acute PAU. Since these patients are more likely to be older and with comorbidities, TEVAR is increasingly being used, with encouraging results [27, 28].

Future Directions

Further studies are required to clarify the association of aortic remodeling with improved mid and long-term outcomes. Newer therapy such as proximal covered stents and distal bare metal stents as used in the STABLE trial, as well as adjunctive techniques like fenestration or branched graft stenting are in development. Consensus regarding optimal timing for endovascular therapy in uncomplicated dissection in terms of patient selection and timing is required.

References

1. Institute of Medicine (US) Committee to Advise the Public Health Service on Clinical Practice Guidelines. Clinical Practice guidelines: directions for a new program. Washington, DC: National Academies Press. 1990. Available from: http://www.ncbi.nlm.nih.gov/books/NBK235751/. Accessed 24 Apr 2020.
2. Svensson LG, Gillinov AM, Weisel RD, et al. The American Association for Thoracic Surgery Consensus Guidelines: reasons and purpose. J Thorac Cardiovasc Surg. 2016;151:935–939.e1.
3. Sundt TM. Guidelines or gospels? J Thorac Cardiovasc Surg. 2016;151:1472–4.
4. Shaneyfelt TM, Mayo-Smith MF, Rothwangl J. Are guidelines following guidelines? The methodological quality of clinical practice guidelines in the peer-reviewed medical literature. JAMA. 1999;281:1900–5.
5. Institute of Medicine (US) Committee on Standards for Developing Trustworthy Clinical Practice Guidelines. Clinical practice guidelines we can trust. Washington, DC: National Academies Press. 2011. Available from: http://www.ncbi.nlm.nih.gov/books/NBK209539/. Accessed 20 June 2020.
6. Hiratzka LF, Bakris GL, et al. 2010 ACCF/AHA/AATS/ACR/ASA/SCA/SCAI/SIR/STS/SVM guidelines for the diagnosis and management of patients with thoracic aortic disease. Circulation. 2010;121:e266–369.
7. Group JJW. Guidelines for diagnosis and treatment of aortic aneurysm and aortic dissection (JCS 2011). Circ J. 2013;77:789–828.
8. Erbel R, Aboyans V, Boileau C, et al. 2014 ESC Guidelines on the diagnosis and treatment of aortic diseases: document covering acute and chronic aortic diseases of the thoracic and abdominal aorta of the adult. The Task Force for the Diagnosis and Treatment of Aortic Diseases of the European Society of Cardiology (ESC). Eur Heart J. 2014;35:2873–926.
9. Appoo JJ, Bozinovski J, Chu MWA, et al. Canadian Cardiovascular Society/Canadian Society of Cardiac Surgeons/Canadian Society for Vascular Surgery joint position statement on open and endovascular surgery for thoracic aortic disease. Can J Cardiol. 2016;32:703–13.
10. Halperin JL, Levine GN, Al-Khatib SM, et al. Further evolution of the ACC/AHA clinical practice guideline recommendation classification system: a report of the American College of Cardiology/American Heart Association Task Force on Clinical Practice Guidelines. J Am Coll Cardiol. 2016;67:1572–4.
11. What is GRADE? BMJ Best Practice Available from: https://bestpractice.bmj.com/info/us/toolkit/learn-ebm/what-is-grade/. Accessed 20 June 2020.
12. Tsai TT, Nienaber CA, Eagle KA. Acute aortic syndromes. Circulation. 2005;112:3802–13.
13. Nienaber CA, Eagle KA. Aortic dissection: new frontiers in diagnosis and management: part I: from etiology to diagnostic strategies. Circulation. 2003;108:628–35.
14. Fattori R, Napoli G, Lovato L, et al. Descending thoracic aortic diseases: stent-graft repair. Radiology. 2003;229:176–83.

15. Fattori R, Tsai TT, Myrmel T, et al. Complicated acute type B dissection: is surgery still the best option? A report from the International Registry of Acute Aortic Dissection. J Am Coll Cardiol Intv. 2008;1:395–402.
16. Tsai TT, Trimarchi S, Nienaber CA. Acute aortic dissection: perspectives from the International Registry of Acute Aortic Dissection (IRAD). Eur J Vasc Endovasc Surg. 2009;37:149–59.
17. Nienaber CA, Rousseau H, Eggebrecht H, et al. Randomized comparison of strategies for type B aortic dissection: the INvestigation of STEnt Grafts in Aortic Dissection (INSTEAD) trial. Circulation. 2009;120:2519–28.
18. Nienaber CA, Kische S, Rousseau H, et al. Endovascular repair of type B aortic dissection: long-term results of the randomized investigation of stent grafts in aortic dissection trial. Circ Cardiovasc Interv. 2013;6:407–16.
19. Brunkwall J, Kasprzak P, Verhoeven E, et al. Endovascular repair of acute uncomplicated aortic type B dissection promotes aortic remodelling: 1 year results of the ADSORB trial. Eur J Vasc Endovasc Surg. 2014;48:285–91.
20. Lombardi JV, Cambria RP, Nienaber CA, et al. Prospective multicenter clinical trial (STABLE) on the endovascular treatment of complicated type B aortic dissection using a composite device design. J Vasc Surg. 2012;55:629–640.e2.
21. Lombardi JV, Gleason TG, Panneton JM, et al. STABLE II clinical trial on endovascular treatment of acute, complicated type B aortic dissection with a composite device design. J Vasc Surg. 2020;71:1077–1087.e2.
22. Bozinovski J, Coselli JS. Outcomes and survival in surgical treatment of descending thoracic aorta with acute dissection. Ann Thorac Surg. 2008;85:965–70. discussion 970-971
23. Takeshi K, Shuichiro K, Atsushi Y, et al. Impact of new development of ulcer-like projection on clinical outcomes in patients with type B aortic dissection with closed and thrombosed false lumen. Circulation. 2010;122:S74–80.
24. Ganaha F, Miller DC, Sugimoto K, et al. Prognosis of aortic intramural hematoma with and without penetrating atherosclerotic ulcer: a clinical and radiological analysis. Circulation. 2002;106:342–8.
25. Tittle SL, Lynch RJ, Cole PE, et al. Midterm follow-up of penetrating ulcer and intramural hematoma of the aorta. J Thorac Cardiovasc Surg. 2002;123:1051–9.
26. Nathan DP, Boonn W, Lai E, et al. Presentation, complications, and natural history of penetrating atherosclerotic ulcer disease. J Vasc Surg. 2012;55:10–5.
27. Botta L, Buttazzi K, Russo V, et al. Endovascular repair for penetrating atherosclerotic ulcers of the descending thoracic aorta: early and mid-term results. Ann Thorac Surg. 2008;85:987–92.
28. Demers P, Miller DC, Mitchell RS, et al. Stent-graft repair of penetrating atherosclerotic ulcers in the descending thoracic aorta: mid-term results. Ann Thorac Surg. 2004;77:81–6.

Part II
Imaging and Initial Management of Acute Aortic Syndromes

Initial Medical Management of Acute Aortic Syndromes

Abigail R. Benkert and Jeffrey G. Gaca

Introduction

Acute aortic syndrome encompasses three life-threatening diseases: aortic dissection, intramural hematoma, and penetrating atherosclerotic aortic ulcer. When symptom onset is within 14 days of inciting event, the presentation is deemed 'acute.' All diseases within the acute aortic syndrome eventually lead to the breakdown of the aortic intima and media [1]. Lesions are classically described based on their location within the thoracic aorta. A lesion involving the ascending aorta is Stanford A (DeBakey type I–II); those not involving the ascending aorta are Stanford B (DeBakey type III). For this chapter, we will use the Stanford nomenclature.

Acute aortic dissection (AAD) occurs when an intimal tear results in formation of a dissection plane and disruption of the medial layer. This results in separation of the aortic wall layers and subsequent formation of true and false lumens [2]. The false channel is contained by the outer medial and adventitial layers. However, the intimal tear (dissection flap) can extend both proximally and distally with each cardiac cycle, potentially compromising flow within branch arteries. When the outer aortic wall weakens, aortic rupture is possible. The International Registry of Acute Aortic Dissection (IRAD) reports that of patients presenting with AAD, 67% presented with type A dissections (TAAD) [3]. The mortality of type A dissection is 1–2% per hour after early symptom onset, and survival appears to depend upon the degree of communication and the wall stress present in the false lumen [4].

Intramural hematoma (IMH) most commonly occurs in the descending aorta and is characterized by rupture of the vaso vasorum into the aortic media, with subsequent hematoma formation [3]. Functionally, the hematoma within the aortic wall does not freely communicate with the lumen and has restricted flow [5]. The absence

A. R. Benkert · J. G. Gaca (✉)
Division of Cardiothoracic Surgery, Department of Surgery, Duke University Medical Center, Durham, NC, USA
e-mail: jeffrey.gaca@duke.edu

J. S. Coselli et al. (eds.), *Aortic Dissection and Acute Aortic Syndromes*,
https://doi.org/10.1007/978-3-030-66668-2_9

of an intimal lesion distinguishes aortic IMH from a peri-aortic hematoma that may be associated with a penetrating aortic ulcer (PAU). IMH accounts for 10–25% of acute aortic syndromes and the overall long-term prognosis is more favorable than that of patients with AAD [2]. However, several studies suggest that 30–40% of IMH evolve into AAD, with the greatest risk at 8 days from symptom onset [2].

Penetrating aortic ulcer (PAU) refers to ulceration of an atherosclerotic plaque, which penetrates through the elastic lamina and into the aortic media. The location of PAU is predominantly in the descending aorta (85–90%). While the true prevalence of the disorder is unknown, it is estimated to represent 2–7% of all acute aortic syndromes [3]. These lesions, left untreated, can lead to progressive aortic enlargement and aneurysm development. Propagation of the ulcerative process may lead to IMH, pseudoaneurysm, AAD, or aortic rupture [2].

Presentation and Diagnosis

Given the high mortality associated with missed and delayed diagnoses of acute aortic syndromes, a high clinical suspicion and diagnosis as early in the disease process as possible is paramount.

Acute Aortic Dissection

The most important risk factor precipitating acute aortic dissection is systemic hypertension, which increases the stress on the aortic wall. Seventy-seven percent of patients presenting with AAD have co-morbid hypertension [3]. Aortic dissection most commonly occurs in men, representing two-thirds of affected patients. Women, when affected, tend to be older (mean 67 vs. 63 years) [3]. Less common precipitating risk factors include atherosclerosis, known aortic aneurysm, previous cardiac surgery, connective tissue disorders (Marfan's, Loeys-Dietz), and cocaine use.

Patients commonly present with a chief complaint of acute onset severe chest or back pain. The pain is typically abrupt in onset and is at its most severe at the time of onset. Most frequently described as sharp [3], it can also be tearing, ripping, and stabbing in nature. In TAAD, the pain is usually retrosternal, whereas in distal dissections the pain is more often localized interscapular and in the back. Of note, symptoms can deceptively be intermittent [1]. Up to 30% of patients later found to have AAD were initially suspected to have other conditions such as myocardial infarctions or pulmonary embolus. Therefore, acute aortic dissection should remain on the differential diagnosis for patients presenting with unexplained syncope, stroke, acute onset congestive heart failure, and acute ischemia of extremities or viscera, even when the typical chest pain is not the leading symptom [4]. Recurrent chest or back pain typically indicates extension, expansion, or rupture of the dissection.

Physical examination should focus on findings that help increase suspicion for dissection and represent high-risk features, as well as signs of end-organ dysfunction. A detailed pulse examination, including carotid, radial, and femoral pulses can indicate the extent of disease. Syncope, stroke, and other neurologic symptoms may occur in up to 40% of patients with proximal aortic dissection, yet these initial symptoms can often mask the diagnosis [3]. Differential upper extremity pulses suggest involvement of the brachiocephalic branch arteries. Iliofemoral involvement can result in lower extremity pulse loss, the most drastic of which is pulseless bilateral lower extremities in the case of complete obstruction of the iliac bifurcation. A complete cardiac exam should be completed, with particular attention to whether there is new-onset diastolic (aortic regurgitation) murmur or signs of pericardial involvement including presence of pericardial friction rub, jugular venous distension, or pulsus paradoxus consistent with tamponade. After aortic rupture, aortic regurgitation is the second most common cause of death, with patients frequently presenting with heart failure and cardiogenic shock [2]. Branch artery compromise can also lead to malperfusion of the bowel (acute abdomen and acidosis) and kidneys (rising blood urea nitrogen/creatinine and oliguria).

Intramural Hematoma

The clinical presentation of IMH is similar to that of AAD. Distinguishing between the two entities cannot be made clinically and requires tomographic imaging [6].

Penetrating Aortic Ulcer

Clinical manifestations of PAU are similar to AAD. However, patients tend to be older and more frequently have a history of tobacco abuse, hypertension, coronary artery disease, chronic obstructive pulmonary disease, and concurrent abdominal aneurysms. Symptoms typically occur once the PAU reaches the adventitia; therefore, symptoms are assumed to indicate an emergency.

Initial Medical Management

There remains a lack of evidence for initial targeted medical management of acute aortic syndromes. As there are no randomized controlled trials or meta-analyses, the recommendations that follow are provided by a consensus of opinions (Class I, Level C).

The aim of medical management in acute aortic syndromes is to prevent aortic rupture, and in the case of IMH and PAU, to prevent progression to AAD. While definitive interventions vary based upon the classification and type of acute aortic syndrome, all patients presenting with acute aortic syndrome are initially managed medically. Upon suspicion of diagnosis, the primary goal is to reduce blood pressure, heart rate, and force of cardiac ejection (dp/dt). Carefully monitored and aggressive management is essential to prevent rupture, as the main cause of death is not the initial tear, but related to the extension of the dissection with ultimate rupture and death due to hemorrhage or cardiac tamponade [1, 7].

Anti-impulse Therapy

Current medical management is largely derived from the seminal work of Wheat et al. [7] as well as Simpson and Taylor [8]. Wheat et al. constructed an *ex vivo* model of aortas using Tygon tubing coated internally with rubber cement to demonstrate the primary goals of pharmacological management of acute aortic syndromes [7]. The contractile force of the myocardium, expressed as change in pressure over time (dp/dt) or as the initial upstroke of the arterial pressure curve, is largely responsible for the initiation and propagation of the dissection. The strength of the pulsation, rather than hypertension or high blood flow alone, leads to progression. Thus, the goals of medical management are to reduce blood pressure, as well as to reduce the left ventricular ejection force (dp/dt) and shear stress [7]. When fed B-aminopropionitrile fumarate (BAPN), a drug that mediates reduction in the tensile strength of the aorta by inhibiting lysyl oxidase, the Broad-Breasted White turkey develops iatrogenic aortic dissection. Simpson et al. investigated the effects of various pharmacologic strategies on the risk of aortic rupture in this model [8]. These studies demonstrate that blood pressure control alone is not adequate to prevent aortic rupture. Rather, beta-blocker therapy acts to reduce both blood pressure as well as chronotropy and inotropy, subsequently reducing dp/dt and the risk of rupture.

Initial medical therapy should aim to decrease wall stress (anti-impulse therapy) in order to limit extension of the dissection and reduce the risk of developing end-organ damage and rupture. Heart rate and blood pressure should be lowered to the lowest tolerable levels while ensuring adequate cerebral, coronary, and renal perfusion; typical heart rate goals are <60 bpm and systolic blood pressure goals are 100–120 mmHg. Intravenous short-acting agents should be administered and titrated using electronic monitoring of blood pressure, heart rate, and EKG. Consistent with European Society of Cardiology Guidelines, IRAD observed that over a period of 17 years, patients with both type A and type B AAD received significantly greater use of beta blockers (88% and 91%, respectively) [9].

First-line management is with intravenous (IV) beta-blocker therapy, with dosing as seen in Table 1. In patients with potential intolerance to beta-blockers (asthma, bradycardia, signs of heart failure), esmolol is a reasonable choice due to its short half-life (9 min) [1]. In patients who are truly beta-blocker intolerant, verapamil or diltiazem may be useful to decrease blood pressure without causing reflex tachycardia. If the systolic blood pressure is still greater than 120 mmHg after beta-blocker therapy, vasodilator therapy is recommended. This should only be done once heart rate is consistently less than 60 bpm. Agent options include nitroprusside and nicardipine, with dosing as seen in Table 1. In patients with an emergent or urgent indication for operation, anti-impulse therapy for hypertensive patients should be continued as the patient progresses to the operating room. In those patients who do not have an indication for immediate intervention and will be treated medically, such as those with an uncomplicated Type B aortic dissection (TBAD), the initial goal of therapy is to eliminate pain. In addition to anti-impulse therapy,

Table 1 Intravenous agents for initial medical management of acute aortic syndromes [1, 10]

Medication	Mechanism of action	Formulation	Bolus dose	Maintenance dose	Notes
First line: beta-blockers					
Esmolol	• Cardio-selective • Negative inotropy and chronotropy	2.5 g/250 mL	250–500 mcg/kg	50–200 mcg/kg/min titrated to maximum dose of 300 mcg/kg/min	• Caution in patients with heart failure, asthma, or concomitant calcium channel blocker therapy • Use cautiously in setting of acute aortic regurgitation as will block compensatory tachycardia • Onset of action: 2 min. Duration of action: 10–20 min
Labetalol	• Both alpha and beta-blockade, plus vasodilation • Negative inotropy and chronotropy	200 mg/200 mL	20 mg over 2 min; then 20–80 mg bolus every 10 min (max 300 mg)	0.5–2 mg/min	• Caution in patients with lung disease or concomitant calcium channel blocker therapy • Adverse events include vomiting, throat burning, heart block, orthostatic hypotension • Onset of action: 5 min. Duration of action: 6 h

(continued)

Table 1 (continued)

Medication	Mechanism of action	Formulation	Bolus dose	Maintenance dose	Notes
If resistant to beta-blockers					
Verapamil	• Reduces SVR • Depresses contractility	120 mg/250 mL	0.1 mg/kg over 2 min	2–5 mcg/kg/min	• Onset of action: 1–5 min
Diltiazem	• Reduces SVR • Negative inotropy	250 mg/250 mL	0.25 mg/kg over 2 min, then 0.35 mg/kg over 2 min	5–15 mg/h	• Caution in patients with heart failure or concomitant beta-blocker therapy • Adverse events include liver dysfunction • Onset of action: 2–5 min
Vasodilators					
Nitroprusside	• Relaxes arterial smooth muscle • Reduces SVR and PVR	50 mg/250 mL		0.25–0.5 mcg/kg/min titrated to maximum 8 mcg/kg/min	• Adverse effects include reflex increase in contractility and dp/dt; in a patient with aortic dissection, this mandates concomitant use of beta-blocker • Caution in patients with hepatic or renal dysfunction • Can cause cyanide toxicity • Effect dissipates in 1–2 min
Nicardipine	• Selectively relaxes arterial smooth muscle • Reduces SVR	50 mg/250 mL	5 mg/h	2.5–5 mg/h titrated to maximum 15 mg/h	• No effect on AV conduction • Has long duration of action: 4–6 h • Can increase V/Q mismatch and produce hypoxemia

proper management of pain is an important factor in management. Morphine sulfate is typically the drug of choice due its reliable and predictable effects, safety profile, ease of reversibility and ease of titration with the intravenous formulation.

A toxicology screen should be considered in all patients presenting with acute aortic syndrome, particularly if there are no known predisposing factors. Patients who develop aortic dissection as a result of cocaine intoxication should not receive non-selective beta blockers alone as this may lead to unopposed alpha stimulation, thus worsening hypertension [2]. Treatment of cocaine-related acute aortic syndromes should aim to reverse the centrally mediated nervous system stimulation.

After initial therapy with IV agents for a period of 12–24 h, the goal of medically managed dissection patients is to transition them to an effective oral anti-hypertensive regimen. The patients are transitioned to an oral regimen consisting of beta blockers, calcium channel blockers, and/or alpha antagonists as the IV regimen is weaned in a monitored setting with the same blood pressure and heart rate goals as above. In addition, all medically managed aortic syndrome patients should undergo repeat cross-sectional imaging (CT scan) at approximately 24–48 h after presentation. A small percentage of aortic pathology managed medically may progress to diagnoses requiring surgical intervention. For example, an ascending IMH may progress to TAAD, or a TBAD may have retrograde extension and evolve into a TAAD. This progression of disease is usually signified by a change in the patient's symptomatology.

While there are no high-quality data on the efficacy of initial medical management for all patients with acute aortic syndrome, anti-impulse therapy remains a Class I recommendation. Anti-impulse therapy addresses the primary precipitating risk factor (hypertension) leading to acute aortic syndromes, as well as reduces the aortic shear stress and risk of disease propagation in the initial period following presentation. Prior to definitive intervention for type A disease, reduction of propagation to further branch arteries reduces associated morbidity and mortality. In-hospital mortality rates are less than 10% for medically managed uncomplicated acute type B dissection [10] and as many as 10% of type B IMH lesions may completely resolve with appropriate beta-blockade [11]. However, long-term data from IRAD demonstrate that the 3-year survival rate for patients managed medically is only 78% [12]. Recently, the trend has favored endovascular intervention even for acute uncomplicated TBAD, though this is not supported by randomized data.

Volume Management

For patients who present with hypotension, the cause should be evaluated prior to fluid volume resuscitation. Alternative causes include hemopericardium with tamponade, valvular dysfunction, or left ventricular systolic dysfunction, all of which require further intervention. Pseudohypotension, which occurs when blood pressure is measured in an extremity with circulation compromised by the dissection, should be ruled-out prior to initiation of medical therapy. In the case of aortic rupture or cardiac tamponade, the initial management includes rapid volume resuscitation as a temporizing measure prior to immediate operative management. Despite high central venous pressure with cardiac tamponade, volume administration will improve cardiac filling against the external pressure within the pericardial space. Pericardiocentesis is associated with adverse outcomes, potentially due to rebound increase in intra-aortic pressure, but may be performed for those who cannot survive until surgery [13].

Complication-Specific Approach

Acute aortic syndromes are described as 'complicated' when there is malperfusion of a vascular bed. Complicated dissections account for approximately 15–20% of cases and can result in malperfusion of the brain, heart, viscera, spinal cord, and limbs [10]. Complicated disease portends a poor prognosis; in patients with limb ischemia or renal/mesenteric malperfusion versus those without, mortality is twice as high [13]. Malperfusion syndromes can be further classified as dynamic or static based on the mechanism of impaired blood flow. Dynamic occlusion occurs when the orifice of the aortic branch vessel is occluded by the mobile aortic dissection flap, thus leading to occlusion of the true lumen by the false lumen. In this case, fenestration of the intimal flap and/or treatment of the primary tear with thoracic endovascular aortic repair (TEVAR) can depressurize the false lumen and restore flow [10]. Static malperfusion occurs when the dissection flap extends into the aortic side branch, thus occluding the distal vessel. Branch vessel stenting in addition to TEVAR is typically necessary in this case to resolve the malperfusion syndrome [10].

In cases of malperfusion, a 'complication-specific approach' is recommended. Patients presenting with an acute TAAD, in whom the associated malperfusion is a more significant threat to life, restoration of flow to the occluded vascular bed is recommended *prior* to repair of the dissection. When considering delay of TAAD repair, all factors related to the presentation must be taken into account in order to judge the risk of rupture and death associated with the delay. These factors include the acuity of symptoms, the presence of continual chest or back pain despite adequate anti-impulse therapy, the degree of aortic insufficiency or tamponade, and the presence of heart failure. In the scenario of complicated acute TBAD, medical management alone is not sufficient, and these dissections should be treated immediately (usually by endovascular therapy or extra-anatomic bypass). Figures 1 and 2 display the algorithms for management of complicated acute aortic syndromes.

Following is a discussion of initial management of patients presenting with various manifestations of complicated dissection.

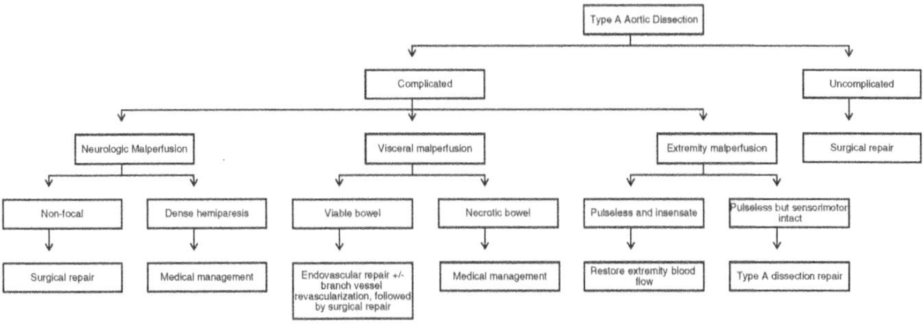

Fig. 1 Management approach for patients presenting with acute type A aortic dissection

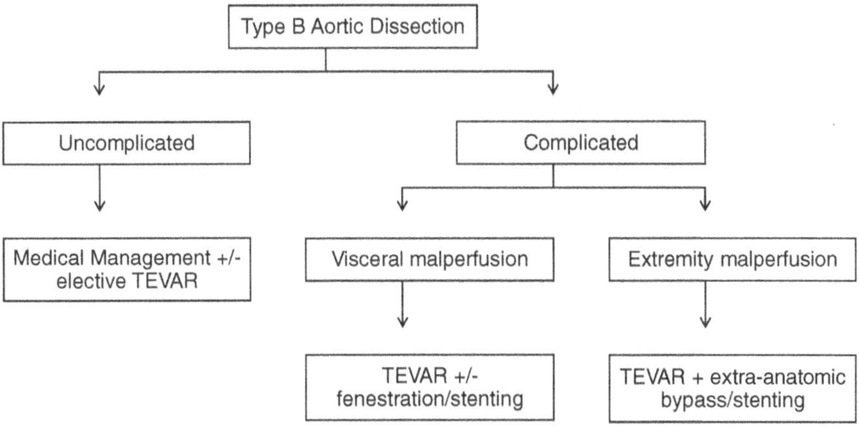

Fig. 2 Management approach for patients presenting with acute type B aortic dissection

Neurologic Complications

Among patients within IRAD, 6% of patients with TAAD also presented with a stroke. These patients commonly presented with syncope, shock, or pulse deficit [3]. Patients presenting with altered sensorium and delirium are common, however these symptoms do not necessarily indicate a cerebrovascular accident (CVA). If these patients have a non-focal neurologic exam, immediate repair of TAAD should not be delayed in order to investigate a possible CVA. However, a dense hemi-paretic CVA is a particularly poor prognostic sign that may make operative repair prohibitively risky. Management of patients with an acute aortic syndrome complicated by CVA remains controversial as immediate surgical repair carries a risk of hemorrhagic conversion, while conservative management is associated with a high incidence of early mortality [14]. Paraplegia and spinal cord malperfusion is a presenting manifestation in 2–5% of patients with AAD [15]. Prior to repair, there is no specific way to revascularize the spinal cord. These patients should undergo immediate repair of TAAD as resolution of paraparesis and even paraplegia after repair is possible. Resolution of paraparesis or paraplegia with immediate endovascular therapy of acute TBAD is less likely but should still be considered.

Visceral Malperfusion

Visceral malperfusion should be suspected in any patient with acute dissection who presents with absent unilateral or bilateral femoral pulses. The presence of intact femoral pulses does not guarantee adequate visceral blood flow, but it does make the presence of visceral malperfusion much less likely. One strategy for management of visceral malperfusion entails taking the patient to a hybrid operating room with both the general and cardiac surgery teams. Exploratory laparotomy is performed first: if the bowel is ischemic and unlikely to recover, no further intervention is performed. If the bowel is viable, blood flow is restored via TEVAR of the thoracic aorta (and potentially branch vessel revascularization). The abdomen is then left open, followed by a second-look operation to assess the bowel integrity. Intensive medical management of systolic blood pressure and resuscitation to correct metabolic abnormalities then allows for resolution of end-organ failure prior to open repair of the acute dissection. This does place the patient at risk for rupture in the intervening period, and is a challenging situation if the patient has severe aortic insufficiency and heart failure associated with the dissection. In a single center, retrospective study of patients with mesenteric malperfusion syndrome, 38% died prior to open repair: 24.4% from organ failure and 13.4% from aortic rupture. A multivariable logistic regression revealed that independent risk factors for death from organ failure were acute stroke, gross bowel necrosis at laparotomy, and serum lactate greater than 6 mmol/L [16].

Isolated renal malperfusion without other visceral malperfusion (intact celiac and superior mesenteric arteries) is exceedingly rare. TAAD repair should not be delayed in this rare scenario as isolated renal malperfusion is not immediately life-threatening. Immediate therapy for TBAD should also be considered in this scenario.

Limb Malperfusion

Lower limb malperfusion syndrome is present in 40% of complicated dissections and in up to 71% of patients with another malperfusion syndrome [17]. The degree of limb ischemia and duration of symptoms are important parameters to consider. A pulseless, cold, and insensate leg with no motor function should be revascularized prior to dissection repair. Traditional approaches include endovascular repairs and extra-anatomic bypass grafting. However, a leg with diminished pulse, but with intact sensorimotor function, will often improve with repair of the dissection. In the latter case, immediate dissection repair is recommended.

References

1. Bojar RM. Aortic dissections. In: Manual of perioperative care in adult cardiac surgery. 5th ed. Oxford: Wiley-Blackwell; 2011. p. 43–8.
2. Erbel R, Aboyans V, Boileau C, et al. 2014 European Society of Cardiology guidelines on the diagnosis and treatment of aortic diseases: document covering acute and chronic aortic diseases of the thoracic and abdominal aorta of the adult. Eur Heart J. 2014;35:2873–926. https://doi.org/10.1093/eurheartj/ehu281.
3. Tsai TT, Trimarchi S, Nienaber CA. Acute aortic dissection: perspectives from the International Registry of Acute Aortic Dissection (IRAD). Eur J Vasc Endovasc Surg. 2009;37(2):149–59. https://doi.org/10.1016/j.ejvs.2008.11.032.
4. Erbel R, Alfonso F, Boileau C, et al. Diagnosis and management of aortic dissection: recommendations of the task force on aortic dissection, European Society of Cardiology. Eur Heart J. 2001;22:1642–81. https://doi.org/10.1053/euhj.2001.2782.
5. Lansman SL, Saunders PC, Malekan R, Spielvogel D. Acute aortic syndrome. JTCVS. 2010;140(6 Suppl):S92–7.
6. Tsai TT, Nienaber CA, Eagle KA. Acute aortic syndromes. Circulation. 2005;112(24):3802–13. https://doi.org/10.1161/circulationAHA.105.534198.
7. Wheat MW Jr, Palmer RF. Dissecting aneurysms of the aorta: present status of drug versus surgical therapy. Prog Cardiovasc Dis. 1968;11(3):198–210. https://doi.org/10.1016/0033-0620(68)90010-8.
8. Simpson CF, Boucek RJ. The B-aminopropionitrile-fed Turkey: a model for detecting potential drug action on arterial tissue. Cardiovasc Res. 1983;17(1):26–32. https://doi.org/10.1093/cvr/17.1.26.
9. Pape L, Awais M, Woznicki EM, et al. Presentation, diagnosis, and outcomes of acute aortic dissection: 17-year trends from the International Registry of Acute Aortic Dissection. J Am Coll Cardiol. 2015;66:350–8.
10. Feldman M, Shah M, Elefteriades JA. Medical management of acute type A aortic dissection. Ann Thorac Cardiovasc Surg. 2009;15(5):286–93.
11. Hughes GC, Andersen ND, McCann RL. Management of acute type B aortic dissection. JTCVS. 2013;145(3 Suppl):S202–7. https://doi.org/10.1016/j.jtcvs.2012.11.078.
12. von Kodolitsch Y, Csösz SK, Koschyk DH, et al. Intramural hematoma of the aorta: predictors of progression to dissection and rupture. Circulation. 2003;107(8):1158–63. https://doi.org/10.1161/01.cir.0000052628.77047.ea.
13. Evangelista A, Isselbacher EM, Bossone E, et al. Insights from the international registry of acute aortic dissection: a 20-year experience of collaborative clinical research. Circulation. 2018;137(17):1846–60. https://doi.org/10.1161/CIRCULATIONAHA.117.031264.
14. Hiratzka LF, Bakris GL, Beckman JA, et al. 2010 ACCF/AHA/AATS/ACR/ASA/SCA/SCAI/SIR/STS/SVM guidelines for the diagnosis and management of patients with thoracic aortic disease: executive summary. A report of the American College of Cardiology Foundation/American Heart Association Task Force on Practice Guidelines, American Association for Thoracic Surgery, American College of Radiology, American Stroke Association, Society of Cardiovascular Anesthesiologists, Society for Cardiovascular Angiography and Interventions, Society of Interventional Radiology, Society of Thoracic Surgeons, and Society for Vascular Medicine. Catheter Cardiovasc Interv. 2010;76(2):E43–86. https://doi.org/10.1002/ccd.22537.
15. Bossone E, Corteville DC, Harris KM, et al. Stroke and outcomes in patients with acute type A aortic dissection. Circulation. 2013;128(11 Suppl 1):S175–9. https://doi.org/10.1161/CIRCULATIONAHA.112.000327.
16. Inamasu J, Hori S, Yokoyama M, Funabiki T, Aoki K, Aikawa N. Paraplegia caused by painless acute aortic dissection. Spinal Cord. 2000;38(11):702–4.
17. Yang B, Norton EL, Rosati CM, et al. Managing patients with acute type A aortic dissection and mesenteric malperfusion syndrome: a 20-year experience. J Thorac Cardiovasc Surg. 2019;158(3):675–687.e4. https://doi.org/10.1016/j.jtcvs.2018.11.127.

Imaging of Aortic Dissection: CT, MRI, and Angiography

Albree Tower-Rader, Lars G. Svensson, and Venu Menon

Imaging is integral to the initial diagnosis, management, and follow-up of patients with a suspected aortic dissection. In contrast to acute coronary syndrome where an ECG and presence of biomarkers indicative of myocardial necrosis can be diagnostic, acute aortic syndrome requires imaging to confirm the diagnosis. The patient with a suspected acute aortic syndrome should undergo immediate imaging with multi-detector computed tomography (MDCT), transesophageal echocardiogram (TEE), or magnetic resonance imaging (MRI) based on the stability of the patient and institutional availability and expertise since there are advantages and disadvantages to each modality [1–3] (Table 1). For most patients MDCT is the diagnostic test of choice to evaluate the aorta. A well-performed study enables immediate confirmation of the suspected diagnosis, as well as information regarding the pathophysiology and prognosis. The use of echocardiography in the evaluation of patients with acute aortic syndrome is discussed in depth in subsequent chapters. The majority of acute aortic syndromes, 80–90%, are aortic dissections [4], with the minority classified as intramural hematoma or penetrating aortic ulcers, the imaging for both of which will be discussed in subsequent chapters. An ideal imaging study would provide a rapid and accurate, noninvasive diagnosis of the presence and extent of an aortic dissection allowing for classification under the DeBakey or more commonly used Stanford system. Patients with involvement of the ascending aorta, Stanford type A, are managed as a surgical emergency; however, it is equally important to identify patients with a complicated type B dissection who are often managed by stent-graft endovascular repair (TEVAR) in the acute setting [5, 6]. Imaging can detect some features of a complicated type B dissection, such as the involvement of aortic branch vessels resulting in end-organ malperfusion, or signs of rupture, such as a pericardial effusion, hemothorax, or mediastinal blood products. Additionally

A. Tower-Rader · L. G. Svensson · V. Menon (✉)
Division of Cardiovascular Medicine, Heart and Vascular Institute, Cleveland Clinic, Cleveland, OH, USA
e-mail: svenssl@ccf.org; menonv@ccf.org

J. S. Coselli et al. (eds.), *Aortic Dissection and Acute Aortic Syndromes*,
https://doi.org/10.1007/978-3-030-66668-2_10

Table 1 Comparison of available imaging techniques of the aorta

	Multidetector computed tomography (MDCT)	Magnetic resonance imaging (MRI)	Angiography	Transesophageal echocardiogram (TEE)
Advantages	• Rapid • Easily accessed and performed • May reveal alternative/additional diagnoses • Able to assess for evidence of end-organ malperfusion	• No radiation exposure • Potential to be performed without gadolinium contrast • Able to assess for aortic regurgitation • Able to assess for left ventricular function and wall motion abnormalities • Able to assess for evidence of end-organ malperfusion	• Often performed during endovascular treatment of a dissection • Able to assess for aortic regurgitation • Possible to evaluate patency of aortic branches	• May be performed at bedside for unstable patients • Immediate interpretation • Able to assess for aortic regurgitation • Able to assess for pericardial effusion with tamponade physiology • Can assess left ventricular function and wall motion abnormalities • Used peri-procedurally in the operating room
Disadvantages	• Radiation exposure • Uses iodinated contrast • Pulsation artifact in aortic root and ascending aorta without ECG-gating	• Longer acquisition time • Difficult to perform hemodynamic monitoring during study • May not be readily accessible • Implanted devices may not be compatible or may create artifacts • May require sedation for claustrophobic patients	• Invasive • Need for an experience operator • Longer acquisition time • Radiation exposure • Uses iodinated contrast • False negatives in setting of intramural hematoma and thrombosed false lumens	• Semi-invasive • Need for an experienced operator • Requires sedation • Distal ascending aorta obstructed from view by airways • Limited assessment of abdominal aorta and branches • Contraindicated in patients with cirrhosis, gastrointestinal bleed or dysphagia • Reverberation artifacts may mimic an intimal flap

the status of blood flow in the false lumen, as well as involvement of other structures including the aortic valve and coronary arteries, or proximity of cardiovascular structures to the sternum for patients with prior sternotomy, is often useful in determining the management strategy. Current guidelines recommend that measurements of the aorta by either MDCT or MRI should be taken at reproducible landmarks in a plane perpendicular to the axis of the flow of blood utilizing either multiplanar reconstruction or the centerline of flow [1, 2, 7] (Fig. 1a, b). The 2015

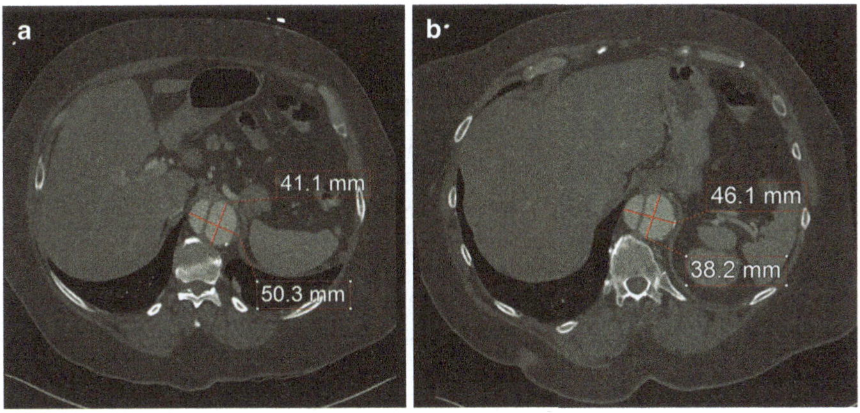

Fig. 1 (**a**) An example of measurement of the descending thoracic aorta at the level of the diaphragmatic hiatus on axial imaging. (**b**) Measurement of the dimensions of the descending thoracic aorta at the level of the diaphragmatic hiatus following multiplanar reconstruction to align the plane of the image to be perpendicular to the axis of blood flow. In this case, failure to reconstruct the plane for measurement of aorta dimensions would result in an erroneous measurement

Multimodality Imaging of Diseases of the Thoracic Aorta guidelines do not specify which technique should be undertaken for measuring the aortic dimensions, though prior guidelines including the 2010 ACC/AHA and the 2014 ESC guidelines had suggested measuring outer edge-to-outer edge on MDCT and MRI, as opposed to the recommendation for echocardiographic measurements of leading edge-to-leading edge [1, 2, 7]. Care should be taken to access available prior imaging, especially for patients who have had prior repairs, because it may be difficult for the medical team to interpret whether acute changes are present without direct comparison to prior images potentially leading to false positive findings of an acute dissection or concerning new aortic dilation [8]. Patients with a confirmed aortic dissection may be transferred to a specialized center and the images obtained at the primary facility need to be able to be rapidly accessible to the receiving care team, either by CD or secure digital image transfer.

Multidetector Computed Tomography

Protocol Considerations

As technology has developed over the past few decades, multidetector computed tomography (≥64 detector rows, MDCT) angiography has evolved as the preferred modality for imaging due to the widespread availability, quality of studies, ease of interpretation, and rapid speed of study acquisition. A meta-analysis examining 16 studies found a very high sensitivity of 100% and specificity of 98–99% for the diagnosis of aortic dissection by MDCT angiography [9]. Standard acquisition times for MDCT with short gantry rotation times are 3–4 s for the chest and <10 s for the chest, abdomen, and pelvis, often accomplished in a single breath-hold [7]. Though protocols vary by institution, ideally they are designed to allow for adequate diagnosis while minimizing radiation if possible. During the cardiac cycle, the aortic root (including the valve and sinuses) and proximal ascending aorta are in motion and thus prone to motion artifacts, which may be erroneously interpreted as intimal flaps [10] (Fig. 2a, b). In fact, studies have shown that the most frequent reason for a false positive diagnosis of an aortic dissection was the use of a non-ECG gated CT [8]. For this reason, synchronizing image acquisition of the chest to the cardiac cycle via ECG-gating should be performed to allow for careful assessment of the aortic root. ECG-gating may be performed either prospectively or retrospectively. With prospective gating, images are acquired only during the desired portion of the cardiac cycle, typically diastole as cardiac motion is limited; however, this requires a fairly regular rhythm. Retrospective gating, however, allows for image acquisition throughout the entire cardiac cycle with subsequent reconstructions at different phases of the cardiac cycle if necessary, which is useful in the setting of arrhythmias, though at the expense of increased radiation exposure. Care should be taken with automated bolus tracking to ensure proper opacification of the aorta. With automated bolus tracking, a region of interest (ROI) is placed on reference image on the descending thoracic aorta and the acquisition is triggered when the predetermined threshold Hounsfield unit (HU) is surpassed. If the ROI spans the true and false lumens, and particularly if the false lumen is thrombosed, the threshold might be reached too late if the operator waits for complete opacification of the false lumen, thus resulting in inadequate opacification of the true lumen. Instead it is recommended that the operator carefully monitor to ensure the location of the ROI is correctly placed over the true lumen as the aorta begins to enhance and be

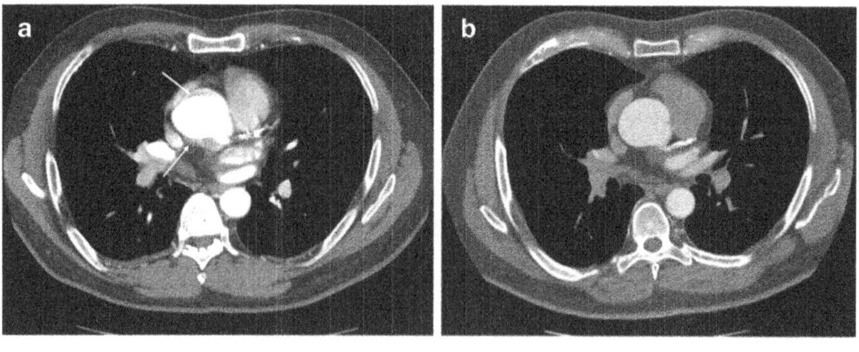

Fig. 2 (**a**) Non-gated CT angiography of the chest demonstrating a central contrast-filled lumen in the ascending aorta with a component of the lumen both anterior and posterior (arrows), which is less intensely opacified. This may be mistaken for a dissection, but the presence of both anterior and posterior segments of the ascending aorta lumen, which are less intensely opacified, is characteristic of a motion artifact. (**b**) ECG-gated CT angiography of the chest performed in the same patient demonstrating the absence of a dissection of the ascending aorta

prepared to manually trigger the scan, if necessary, when the true lumen is well opacified with a goal of ≥250 HU [3]. Use of a saline flush is recommended to help tighten the contrast bolus, resulting in a higher peak contrast opacification [3, 4]. Contrast should be administered via the right arm to limit the appearance of streak artifacts obscuring the head and neck vessels, including the left subclavian artery. Following acquisition of an ECG-gated chest, a continuous scan extending from the lung apices to the groin should be performed in order to obtain a continuous dataset, which is often necessary when planning for an endovascular repair, instead of subsequently obtaining a separate acquisition of the abdomen and pelvis, effectively splitting the aorta into two separate datasets. Acquisition of thin slice axial images (0.5–2.0 mm) is recommended [11]. A triple-rule-out (TRO) protocol is intended to assess the aorta, coronary arteries, and pulmonary arteries in a single ECG-gated scan utilizing a biphasic contrast injection designed for simultaneous arterial (>300 HU) and pulmonary arterial (>200 HU) enhancement [12]. In practice, TRO scans have been shown to be associated with higher radiation exposure and contrast doses and non-diagnostic images, and thus for patients with a high-risk feature of aortic dissection, a dedicated study should be performed for instead [7, 13]. In general, careful attention should be paid to adjusting the tube voltage and current, as well as any other scanner-specific features in order to minimize the radiation dose to the patient.

CT Findings of Aortic Dissections

Non-contrast CT Findings

Non-contrast CT is not diagnostic for aortic dissection, though it may be performed in some centers prior to CTA to aid in the detection of an intramural hematoma or may have been performed for another indication. Findings on non-contrast CT, which are suggestive of aortic dissection, include displacement of intimal calcifications into the lumen (Fig. 3a, b), as well as a hyperattenuating fluid collection within the pericardium, pleural cavity, or mediastinum suggestive of aortic rupture.

CTA Findings

Diagnosis of an aortic dissection includes identification of a true and false lumen separated by an intimal flap. The true lumen is often smaller, while the false lumen is often crescent-shaped with a "beak" sign, or acute angle between the intimal flap and the aortic wall. The typical appearance of an intimal flap or "double barrel" is noted in approximately 70% of cases, thoughif there is circumferential separation of the intima, the true lumen may have a more cylindrical or "windsock" appearance due to intussusception of the flap [14] (Fig. 4a, b). The true lumen typically will run along the inferomedial aspect of the arch and descending thoracoabdominal aorta,

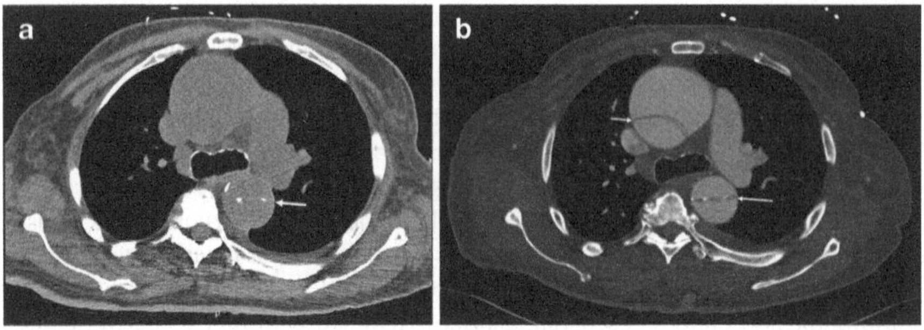

Fig. 3 (**a**) Non-contrast gated CT chest with a dilated ascending aorta and evidence of intimal calcifications within the lumen of the descending thoracic aorta (arrow) concerning for possible aortic dissection. (**b**) ECG-gated CT angiography of the chest in the same patient confirming the presence of a Type A dissection with an intimal flap present in the ascending and descending thoracic aorta (arrows)

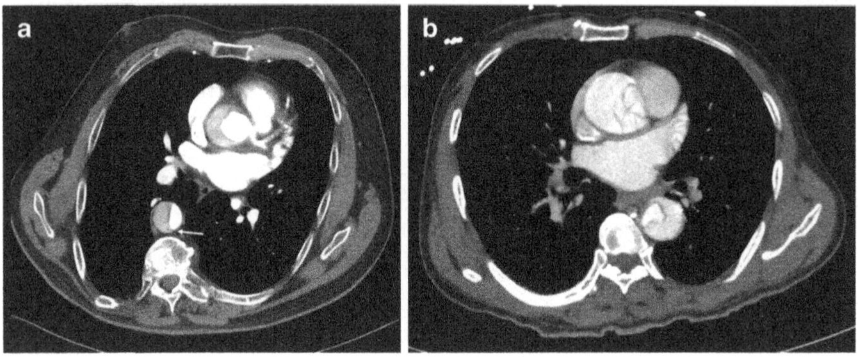

Fig. 4 (**a**) ECG-gated CT angiography of the chest demonstrating a Type A aortic dissection with an intimal flap present in the ascending and descending thoracic aorta with a typical "double barrel" lumen appearance of the descending thoracic aorta with a less intensely opacified false lumen with a "beak" appearance at the intersection of the intimal flap and aorta wall (arrow). (**b**) ECG-gated CT angiography of the chest demonstrating a Type A aortic dissection with an intimal flap present in the ascending and descending thoracic aorta with near complete separation of the intima within the descending thoracic aorta, which results in a "windsock" appearance

though variation is common [15]. Identification of the true lumen may be difficult in the setting of an extensive dissection, but can be determined with the aid of the pattern of intimal calcifications and tracking the lumens. By scrolling through the axial images, or using reconstructions, a reader can identify and track a portion of unaffected aorta to identify the true lumen since they remain in continuity. Additionally, the false lumen may be less intensely opacified than the true lumen due to either differential timing of contrast opacification, a finding that can be confirmed by delayed imaging. Thrombus may be present within the false lumen at the time of presentation in approximately 40% of patients with a type B dissection [16]. Depending on the pressure differential between the true and false lumens, the false lumen may compress the true lumen. Compression of the true lumen by an expanding false lumen is more likely to occur in the absence of distal reentry tears. The location of calcifications in relation to the intimal flap may also aid in differentiating the true and false lumens because in the acute setting, intimal calcifications will remain on the true lumen side of the displaced intimal flap, whereas in the setting of a chronic dissection, calcifications may be seen on either side because mural calcifications may form within the false lumen in the setting of a chronic dissection [14]. Additionally, the intimal flap is often curved in the setting of an acute dissection due to mobility, whereas in chronic dissections, the intimal flap is often flat and fixed [14]. These features, which can help to distinguish an acute from a chronic dissection, are important to note, since it is possible for patients to present with a different etiology for their symptoms in the setting of either a known chronic dissection, or a previously unknown chronic dissection.

In addition to identifying of the presence of an acute dissection and the status of the true and false lumens, one must next determine whether there is involvement of the ascending aorta and the site of the entry tear. In practice, identification of the true and false lumens often occurs at the same time as identification of the proximal and distal aspects of the dissection. The most common sites of entry tears, accounting for ~90% of cases, are within the first 2 cm of the ascending aorta and at the isthmus near the ligamentum arteriosum, which is thought to be because these two areas are under the greatest hemodynamic stress [17]. The entry tear is found by tracing the intimal flap and looking for an area where the flap is interrupted, often in a transverse orientation to the lumen. The ends of the discontinuous intimal flap are often visible at the site of the entry tear with the ends pointed in the direction of flow between the lumens. Often the ends are oriented from the true into the false lumen, and with variation, may occur throughout the cardiac phase or due to the relative pressure differences between the lumens. The site of the entry tear is important to note since it can affect the type of repair, especially if the tear is located in the arch with retrograde extension into the ascending aorta [15]. Identification of the head and neck vessel branching pattern and involvement by the dissection flap is important because it may affect procedural planning in regards to the cannulation site for cardiopulmonary bypass or endovascular stent graft placement (Fig. 5). During cardiopulmonary bypass, antegrade cerebral perfusion is often performed by cannulating of the right axillary or subclavian artery and clamping the brachiocephalic trunk, diverting blood flow to the right common carotid artery [18]; however, an alternative mechanism must be considered in the presence of an aberrant right subclavian artery since the right common carotid artery instead has a separate origin from the aortic arch. Extension of the dissection flap into the iliac or femoral arteries should also be noted, as this may affect arterial access for procedural planning, especially endovascular stent graft repair. Reports should include details regarding the location of the intimal tear, extent of aortic involvement, dimensions of the aorta, status of the false lumen (i.e., patent or thrombosed), and whether the true lumen is compressed (Table 2).

For patients with involvement of the ascending aorta, particular attention should also be paid to the ostia of the coronary arteries, the relation of the flap to the aortic

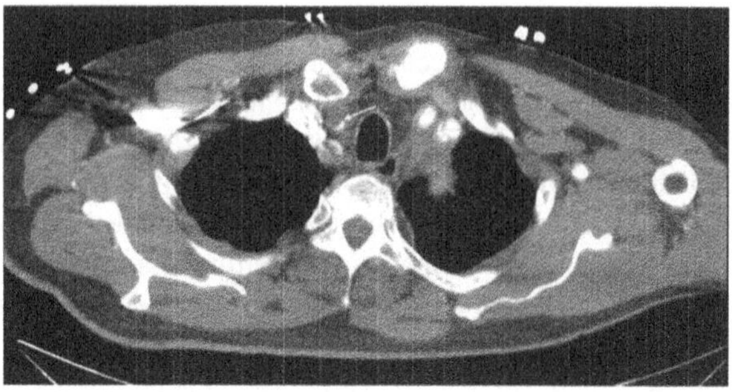

Fig. 5 ECG-gated CT angiography of the chest in a patient with a Type A aortic dissection demonstrating extension of the intimal flap into the aortic branch vessels, in particular with compression of the true lumen of the innominate artery by a thrombus-filled false lumen. In this case, the operative plan was adjusted to provide antegrade cerebral perfusion via an interposition graft

Table 2 Features to include in imaging reports in an Acute Aortic Dissection

• Extent of dissection
– Proximal and distal aspects of the dissection
– Involvement of the ascending aorta
• Dimensions of the aorta
• Status of the true and false lumens
– i.e., perfused, partial/complete thrombosis, compression
• Site of the entry tear
• Evidence of rupture
– i.e., hemorrhagic pericardial effusion, pleural effusion, mediastinal hematoma
• Involvement of the coronary arteries
• Arch and abdominal branch vessel pattern and patency
• Evidence of end-organ malperfusion
– Origin of each branch from true or false lumen
– Evidence of dissection flap extending into the ostium
– Evidence of static or dynamic obstruction
– Decreased organ perfusion
• Patency and/or dissection involvement of the iliac and femoral arteries
• Proximity of cardiovascular structures to the sternum with prior sternotomy
• Presence/location of reentry tears (if present)
• Type of aortic valve, and presence/mechanism of aortic regurgitation (if possible)
• Features associated with underlying connective tissue disease

valve, and the pericardium, all which are best examined on an ECG-gated study. Aortic regurgitation has been reported in approximately 40–70% of cases of a type A dissection [1]. Aortic regurgitation may occur in a dissection due to one of three possible mechanisms: (1) acute enlargement of the aortic root, resulting in lack of coaptation, (2) extension of the dissection into the aortic root, resulting in leaflet prolapse from disruption of the commissures, or (3) prolapse of the dissection flap through the aortic valve in diastole, preventing valve closure [19]. Myocardial ischemia may occur due to extension of the dissection into the coronary artery ostia, or due to external compression by the false lumen (Fig. 6a–c). As previously noted, the

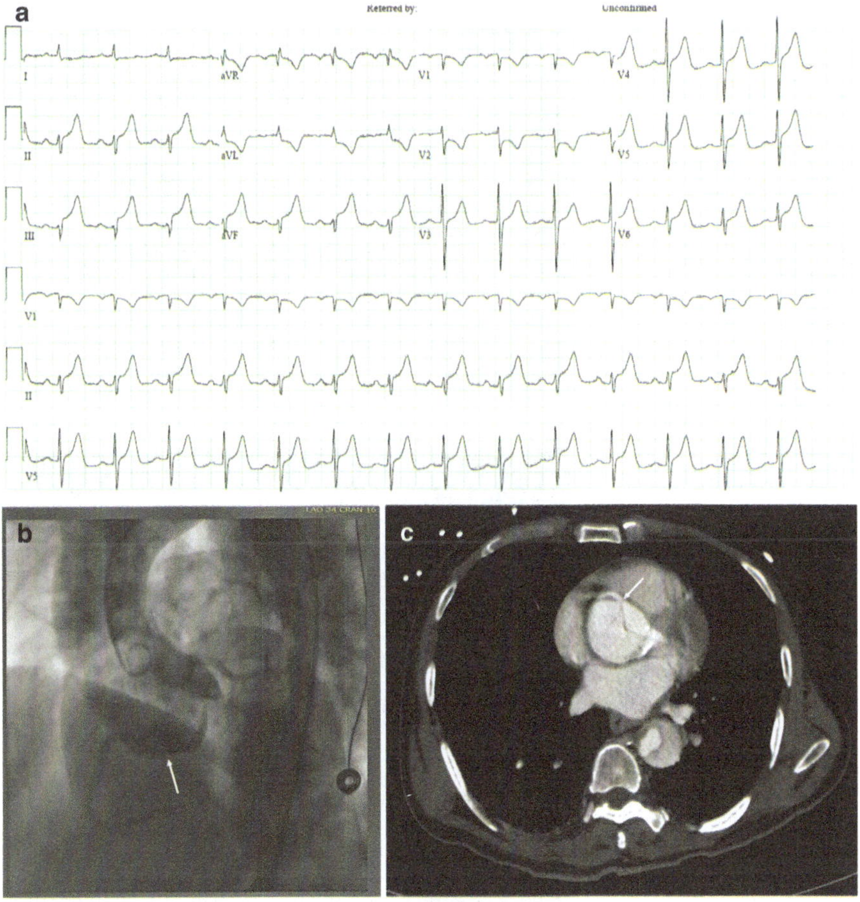

Fig. 6 (**a**) ECG demonstrating an inferoposterior ST elevation myocardial infarction in a patient presenting with chest pain. (**b**) Invasive aortography was performed following activation of the cardiac catheterization lab for an ST elevation myocardial infarction and non-obstructive coronary angiography. In this case, aortography demonstrated a double lumen with an intimal flap (arrow) and differential opacification of the two lumens within the ascending aorta. (**c**) ECG-gated CT angiography of the chest (shown), abdomen, and pelvis was subsequently performed to confirm the diagnosis and evaluate the extent of the dissection. An intimal flap is present in the aortic root extending into the ostium of the right coronary artery

presence of a hyperattenuating (>40 HU) fluid collection within the pericardium, pleural space, or mediastinum is suggestive of aortic rupture on both non-contrast and contrast studies (Figs. 7 and 8) [4]. With contrast administration, irregularity of the aortic wall may be noted, or frank extravasation of vascular contrast into the fluid collection [20].

The identification of features suggestive of a complicated dissection with end-organ malperfusion or evidence of rupture is of almost equal importance to diagnosing the presence of an aortic dissection. In up to 30% of patients with an aortic

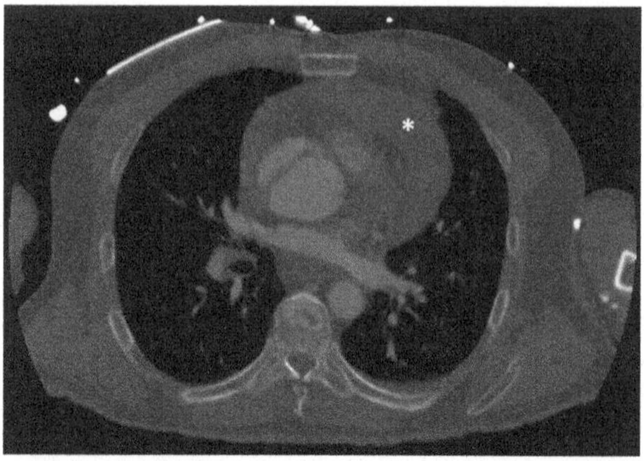

Fig. 7 ECG-gated CT angiography of the chest with a large hyperattenuating (~54 Hounsfield units) pericardial effusion (asterisk), concerning for hemopericardium and aortic rupture in the setting of a Type A aortic dissection

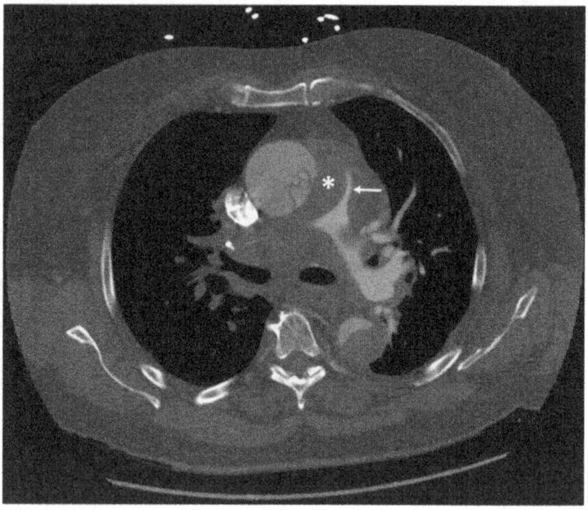

Fig. 8 ECG-gated CT angiography of the chest with a large hyperattenuating (~62 Hounsfield units) mediastinal fluid collection (asterisk) compressing the main pulmonary artery (arrow), concerning for mediastinal blood products due to aortic rupture in the setting of a Type A aortic dissection

dissection, and approximately 10% of patients with a type B aortic dissection, evidence of end-organ malperfusion is apparent at the time of initial presentation [2, 5]. While the most common description is of the celiac trunk, superior mesenteric and right renal arteries arising from the true lumen, and the left renal artery arising from the false lumen, significant variation has been noted in the pattern of abdominal branch vessel involvement [15]. It is important to examine whether each branch, including the head and neck vessels, arises from the true or false lumen, as well as the presence and mechanism of end-organ malperfusion for each branch vessel territory. End-organ malperfusion may be due to one of four mechanisms: (1) static occlusion of the branch artery by extension of the dissection flap into the ostium or proximal segment, (2) dynamic due to the dissection flap prolapsing over and intermittently occluding the ostium of the non-dissected branch vessel, (3) mixed static and dynamic, or (4) ostial disconnection and avulsion from the true lumen [10, 14, 21]. The mechanism of occlusion is important to identify since it influences management: static occlusion is often treated with a stent, whereas dynamic occlusion may be managed by creating fenestrations in the intimal flap to reduce the pressure within the false lumen [10, 14]. Additionally, the evaluation of the ostia and proximal segment of each branch vessel of the aorta is crucial to understanding which organs may be at risk for ischemia. Regardless, careful inspection of the abdominal organs for evidence of decreased perfusion should also be performed (Fig. 9). Delayed phase imaging may be helpful in differentiating complete versus delayed perfusion of a vascular territory in the setting of a chronic dissection; however, in the setting of acute symptoms, organ hypoperfusion on arterial phase imaging is presumed to represent an area at risk and delayed phase imaging is typically not included in the protocol in order to decrease both the acquisition time and radiation dose of the study. Reports should include a detailed description of whether the aortic branch vessels are involved in the dissection, patency of the ostia and proximal aortic branch vessels, and evidence of decreased organ perfusion or infarction (Table 2).

Additional Findings on CT Imaging

In addition to obtaining data regarding the aorta itself, additional information is obtained regarding both cardiovascular and non-cardiovascular structures, which may give clues to an underlying syndrome or predisposition for aortic dissection, alternative diagnosis, or may help guide surgical planning. As is discussed in depth in the sections regarding long-term imaging of the aorta and management of chronic

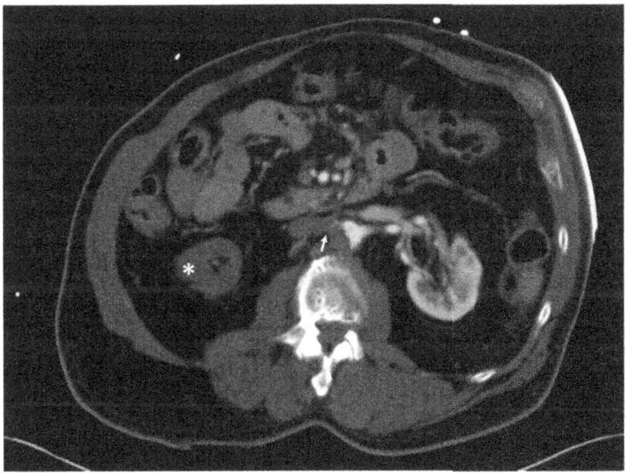

Fig. 9 CT angiography of the abdomen demonstrating an aortic dissection with the left renal artery arising from the true lumen and an intimal flap extending to the ostium of the right renal artery, resulting in occlusion by the false lumen (arrow). Additionally there is hypoperfusion of the right kidney (asterisk), which is readily apparent, especially in comparison to the well-perfused left kidney

dissections, several imaging features have been identified that are predictive of future aortic dilation and adverse aortic events (Table 3). With the use of ECG-gating MDCT, it is possible to identify the aortic valve as well as the anatomy of the sinotubular junction. The identification of a bicuspid aortic valve carries additional implications for follow-up for the patient, as well as first degree relatives. In the case of syndromic connective tissue disorders, including Marfan, vascular type Ehlers-Danlos and Loeys-Dietz syndromes, additional associated features may be identified including pectus deformity of the chest wall, scoliosis or kyphosis, dural ectasia, or lung bullae. One of the other main benefits of MDCT in comparison to other imaging modalities is that in the absence of an aortic dissection other etiologies of chest pain may be identified, including pulmonary embolus, pneumothorax, or pulmonary or chest wall mass. In patients who have undergone prior sternotomy it is important to detail the proximity of cardiovascular structures to the sternum, particularly bypass grafts and whether they cross the midline, since this may affect planning for a redo sternotomy. Reports should include information regarding proximity of cardiovascular structures to the sternum, as well as features that may suggest an underlying syndrome since the management of these patients in the acute and chronic phases, and the implications for screening of family members varies (Table 2).

Magnetic Resonance Imaging

Magnetic resonance imaging (MRI) is best reserved for stable patients, or those with chronic dissections. Prior studies have demonstrated a sensitivity and specificity of 95–98% and 94–98%, respectively, for the detection of an aortic dissection [9]. Several different types of MRI sequences are available for imaging the aorta including cine (dynamic) imaging, MR angiography, and respiratory navigator-gated 3D acquisitions. In addition to assessment of the aorta, cine MRI imaging allows for the assessment of aortic regurgitation, left ventricular function, and pericardial effusions, offering the potential to obtain additional data regarding cardiac function and potential complications of a type A dissection as part of the study.

Table 3 Imaging features predictive of aortic dilation and adverse aortic events

• Partially thrombosed false lumen > patent false lumen > thrombosed false lumen
• Maximal aortic diameter ≥ 40 mm
• Fusiform index ≥ 0.64
• False lumen diameter ≥ 22 mm in the proximal descending aorta
• Crescent shape of the true lumen
• Thrombosed false lumen with ulcer-like projections (especially in the proximal descending aorta)
• Entry tear ≥ 10 mm in the proximal descending aorta

Fusiform index = Maximum diameter of descending aorta/(diameter of the distal aortic arch + diameter of the descending aorta at the level of the pulmonary artery)

Unfortunately, despite these benefits, the relatively long acquisition time (approximately 20–30 min), as well as the inability to adequately monitor patients who are potentially hemodynamically unstable, makes the use of MRI for diagnosing an acute dissection far less appealing [3]. However, MRI may be used in select scenarios where an acute aortic dissection is suspected, for instance in a hemodynamically stable patient with a severe allergy to iodinated contrast, or in a facility that does not have immediate access to transesophageal echocardiography. Instead, MRI is often used for monitoring patients with a chronic dissection due to the lack of radiation exposure, and, with newer techniques, the ability to avoid contrast administration altogether. MR angiography is also ill-suited for patients with advanced renal dysfunction and pregnancy since gadolinium chelate contrast agents are contraindicated. Implantable medical devices may be problematic either because the device is not MRI compatible, or due to artifacts created by the device interfering with image interpretation.

MRI Findings

As with CT, a dissection is often identified on MRI with the presence of a double-barrel lumen on axial images. In particular, spin-echo black-blood sequences allow for the rapid identification of an intimal flap [22] (Fig. 10). The true lumen can be identified using the same anatomic considerations as with MDCT; the true lumen is usually smaller and in continuity with the unaffected aorta. Thrombus within the false lumen is hypointense on T1 and T2 imaging [22]. Again, the status of all of the aortic arch and abdominal aortic branches should be described. Pericardial and pleural effusions may be recognized by their high signal intensity on axial imaging. ECG-gated gradient echo sequences can be displayed as cine images with areas of

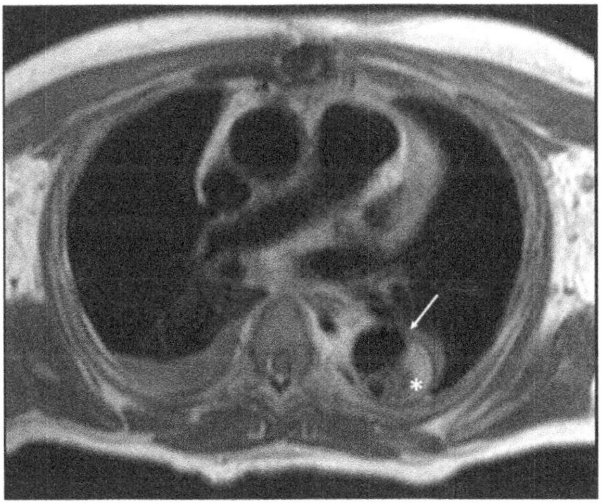

Fig. 10 Magnetic resonance imaging with spin-echo black blood imaging demonstrating an intimal flap (arrow) with partial thrombosis of the false lumen (asterisk)

turbulent flow creating dephasing and resulting in a signal void, which may be useful in identifying aortic regurgitation or flow between the true and false lumens. MR angiography utilizes 3D spoiled gradient echo sequences and a gadolinium-chelate contrast agent and is rapidly acquired during a single breath-hold with high-intensity signal localized to the intravascular space (Fig. 11). Typically unenhanced, arterial and delayed phase images are obtained. MR angiography results in the reconstruction of a 3D dataset, which may then be manipulated to allow for multiplanar reconstruction of cross-sectional sections to the lumen to measure aortic dimensions in a similar fashion to CT [11]. Non-contrast techniques for acquisition and reconstruction of a 3D dataset, including respiratory navigator-gated, ECG-gated 3D whole heart balanced steady state free precession, have a long acquisition time (10–12 min) and are thus ill-suited for imaging in the acute setting [23].

Angiography

Prior to the advent of non-invasive techniques for evaluating the aorta, aortography was considered the standard for diagnosis for an aortic dissection. As a primary diagnostic tool angiography has fallen out of favor compared to other modalities because it is invasive, time-consuming, requires an experienced operator, and exposes the patient to both iodinated contrast and radiation. Digital subtraction angiography (DSA) is still utilized in a few clinical scenarios and thus, it is still important to understand the appearance of a dissection on DSA, as well as the disadvantages of the technique. For instance, DSA is often utilized during endovascular treatment of a dissection, and may be useful as a diagnostic tool for patients presenting to the cardiac catheterization lab for chest pain with a suspected acute coronary syndrome who are found to have non-obstructive coronary arteries and an alternative diagnosis of aortic dissection is suspected. Aortography may also be

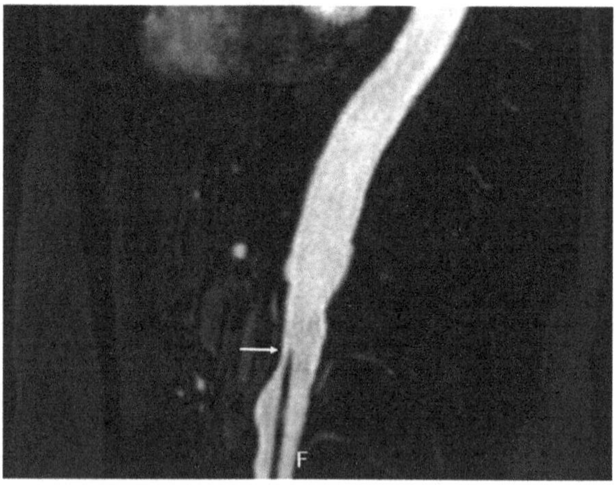

Fig. 11 Magnetic resonance imaging with contrast enhanced angiography, revealing an intimal flap (arrow) and double barrel lumen in the abdominal aorta

necessary to diagnose an aortic dissection for institutions without access to noninvasive imaging (MDCT or MRI) or transesophageal echocardiography. Aortography involves the placement of a pigtail catheter placed within the aortic lumen, with injection of iodinated contrast initially by hand to confirm catheter placement followed by injection via a hydraulic power injector with digital subtraction cine fluoroscopic imaging [24]. Initially aortography was thought to be associated with a risk for propagation of the dissection, but further study demonstrated the procedure to be relatively safe, thus becoming the standard for diagnosis around 1970 [25]. The sensitivity and specificity of angiography are also lower than with MDCT and MRI at 88% and 94%, respectively [26].

Angiography Findings

Following injection of iodinated contrast within the aorta lumen, the lumen of the aorta, as well as its branches, become opacified. The presence of double lumen with an intimal flap and communication between the two lumens is diagnostic for an aortic dissection [24] (Fig. 6a–c). Either flow reversal or stasis of contrast within the false lumen is often seen. Indirect signs of an aortic dissection include compression of the true lumen, thickening of the aortic wall, out-pouchings along the aortic wall, failure of aortic branches to fill, and aortic regurgitation [24, 26–28]. Injection of contrast alters the pressure dynamics between the true and false lumen and thus the assessment of malperfusion syndromes proves more complicated. False positives may occur when the true and false lumens opacify simultaneously [29]. Additionally, angiography is not capable of identifying intramural hematoma or patients with a completely thrombosed false lumen, especially if there is no aortic branch vessel involvement [27].

Conclusions

In conclusion, the sensitivity and specificity of MDCT and MRI for the detection of an aortic dissection are similar [9], though the relative length of MRI and inability to fully monitor patients hemodynamically make it less ideal for the evaluation of an acute aortic dissection unless the patient is stable and unable to receive iodinated contrast. Angiography, previously the standard for diagnosis, is less sensitive and specific for aortic dissection, though it does still play a role during endovascular procedures, or for further evaluation of patients with chest pain who are already in the cardiac catheterization laboratory for assessment of chest pain. Choice of imaging modality is influenced by institutional accessibility and expertise, though the advantages and disadvantages of each modality should be recognized by providers.

References

1. Hiratzka LF, Bakris GL, Beckman JA, et al. 2010 ACCF/AHA/AATS/ACR/ASA/SCA/SCAI/SIR/STS/SVM Guidelines for the diagnosis and management of patients with thoracic aortic disease. A Report of the American College of Cardiology Foundation/American Heart Association Task Force on Practice Guidelines, American Association for Thoracic Surgery, American College of Radiology, American Stroke Association, Society of Cardiovascular Anesthesiologists, Society for Cardiovascular Angiography and Interventions, Society of Interventional Radiology, Society of Thoracic Surgeons,and Society for Vascular Medicine. J Am Coll Cardiol. 2010;55(14):e27–e129.
2. Erbel R, Aboyans V, Boileau C, et al. 2014 ESC Guidelines on the diagnosis and treatment of aortic diseases: document covering acute and chronic aortic diseases of the thoracic and abdominal aorta of the adult. The Task Force for the Diagnosis and Treatment of Aortic Diseases of the European Society of Cardiology (ESC). Eur Heart J. 2014;35(41):2873–926.
3. Vardhanabhuti V, Nicol E, Morgan-Hughes G, et al. Recommendations for accurate CT diagnosis of suspected acute aortic syndrome (AAS)—on behalf of the British Society of Cardiovascular Imaging (BSCI)/British Society of Cardiovascular CT (BSCCT). Br J Radiol. 2016;89(1061):20150705.
4. Baliga RR, Nienaber CA, Bossone E, et al. The role of imaging in aortic dissection and related syndromes. JACC Cardiovasc Imaging. 2014;7(4):406–24.
5. Fattori R, Cao P, De Rango P, et al. Interdisciplinary expert consensus document on management of type B aortic dissection. J Am Coll Cardiol. 2013;61(16):1661–78.
6. Grabenwoger M, Alfonso F, Bachet J, et al. Thoracic Endovascular Aortic Repair (TEVAR) for the treatment of aortic diseases: a position statement from the European Association for Cardio-Thoracic Surgery (EACTS) and the European Society of Cardiology (ESC), in collaboration with the European Association of Percutaneous Cardiovascular Interventions (EAPCI). Eur Heart J. 2012;33(13):1558–63.
7. Goldstein SA, Evangelista A, Abbara S, et al. Multimodality imaging of diseases of the thoracic aorta in adults: from the American Society of Echocardiography and the European Association of Cardiovascular Imaging: endorsed by the Society of Cardiovascular Computed Tomography and Society for Cardiovascular Magnetic Resonance. J Am Soc Echocardiogr. 2015;28(2):119–82.
8. Raymond CE, Aggarwal B, Schoenhagen P, et al. Prevalence and factors associated with false positive suspicion of acute aortic syndrome: experience in a patient population transferred to a specialized aortic treatment center. Cardiovasc Diagn Ther. 2013;3(4):196–204.
9. Shiga T, Wajima Z, Apfel CC, Inoue T, Ohe Y. Diagnostic accuracy of transesophageal echocardiography, helical computed tomography, and magnetic resonance imaging for suspected thoracic aortic dissection: systematic review and meta-analysis. Arch Intern Med. 2006;166(13):1350–6.
10. Valente T, Rossi G, Lassandro F, et al. MDCT evaluation of acute aortic syndrome (AAS). Br J Radiol. 2016;89(1061):20150825.
11. Expert Panels on Vascular Imaging and Interventional Radiology, Bonci G, et al. ACR appropriateness criteria((R)) thoracic aorta interventional planning and follow-up. J Am Coll Radiol. 2017;14(11S):S570–83.
12. Halpern EJ. Triple-rule-out CT angiography for evaluation of acute chest pain and possible acute coronary syndrome. Radiology. 2009;252(2):332–45.
13. Burris AC 2nd, Boura JA, Raff GL, Chinnaiyan KM. Triple rule out versus coronary CT angiography in patients with acute chest pain: results from the ACIC consortium. JACC Cardiovasc Imaging. 2015;8(7):817–25.
14. McMahon MA, Squirrell CA. Multidetector CT of aortic dissection: a pictorial review. Radiographics. 2010;30(2):445–60.
15. Swee W, Dake MD. Endovascular management of thoracic dissections. Circulation. 2008;117(11):1460–73.

16. Tsai TT, Evangelista A, Nienaber CA, et al. Partial thrombosis of the false lumen in patients with acute type B aortic dissection. N Engl J Med. 2007;357(4):349–59.
17. Hirst AE Jr, Johns VJ Jr, Kime SW Jr. Dissecting aneurysm of the aorta: a review of 505 cases. Medicine (Baltimore). 1958;37(3):217–79.
18. Angeloni E, Benedetto U, Takkenberg JJ, et al. Unilateral versus bilateral antegrade cerebral protection during circulatory arrest in aortic surgery: a meta-analysis of 5100 patients. J Thorac Cardiovasc Surg. 2014;147(1):60–7.
19. Movsowitz HD, Levine RA, Hilgenberg AD, Isselbacher EM. Transesophageal echocardiographic description of the mechanisms of aortic regurgitation in acute type A aortic dissection: implications for aortic valve repair. J Am Coll Cardiol. 2000;36(3):884–90.
20. Castaner E, Andreu M, Gallardo X, Mata JM, Cabezuelo MA, Pallardo Y. CT in nontraumatic acute thoracic aortic disease: typical and atypical features and complications. Radiographics. 2003;23 Spec No:S93–110.
21. Williams DM, Lee DY, Hamilton BH, et al. The dissected aorta: part III. Anatomy and radiologic diagnosis of branch-vessel compromise. Radiology. 1997;203(1):37–44.
22. Lichtenberger JP 3rd, Franco DF, Kim JS, Carter BW. MR imaging of thoracic aortic disease. Top Magn Reson Imaging. 2018;27(2):95–102.
23. Amano Y, Takahama K, Kumita S. Non-contrast-enhanced MR angiography of the thoracic aorta using cardiac and navigator-gated magnetization-prepared three-dimensional steady-state free precession. J Magn Reson Imaging. 2008;27(3):504–9.
24. Cigarroa JE, Isselbacher EM, DeSanctis RW, Eagle KA. Diagnostic imaging in the evaluation of suspected aortic dissection. Old standards and new directions. N Engl J Med. 1993;328(1):35–43.
25. Kirschner LP, Twigg HL, Conrad PW, Hufnagel C. Retrograde catheter aortography in dissecting aortic aneurysms. Am J Roentgenol Radium Therapy, Nucl Med. 1968;102(2):349–53.
26. Erbel R, Engberding R, Daniel W, Roelandt J, Visser C, Rennollet H. Echocardiography in diagnosis of aortic dissection. Lancet. 1989;1(8636):457–61.
27. Bansal RC, Chandrasekaran K, Ayala K, Smith DC. Frequency and explanation of false negative diagnosis of aortic dissection by aortography and transesophageal echocardiography. J Am Coll Cardiol. 1995;25(6):1393–401.
28. Earnest F, Muhm JR, Sheedy PF 2nd. Roentgenographic findings in thoracic aortic dissection. Mayo Clin Proc. 1979;54(1):43–50.
29. Shuford WH, Sybers RG, Weens HS. Problems in the aortographic diagnosis of dissecting aneurysm of the aorta. N Engl J Med. 1969;280(5):225–31.

Imaging of Intramural Hematoma and Penetrating Atherosclerotic Ulcer by CT and MRI

Zachary Hartley-Blossom, Saurabh Agarwal, and Michael K. Atalay

Introduction

Intramural hematomas (IMH) and penetrating atherosclerotic (or aortic) ulcers (PAU) are two lesions on the spectrum of acute aortic syndromes (AAS), and their timely, accurate diagnosis is paramount for appropriate triage and management. Among all AAS, IMH constitutes ~4–11% of cases in North American and European populations and ~ 28–32% of cases in Asian populations—highlighting geographic differences—while PAU accounts for less than 10% of such injuries [1–5]. Aortic dissection remains the leading cause of AAS, accounting for 65–75% of all cases [4–7], and is discussed in another chapter.

Imaging is essential for the prompt diagnosis of IMH and PAU. This chapter aims to describe the imaging protocols, lesion characteristics, and diagnostic challenges regarding both IMH and PAU, specifically focusing on computed tomography (CT) and magnetic resonance imaging (MRI). These two cross-sectional imaging modalities provide complementary approaches to the diagnosis and management of AAS including the identification of associated findings and complications. CT is generally preferred in the acute setting due to its high accuracy, ease of use, speed, and ready-access in most emergency departments.

This chapter will: (1) briefly review normal aortic anatomy, (2) discuss the basic pathophysiology of IMH and PAU, (3) describe pertinent MRI and CT techniques and the salient imaging findings of PAU and IMH—along with potentially useful prognostic features and diagnostic pitfalls—and finally (4) briefly mention management options that are covered in greater detail elsewhere.

Z. Hartley-Blossom · S. Agarwal · M. K. Atalay (✉)
Department of Diagnostic Imaging, Rhode Island Hospital, Warren Alpert School of Medicine of Brown University, Providence, RI, USA

J. S. Coselli et al. (eds.), *Aortic Dissection and Acute Aortic Syndromes*,
https://doi.org/10.1007/978-3-030-66668-2_11

Normal Aortic Anatomy

Familiarity with aortic anatomy is important to understanding the pathophysiology and in turn the imaging appearances of AAS. There are three discrete layers of the aortic wall: the tunica intima (or intima), tunica media (or media), and the adventitia (Fig. 1a). The intima is the luminal layer of the aorta and is in direct contact with the blood pool by which it is nourished. It is the thinnest of the three layers, consisting of only a single layer of endothelial cells, supporting connective tissue, and a very thin internal elastic lamina that separates it from the media. The media (middle layer) is the thickest of the three layers and consists of smooth muscle, collagen, and elastic tissue, and is responsible for the vascular tone of the aorta. Consisting chiefly of connective tissue, the outermost layer, the adventitia, provides additional structural support [3, 8]. The blood supply to the mid and outer aortic wall comes by way of the vasa vasorum which is a network of small arteries that enter through the adventitia before terminating in the media [8–10]. Coronary and brachiocephalic arteries supply the vasa vasorum of the ascending aorta and intercostal arteries supply those of the descending thoracic aorta. Lumbar and mesenteric arteries supply the vasa vasorum of the abdominal aorta [3, 11]. Normal aortic wall thickness is <3 mm [8]. The cross-sectional imaging methods described in this chapter and routinely used in clinical imaging are not typically able to resolve these layers in the normal aorta.

For descriptive purposes, the aorta is typically divided into longitudinal segments (Fig. 2). The ascending segment extends from the aortic annulus to the origin of the brachiocephalic artery. The aortic root is the most proximal portion of the ascending segment and spans from the annulus through the sinuses of Valsalva to the

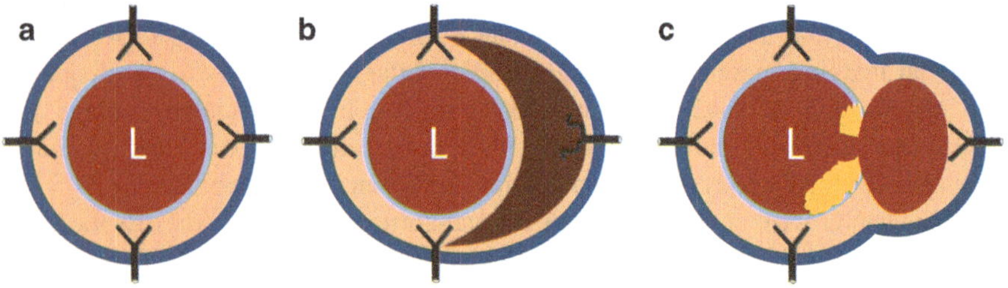

Fig. 1 Diagram of the aortic wall in cross-section. (**a**) Normal. The innermost layer—the thin tunica intima (light blue)—is nourished directly from luminal blood (L). The middle layer—or tunica media (light brown)—is the thickest of the 3 layers, contains smooth muscle cells, and provides vasomotor tone to the wall. The outer adventitial layer (dark blue) consists chiefly of connective tissue and provides structural support. Vasa vasorum (branching black lines) are small blood vessels that provide blood flow to the mid and outer wall. These small vessels penetrate through the adventitia and terminate in the media. (**b**) Intramural hematoma (IMH). A proposed mechanism of IMH is rupture of the vasa vasorum with the formation of crescentic or circumferential hematoma (burgundy crescent). Typically, both the lumen and the outer wall of the aorta remain smooth at imaging. (**c**) Penetrating atherosclerotic ulcer (PAU). Rupture through an atheromatous plaque (yellow) leads to a focal outpouching through the intima and into the media of the aortic wall. This results in focal outward bulging of the outer wall, often with surrounding periaortic edema and inflammation. IMH and PAU may coexist

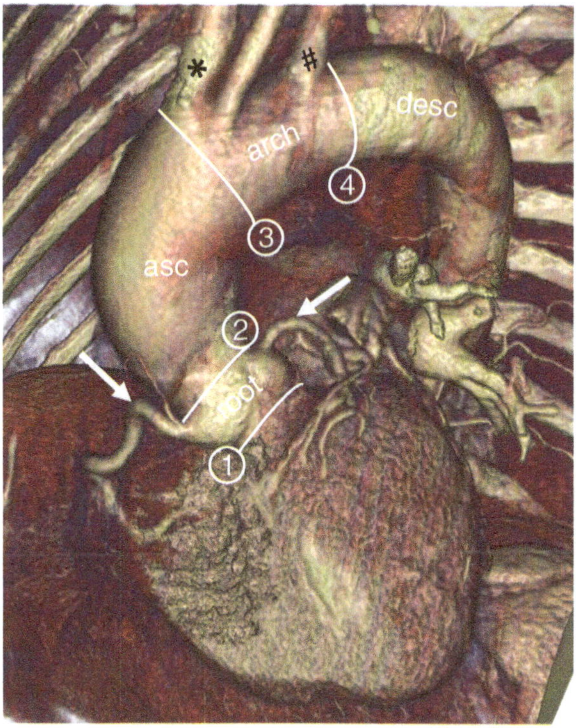

Fig. 2 Oblique views of the heart and aorta using reconstructed data from computed tomography. Segments of the thoracic aorta are delineated as follows: The root extends from the virtual basal ring of the aortic valve (1) to the sinotubular junction (2). The ascending aorta (asc) extends above this to the origin of the brachiocephalic artery (*) (3). The aortic arch consists of the short segment between the brachiocephalic artery and left subclavian (#) arteries. The remainder of the aorta—the descending (desc) aorta—extends to the iliac bifurcation and is divided by the diaphragm into thoracic and abdominal components. The coronary arteries (arrows) arise from the aortic root. This patient has an ectactic ascending aorta measuring 44 cm in diameter

sinotubular junction just distal to the coronary artery origins. The aortic arch is a short segment that gives rise to the vessels of the head, neck, and upper extremities and extends from the brachiocephalic artery to the left subclavian artery. The descending aorta continues from the left subclavian artery to the iliac bifurcation and is further subdivided by the diaphragm into thoracic and abdominal components.

Pathophysiology of IMH and PAU

Aortic intramural hematoma was first described in 1920 as "dissection without an intimal tear" [12], yet a century later our understanding of its pathophysiology continues to evolve. It has historically been attributed to the spontaneous rupture of the vascular supply to the aorta itself, the vasa-vasorum (Fig. 1b). This in turn has been felt to result from a combination of factors including hypertension, chronic inflammation, wall stress, and connective tissue weakening [2, 13]. While in some cases this may be an accurate representation of the underlying pathophysiology, there is an emerging body of literature suggesting that micro-intimal tears may represent a sentinel event for these lesions, and rupture of the vaso-vasorum a secondary process [14–17]. In any case, a common denominator across a broad range of non-traumatic aortic injuries seems to include medial degeneration (formerly 'cystic medial necrosis'), characterized by fragmentation of elastic fibers, increased deposition of proteoglycans, and loss of smooth muscles cells in the media [18–20].

Penetrating atherosclerotic (or aortic) ulceration is caused by a rupture of an atheromatous plaque that compromises the intima, probably through local inflammatory factors, and creates a focal communication between the lumen and the media (Fig. 1c). This resulting outpouching or ulceration into the weakened wall causes a focal outward bulge of the aorta, often with surrounding periaortic edema and inflammation. The injury to the media may propagate locally or distally in the form of an IMH or a frank dissection. In fact, all three lesions may coexist and PAU often has at least a small associated IMH. Conversely, IMH may be seen in the absence of significant atherosclerosis—a prerequisite of PAU—and may demonstrate small luminal outpouchings that protrude into the media. These lesions are referred to as intramural blood pools (IBP) and ulcer-like projections (ULP). The former are pseudoaneurysms of intercostal, bronchial, or lumbar artery origins *within* the aortic wall. Although a ULP demonstrates a clear communication with the lumen owing to a frank intimal disruption, direct continuity of the lumen with IBPs, which are usually small, are typically not evident at imaging. ULPs may also be referred to as focal intimal disruptions (FIDs). These IMH-associated microlesions are mimickers of PAU but are not related to atheroma.

The typical patient risk factors, demographics, aortic location, and basic imaging characteristics of IMH and PAU are presented in Table 1. In addition to characterizing the primary lesion, the imaging description of acute aortic syndromes is based on the layer(s) and segment(s) involved (including the presence and size of intimal tears and intramural blood sacs such as ULPs and IBPs), the aortic diameter and wall thickness, and associated complications.

Stanford Classification

All acute aortic syndromes are classified according to the Stanford classification scheme. This system is based on lesion location and helps guide management decisions. According to the original description, any lesion involving the ascending aorta was recognized as Stanford Type A, and any lesion limited to the descending aorta was classified as Stanford Type B [21]. This description left unclassified those lesions confined to or originating in the aortic arch. The surgical repair of Type A lesions involves interposition graft replacement of the ascending aorta to prevent complications related to coronary artery and aortic valve involvement or rupture

Table 1 Pertinent features and associations of aortic intramural hematoma (IMH) and penetrating atherosclerotic ulcer (PAU) gleaned from multiple sources [1–7].

Lesion	Layer Affected	Demo.	Risk Factors	Presentation	Location	Appearance	Complications
IMH	Medial	65 y + Males	• HTN	Acute aortic syndrome	Descending > Ascending > Arch	• Crescentic or circumferential thickening	• Rupture
			• Trauma			• No intimal flap	• Dissection
			• Iatrogenic			• No false lumen	• Aneurysm
PAU	Intimal	70 y + Males	• HTN	Acute aortic syndrome	Descending >>> Arch >> Ascending	• Irregular surface	• IMH
			• Tobacco			• Focal luminal outpouching	• Aneurysm
			• COPD			• No intimal flap	• Embolization
			• CAD				• Dissection
							• Rupture

Demo Demographics; *HTN* Hypertension; *COPD* Chronic Obstructive Pulmonary Disease; *CAD* Coronary artery disease into the pericardium. In this context, a lesion beginning in the arch has come to be recognized as a Type B lesion since surgery is not usually warranted. Despite this, the controversy has lingered with many manuscripts, book chapters, and textbooks adhering to the original classification description. Offering recognition of this controversy and a descriptive remedy, some authors have suggested an additional classification of "type B with arch involvement" [22]. In general, the simplest distinction is 'Type A' or 'not Type A'. The majority of IMH lesions are type B (up to 63%) and similarly for PAU [3, 4, 19, 23].

CT and MRI for AAS: Imaging Techniques and Findings

Imaging for AAS needs to be fast, readily available, and straightforward to perform and interpret. Imaging these lesions is critical for prompt, accurate diagnosis, identification of associated complications, risk stratification, and ultimately formulating a management plan. While there are several imaging modalities available for imaging the aorta, CT and MRI are the primary tools used for the initial diagnosis, risk-stratification, and subsequent follow-up of AAS. Initial diagnosis of AAS by CT and MRI have sensitivities and specificities ranging from 90% to 100% [6, 24–26]. Owing to their 3-dimensional nature these modalities permit multi-planar reconstruction, and as warranted a more complete assessment of the entire aorta and surrounding structures.

Computed Tomography: Techniques

Although CT and MRI are generally complementary techniques, CT is usually preferred over MRI for the initial evaluation of suspected AAS in the acute setting as it is faster, more straightforward to perform, and more widely available, usually within or a short distance from an emergency department. Radiation is an inevitable concern associated with any CT scan, especially in young patients, but widely available and ever-improving dose reduction strategies are usually implemented to minimize patient risk. As an additional concern, a small percentage of patients are allergic to iodinated contrast, with an incidence of approximately 0.2–0.7% [27]. The administration of intravenous contrast to patients with impaired renal function has historically been controversial owing to a possible contrast-associated exacerbation. However, according to the most recent literature and joint statements from the American College of Radiology (ACR) and National Kidney Foundation (NKF) intravenous iodinated contrast is not felt to cause nephrotoxicity, and this should not be a principle consideration in the imaging of AAS [28]. This is particularly true given the necessity of a timely and accurate diagnosis. The sensitivity and negative predictive value of CT for the diagnosis of AAS are very high, both approaching 100% in optimal settings [29–31]. As will be discussed, in some cases subtle abnormalities may be missed and normal findings may be misinterpreted due to a variety of patient and technical factors (such as motion artifact and poor contrast opacification). These constitute diagnostic pitfalls of which an interpreting physician must be aware.

A CT protocol for suspected AAS virtually always includes a contrast enhanced CT angiography (CTA) acquisition. This is typically obtained as a standard helical (or 'spiral') acquisition conducted without ECG-gating and with exogenous intravenous iodinated contrast injected at a relatively high rate (~4–5 cc/s) to densely opacify vascular structures of interest. Contrast opacification will ultimately be determined by a host of imaging and injection parameters that are typically preset in the protocol and include X-ray tube current (mA) and voltage (kVp), scanner table speed, contrast injection rate and timing strategy (e.g. bolus tracking, bolus trigger, or fixed delay), as well as by patient-related parameters such as body-mass index, cardiac output, and breath-holding capability. Imaging data are then reconstructed in multiple imaging planes for improved diagnostic clarity. Additional reconstructions methods, such as maximum intensity projection and volume-rendering, can be implemented as needed. A comprehensive CT protocol may benefit from an initial noncontrast scan, but it comes at the cost of additional radiation. Importantly, the specific diagnosis of intramural hematoma can commonly be made on noncontrast CT imaging (as will be discussed), and the lesion can often be seen to better advantage on the noncontrast series than on the post-contrast series. Therefore, in the setting of suspected AAS, a noncontrast series is usually advised [32].

Since the imaging acquisition of standard helical CT is not synchronized to the ECG, some degree of cardiac-related motion will be present around the heart and the aortic root, potentially reducing the accuracy for detecting short or subtle lesions in the ascending aorta. If the initial CT study is inconclusive or demonstrates spurious findings, a repeat CT with ECG-gating or an MRI with ECG-gating may be performed. (ECG-gating is not typically performed at the outset because of slightly increased technical complexity and increased radiation dose relative to a non-gated helical acquisition.)

An ECG-gated CT can be performed using a non-helical, *prospective* acquisition—also colloquially referred to as 'step-and-shoot'—during which the x-ray tube is active for only a short period of the cardiac cycle and sequential sections have no or minimal irradiation overlap, or a helical, *retrospective* acquisition during which the X-ray tube output peaks during a predetermined phase of the cardiac cycle, but is active at a nominal output throughout the remainder of the acquisition. In retrospective mode, scanners usually use low pitch meaning that there is substantial overlap of sequential acquisition volumes. Broadly, this means that the radiation dose of the former method is considerably less than that of the latter, but the latter permits image reconstruction at multiple cardiac phases throughout the cardiac cycle. Multiphase availability enables cine imaging if desired or simply evaluation of different regions of the aorta at different points in the cardiac cycle, potentially confirming pathology or reducing artifact. Moreover, unlike non- or even prospectively ECG-gated CT, retrospectively gated CT can provide limited functional information regarding the ventricles and valves, like echocardiography and MRI, but with poorer temporal resolution—akin to a slower camera shutter speed. Typically, patients with tachycardia or high normal heart rates are better served with retrospective gating (versus prospective gating) to reduce motion-related artifacts. Newer scanner technology, such as that offered by dual-source scanners employing ultra-high pitch acquisition, overcomes some of these motion and radiation dose related issues.

Magnetic Resonance Imaging: Techniques

For reasons stated above, CT is preferred for suspected AAS in the acute setting. However, for stable patients, patients with iodinated contrast allergy, those with questionable imaging findings on initial CT, or patients requiring follow-up, MRI is often the modality of choice. MRI offers improved soft tissue contrast compared to CT, does not involve ionizing radiation, and has sensitivity and negative predictive values comparable to that of CT [13, 30, 31]. Unfortunately, MRI is not as widely available, takes longer, and is more technically challenging than CT, usually requiring patient cooperation for compliance with breath-holding and staying-still. Furthermore, monitoring unstable to marginally stable patients or those with MRI compatible instruments/hardware can be cumbersome and challenging. An additional consideration is that gadolinium based contrast agents have been linked to cases of nephrogenic systemic fibrosis (NSF). It is important to recognize that for the newer contrast agents there have been no reported cases of NSF across patients with a wide range of renal function [33]. Nevertheless, it remains a consideration and the ACR guidelines advise caution and thoughtful risk-benefit analysis for patients with impaired renal function (GFR < 30) [34]. Finally, there is also a risk of MRI contrast allergy, but this risk is very low, occurring in approximately 0.08% of administrations [35]. Importantly, it is even possible to diagnose AAS by MRI *without* contrast using standard imaging methods as described below.

While the specifics of MRI methodology are beyond the scope of this text, there are important imaging techniques that when utilized appropriately can substantially assist in the diagnosis and management of AAS. MRI uses 'bright-blood' and 'dark-blood' pulse sequences with ECG-gating (and with and without fat-suppression) in combination with 3-D MR angiography (MRA) to optimally visualize the aorta and branch vessels. Often patients have been imaged by other modalities prior to MRI, allowing the MRI to focus on a specific area of interest. As with CTA, MRA requires a high contrast injection rate and specifically timed data acquisition to best visualize the vascular region in question. MRA is performed over several seconds without ECG-gating. (ECG-gating cannot be employed with MRA because of the necessity for acquiring a large volume of 3-D data during a single breath-hold as the contrast bolus transits the vascular system.) As a consequence, motion artifacts in the aortic root are again a common problem. However, although MRA with its high spatial resolution is preferred for detailing branch vessel pathology and identifying intramural outpouchings/ulcerations, AAS can frequently be diagnosed and accurately characterized using noncontrast MR techniques. ECG-gated MRI can reveal intramural aortic injuries such as hematomas, ulcerations, and intimomedial flaps with high accuracy. Importantly, bright-blood cine MR imaging, like that used in cardiac imaging and generically referred to as 'steady-state free precision' (SSFP), can be readily implemented for visualization of the aorta and adjacent structures throughout the cardiac cycle. If present a dissection flap can be identified and distinguished from common artifacts that are typically associated with cardiac pulsation or blood flow. There is a limited, possibly beneficial role for cine imaging in the detection of IMH and PAU. These particular lesions are frequently best visualized using dark-blood pulse sequences ("T1-" and "T2-weighted fast spin-echo") that are sensitive to intramural blood, and by virtue of the changing magnetization states of hemoglobin over time may even assist in IMH dating. As with CT, ECG-gated MRI provides more optimal visualization of the aortic root.

Imaging Findings

Both noncontrast and postcontrast CT images can be helpful when diagnosing IMH and distinguishing it from other acute aortic pathologies. Noncontrast images demonstrate smooth crescentic or circumferential thickening of the aortic wall with increased mural attenuation relative to the vessel lumen (Fig. 3). The thickened hyperdense wall is virtually diagnostic of IMH. Visualization of this hyperdense crescent may be aided through the use of thicker slice reconstruction (e.g. 5 mm)—due to reduced image noise—and a narrow display window (e.g. width 100–200 HU, level 40 HU). Although the wall density is the same on pre- and postcontrast imaging, increased lumen density on postcontrast images may visually obscure the intramural hyperattenuation rendering it less conspicuous, especially in subtle cases

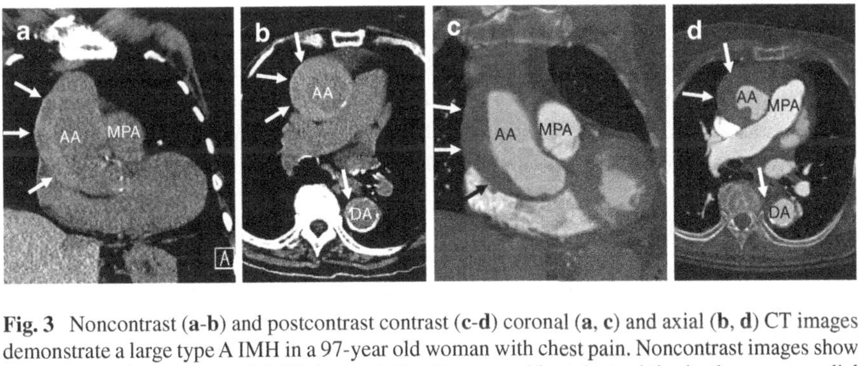

Fig. 3 Noncontrast (**a**-**b**) and postcontrast contrast (**c**-**d**) coronal (**a**, **c**) and axial (**b**, **d**) CT images demonstrate a large type A IMH in a 97-year old woman with chest pain. Noncontrast images show the high-density crescent of IMH (arrows) that is even evident, but subtle, in the anteromedial descending aorta (DA) (**b**, **d**). As noted in the text section 'Predictors of Outcome', the maximal wall thickness of 17 mm and maximum ascending aortic diameters of 56 mm seen in this case would generally be considered high risk features of IMH. *AA* ascending aorta; *DA* descending aorta; *MPA* main pulmonary artery

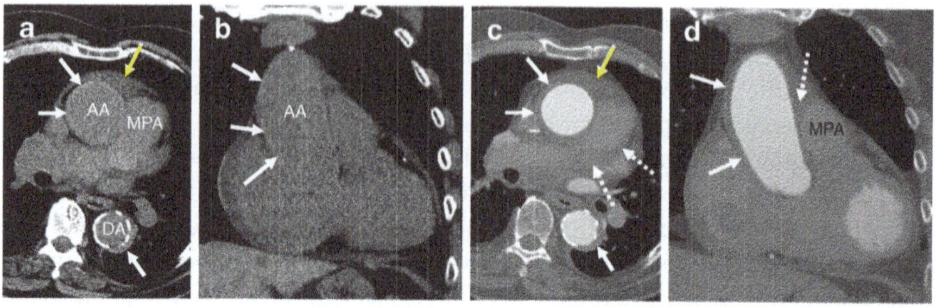

Fig. 4 Noncontrast (**a**, **b**) and postcontrast (**c**, **d**) axial (**a**, **c**) and coronal (**b**, **d**) CT images demonstrate a type A IMH in a 76-year old man with chest pain. Noncontrast images show a subtle, thin high-density crescent of IMH (white arrows) that is even evident in the posterolateral descending aorta (DA) (**a**, **c**). Addition findings of hemopericardium (yellow arrow) and blood in the mediastinum around the main pulmonary artery (MPA) (dotted arrows) are consistent with rupture. *AA* Ascending aorta

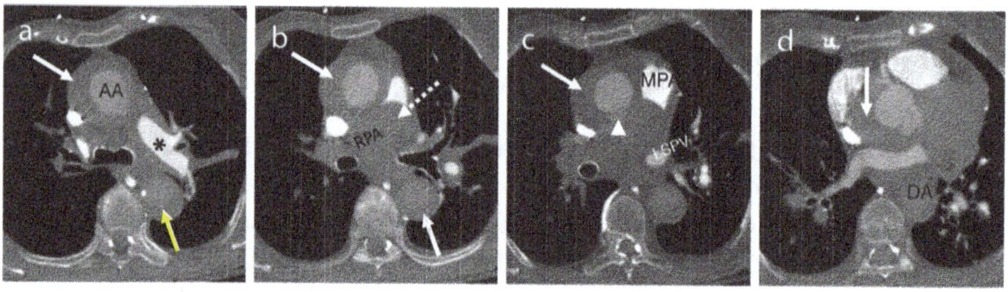

Fig. 5 Sequential transaxial CTA images (**a**–**d**) demonstrate a ruptured type A IMH (arrows) in an 88-year old woman with chest pain. Mediastinal hemorrhage (dotted arrow) tracks into the shared adventitia between the aorta and pulmonary arteries causing severe narrowing of the main pulmonary artery (MPA) and occlusion of the right PA (RPA). The left PA (*) is narrowed but patent. Poor cardiac output results in diminished contrast in the descending aorta (DA). Note the ulcerlike projection arising from the posterior ascending aorta (AA)(arrowhead) and the displaced intimal calcification in the DA (yellow arrow) (**a**). LSPV Left superior pulmonary vein

(Fig. 4). In addition, the postcontrast appearance of IMH may appear similar to mural atheroma, though the latter is usually irregular and demonstrates a lower density. Attenuation in the aortic wall of >45 HU on postcontrast CTA images has been proposed as an accurate threshold for IMH diagnosis [36]. Medial displacement of intimal atheromatous calcification in IMH may aid in this distinction (Figs. 5a and 6e).

Although intimal injuries have not classically been a hallmark of IMH, improvements in imaging techniques—especially spatial resolution—combined with careful scrutiny at surgery have revealed micro-intimal tears in up to 80% of IMH cases. These small injuries may in some cases represent a sentinel insult [14, 17, 23, 37]. There has been a growing consideration in fact that IMH may represent a subset of aortic dissection, with little or no flow within the false lumen, rather than a discretely separate entity [14, 37–39]. On the other hand, intimal defects not apparent on initial imaging may develop and become evident at follow-up. Noting

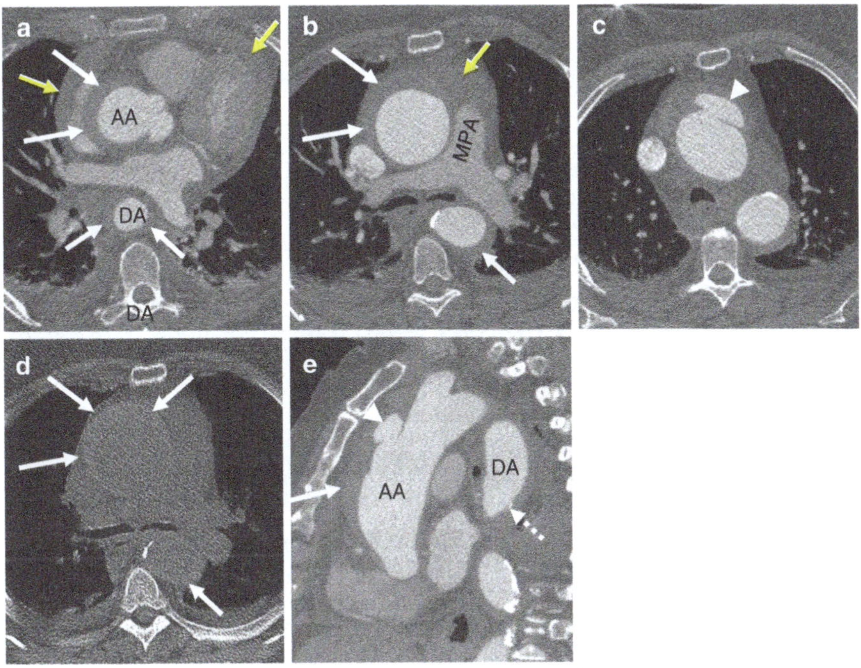

Fig. 6 Noncontrast (**d**) and postcontrast (**a-c**, **e**) axial (**a-d**) and sagittal (**e**) CT images demonstrate a type A IMH in a 79-year old woman with chest pain. The noncontrast image shows a thin high-density crescent of IMH (white arrows) in both the ascending aorta (AA) and the descending aorta (DA). An ascending aneurysm is evident (52 mm). A large ulcer-like projection (ULP) arises from the anterior AA (arrowheads). Note the displaced intimal calcification in the DA (dotted arrow). Mild hemopericardium (yellow arrows) is present. *MPA* Main pulmonary artery

the presence and size of these defects may be important for prognosis (Figs. 5, 6, and 7). ULPs (or FIDs) occurring in the first two weeks of diagnosis in type B IMH and a broad neck >3 mm are associated with a higher risk of pseudoaneurysm formation and rupture than those lesions with tiny intimal defects (TIDs) < 3 mm, no defects at all, or larger defects occurring after two weeks [40, 41]. Moreover, the likelihood for progression to aneurysm, dissection, and rupture increases with lesion size, and lesions having a diameter of >20 mm and a depth of >10 mm, as well as those in the ascending aorta and arch, are particularly ominous [42, 43]. ULPs can resemble PAUs but can usually be distinguished by the appearance of the surrounding aorta. Unlike the latter, ULPs commonly protrude through a smooth intima and are not specifically associated with ulceration through an atheromatous plaque (Fig. 7).

As mentioned earlier, intramural blood pools (IBPs) are small, blood containing sacs that represent pseudoaneurysms of intercostal, bronchial, and lumbar arteries at their origins *within* the aortic wall (43,44) (Figs. 8, 9, and 10). Curiously, they frequently do not appear to communicate with the aortic lumen, probably due to their small size, local mechanical effects, and the spatial resolution of imaging [14, 44]. Occasionally, a series of IBPs will be present in the descending aorta generating

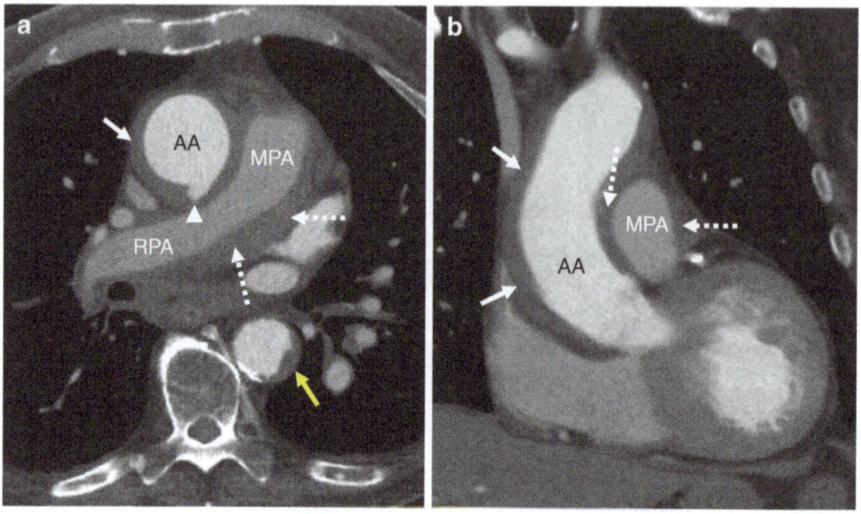

Fig. 7 Axial (**a**) and coronal (**b**) postcontrast CT images of a 75-year old man with chest pain demonstrating a ruptured type A IMH (white arrows) with an ulcer-like projection in the posterior ascending aorta (arrowhead). Soft tissue density material surrounding the main and right pulmonary arteries (MPA, RPA) represents mediastinal blood tracking into the shared adventitia between the aorta and pulmonary arteries—a 'shared-sheath' hematoma (dotted arrows). Note that the irregular mural atheroma in the mid descending aorta (yellow arrow) is slightly lower density than the IMH and lacks its smooth crescentic morphology. *AA* Ascending aorta

an imaging appearance referred to as the "Chinese ring-sword sign" [45] (Figs. 9 and 10). IBPs are most commonly identified in the descending aorta, and do not confer any specific increased risk for progression or complication, however those hematomas are less likely to completely resolve [44, 46].

IMH typically results in smooth thickening of the aortic wall. PAU in contrast has an irregular lumen—due to atheroma—with a focal luminal outpouching, mural thickening, and bulging of the overlying adventitia (Figs. 11 and 12). The appearance is characteristically mushroom-like, especially at angiography. The location of the lesion can help differentiate between IMH and PAU if imaging characteristics are not clear (as can often be the case). PAU is overwhelmingly (>90%) found in the mid-descending aorta, while IMH lesions can be found anywhere throughout the aorta [8, 47]. Finally, at least a small IMH is commonly seen with PAU. In these cases, it can often be best to describe and localize the findings rather than trying to specifically categorize the lesion.

MRI findings of IMH and PAU are morphologically similar to CT, with a crescentic region of abnormal signal within the aortic wall with IMH, and a focal atheroma-associated luminal outpouching and accompanying outer wall bulging with PAU. As discussed previously, cine imaging can offer dynamic visualization of intimal flaps in the setting of dissection. With its excellent soft-tissue contrast, MRI can detect small regions of intramural blood confirming the diagnosis of IMH/PAU in questionable cases and dynamic postcontrast T1-weighted imaging will reveal the

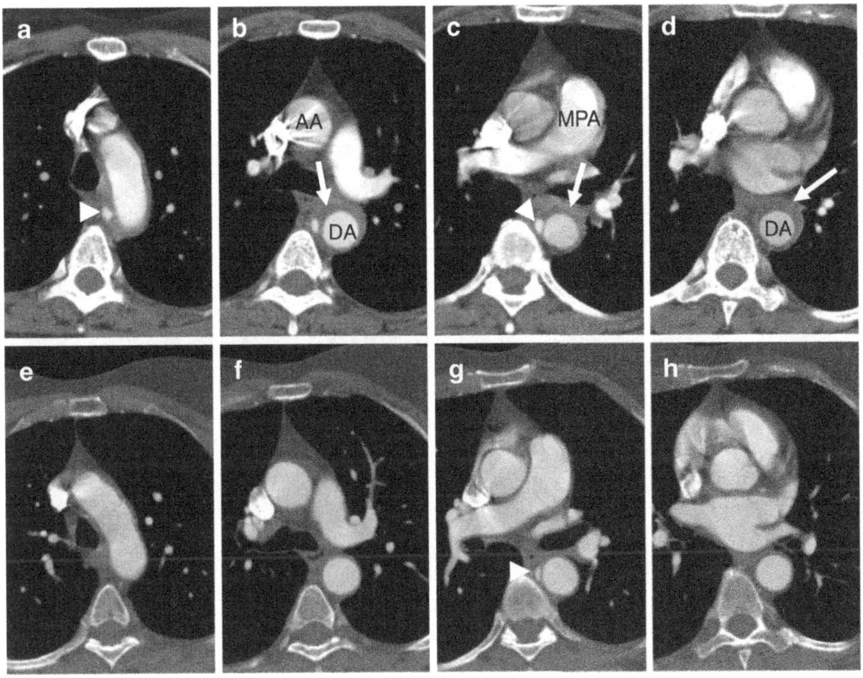

Fig. 8 Type B IMH in a 57-year old woman with a few days of chest and back pain. Transaxial CT images (**a–d**) obtained on the same day as the MRI study in figure 9 and 3 years later (**e–h**). There is a relatively smooth low-density crescent of intramural hemorrhage (arrows) with a few intramural blood pools (IBPs) (arrowheads). Except for minimal mural thickening and a single IBP, there has been near complete resolution of the lesion on follow-up imaging. *AA* Ascending aorta; *DA* Descending aorta; *MPA* Main pulmonary artery

absence of enhancement in such cases (Figs. 9, 10, and 16). Wall-thickening due to vasculitis—an occasional IMH mimicker—will on the other hand show mural enhancement. Moreover, the varying magnetic states of hemoglobin allow MRI to better date a lesion's chronicity. Hyperacute hemorrhage (oxyhemoglobin), acute (deoxyhemoglobin), early subacute (intracellular methemoglobin), late subacute (extracellular methemoglobin), and chronic (hemosiderin), all have different signal characteristics on T1- and T2- weighted MRI which aids in ascertaining lesion acuity (Figs. 9 and 10).

Diagnostic Pitfalls

As noted in the preceding section IMH and PAU share imaging features and may in fact co-exist. Other conditions may mimic these lesions, and imaging findings must therefore be clearly interpreted in the appropriate clinical context. For example, large vessel vasculitides such as Takayasu aortitis and giant cell arteritis can result

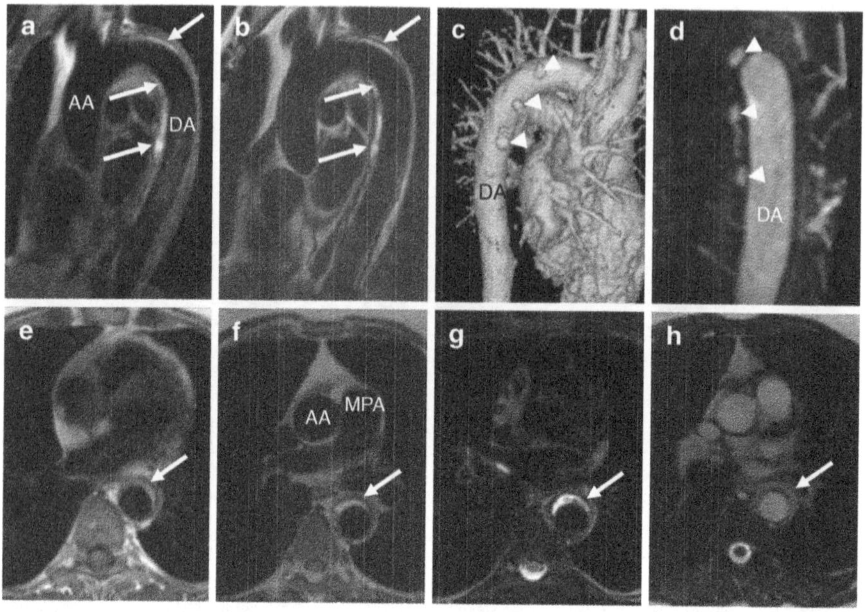

Fig. 9 Same patient as in Fig. 8. Candy cane (**a** & **b**) and transaxial (**e-h**) magnetic resonance images using T1-weighted fast spin echo (FSE) with fat saturation (FS) (**a**) without FS (**e**), T2-weighted FSE without (**b** & **f**) and with FS (**g**), and a single frame from a cine acquisition using steady-state free precession (SSFP) (**h**). In addition shaded surface display (SSD) (**c**) and maximum intensity projection (MIP) images (**d**) from an MR angiogram are shown. Arrows identify IMH in the descending thoracic aorta. Bright signal on both T1- and T2-weighted images indicated blood products chiefly in the extracellular methemoglobin phase consistent with a subacute to chronic lesion. Small outpouchings seen on the MRA images (arrowheads) represent intramural blood pools (IBP) that are pseudoaneurysms of small branching vessels, in this case intercostal arteries, within the aortic wall. When multiple IBPs are present the appearance resembles a so-called Chinese ring-sword. *AA* Ascending aorta; *DA* Descending aorta; *MPA* Main pulmonary artery

in smooth thickening of the aorta that strongly resembles IMH (Figs. 13 and 14). Here, the clinical scenario and laboratory biomarkers may be critical in rendering a prompt and accurate diagnosis. Heaped-up atheroma with extensive irregularity and fissuring can mimic PAU (Fig. 15). However, non-calcified atheroma has uniformly low density and does not lead to outward bulging of the adventitia. Moreover, the periaortic fat should be easily demarcated from the aortic wall, in contrast to the indistinct appearance typically seen in PAU. On postcontrast CT imaging felt pledgets commonly used in aortic surgery have a density at CT that is often indistinguishable from intravascular contrast and may also mimic a PAU (Fig. 16). Correlation with prior surgical history is usually adequate to assuage any concerns, but if there is lingering question noncontrast CT imaging or MRA will readily resolve the issue. Uncommonly, fluid in the superior aortic pericardial recess may resemble an IMH. Although familiarity with this and other recesses usually suffices to avoid any confusion, in rare cases, additional imaging may be necessary. Finally, motion related artifacts are commonly seen near the aortic root. Here again, while

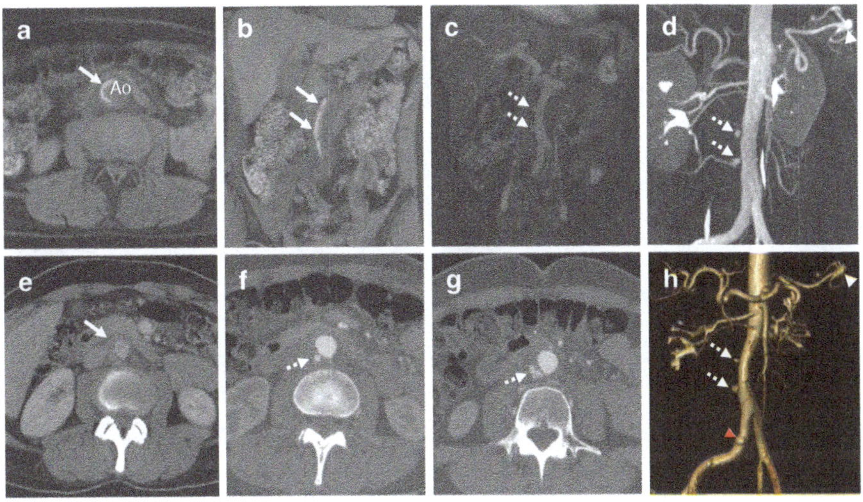

Fig. 10 IMH of the abdominal aorta in a 45-year old woman with acute abdominal pain by MRI (**a-d**, **h**) and CT (**e-g**). Axial (a) and coronal (b) T1-weighted noncontrast MRI demonstrate crescentic high T1-signal in aortic wall (arrows) consistent with IMH. Subtraction postcontrast coronal T1-weighted imaging (**c**) shows no enhancement of the wall as well as small outpouchings (dotted arrows) representing intramural blood pools (IBP) which are pseudoaneurysms of lumbar arteries within the aortic wall. These IBPs are also evident on coronal oblique MRA maximum intensity projection (MIP) (**d**) and shaded-surface display (SSD) (**h**) reconstructions that also show aortic narrowing but that—as luminograms—do not show the IMH itself. Also noted on the MRA images is an incidental 1.8 cm splenic artery aneurysm (arrowheads). Note also that a right common iliac artery ulcer-like projection (ULP) is evident on the SSD (red arrowhead). CT images obtained a few days earlier also show the IMH (arrow) and IBPs (dotted arrows)

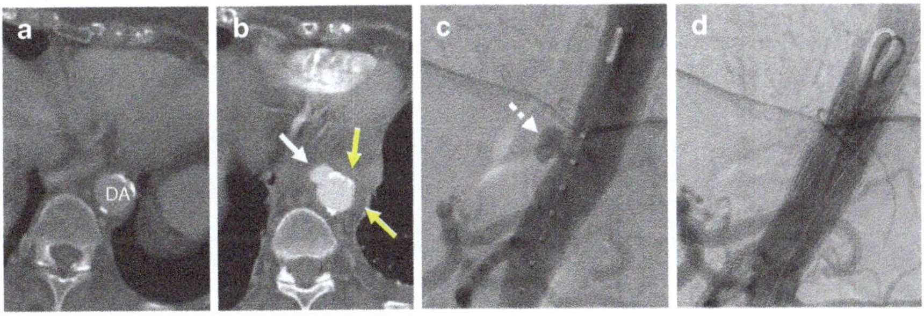

Fig. 11 Penetrating atherosclerotic ulcer. Ten months after a CT scan demonstrated a normal caliber, atherosclerotic descending thoracic aorta (**a**), this patient presented with acute back pain and evidence at repeat CT (**b**) of a new focal aortic ulceration at the site of atheroma consistent with a PAU (white arrow). There is circumferential high-density thickening of the wall (yellow arrows) likely due to a component of short-segment IMH, and the aortic wall is indistinct. Images (**c**) and (**d**) demonstrate the lesion at angiography (white arrow) before and after stenting. Notice on (**c**) the characteristic mushroom-like outpouching. *DA* Descending aorta

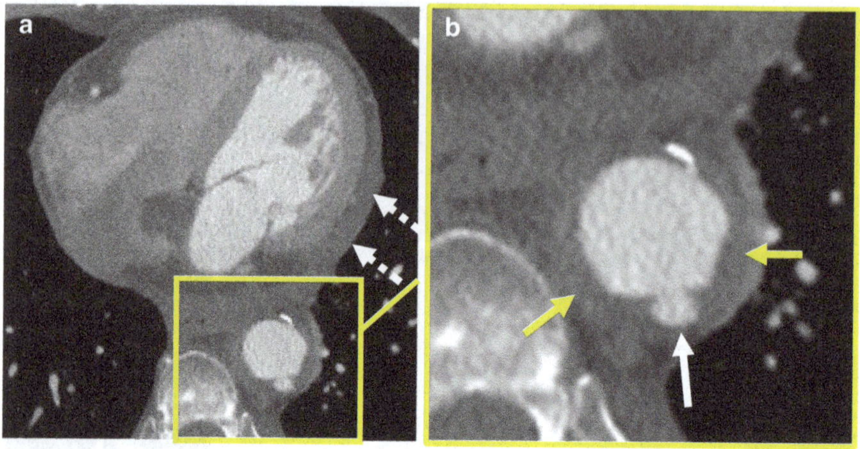

Fig. 12 Penetrating atherosclerotic ulcer in a patient with acute chest and back pain. Image (**b**) is a zoomed in view of the descending thoracic aorta shown in image (**a**). A small PAU is seen in the posterior aspect of the atherosclerotic aorta (white arrow). There is circumferential high-density thickening of the indistinct aortic wall (yellow arrows) likely due to a component of short-segment IMH. A small reactive pericardial effusion is seen adjacent to the aorta (dotted white arrows)

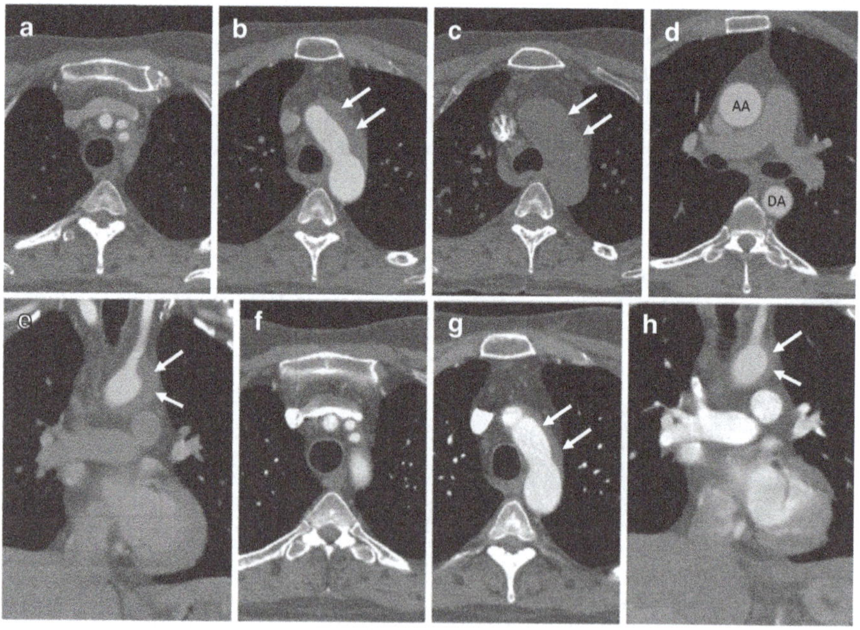

Fig. 13 Aortitis confined to the aortic arch in a 53-year old man with chest pain. Transaxial (**a-d**) and coronal (**e**) images demonstrate asymmetric thickening of the lateral aspect of the aortic arch (arrows) without increased density on noncontrast imaging (**c**) confirming that this lesion was not an acute IMH. Laboratory studies confirmed the diagnosis of vasculitis and follow-up imaging 4 months later (**f-h**) confirmed improvement after appropriate medical management

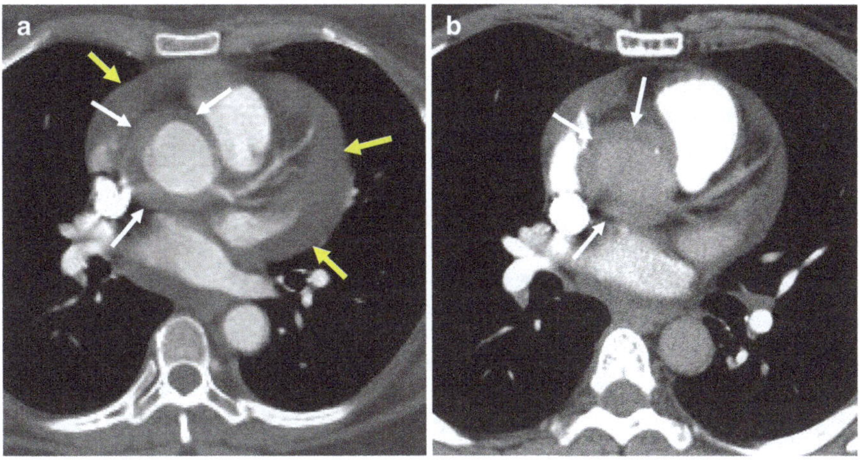

Fig. 14 Aortitis of the ascending aorta seen on abdomen CT (**a**) and unchanged 4 months later (**b**). Images demonstrate near circumferential thickening of the ascending aorta. This appearance may be indistinguishable from type A IMH at imaging and careful history and clinical examination must be undertaken to help differentiate the two entities. A small pericardial effusion present on the first study has essentially resolved by the second

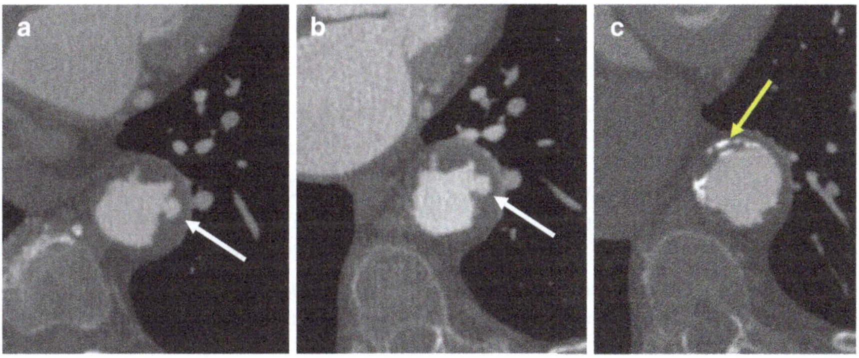

Fig. 15 Axial CT images in a patient with no pertinent symptoms demonstrate irregular atheroma mimicking a PAU (white arrows). Images (**a**) & (**c**) are from the same study and image (**b**) from a study 5 months later. Notice the similarity of appearance of the fissured and excavated atheroma in images (**a**) and (**c**). Also, note the similarity of appearance to the lesion in Fig. 11. The plaque at this level has uniform low-density. Image (**b**) demonstrates calcification on both sides of the plaque in the anterior aorta (arrow). This should not be confused with the medially displaced plaque of IMH or dissection

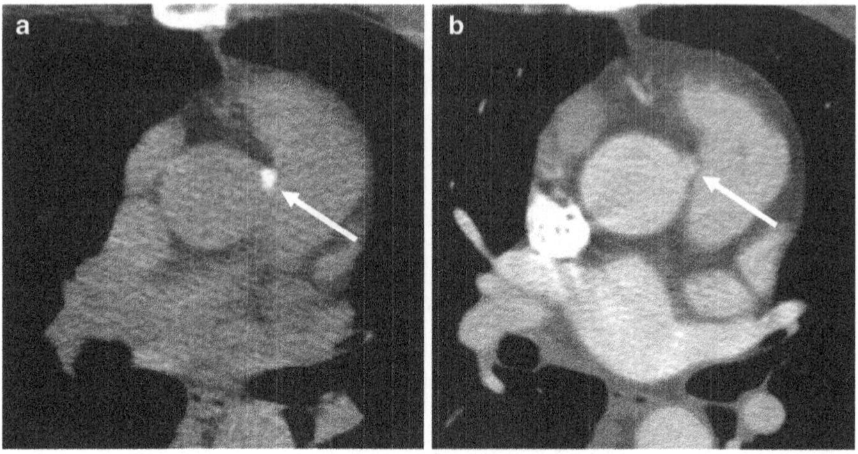

Fig. 16 Axial CT images of a patient who had a prior aortotomy. High density felt pledgets that are easy to recognize and dismiss on noncontrast CT (**a**) (arrow) can mimic a PAU on postcontrast imaging owing to a similar density to luminal contrast (**b**). Note however that there are no ancillary findings such as mural thickening or adjacent fat stranding to suggest an acute aortic injury

familiarity with the appearance of these artifacts is usually sufficient to rule in or rule out pathology, persistent concerns should be managed with additional imaging, including ECG-gated CT, ECG-gated MRI, or echocardiography.

Predictors of Outcome

The natural history of IMH and PAU is variable. IMH may resolve, stabilize, enlarge, or progress to aneurysm, dissection, or frank rupture. Hemopericardium may result in cardiac tamponade; hemorrhage across the shared adventitia of the ascending aorta and main pulmonary artery gives rise to a so-called 'shared-sheath' or 'pulmonary sheath' hematoma that can compromise pulmonary blood flow (Figs. 5 and 7); coronary artery involvement may result in myocardial ischemia and infarction [48]. Various vignettes and outcomes are provided in Figs. 8, 11, 13, 17, 18, 19, 20, and 21.

In addition to the presence and size of ULPs described earlier, other imaging biometrics of IMH are known to correlate with risk of complications. Maximum aortic diameter (MAD) and maximum aortic wall/IMH thickness have been shown to correlate with outcomes. A MAD of ≥45–55 mm for the ascending aorta and of >40–41 mm for the descending aorta are associated with lesion progression [15, 49–52]. Maximum aortic wall/IMH thickness > 10–16 mm is also considered high risk for progression/complications [15, 44, 51, 53] (Fig. 16). Finally, a ratio of the

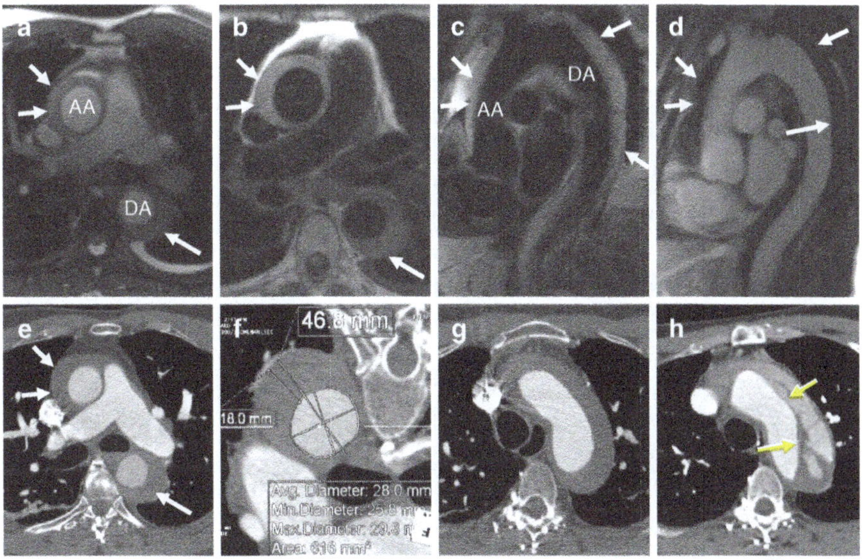

Fig. 17 Near concurrent MRI (**a-d**) and CT (**e-h**) images of a 65-year old man with chest and back pain demonstrate acute type A IMH (white arrows). Transaxial (**a**, **b**) and candy-cane (**c**, **d**) magnetic resonance images using single frame from a cine acquisition using steady-state free precession (SSFP) (**a**), T1-weighted fast spin echo (FSE) with fat saturation (FS) (**b**), T2-weighted FSE with FS (**c**), and T1-weighted gradient echo (GRE) with contrast (**d**). As expected, there is no enhancement of the lesion after contrast. The maximum thickness of the IMH is 18 mm (**g**) which is believed to be a high-risk feature (>10–16 mm). The patient was initially treated medically. He returned with chest pain one month later and CT revealed (**h**) that the lesion had converted to a dissection with a complex dissection flap in the aortic arch (yellow arrows). He was subsequently operated on. *AA* Ascending aorta; *DA* Descending aorta

minimum and maximum luminal diameters at the site of maximum IMH thickness—referred to as the luminal compression ratio—of <0.75 is associated with worse outcomes [54].

Management/Outcomes of IMH and PAU

Detailed medical and surgical management strategies for IMH and PAU are discussed elsewhere. In general, the management of these lesions is chiefly determined by the location of the lesion (Type A or Type B), any associated active or impending complications, prognostic factors described above, and patient status including their frailty or robustness for surgery. Historically, surgery is indicated for Type A lesions and medical therapy or endovascular stenting for Type B lesions. The necessity for urgent or emergent surgery for Type A IMH has been

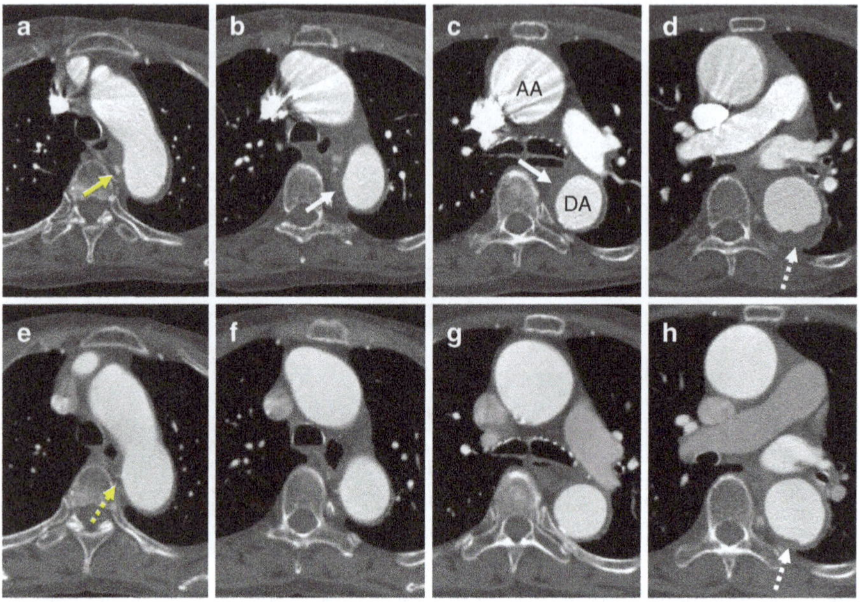

Fig. 18 95-year old woman with chest pain and known ascending aortic (AA) aneurysm. Axial CT images with contrast (**a-d**) show a subtle type B IMH involving the proximal descending aorta (DA) (arrows). A small intramural blood pool associated with an intercostal arrow is evident (solid yellow arrow) (**a**). Images from 9 months prior (**e-h**) confirm that the AA aneurysm is stable, but that the IMH is new. Also note the normal appearance of the intercostal artery in question (dotted yellow arrow) and the interval increase in mural atheroma (dotted arrows) which has a slightly lower density than the hemorrhage

challenged by the observation that stabilization and regression are possible in an appropriately selected subgroup of patients whose imaging biometrics are favorable and whose blood pressure and pain control are adequate. In this population, a conservative approach has been found to be safe and feasible—though surgery may at some point be necessary—and outcomes appear to be very good and comparable to surgery [52, 55]. In the acute setting, medical management is virtually always initiated emergently—including aggressive blood pressure (systolic <110–120 mmHg), heart rate (<70 beats/min), and pain control—while the decision on whether and when to proceed to surgery is considered [1, 37, 51]. For those IMH and PAU patients who are managed medically, close clinical and imaging surveillance over the first few days—and temporally more spread-out thereafter—may therefore represent a reasonable initial management strategy. A potential follow-up strategy includes imaging multiple times in the first week, then weekly for 2–4 weeks, monthly for the next 3–6 months, and at 6–12 months thereafter, unless complications are suspected [53]. Overall, patients with type A IMH are considerably more likely to progress (88%) than patients with type B IMH (3–15%) [1, 23, 56].

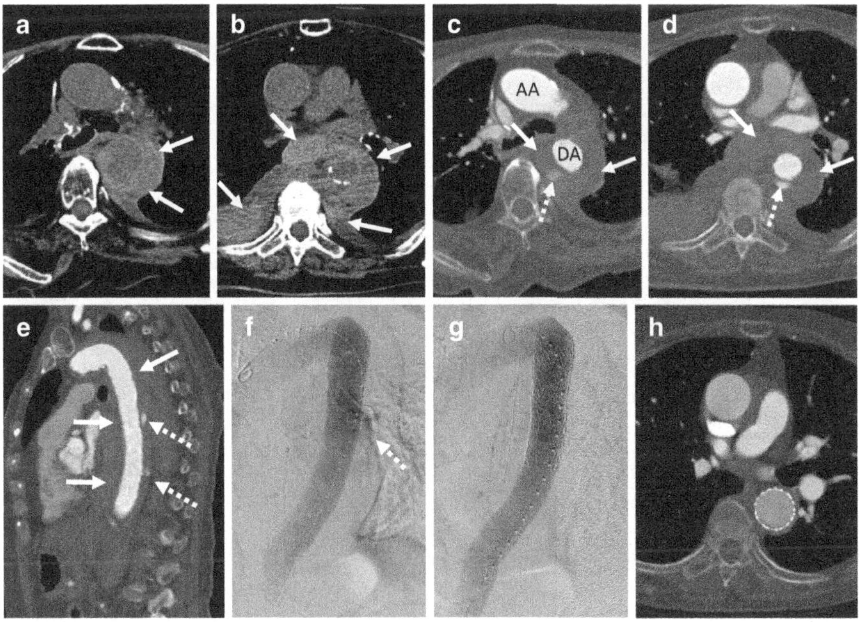

Fig. 19 Axial (**a-d**) and sagittal (**e**) postcontrast CT images demonstrate a ruptured type B IMH in an 80-year old woman with acute chest and back pain. High density material consistent with acute hemorrhage (arrows) is seen around the descending aorta (DA), throughout the posterior mediastinum, and in the pleural spaces bilaterally, right more than left. Intramural blood pools (IBPs) are present (dotted arrows). Angiographic views pre- (**f**) and post- (**g**) endovascular stent placement show successful coverage of IBPs and resolution of contrast extravasation. Single axial postcontrast CT image 18 months later (**h**) reveals resolution of IMH and hemorrhage. *AA* Ascending aorta

Conclusions

Aortic IMH and PAU are two lesions in the spectrum of acute aortic syndromes and their timely diagnosis is crucial for optimizing patient outcomes. CT is the primary initial imaging modality because of its accuracy, speed, and widespread and rapid availability. MRI demonstrates comparable accuracy and is generally used for problem solving and imaging follow-up. Pitfalls in accurate imaging diagnosis are important to consider but can usually be resolved with careful scrutiny and repeat or additional imaging when appropriate.

Management decisions for IMH and PAU are guided by clinical and imaging findings, the latter including Stanford classification, maximum aortic diameter, maximal hematoma thickness, the presence, size, and location of an intimomedial injury (ULP/FID), and the presence and size of extra-aortic complications such as pleural and pericardial effusions and mediastinal hematomas. The majority of type A lesions are treated surgically, although there has been a growing body of literature showing that medical management may be equally efficacious in appropriately

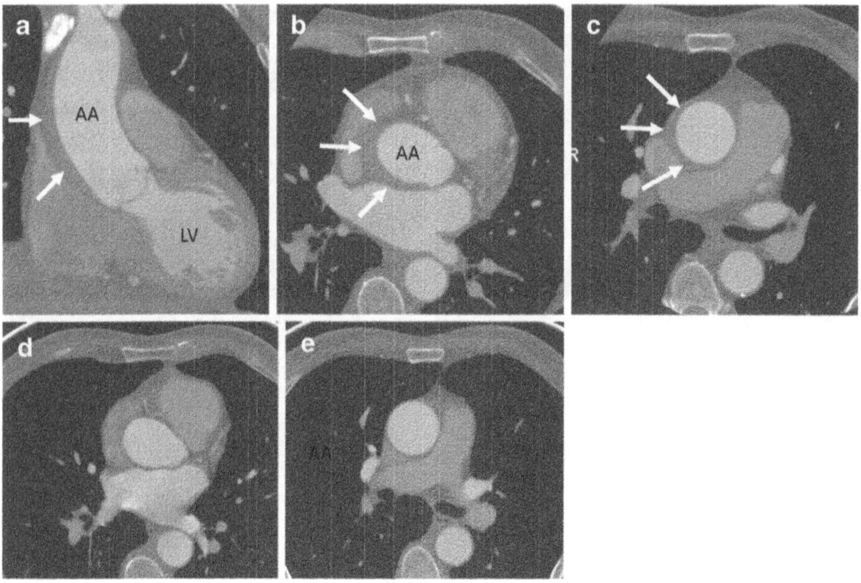

Fig. 20 Postcontrast CT images demonstrate an 8 mm thick type A IMH in a 54-year old man with chest pain (**a-c**) that is found to have resolved at 3 month follow up (**d**, **e**) with medical management only. *AA* Ascending aorta; *LV* Left ventricle

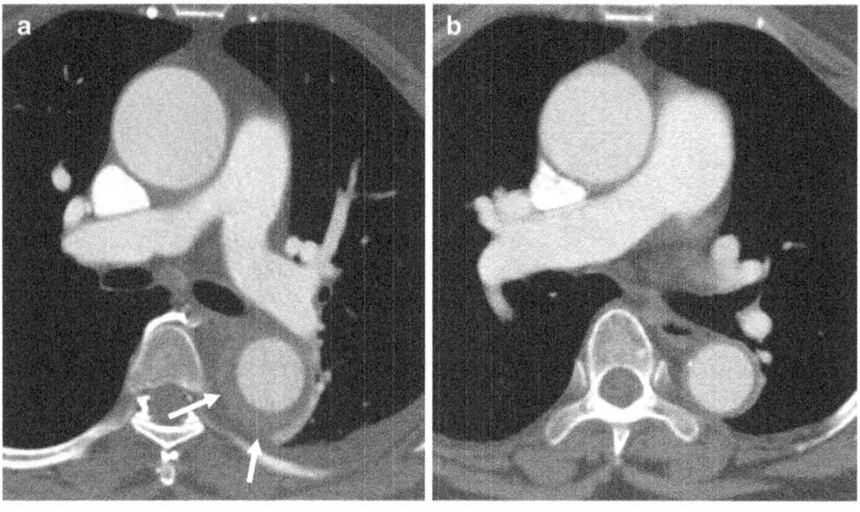

Fig. 21 Axial CT images with contrast demonstrate a type B IMH (arrows) in a middle-aged woman (**a**) that resolved on follow-up imaging 8 months later (**b**)

selected subgroups. Conversely, type B lesions are typically treated medically or with endovascular stenting with surgery being reserved for those patients in which serious complications are identified. Outcomes are favorable for those patients that are appropriately managed, and identifying harbingers for potential complications are crucial in the successful management of IMH.

References

1. Masip AE. Progress in the acute aortic syndrome. Rev Esp Cardiol. 2007. 60 428–439 https://doi.org/10.1016/s1885-5857(07)60175-3.
2. Alomari IB, Hamirani YS, Madera G, Tabe C, Akhtar N, Raizada V. Aortic intramural hematoma and its complications. Circulation. 2014;129(6):711–6.
3. Gutschow SE, Walker CM, Martínez-Jiménez S, Rosado-de-Christenson ML, Stowell J, Kunin JR. Emerging concepts in intramural hematoma imaging. Radiographics. 2016;36(3):660–74.
4. Harris KM, Braverman AC, Eagle KA, et al. Acute aortic intramural hematoma: an analysis from the international registry of acute aortic dissection. Circulation. 2012;126(11 Suppl 1):S91–6.
5. Jánosi RA, Erbel R, Konorza TFM. Recent advances in the diagnosis of acute aortic syndromes. Expert Opinion on Medical Diagnostics. 2012. 6 529–540 https://doi.org/10.1517/17530059.2012.704362.
6. Erbel R. Diagnosis and management of aortic dissection task force on aortic dissection, European Society of Cardiology. Eur Heart J. 2001. 22 1642–1681 https://doi.org/10.1053/euhj.2001.2782.
7. Maslow A, Atalay MK, Sodha N. Intramural Hematoma. J Cardiothorac Vasc Anesth. 2018;32(3):1341–62.
8. Hiratzka LF, Bakris GL, Beckman JA, et al. ACCF/AHA/AATS/ACR/ASA/SCA/SCAI/SIR/STS/SVM guidelines for the diagnosis and management of patients with thoracic aortic disease. Circulation. 2010;121:e266–369.
9. Lin FY, Devereux RB, Roman MJ, et al. Assessment of the thoracic aorta by multidetector computed tomography: age- and sex-specific reference values in adults without evident cardiovascular disease. J Cardiovasc Comput Tomogr. 2008;2(5):298–308.
10. Federspiel JM, Tschernig T, Laschke MW, Wagenpfeil S, Schnabel P, Schäfers H-J. The vasa vasorum reach deep into the human thoracic aorta. Annals of Anatomy–Anatomischer Anzeiger. 2019. 225 54–56 https://doi.org/10.1016/j.aanat.2019.06.001.
11. Tanaka H, Zaima N, Sasaki T, et al. Adventitial vasa vasorum arteriosclerosis in abdominal aortic aneurysm. PLoS One. 2013;8(2):e57398.
12. Krukenberg E. Beitrage Zur Frage Des Aneurysma Dissecans. Beitr Pathol Anat. 1920;67:329–51.
13. Chao CP, Walker TG, Kalva SP. Natural history and CT appearances of aortic intramural hematoma. Radiographics. 2009;29(3):791–804.
14. Park K-H, Lim C, Choi JH, et al. Prevalence of aortic intimal defect in surgically treated acute type a intramural hematoma. Ann Thorac Surg. 2008;86(5):1494–500.
15. Sawaki S, Hirate Y, Ashida S, Takanohashi A, Yagami K, Usui M. Clinical outcomes of medical treatment of acute type a intramural hematoma. Asian Cardiovasc Thorac Ann. 2010;18(4):354–9.
16. Kitai T, Kaji S, Yamamuro A, et al. Detection of intimal defect by 64-row multidetector computed tomography in patients with acute aortic intramural hematoma. Circulation. 2011;124(11 Suppl):S174–8.
17. Estrera AL, Sandhu HK, Leake SS, et al. Early and late outcomes of acute type a aortic dissection with intramural hematoma. J Thorac Cardiovasc Surg. 2015;149(1):137–42.

18. Milewicz DM, Guo D-C, Tran-Fadulu V, et al. Genetic basis of thoracic aortic aneurysms and dissections: focus on smooth muscle cell contractile dysfunction. Annu Rev Genomics Hum Genet. 2008. 9. 283–302 https://doi.org/10.1146/annurev.genom.8.080706.092303.
19. Hagan PG, Nienaber CA, Isselbacher EM, et al. The international registry of acute aortic dissection (IRAD): new insights into an old disease. JAMA. 2000;283(7):897–903.
20. Nienaber CA, Powell JT. Management of acute aortic syndromes. Eur Heart J. 2012. 33 26–35 https://doi.org/10.1093/eurheartj/ehr186.
21. Daily PO, Ward Trueblood H, Stinson EB, Wuerflein RD, Shumway NE. Management of Acute Aortic Dissections. Ann Thorac Surg. 1970. 10 237–247 https://doi.org/10.1016/s0003-4975(10)65594-4.
22. Lempel JK, Frazier AA, Jeudy J, et al. Aortic arch dissection: a controversy of classification. Radiology. 2014;271(3):848–55.
23. Ferrera C, Vilacosta I, Gómez-Polo JC, et al. Evolution and prognosis of intramural aortic hematoma. Insights from a midterm cohort study. Int J Cardiol 2017. 249:410–413 https://doi.org/10.1016/j.ijcard.2017.09.170.
24. Erbel R, Aboyans V, Boileau C, et al. ESC Committee for practice guidelines. 2014 ESC guidelines on the diagnosis and treatment of aortic diseases: document covering acute and chronic aortic diseases of the thoracic and abdominal aorta of the adult. The task force for the diagnosis and treatment of aortic diseases of the European Society of Cardiology (ESC). Eur Heart J. 2014;35(41):2873–926.
25. Mussa FF, Horton JD, Moridzadeh R, Nicholson J, Trimarchi S, Eagle KA. Acute aortic dissection and intramural hematoma. JAMA 2016. 316(7):754 https://doi.org/10.1001/jama.2016.10026.
26. Shiga T, Wajima Z, Apfel CC, Inoue T, Ohe Y. Diagnostic accuracy of transesophageal echocardiography, helical computed tomography, and magnetic resonance imaging for suspected thoracic aortic dissection. Arch Intern Med 2006. 166(13):1350 https://doi.org/10.1001/archinte.166.13.1350.
27. Beckett KR, Moriarity AK, Langer JM. Safe use of contrast media: what the radiologist needs to know. Radiographics. 2015;35(6):1738–50.
28. Davenport MS, Perazella MA, Yee J, et al. Use of intravenous iodinated contrast Media in Patients with kidney disease: consensus statements from the American College of Radiology and the National Kidney Foundation. Radiology. 2020;294(3):660–8.
29. Nienaber CA, Rousseau H, Eggebrecht H, et al. Randomized comparison of strategies for type B aortic dissection. Circulation 2009. 120(25):2519–2528 https://doi.org/10.1161/circulationaha.109.886408.
30. Alkadhi H, Wildermuth S, Desbiolles L, et al. Vascular emergencies of the thorax after blunt and iatrogenic trauma: multi–detector row CT and three-dimensional imaging. Radiographics Radiological Society of North America. 2004;24(5):1239–55.
31. Hayter RG, Rhea JT, Small A, Tafazoli FS, Novelline RA. Suspected aortic dissection and other aortic disorders: multi–detector row CT in 373 cases in the emergency setting. Radiology 2006. 238(3):841–852 https://doi.org/10.1148/radiol.2383041528.
32. Lemos AA, Pezzullo JC, Fasani P, et al. Can the unenhanced phase be eliminated from dual-phase CT angiography for chest pain? Implications for diagnostic accuracy in acute aortic intramural hematoma. AJR Am J Roentgenol. 2014;203(6):1171–80.
33. Woolen SA, Shankar PR, Gagnier JJ, MacEachern MP, Singer L, Davenport MS. Risk of nephrogenic systemic fibrosis in patients with stage 4 or 5 chronic kidney disease receiving a group II gadolinium-based contrast agent. JAMA Intern Med 2020. 180(2):223 https://doi.org/10.1001/jamainternmed.2019.5284.
34. ACR Committee on Drugs and Contrast Media. ACR manual on contrast media. 2020;https://www.acr.org/-/media/ACR/files/clinical-resources/contrast_media.pdf.
35. Jung J-W, Kang H-R, Kim M-H, et al. Immediate hypersensitivity reaction to gadolinium-based MR contrast media. Radiology 2012;264(2):414–422.

36. Knollmann FD, Lacomis JM, Ocak I, Gleason T. The role of aortic wall CT attenuation measurements for the diagnosis of acute aortic syndromes. Eur J Radiol. 2013;82(12):2392–8.
37. Tanaka A, Leake S, Estrera AL. Management strategies in acute type B aortic intramural hematoma. Curr Opin Cardiol. 2017;32(6):687–91.
38. Uchida K, Imoto K, Karube N, et al. Intramural haematoma should be referred to as thrombosed-type aortic dissection†. Eur J Cardiothorac Surg 2013. 44:366–369 https://doi.org/10.1093/ejcts/ezt040.
39. Song J-K. Update in acute aortic syndrome: intramural hematoma and incomplete dissection as new disease entities. J Cardiol 2014. 64(3):153–161 https://doi.org/10.1016/j.jjcc.2014.05.005.
40. Moral S, Ballesteros E, Roque M, et al. Intimal disruption in type B aortic intramural hematoma. Does size matter? A systematic review and meta-analysis Int J Cardiol 2018. 269:298–303 https://doi.org/10.1016/j.ijcard.2018.07.111.
41. Moral S, Cuéllar H, Avegliano G, et al. Clinical implications of focal intimal disruption in patients with type B intramural hematoma. J Am Coll Cardiol. 2017;69(1):28–39.
42. Sueyoshi E, Matsuoka Y, Imada T, Okimoto T, Sakamoto I, Hayashi K. New development of an ulcerlike projection in aortic intramural hematoma: CT evaluation. Radiology. 2002;224(2):536–41.
43. Kruse MJ, Johnson PT, Fishman EK, Zimmerman SL. Aortic intramural hematoma: review of high-risk imaging features. J Cardiovasc Comput Tomogr 2013. 7(4):267–272 https://doi.org/10.1016/j.jcct.2013.04.001.
44. Wu M-T, Wang Y-C, Huang Y-L, et al. Intramural blood pools accompanying aortic intramural hematoma: CT appearance and natural course. Radiology. 2011;258(3):705–13.
45. Wu M-T, Wu T-H, Lee D. Multislice computed tomography of aortic intramural hematoma with progressive intercostal artery tears. Circulation 2005. 111:e92–e93 https://doi.org/10.1161/01.cir.0000154547.65893.45.
46. Schlatter T, Auriol J, Marcheix B, et al. Type B intramural hematoma of the aorta: evolution and prognostic value of intimal erosion. J Vasc Interv Radiol. 2011;22(4):533–41.
47. Coady MA, Rizzo JA, Elefteriades JA. Pathologic variants of thoracic aortic dissections. Cardiol Clin 1999. 17:637–657 https://doi.org/10.1016/s0733-8651(05)70106-5.
48. Herrán FL, Bang TJ, Restauri N, et al. CT imaging of complications of aortic intramural hematoma: a pictorial essay. Diagn Interv Radiol. 2018;24(6):342–7.
49. Sueyoshi E, Sakamoto I, Uetani M, Matsuoka Y. CT analysis of the growth rate of aortic diameter affected by acute type B intramural hematoma. AJR Am J Roentgenol. 2006;186(6 Suppl 2):S414–20.
50. Sueyoshi E, Imada T, Sakamoto I, Matsuoka Y, Hayashi K. Analysis of predictive factors for progression of type B aortic intramural hematoma with computed tomography. J Vasc Surg 2002. 35:1179–1183 https://doi.org/10.1067/mva.2002.123683.
51. Song J-K, Yim JH, Ahn J-M, et al. Outcomes of patients with acute type a aortic intramural hematoma. Circulation. 2009;120(21):2046–52.
52. Chow SCY, Wong RHL, Lakhani I, et al. Management of acute type a intramural hematoma: upfront surgery or individualized approach? A retrospective analysis and meta-analysis. J Thorac Dis. 2020;12(3):680–9.
53. Lee YK, Seo JB, Jang YM, et al. Acute and chronic complications of aortic intramural hematoma on follow-up computed tomography. J Comput Assist Tomogr 2007. 31:435–440 https://doi.org/10.1097/01.rct.0000250112.87585.8e.
54. Choi SH, Choi SJ, Kim JH, et al. Useful CT findings for predicting the progression of aortic intramural hematoma to overt aortic dissection. J Comput Assist Tomogr. 2001;25(2):295–9.
55. Evangelista A, Maldonado G, Moral S, Rodriguez-Palomares J. Uncomplicated type a intramural hematoma: surgery or conservative approach?—surgery. Ann Cardiothorac Surg. 2019. 8 556–557 https://doi.org/10.21037/acs.2019.07.04.
56. Evangelista A, Dominguez R, Sebastia C, et al. Long-term follow-up of aortic intramural hematoma. Circulation. 2003. 108. 583–589 https://doi.org/10.1161/01.cir.0000081776.49923.5a.

Echocardiography for the Diagnosis and Management of Acute Aortic Syndromes

Sumbal Janjua, Andrew D. Maslow, and Athena Poppas

Introduction: Definitions

The aorta consists of five main anatomic segments: the aortic root, the tubular portion of the ascending aorta (the proximal ascending aorta), the aortic arch, the descending thoracic aorta, and the abdominal aorta. The aortic root includes the aortic valve annulus, aortic valve cusps, coronary ostia, and sinuses of Valsalva. The aortic root joins the proximal ascending aorta at the sinotubular junction (STJ). The proximal portion of the ascending aorta extends from the STJ to the origin of the brachiocephalic artery. The aortic arch extends from the brachiocephalic artery to the left subclavian artery. The descending thoracic aorta consists of the proximal part (from the left subclavian artery to the level of the pulmonary artery) and the distal part (from the level of the pulmonary artery to the diaphragm). The abdominal aorta consists of the proximal part, which extends from the diaphragm to the ostia of the renal arteries; and the distal part, which extends from the renal arteries to the iliac bifurcation.

S. Janjua
Department of Cardiology, MedStar Washington Hospital Center, Georgetown University, Washington, DC, USA
e-mail: sumbal.a.janjua@medstar.net

A. Poppas (✉)
Division of Cardiology, Lifespan Cardiovascular Institute, Brown University Warren Alpert School of Medicine, Providence, RI, USA
e-mail: apoppas@lifespan.org

A. D. Maslow
Department of Anesthesiology, Rhode Island Hospital, Brown University Warren Alpert School of Medicine, Providence, RI, USA
e-mail: amaslow@rcn.org

J. S. Coselli et al. (eds.), *Aortic Dissection and Acute Aortic Syndromes*,
https://doi.org/10.1007/978-3-030-66668-2_12

Transthoracic Approach

Echocardiographic Imaging

The aortic root is best visualized in the parasternal long-axis view by TTE [1–8] (Fig. 1). Measurement of the aortic root diameter should be made perpendicular to the axis of the proximal aorta. The standard measurement is taken as the largest diameter from the right coronary sinus of Valsalva to the posterior (usually noncoronary) sinus. Most studies report aortic root diameter measurements at end-diastole using the leading edge–to–leading edge technique [2, 7, 9, 10]. The aortic annulus is generally elliptical in older adults and, hence, most reliably measured with 3D echocardiography. The proximal ascending aorta is best seen in parasternal long and short-axis views or right upper sternal border. Once again, the measurements are made from leading edge to leading edge. The aortic arch is imaged from a suprasternal notch or supraclavicular approach. Only a short segment of the ascending aorta is visible from the suprasternal notch, in most adults (Fig. 2). The descending thoracic aorta is seen in cross section posterior to the left atrium in the parasternal long-axis view. From the subcostal view, the distal thoracic and proximal abdominal aorta is seen as it traverses the diaphragm.

Doppler Flows

Color Doppler interrogation of the ascending aorta from the parasternal approach allows evaluation of the flow pattern in the proximal aorta and assessment of any concomitant aortic regurgitation and grading of severity. Pulsed- wave (PW) or continuous-wave (CW) Doppler recordings of descending aortic flow from the suprasternal notch show systolic flow away from the transducer. Normal flow in the descending aorta shows brief, low-velocity, early diastolic flow reversal,

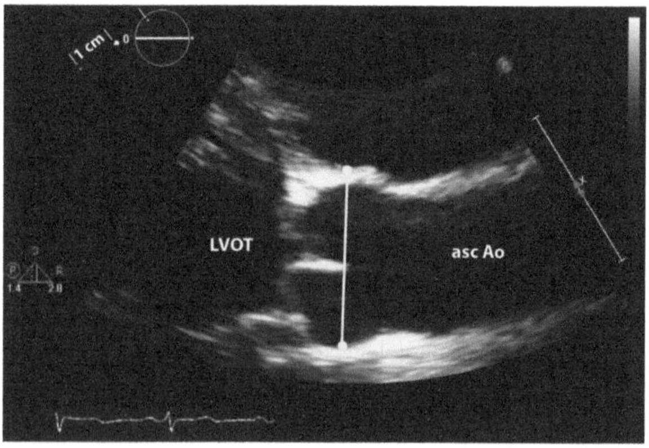

Fig. 1 Normal aortic root morphology and dimensions on transthoracic imaging parasternal long axis view. Yellow line is proper root measurement in mid sinus of Valsalva

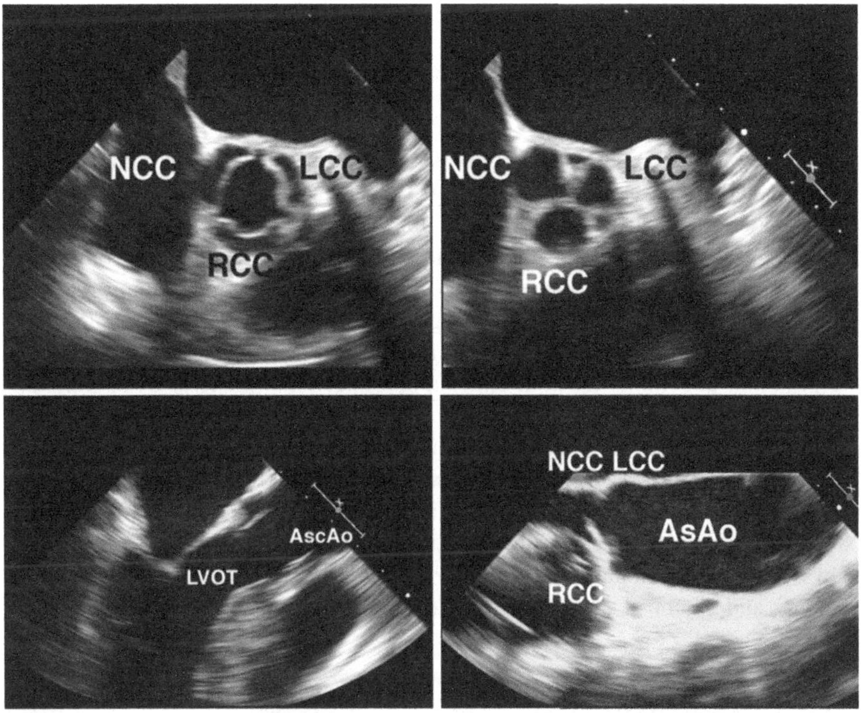

Fig. 2 Normal Transesophageal images of aortic root, valve and ascending aorta. Upper panel is short axis view of the aortic valve in systole and diastole. NCC-noncornary cusp, LCC-left coronary cusp, RCC-right coronary cusp. Lower panel is long axis view of the aorta showing the relationship of the ascending aorta (AscAo) to the left ventricular outflow tract (LVOT) and the coronary cusps

low-velocity antegrade flow in mid-diastole, low-velocity flow reversal at end-diastole. Flow patterns in the proximal abdominal aorta are similar to those seen in the descending thoracic aorta.

Limitations of Transthoracic Imaging

The major limitations of TTE evaluation of the aorta are acoustic access and image quality. Acoustic access maybe suboptimal from one or more of the windows needed for full evaluation of the aorta. Image quality maybe poor due to beam width at the depth of the aorta. Beam-width artifact, noise, and poor lateral resolution make differentiation of intraluminal defects from artifacts difficult. Evaluation by TEE is more sensitive and specific for diagnosing pathology, and hence, is the appropriate modality in most patients with acute aortic disease.

Transesophageal Approach

Echocardiographic Imaging

The aortic valve and sinuses of Valsalva are best seen in short-axis with the image plane rotated to approximately 45°. The aortic valve, sinuses of Valsalva, and ascending aorta are then obtained in the long axis by rotating the image plane to approximately 120° (Fig. 3a and b). The aortic arch is best imaged from a high esophageal transducer position. Presence of the trachea/left bronchus impedes complete visualization of the distal ascending aorta and proximal aortic arch. Posterior rotation of the probe provides excellent images of the descending thoracic aorta and the proximal abdominal aorta in either a cross-sectional plane at 0° or long-axis plane at 90° to 120°. From a transgastric position, the proximal abdominal aorta is seen posterior to the stomach. The entire length of the aorta can be examined in cross-sectional views as the probe is slowly withdrawn from the stomach into the esophagus, with imaging of the aortic arch just prior to removal of the probe. X-plane or biplane feature can allow simultaneous images in the long and short axis views. Three-dimensional (3D) TEE provides additional information in defining the anatomy and extent of abnormalities such as a dissection flap or identifying the

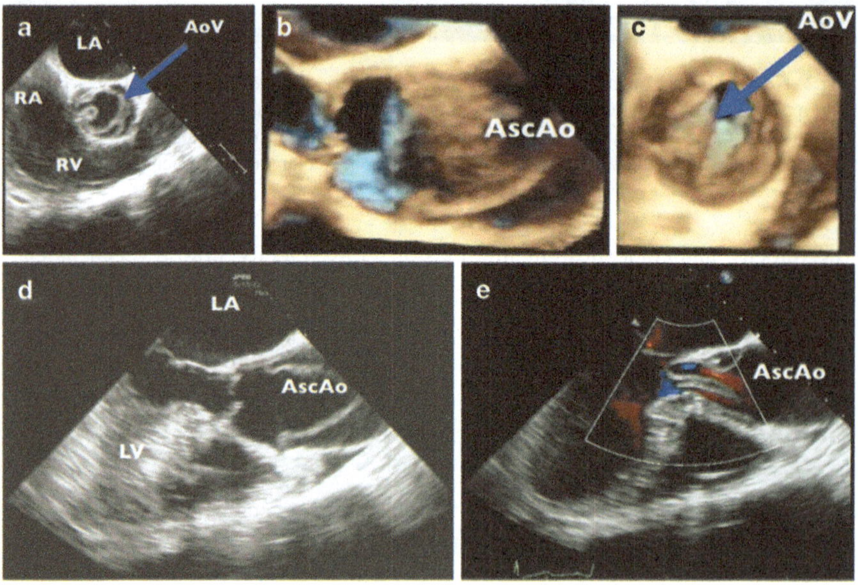

Fig. 3 2D and 3D TEE imaging of Aortic Dissection. (**a**) 2D SAX view of dissection flap prolapsing across the aortic valve (AoV). Surrounding structures: LA-left atrium, RA-right atrium, RV-right ventricle. (**b**) 3D LAX view of the dissection flap in the ascending aorta (AscAo) (**c**) 3D SAX view of the dissection flap prolapsing across the trileaflet aortic valve. (**d**) 2D LAX view of the circumferential dissection flap with insertion at the sinotubular junction. (**e**) Color Doppler of LAX showing differential flow in large false and small true lumen

location and size of the entry site. The origins and course of the coronary arteries are visible in both short- and long-axis views on some TTE and all TEE images.

Doppler Flows

TEE color flow imaging of the aorta shows the normal antegrade flow pattern in the ascending aorta, arch, and descending aorta and is essential in the evaluation of abnormal blood flow patterns in the presence of aortic dissection. Color Doppler evaluation of the aortic valve is essential since aortic valve regurgitation can result from commissural involvement by aortic dissection resulting in inadequate support of the leaflets or a flail aortic leaflet due to extension of a dissection flap into the valve tissue.

Acute Aortic Syndromes

Acute aortic syndromes (AAS) include a spectrum of life-threatening aortic conditions.

The term AAS includes classic aortic dissection, intramural hematoma (IMH), penetrating aortic ulcer (PAU), aortic aneurysm rupture (contained or not contained) [11]. Aortic pseudoaneurysm, traumatic aortic disease and sinus of valsalva aneurysm will also be briefly discussed given their clinical relevance and the need to differentiate pathological processes.

Aortic Dissection

Transthoracic Imaging

Advances in echocardiography have improved the sensitivity of TTE for diagnosis of aortic dissection to approximately 85 percent or more [12, 13]. The echocardiographic diagnosis of aortic dissection is highly secure when there is a dilated aortic lumen, a linear, mobile echogenic structure with a pattern of motion different than the aortic wall and different color Doppler flow patterns in the true and false lumen. The role of TTE in suspected aortic dissection also includes diagnosis of cardiac complications of dissection, including aortic insufficiency, pericardial effusion/tamponade and regional left ventricular systolic function. Importantly, TTE remains less sensitive for detection of aortic dissection than TEE, CT, and MRI. Thus, absence of a dissection flap on TTE should not be used to exclude aortic dissection but prompt further assessment.

Transesophageal Imaging

TEE is highly accurate for establishing the diagnosis of both type A and type B acute.

aortic dissection. Several studies have demonstrated the high accuracy of TEE, with sensitivity approaching 100% [14–16]. TEE images of the aorta are superior to TTE images because of the shorter distance between the transducer and the aorta, the use of a higher-frequency transducer, and better ultrasound tissue penetration (Fig. 4). Features of aortic dissection seen on TEE imaging include a dissection flap that appears as a thin, linear, echogenic structure in the aortic lumen with undulating motion different than the normal systolic pulsations, Color Doppler evidence of blood flow in both the true (bounded by endothelium) lumen and the false (bounded by media) lumen, the entry site into the false lumen, other communications between the two channels, thrombosis of the false lumen or a hematoma in the wall of the aorta (Table 1). TEE imaging of the integrity of the aortic valve apparatus can help guide the surgeon of the potential for aortic valve-sparing operations as well (Table 2).

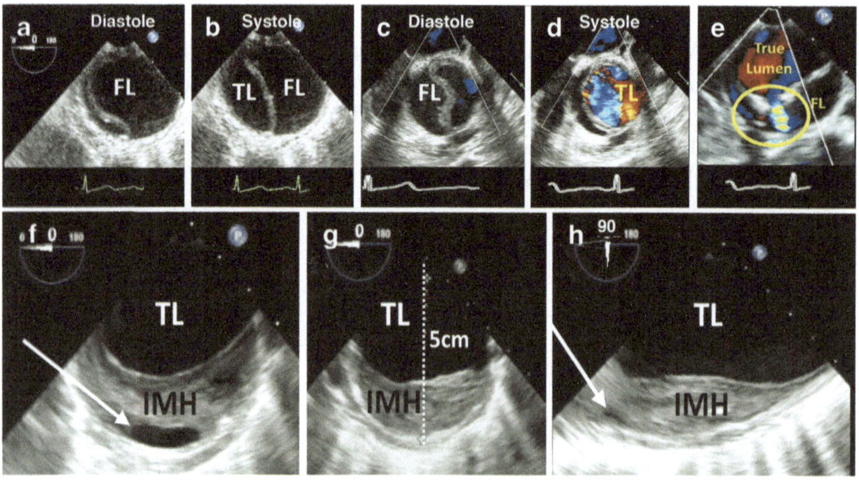

Fig. 4 Aortic Dissection compared with Intramural Hematoma on TEE imaging. The top panel is a SAX of aortic dissection. (**a** and **b**). Diastole and systole showing the thin intimal flap with a larger false lumen (FL). (**c** and **d**). Diastole and systole with color flow revealing flow in true lumen (TL). (**e**). Color flow with circle highlighting the entry tear with flow from true to false lumen. The lower panel is a different patient with an intramural hematoma (IMH) seen as echo density contained within the media (with permission from Maslow et al. Journal of Cardiothoracic and Vascular Anesthesia, Vol. 32, Issue 3, p1341–1362)

Table 1 Mortality Trends Among Patients with Acute Aortic Dissection Over Time from IRAD. (IRAD: International Registry of Acute Aortic Dissection)

a

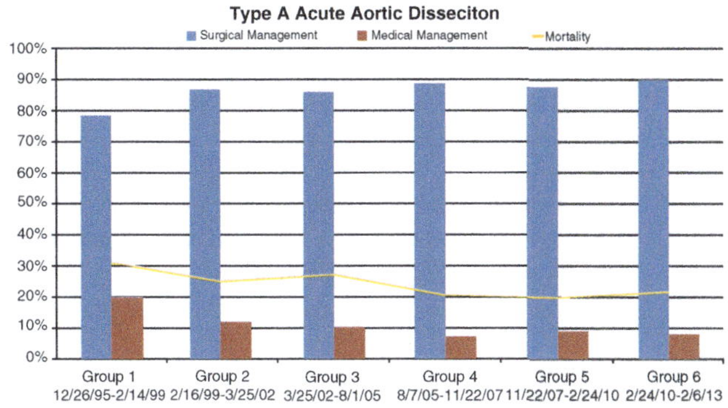

	Group 1	Group 2	Group 3	Group 4	Group 5	Group 6	p-value	Trend p-value
Overall Mortality	154 (31.4%)	119 (25.3%)	140 (27.6%)	99 (20.8%)	103 (19.8%)	106 (21.7%)	<0.001	<0.001
Surgical Mortality	96 (25.0%)	80 (19.6%)	97 (22.1%)	76 (17.9%)	72 (15.8%)	81 (18.4%)	0.015	0.003
Medical Mortality	54 (54.5%)	37 (64.9%)	34 (64.2%)	17 (48.6%)	24 (52.2%)	22 (56.4%)	0.512	0.626

b

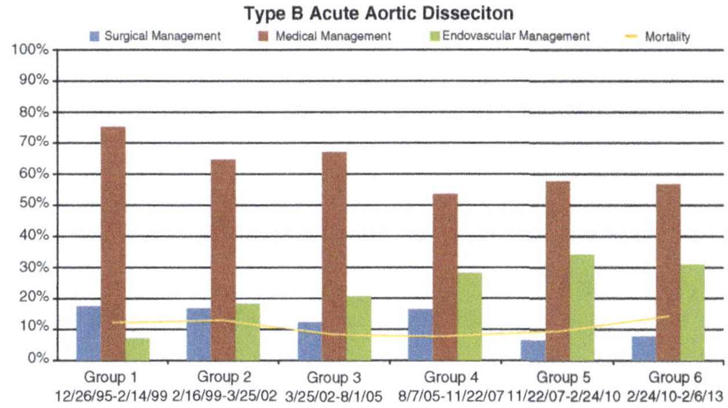

	Group 1	Group 2	Group 3	Group 4	Group 5	Group 6	p-value	Trend p-value
Overall Mortality	30 (12.1%)	34 (12.7%)	19 (8.2%)	20 (7.7%)	20 (9.1%)	35 (14.1%)	0.103	0.915
Surgical Mortality	13 (30.2%)	12 (26.7%)	1 (3.6%)	3 (7.0%)	0 (0.0%)	4 (21.1%)	0.003	0.007
Medical Mortality	17 (9.1%)	16 (9.2%)	11 (7.1%)	10 (7.1%)	9 (7.1%)	17 (12.1%)	0.630	0.705
Endovascular Mortality	0 (0.0%)	6 (12.2%)	7 (14.6%)	7 (9.5%)	10 (13.3%)	12 (15.6%)	0.528	0.216

***Reference for the Table 1:**
Evangelista et al. Circulation April 2018- Insights from the IRAD registry

Aortic Intramural Hematoma (IMH)

Aortic intramural hematoma is a variant of aortic dissection and defined by a localized collection of blood within the aortic wall, but without a discrete intimal tear or false lumen. This pathology accounts for approximately 10–25% of patients with an acute aortic syndrome [17]. Putative mechanisms of intramural hematoma include rupture of the vasa vasorum vessels into an area of medial degeneration or a penetrating atherosclerotic ulcer without an intimal tear and with subsequent blood flow

Table 2 Role of echocardiography in detecting evidence of aortic dissection and echocardiographic definitions of main findings

Diagnostic goals	Definition by echocardiography
Identify presence of a dissection flap	Flap dividing two lumens
Define extension of aortic dissection	Extension of the flap and true/false lumens in the aortic root(ascending/arch/descending abdominal aorta)
Identify true lumen	Systolic expansion, diastolic collapse, systolic jet directed away from the lumen, absence of spontaneous contrast, forward systolic flow)
Identify false lumen	Diastolic diameter increase, spontaneous contrast and or thrombus formation, reverse/delayed or absent flow
Identify presence of false luminal thrombosis	Mass separated from the intimal flap and aortic wall inside the false lumen
Localize entry tear	Disruption of the flap continuity with fluttering or ruptured intimal borders; color Doppler shows flow through the tear
Assess presence, severity and mechanisms of AR	Anatomic definition of the valve (bicuspid, degenerated, normal with/without prolapse of one cusp); dilation of different segments of the aorta; flap invagination into the valve; severity by classic echocardiographic criteria
Assess coronary artery involvement	Flap invaginated into the coronary ostium; flap obstructing the ostium; absence of coronary flow; new regional wall motion abnormalities
Assess side-branch involvement	Flap invaginated into the aortic brandies
Detect pericardial and/or pleural effusion	Echo-free space in the pericardium/pleura
Detect signs of cardiac tamponade	Classic echocardiographic and Doppler signs of tamponade

*Reference for Table 2:
Source: [9]

from the lumen into the vessel wall [18]. Importantly, this is a dynamic condition; 12% of patients with an aortic intramural hematoma progress to a frank dissection with adverse clinical outcomes analogous to patients presenting initially with a clearly delineated dissection flap [19].

Though TTE is less sensitive for the diagnosis, an aortic intramural hematoma is suggested by an echogenic thickening of the aortic wall. Intramural hematoma of the ascending aorta may be visualized on TTE by the following features: focal wall thickening and or echolucent regions, preservation of the shape and smooth border of the lumen, central/luminal displacement of intimal atherosclerosis [9].

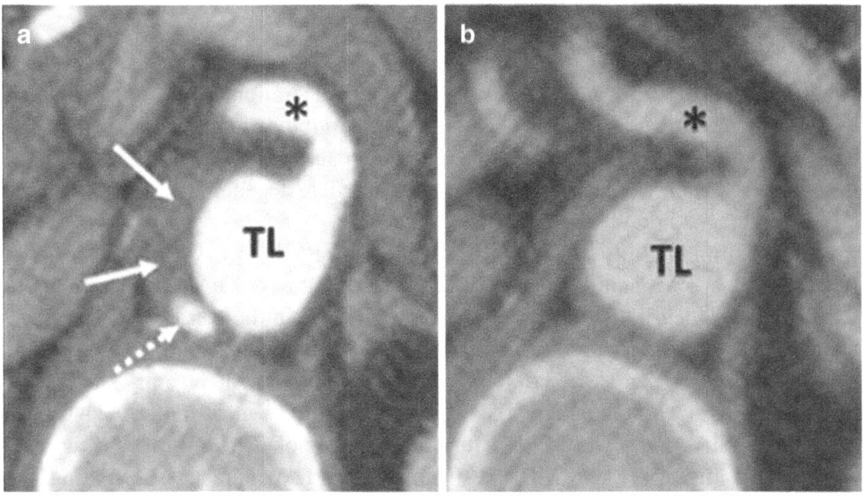

TEE is needed for the diagnosis of all aortic segments, outside of the ascending aorta. On short axis imaging, an intramural hematoma of the descending thoracic aorta appears as a crescent-shaped mass adjacent to the aortic lumen and bounded by the bright adventitial echo signal. Long-axis imaging then allows evaluation of the extent of the hematoma (Fig. 5). Notably, the imaging hallmarks of classic aortic dissection; dissection flap and double channel aorta are both absent in IMH.

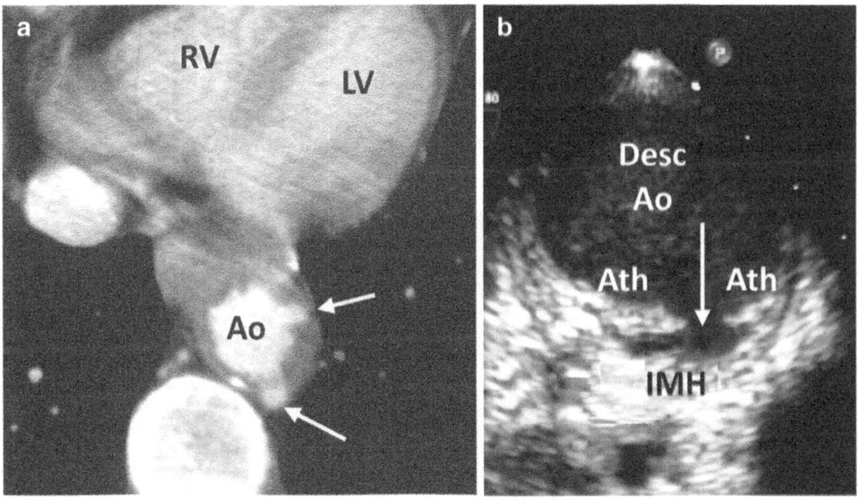

Fig. 5 CT compared with TEE for Penetrating Aortic Ulcer. (**a**) CT scan showing two penetrating ulcers (white arrows) of the descending aorta (Desc Ao) (**b**) TEE showing penetrating ulcer (white arrow) through atherosclerotic intimal plaque (Ath) with intramural hematoma (IMH) in the Descending Aorta (Desc Ao). (with permission from Maslow et al. Journal of Cardiothoracic and Vascular Anesthesia, Vol. 32, Issue 3, p1341–1362)

Penetrating Aortic Ulcer (PAU)

Penetrating aortic ulcer is a condition in which ulceration of an atherosclerotic lesion penetrates the aortic internal elastic lamina into the aortic media [20]. PAU is considered to be a disease of the intima (i.e., atherosclerosis), whereas aortic dissection and its variant (IMH) are diseases of the media (degenerative changes of the elastic fibers and smooth muscle cells).

There is limited utility of TTE in the diagnosis of PAU. TEE, CT or MRI is better suited to detect PAU and its complications. The diagnosis of PAU requires demonstration of an "ulcerlike" or "craterlike" out-pouching in the aortic wall. PAUs can be detected only when they protrude outside the contour of the aortic lumen. The maximum depth of penetration of the ulcer, maximum width at the entry site and the axial length of any associated medial hematoma should be measured. TEE has been less well studied than CT and MRI for the diagnosis of PAU but may be of value when the results of CT and MRI are inconclusive. The characteristic finding is a craterlike out-pouching of the aortic wall, often with jagged edges and usually associated with extensive aortic atheroma [20] (Fig. 6). A localized aortic dissection may occur, but the dissection flap, if present, tends to be thick, irregular, non-oscillating, and usually of limited length. The reason for the limited length of the dissection may be that the dissection plane is lost because of scarring or atrophy of the media and secondary to the atherosclerotic process.

Aortic Aneurysm Rupture

Aneurysm is defined as a permanent focal dilatation of an artery having a 50% increase in diameter compared with the expected normal diameter of the artery [21]. Aneurysms of the aorta can be classified into two main morphologic types: fusiform

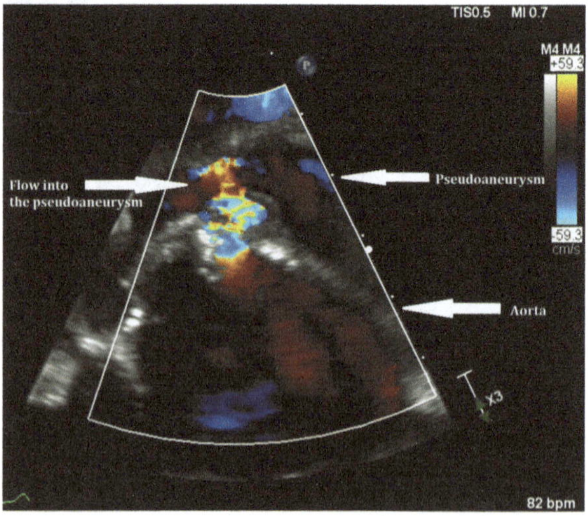

Fig. 6 Aortic Pseudo Aneurysm. The TEE shows color Doppler flow from the aorta into the pseudo aneurysm (white arrows)

and saccular. Fusiform aneurysms result from diffuse weakening of the aortic wall leading to dilatation of the entire circumference of the aorta, producing a spindle-shaped deformity with a tapered beginning and end while saccular aneurysms result when only a portion of the aortic circumference is weakened, producing an asymmetric, relatively focal balloon-shaped out-pouching.

TTE can be utilized for sequential follow-up of aortic root dilatation. Diameter expansion, severity of aortic regurgitation and left ventricular size and function can be evaluated. When dilatation involves the ascending aorta above the STJ, TTE may not adequately visualize the affected segment, in which case other modalities including TEE, CT or MRI should be utilized.

TEE is most often utilized to help guide surgical decision-making. A detailed understanding of the entire aortic valve apparatus is crucial for determining the need for and type of aortic valve repair or valve replacement. TTE and TEE are not tomographic imaging and hence have some limitations for reliable measurements of distal ascending aorta, aortic arch, descending aorta diameters, especially in the presence of a tortuous aorta.

Aortic Pseudoaneurysm

An aneurysm involves all the layers of the aortic wall, whereas a pseudoaneurysm is actually a contained rupture due to loss of integrity of the aortic wall, with a blood collection outside the aorta. Following surgery for aortic disease, blood can escape from the graft lumen or prosthetic valve sewing ring into an area contained by surrounding scar tissue or the native aorta at the proximal or the distal graft anastomoses to the aorta or at the coronary reimplantation sites resulting in pseudoaneurysm formation.

Transthoracic/Transesophageal Imaging

On TTE or TEE, a pseudoaneurysm appears as an echolucent area adjacent to the aortic graft. Flow in this area can be demonstrated with color flow imaging, although a TEE study is often necessary for adequate image quality. The pseudoaneurysm may rupture back into the left ventricle (LV) underneath the aortic annulus and creating a fistula with flow in both systole and diastole. The pseudoaneurysm may form underneath the valve creating "pseudo-aortic regurgitation" with flow from the pseudoaneurysm into the LV in diastole, and from the LV into the pseudoaneurysm in systole. The characteristics of the latter paravalvular flow signal on PW and CW Doppler are similar to those of transvalvular aortic regurgitation with color flow *around,* rather than through, the prosthetic aortic valve.

Traumatic Aortic Disease

Blunt force trauma, most often due to motor vehicle accidents, can result in aortic injury and rupture and is the most common form of traumatic aortic injury. The most vulnerable site, is the aortic isthmus [22]. The second most common location is the supravalvular portion of the ascending aorta [23] (Fig. 7a and b).

Transthoracic/Transesophageal Imaging

TEE findings in patients with blunt force trauma are variable and include dilatation in the region of the isthmus, an abnormal aortic contour, a thick intraluminal medial flap, a pseudoaneurysm, a crescentic or circumferential thickening of the aortic wall (IMH), and mobile linear echodensities attached to the aortic wall consistent with an intimal tear or a thrombus. In differentiating from a spontaneous aortic dissection, the medial flap tends to be thicker, has greater mobility, and is typically perpendicular (rather than parallel) to the aortic wall so that there is an absence of two channels. The aortic contour is usually deformed because of the presence of a localized pseudoaneurysm and the findings are confined to the isthmus, rather than propagating distally all the way to the iliac arteries (Fig. 8).

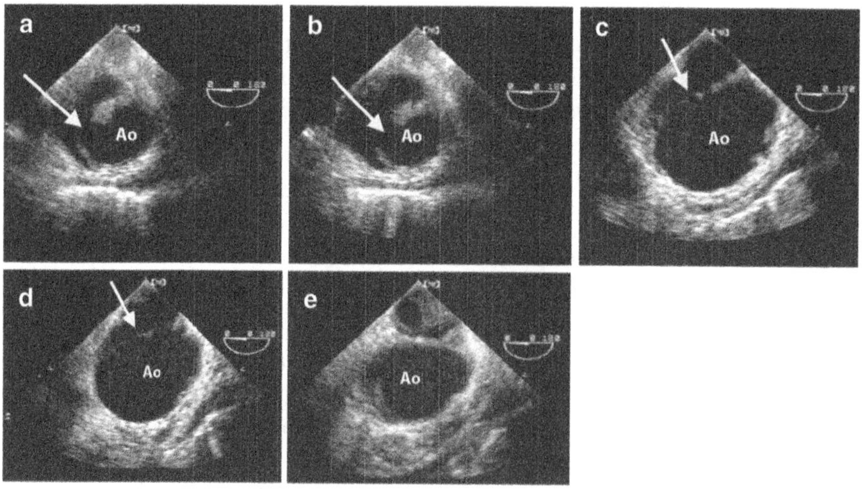

Fig. 7 Traumatic Aortic Disruption. Top panels (**a-d**) are descending aorta progression showing loss of continuity which appears as a step off (white arrows). The final panel (**e**) is the normal descending aorta integrity just below the transsection. Note the thicker flap consisting of both intima and media

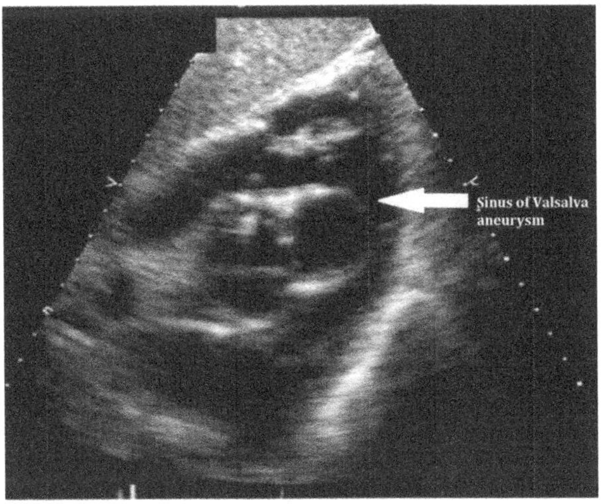

Fig. 8 Sinus of Valsalva Aneurysm. On transthoracic imaging, subcoastal view, there is an enlargement of the right coronary sinus (white arrow) consistent with aneurysm. There was no color flow detected to suggest rupture

Sinus of Valsalva Aneurysm

Sinus of Valsalva aneurysms may be seen on long- and short-axis views of the 2D echocardiogram. Generally, a diameter from the widest portion of the asymmetric sinus to the opposing wall of greater than 4 cm in adults is used as the definition.

Transthoracic/Transesophageal Imaging

A dilated and distorted sinus of Valsalva is seen both in long- and short-axis views at the aortic valve level either from a TEE or TTE approach. A congenital aneurysm may have a complex shape with a "wind sock" appearance of a mass of irregular, mobile echoes protruding from the aortic sinus into adjacent cardiac structures. There may be a communication with multiple fenestrations, with high-velocity turbulent flow from the high-pressure aorta to the low-pressure adjacent chambers detectable by CW, PW, and color flow Doppler techniques. Doppler flow examination is unremarkable in the absence of communication. Contrast echocardiography maybe helpful in delineating the aneurysm, however, color flow Doppler imaging is the technique of choice for identifying a ruptured sinus of Valsalva aneurysm.

References

1. Vriz O, et al. Aortic root dimensions and stiffness in healthy subjects. Am J Cardiol. 2013;112(8):1224–9.
2. Vasan RS, et al. Echocardiographic reference values for aortic root size: the Framingham heart study. J Am Soc Echocardiogr. 1995;8(6):793–800.

3. Soewarto J, et al. Transcriptome data from three endemic Myrtaceae species from New Caledonia displaying contrasting responses to myrtle rust (Austropuccinia psidii). Data Brief. 2019;22:794–811.
4. Roman MJ, et al. Two-dimensional echocardiographic aortic root dimensions in normal children and adults. Am J Cardiol. 1989;64(8):507–12.
5. Lin FY, et al. Assessment of the thoracic aorta by multidetector computed tomography: age- and sex-specific reference values in adults without evident cardiovascular disease. J Cardiovasc Comput Tomogr. 2008;2(5):298–308.
6. Burman ED, Keegan J, Kilner PJ. Aortic root measurement by cardiovascular magnetic resonance: specification of planes and lines of measurement and corresponding normal values. Circ Cardiovasc Imaging. 2008;1(2):104–13.
7. Devereux RB, et al. Normal limits in relation to age, body size and gender of two-dimensional echocardiographic aortic root dimensions in persons >/=15 years of age. Am J Cardiol. 2012;110(8):1189–94.
8. Hager A, et al. Diameters of the thoracic aorta throughout life as measured with helical computed tomography. J Thorac Cardiovasc Surg. 2002;123(6):1060–6.
9. Goldstein SA, et al. Multimodality imaging of diseases of the thoracic aorta in adults: from the American Society of Echocardiography and the European Association of Cardiovascular Imaging: endorsed by the Society of Cardiovascular Computed Tomography and Society for cardiovascular magnetic resonance. J Am Soc Echocardiogr. 2015;28(2):119–82.
10. Vasan RS, Larson MG, Levy D. Determinants of echocardiographic aortic root size. The Framingham Heart Study. Circulation. 1995;91(3):734–40.
11. Vilacosta I, San Roman JA. Acute aortic syndrome. Heart. 2001;85(4):365–8.
12. Cecconi M, et al. The role of transthoracic echocardiography in the diagnosis and management of acute type a aortic syndrome. Am Heart J. 2012;163(1):112–8.
13. Evangelista A, et al. Impact of contrast-enhanced echocardiography on the diagnostic algorithm of acute aortic dissection. Eur Heart J. 2010;31(4):472–9.
14. Erbel R, et al. Echocardiography in diagnosis of aortic dissection. Lancet. 1989;1(8636):457–61.
15. Nienaber CA, et al. The diagnosis of thoracic aortic dissection by noninvasive imaging procedures. N Engl J Med. 1993;328(1):1–9.
16. Adachi H, et al. Emergency surgical intervention of acute aortic dissection with the rapid diagnosis by transesophageal echocardiography. Circulation. 1991;84(5 Suppl):III14–9.
17. Ganaha F, et al. Prognosis of aortic intramural hematoma with and without penetrating atherosclerotic ulcer: a clinical and radiological analysis. Circulation. 2002;106(3):342–8.
18. Yamada T, Tada S, Harada J. Aortic dissection without intimal rupture: diagnosis with MR imaging and CT. Radiology. 1988;168(2):347–52.
19. Evangelista A, et al. Long-term follow-up of aortic intramural hematoma: predictors of outcome. Circulation. 2003;108(5):583–9.
20. Stanson AW, et al. Penetrating atherosclerotic ulcers of the thoracic aorta: natural history and clinicopathologic correlations. Ann Vasc Surg. 1986;1(1):15–23.
21. Hiratzka LF, et al. 2010 ACCF/AHA/AATS/ACR/ASA/SCA/SCAI/SIR/STS/SVM guidelines for the diagnosis and management of patients with thoracic aortic disease. A report of the American College of Cardiology Foundation/American Heart Association task force on practice guidelines, American Association for Thoracic Surgery, American College of Radiology, American Stroke Association, Society of Cardiovascular Anesthesiologists, Society for Cardiovascular Angiography and Interventions, Society of Interventional Radiology, Society of Thoracic Surgeons, and Society for Vascular Medicine. J Am Coll Cardiol. 2010;55(14):e27–e129.
22. Steenburg SD, Ravenel JG. Multi-detector computed tomography findings of atypical blunt traumatic aortic injuries: a pictorial review. Emerg Radiol. 2007;14(3):143–50.
23. Mirvis SE. Thoracic vascular injury. Radiol Clin N Am. 2006;44(2):181–97. vii

Long-Term Imaging of the Aorta: Considerations and Comparison of Modalities

Nicholas S. Burris, Bradley D. Allen, and David M. Williams

Introduction

Despite the importance of cross-sectional imaging in acute aortic disease, the majority of imaging utilization occurs in the chronic phase as part of imaging surveillance. Whereas imaging protocols for acute aortic disease are more standardized, and rely heavily on CT angiography (CTA), protocols for long-term imaging surveillance are less uniform and often vary significantly across centers and between individual physicians. The choice of imaging modality may depend on patient-specific factors, and institutional and physician preferences often play a role. Knowledge of the strengths and limitations of each technique is important for selecting the optimal imaging modality, understanding disease-specific variations in imaging protocols, and appropriately interpreting imaging results. Beyond simply acquiring the images, there exists multiple challenges related to image analysis and measurement technique that can affect the clear assessment of disease progression.

N. S. Burris (✉) · D. M. Williams
Department of Radiology, University of Michigan School of Medicine, Ann Arbor, MI, USA
e-mail: nburris@med.umich.edu

B. D. Allen
Department of Radiology, University of Wisconsin School of Medicine and Public Health, Madison, WI, USA

Department of Radiology, Northwestern University Feinberg School of Medicine, Chicago, IL, USA

J. S. Coselli et al. (eds.), *Aortic Dissection and Acute Aortic Syndromes*,
https://doi.org/10.1007/978-3-030-66668-2_13

Indications and Frequency of Imaging Follow-Up

Aortic Dissection

Patients with medically managed aortic dissection have a high rate of long-term morbidity and mortality, largely owing to the false lumen's propensity to undergo aneurysmal degeneration [1, 2]. Imaging surveillance is a central component of long-term management of patients with aortic dissection and is used to detect aortic growth and identify dissection related complications. Despite the importance of imaging surveillance, there are few data to support any specific long-term imaging surveillance strategy, and even official guidelines state the level of evidence for specific long-term imaging recommendations is "C" (i.e., very limited populations evaluated; only consensus opinions of experts) [3].

There is general recognition that more frequent imaging is needed during the first 6 to 12 months post-dissection to identify patients who develop rapid growth or other complications during the subacute to early chronic phase of aortic remodeling, and may require earlier surgical repair [3]. Early post-operative imaging surveillance is particularly important in patients with Marfan syndrome or other aortic-related connective tissue disorders considering that such patients have been reported to be at higher risk for complications after type A dissection repair [4]. The 2010, multi-disciplinary "Guidelines for the Diagnosis and Management of Patients With Thoracic Aortic Disease" recommends CTA/MRA imaging at 1, 3, 6, and 12 months post-dissection [3]. The authors also state that CTA/MRA imaging is reasonable prior to the patient's discharge from the hospital to establish a clear anatomic baseline to be used for subsequent follow-up. Lastly, it is generally agreed that once patients have demonstrated relatively stable aortic dimensions over a period of 6 or 12 months, that imaging surveillance can be performed on an annual basis in the absence of the development of complications or significant growth.

The definition of aortic "growth" is poorly defined, but is generally considered to be present when aortic diameters increased by ≥3 mm per year, based on the observation that mean growth rates of TBAD are around 3–4 mm per year and measurement variability alone frequently results in 1–2 mm of increase in aortic dimensions [5, 6]. Furthermore, "rapid growth" is often used to suggest a growth rate of 5 mm per year or greater [3]. A study of long-term outcomes in patients with aortic dissection demonstrated that growth of ≥5 mm within the first 6 months confers a greater than two-fold increased risk of future complications, emphasizing the importance of frequent imaging in the early post-dissection period [7]. If a patient with previously stable aortic dimensions develops growth during the surveillance interval, but is not yet deemed a candidate for surgical repair, more frequent imaging follow-up should be considered to detect and prevent the development of complications. While CT is generally the preferred method for imaging surveillance in the acute phase given its superior spatial resolution and better ability to detect mediastinal/periaortic soft tissue abnormalities associated with leak/contained rupture, magnetic resonance angiography (MRA) is a reasonable alternative for long-term annual imaging surveillance of patients with stable and uncomplicated dissections, and avoids the cumulative risk of repeated radiation exposure.

Intramural Hematoma (IMH) and Penetrating Atherosclerotic Ulcer (PAU)

Published recommendations for imaging surveillance of patients with IMH and PAU largely mirror those for patients with aortic dissection, although data on long-term imaging are even more limited than for dissection. Frequent imaging follow-up in the early phase is of particular importance to patients with IMH, as the majority of the complications occur within the first year, and patients with non-resolving IMH have been shown to be at the greatest risk [7]. In addition to maximal aortic dimeter of the affected segment, the degree of mural thickness should be assessed to track IMH evolution. PAUs are occasionally incidentally detected in asymptomatic patients, and in this setting annual imaging surveillance is generally performed. While many PAUs can be managed non-operatively, lesions that are painful or associated with other complications such as intramural hematoma, pseudoaneurysm or signs of rupture, open or endovascular repair may be necessary [8, 9]. Long-term imaging follow-up is important in PAUs as approximately 43% of symptomatic PAUs and 16% of asymptomatic PAUs were noted to progress on follow-up imaging [10]. Although specific imaging surveillance recommendations are not supported by strong evidence and are subject to significant variability, a general summary of standard imaging follow-up intervals in several clinical scenarios is presented in Table 1.

Comparison of Imaging Modalities

The three primary imaging modalities for long-term monitoring and follow-up imaging in the thoracic aorta are CT angiography (CTA), MR angiography (MRA), and echocardiography. Each modality has strengths and weaknesses for imaging the thoracic aorta. The selection of the appropriate imaging test should be driven by specific aortic pathology, surgical history, co-morbidities such as aortic valve disease or extension of dissection or aneurysm into the abdominal aorta, and patient related factors, particularly renal function and age.

Table 1 Summary of standard imaging surveillance intervals

Clinical Scenario	Early Follow-Up (0–12 months)	Long-Term Follow-up (12 months +)
Aortic dissection	—	—
Type A (repaired)	Before discharge **or** @1 month* – *If enlarging*: 3, 6 & 12 months* – *If stable*: 6 & 12 months	*If stable*: Annual intervals† *If enlarging*: 6 month intervals – After ≥3 years stability, consider change to 2 or 3 year intervals†.
Type B (OMT)	Before discharge **and** @1 month* – *If enlarging*: 3, 6 & 12 months* – *If stable*: 6 & 12 months	*If stable*: Annual intervals† *If enlarging*: 6 month intervals – After ≥3 years stability, consider change to 2 year intervals†.
Post-Endograft	Before discharge **or** @1 month*‡ – *If enlarging and/or significant endoleak*: 3, 6 & 12 months*‡ – *If stable/no endoleak*: 6 & 12 months	*If stable/FL regression*: Annual intervals† *If enlarging*: 6 month intervals – After ≥3 years stability, consider change to 2 or 3 year intervals†.
IMH/PAU	Before discharge **and** @1 month* – *If non-resolving*: 3, 6 & 12 months* – *If resolving*: 6 & 12 months Recommend careful image analysis for development of intimomedial defects or ULP [11]	In the absence of indications for repair: *If non-resolving IMH*: 6–12 months intervals *If resolved IMH*: – Annual intervals if residual aortic dilation† – Unclear role of continued imaging if no residual aortic dilation

† Consider MRI/MRA if appropriate for patient-specific factors
‡ Addition of delayed phase imaging is recommended
[a]CTA is preferred modality
Abbreviations: *OMT* optimal medical therapy, *IMH* intramural hematoma, *PAU* penetrating atherosclerotic ulcer, *ULP* ulcerlike projection

Echocardiography Versus Cross-Sectional Imaging

While echocardiography is not the preferred modality for comprehensive thoracic aorta evaluation, all standard echocardiography examinations can provide information on multiple aortic segments and it has been recommended as a primary screening tool in aortic disease. The aortic valve, sinuses and proximal ascending aorta can usually be well assessed with transthoracic echocardiography (TTE), while evaluation of the descending aorta requires transesophageal echo for evaluation (TEE). On TTE, using a combination of left and right parasternal long axis views and basal short axis views, it is possible to measure the aortic annulus, sinuses of Valsalva (SOV), and sinotubular junction (STJ). Right parasternal and apical long axis views are used to measure ascending aorta diameters (AAo). Suprasternal views allow visualization of the aortic arch and branch vessels although this sonographic window can be limited due to patient body habitus or emphysema. TEE allows for short- and long-axis evaluation of the descending aorta, but the invasive nature of this test limits its usefulness as a standard follow-up or monitoring tool [12].

An important advantage of the TTE compared to other cross-sectional modalities is the relative ease of acquisition without the need for intravenous contrast or exposure to ionizing radiation. This feature makes TTE a useful tool in serial monitoring post-operative complications following ascending aorta repair. Additional key advantages of echocardiography for aortic evaluation include the opportunity to assess any co-morbid aortic valve disease and measure biophysical properties such as aortic distensibility and pulse wave velocity with Doppler echocardiography [13]. For follow-up imaging in ascending aortic disease, an important disadvantage of TTE is that aortic diameters are measured only in the long-axis plane, and this approach has been shown to underestimate aortic diameter when compared to double-oblique measurements [14]. While there are several possible measurement techniques, the "leading edge to leading edge" technique has been shown to have excellent reproducibility and the best agreement with CTA measurements [15].

CTA Acquisition

CT Angiography is considered the primary imaging modality for diagnosing and monitoring thoracic aorta disease and for follow-up imaging after aortic interventions. Key advantages of CTA are that image acquisition is fast, less complex than MRI/MRA and yields high resolution images. CTA is generally performed with spatial resolutions on the order of 0.7 mm^3, and its volumetric nature allows for 3D analysis and multi-planar reformats of aortic anatomy. Depending on scanner specific features such as detector size, CTA acquisitions of the chest can be performed in a single breath-hold of 5–10 seconds, with some modern scanners in 1–2 seconds [16]. An important disadvantage of CTA is that the exam most often provides static snapshot of the anatomy and lacks hemodynamic information. CTA can generate dynamic "cine" images with the use of retrospective electrocardiograph (ECG) gating techniques, however, this comes at the cost of higher radiation dose and should thus be used sparingly.

CTA requires intravenous injection of iodinated contrast with timing of image acquisition such that aortic opacification is maximal. Poor contrast timing can significantly limit the diagnostic performance of the test. Patients are generally asked to hold their breath during the scan to minimize respiratory motion. For evaluation of aortic root size or ascending aorta diameter, ECG gating is usually employed. ECG-gating limits cardiac and aortic root motion to decrease motion-related artifacts which can result in inaccurate measurements and limit the assessment of the dissection flaps. Prospective ECG gating involves only acquiring images during a portion of the cardiac cycle, most often in mid-late diastole (70–75% R-R interval), and this approach requires significantly less radiation than retrospective gating. ECG-gating can fail in the setting of arrhythmia due to inconsistent R-R intervals resulting in motion/pulsation artifact. ECG-gating is generally not required for evaluation of the arch and descending aorta where pulsatile motion is less pronounced.

MRI/MRA Acquisition

MR angiography has similar spatial resolution to CTA, usually in the range of 0.7–1.2 mm^3, but patient related factors such as body habitus may necessitate changing the field of view which can lower image resolution. Scan times for MRA tend to be longer, usually due to the acquisition of multiple sequences during each study. However, MRA offers several advantages relative to CTA including lack of ionizing radiation, opportunity to acquire hemodynamic information through time-resolved techniques, and ability to evaluate luminal/intraluminal structures with non-contrast MRA techniques.

Similar to CTA, contrast-enhanced MRA (CE-MRA) acquisition requires image acquisition timing to be optimized to contrast opacification of the aorta. The CE-MRA technique employs a 3D T1 weighted sequence which leverages the T1 shortening properties of gadolinium—rather than the x-ray attenuating properties of iodine—to provide high contrast within the aortic lumen. Similar to CTA, MRA of the aorta is ECG-gated to reduce artifacts at the root and ascending aorta due to cardiac motion. Breath-holding is also necessary at MRA to limit respiratory motion artifact. In addition to CE-MRA images, most studies will include pre- and/or post-contrast T1 and T2 weighted sequences, which can help with identification of intramural hematoma, mediastinal abnormalities, and vessel wall inflammation [17].

Multiple non-contrast MRA techniques have been developed that can be useful in patients where contrast imaging is either limited or not possible. Steady-state free precession (SSFP) is an MR acquisition technique which results in high signal intensity of the blood without the need for intravenous contrast. Three-dimensional, ECG-gated, non-contrast SSFP MRA provides excellent image quality and accurate aorta measurements relative to CE-MRA, but requires significantly longer scan times [18, 19]. Other options for non-contrast assessment of the thoracic aorta include spin-echo, time-of-flight (TOF), and phase contrast techniques.

MRI/MRA also provides the ability to evaluate aortic hemodynamics using time-resolved MRA (TR-MRA), as well as two-dimensional and three-dimensional ("4D Flow") phase contrast techniques (Fig. 1). Time-resolved MRA is a contrast-enhanced technique which acquires images rapidly during contrast injection yielding dynamic images of contrast transit similar to angiography, and can provide information such as the location of endoleaks after TEVAR and false lumen filling patterns in aortic dissection. Phase-contrast MRA can be used as a non-contrast technique which measures differences in magnetic spin phase shifts that occur with flowing blood. These phase shifts are proportional to flow velocity, thus allowing for quantification of aortic blood velocity and flow rates. This technique can be

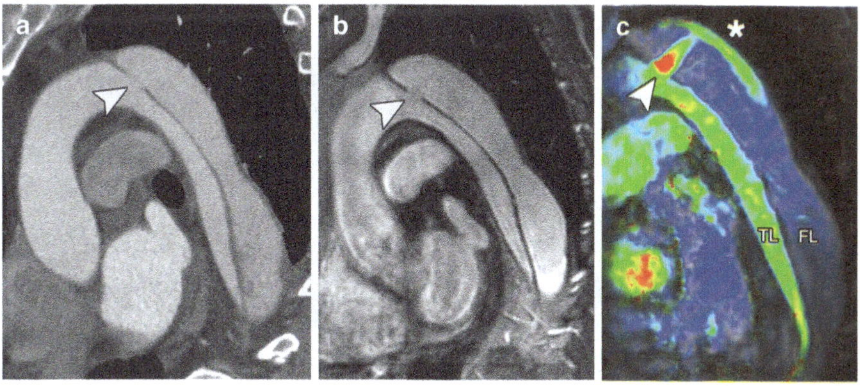

Fig. 1 *Anatomic Versus Hemodynamic Assessment with Computed Tomography Angiography (CTA) and Magnetic Resonance Angiography (MRA):* Sagittal view of a patient with TBAD using CTA (**a**) demonstrates a proximal entry tear (arrow head) and distinct true and false lumen. Similarly, sagittal MRA images also clearly depict the entry tear with similar anatomic detail to CTA (**b**). MRI also allows for measurement of blood flow velocity, and three-dimensional maps of blood flow can be generated using 4D Flow MRI techniques, allowing for clear visualization of the flow jet at the proximal entry tear (**c**), which impacts the opposite wall of the false lumen (asterisk)

applied in 2D or 3D and has been used to assess valve-related aortopathy, pulse-wave velocity and many other advance hemodynamic parameters [20].

Artifacts and Technical Limitations

Several imaging related artifacts can limit CTA image quality. One of the most commonly encountered CT artifacts is beam-hardening or "streak" artifact which results from dense structures (bones, surgical implants, wires, pacemaker/defibrillator generators, iodinated contrast in the superior vena cava) interfering with normal image formation [21]. Newer dual-energy CT scanners have metal artifact reduction algorithms which can be employed to reduce the impact of such artifacts [22]. To image the entire chest with CTA, the CT table must translate during the scan, and with ECG-gating this can mean different portions of the chest are imaged at different R-R intervals. Motion during imaging can lead to a linear "step-off" or "stair step" artifact, which is most visible on coronal or sagittal reformatted series. Such step-offs can blur the aortic wall, lead to inaccurate aortic measurements and be mistaken for dissection (Fig. 2) [23].

With MRA, distortions in the magnetic field caused by metallic objects in the body often can produce susceptibility artifact, which present as areas of dark signal void surrounding the metallic object and are worse in 3 T compared to 1.5 T scanners. Potential sources of artifact include pacemaker/ICD generators or electrodes, spinal hardware, and sternal wires. Endografts composed of nitinol can be imaged with MRI/MRA, whereas stainless-steel endografts result significant

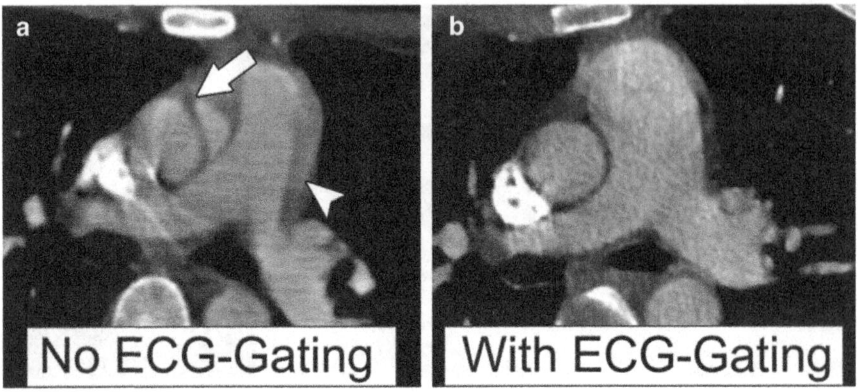

Fig. 2 Motion/pulsation artifact on non-ECG gated CT scans can result in blurring of the margins of the aorta and main pulmonary artery (**a**, arrow head) and image artifacts that simulate aortic dissection. In this representative case, a dissection flap in the ascending aorta (**a**, arrow) was described at an outside hospital CT performed without ECG-gating, however, on repeat CT scan with ECG-gating the flap was confirmed to be artifactual in nature (**b**)

artifacts and are poorly evaluated [24]. Patient specific factors can degrade image quality, with the most important factors being arrhythmia (failure of ECG-gating), difficulty with breath holding, and claustrophobia. Claustrophobia and breath-holding difficulties tend to be more severe in MRA than CTA due to longer image acquisition times, a longer scanner bore, and need for multiple breath-holds during the exam.

CTA Radiation Exposure

Radiation exposure if a common concern of patients and physicians, and it is well documented that ionizing radiation is associated with a risk of malignancy, particularly in radiosensitive organs in the chest such as the breasts, lungs, and thyroid. Estimates of cancer risks due to radiation doses below 100 millisievert (mSv), a dose corresponding to approximately 1000 chest radiographs or 10 CTAs, are not well validated but are estimated at approximately 1% lifetime risk [25]. As scanner technology and imaging processing algorithms have improved, CT doses have dramatically decreased. Currently, an ECG-gated CTA of the chest has an effective radiation dose of ~5–8 mSv. In most patients with thoracic aortic disease, the benefit of undergoing optimal imaging far outweighs the risk of radiation-induced malignancy. Considering the typical latency period of ≥10 years, the significance of radiation-induced malignancy should be considered in the context of patient life expectancy [26]. However, children, younger adults and pregnant patients exposed to similar doses of radiation have a considerably higher risk, and alternative imaging strategies should be considered in these groups [27].

Contrast Safety Concerns

Both iodinated contrast for CTA and gadolinium contrast for MRA have patient safety concerns that may determine which modality is should be considered when selecting the best imaging modality for a given patient. Iodinated contrast has historically been associated with acute kidney injury, a phenomenon termed contrast induced nephropathy (CIN), with guidelines suggesting reduced contrast dose or the withholding contrast in patients with renal insufficiency to reduce the risk of renal failure in these patients. Increasingly, data has suggested that the risk of CIN, even in patients with GFR < 30 mL/min is very low or possibly non-existent [28]. Institutional guidelines should be reviewed to determine the locally accepted iodinated contrast dosing practice.

Gadolinium-related nephrogenic systemic fibrosis (NSF) has been a concern in patients with low renal function (GFR < 30 ml/min) undergoing contrast-enhanced MRI/MRA. However, gadolinium-based contrast agents have now been developed with safety profiles which make the likelihood of NSF exceedingly low and routinely checking renal function prior to contrast enhanced MRI is not required in most patients [29]. Over the last several years there has been increasing evidence of MRI-related gadolinium deposition in the brain and other organs. While the significance of this finding remains uncertain and no clear clinical sequela have been identified, it is a dose dependent phenomenon, and therefore patients undergoing frequent MR studies, particularly younger patients, should carefully consider the potential risks and benefits of contrast administration [30]. This phenomenon may increase the importance of non-contrast MRA techniques in the future. The strengths and limitations of CTA and MRA are summarized in Table 2.

Post-Endograft Imaging

Imaging Follow-Up

There are no standardized guidelines for imaging follow-up of patients after endovascular repair of aortic dissection or other acute aortic syndromes, partly owing to the wide degree of variability in repair complexity and the rapidly evolving nature of endovascular techniques. However, there are some principles of post-endograft surveillance that are widely accepted and have been summarized in recently published appropriateness criteria [31]. CTA is generally considered the optimal modality for imaging surveillance, at least within the first 6–12 months after repair, given the superior imaging resolution, ability to evaluate the integrity of metallic stent frames, and improved evaluation for potential mediastinal or other intra-thoracic complications. Assessment of aortic remodeling after TEVAR is most commonly performed by aortic diameter measurement (either overall diameter or false lumen

Table 2 Comparing CTA and MRI

Characteristic	CT Angiography (CTA)	MR Angiography (MRA)
Radiation	Ionizing radiation (X-ray) – DNA damage	Non-ionizing (radiofrequency) – No DNA damage
Spatial resolution	0.5 mm^3 (minimal)	~ 0.7–1.2 mm^3 (variable)
Number of acquisitions	Usually single	Usually multiple
Set-up and scan time	Short (5–10 min)	Long (45–60 min)
Acquisition complexity	Easy	More difficult
Patient participation	Minimal – Single breath hold – Hold still for ~10–30 seconds	Significant—Multiple breath hold – Multiple breath holds – Hold still for at least 5–10 minutes
Strength	Anatomy	Soft tissue characterization and hemodynamic/functional assessment
Contrast risk	*Iodinated contrast:* 1. Contrast-induced nephropathy (CIN) – Rare 2. Severe allergy (~1:1000)	*Gadolinium contrast:* 1. Nephrogenic systemic fibrosis (NSF) – Extremely rare 2. Gadolinium deposition in brain (unclear significance) 2. Severe allergy (~1:100,000)

diameter). False lumen volumetric assessment has been proposed as a more sensitive marker of false lumen remodeling in a variety of studies and trials, and while there are clear theoretical benefits of volumetric measurements, such measurement techniques remain poorly standardized and the benefit over diameter measurements has not been formally established [32].

Imaging surveillance in the post-endograft generally involves the first post-operative study being performed before discharge or at least within the first month, with subsequent studies typically occurring at 3–6 and 12 months and annually thereafter in the absence of growth or other complications. Long-term follow-up studies of TEVAR patients have shown that late complications can occur (e.g. development of endoleaks, stent fracture, stent graft migration), and lifelong imaging surveillance of patients with aortic endografts is therefore recommended [33]. Imaging protocols for CTA/MRA vary by institution, however, generally post-endograft studies are performed with multiple phases of contrast including noncontrast, arterial phase and delayed phase (30–60 seconds after arterial phase) (Fig. 3). Delayed phase imaging is a unique feature of post-endograft studies, and is necessary for the detection of low flow endoleaks [34].

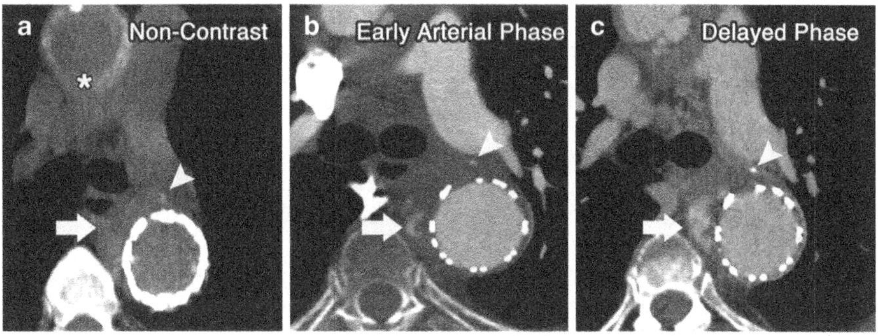

Fig. 3 *Post-Endograft CTA Technique*: Standard post-endograft CTA consists of a 3-phase imaging protocol. First, a non-contrast scan is performed (**a**) to clearly identify any dense objects such as the metallic endograft, surgical material (asterisk) or calcium (arrowhead). Second, contrast is administered and images are acquired in the early arterial phase (**b**), producing maximal aortic opacification and allowing identification of endoleaks (arrow). Lastly, a delayed phase is acquired (30–60 seconds after arterial phase) to allow detection of slow filling endoleaks and better depict the full extent of any endoleaks (arrowhead)

Patient-Specific Considerations for Post-Endograft Imaging Surveillance

Two common patient-specific considerations that arise with post-endograft imaging surveillance are the cumulative radiation exposure of CT among young patients (<50–60), particularly those with connective tissue disease or traumatic aortic injury, and contrast-induced nephropathy among patients with renal insufficiency. Both of these situations can often be managed effectively by utilizing noncontrast imaging, MRI/MRA or a combination of both. Studies have shown that cumulative radiation doses accrued during post-endograft CT imaging surveillance can often reach the level of 350 mSieverts, a level at which the estimated rate of radiation-induced malignancy would be 2.5% [35]. Radiation concerns are less over 65–70 years of age or when the expected lifespan is less than 10–15 years, given the latency period of radiation-induced malignancy. Options to limit radiation dose include limiting the number of phases acquired (e.g. noncontrast phase if already acquired in prior studies) or utilizing MRI/MRA techniques, which do not utilize employ ionizing radiation. Magnetic artifact prevents MR imaging of stainless steel endografts, however, newer nitinol endografts do not produce significant artifact and can be adequately assessed with MRI/MRA (Fig. 4) [36]. In the setting of renal insufficiency, noncontrast CT imaging can be performed to assess the overall aortic dimensions and device stability/integrity, although assessment of endoleaks and individual lumen dimensions and intraluminal pathology is not possible. Noncontrast

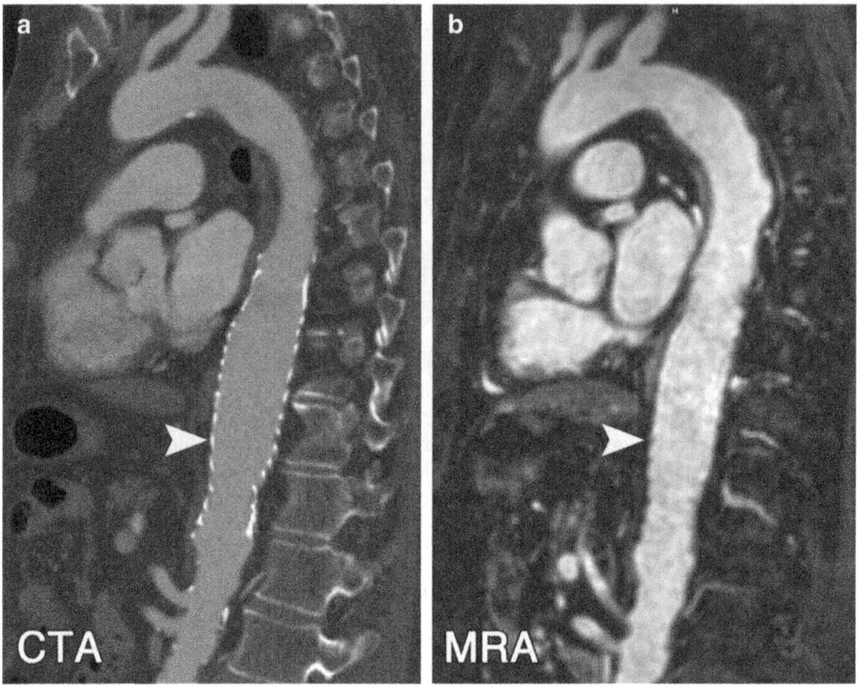

Fig. 4 *Post-Endograft Surveillance with MRA*: Sagittal images of a patient with penetrating atherosclerotic ulcer of the descending aorta who underwent TEVAR using a nitinol endograft. The metallic endograft can be clearly seen on CTA images (**a**, arrow head). While the endograft material appears dark/black on MRA images (**b**), the nitinol doesn't create any significant artifact in the image and detailed evaluation of the lumen and surrounding anatomy is possible

MRI/MRA techniques have the unique ability to delineate blood, thrombus and the aortic wall, and can thus be a powerful tool for long-term imaging surveillance for patients with nitinol-based endografts.

Post-Processing and Measurement

Measurement Techniques and Limitations

Maximal aortic diameter is the primary metric of aortic disease severity, and is measured in imaging surveillance to monitor disease progression, estimate risk of complications and to determine surgical candidacy [37]. While aortic diameter is simple to measure and has a well-defined biomechanical relationship with wall tension (i.e., Laplace's law), accurate and reproducible diameter measurements can be challenging for technical and anatomic reasons. Traditionally aortic diameter measurements were performed on axial CT images; however, it is well-recognized that this approach can lead to significant measurement variability (on the order of 5–10 mm) related to the degree of aortic obliquity, particularly at the root and arch segments [38]. With the advent of medical image analysis software, multi-planer reformats (MPR) can be generated that allow for measurement of the aortic diameter orthogonal to the vessel axis (i.e. double-oblique plane), and these orthogonal measurement planes can be generated either manually, or more recently with the assistance of semi-automated image analysis software that first generates a centerline through geometric center of the vessel lumen (Fig. 5). However, despite optimal centerline assessment technique, measurement variability remains within the ±2 mm range for TAA even in the setting of highly standardized measurement protocols [39, 40]. Measurement variability is further increased when the aortic wall geometry is non-circular/ovoid or the aortic wall is difficult to clearly visualize, as is often the case with aortic dissection. Measurement variability alone often precludes confident determination of aortic enlargement considering that aortic growth rates commonly fall within the range of 1–3 mm per year.

Methods to Improve Quality of Imaging Surveillance

Considering that aortic diameter is the gold standard metric for assessment of aortic disease, it is important for both imagers and surgeons to understand and utilize best practices for aortic measurement in order to ensure the most reliable aortic growth

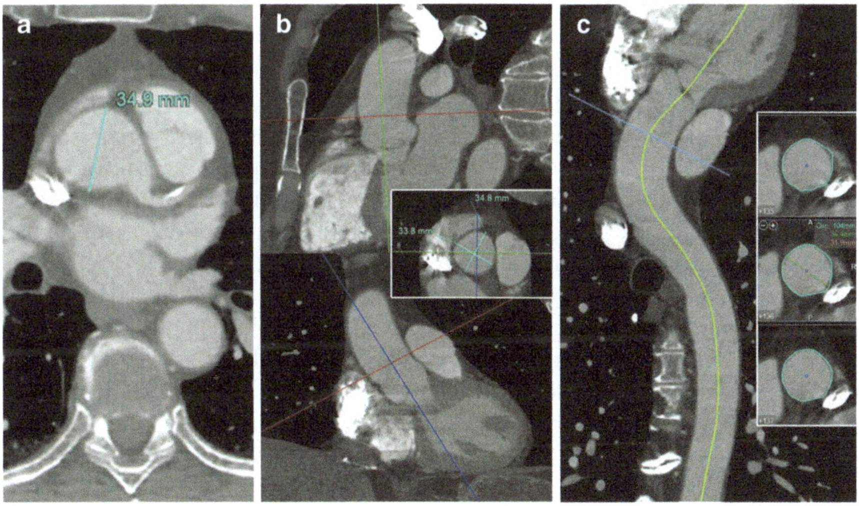

Fig. 5 *Aortic Measurement Techniques*: The simplest method of measurement involves measuring the shortest dimension of the aorta on standard axial images (**a**), although this method can lead to significant measurement variability. Double-oblique measurement technique minimize inaccuracy related to measurement plane obliquity and can either be performed manually using multi-planar reformats (**b**) or using a semi-automated centerline approach (**c**)

assessment possible. The key to minimizing measurement variability is to minimize any differences in measurement technique between two different scans. Specifically, it is ideal to have both prior and current scans measured using the same measurement technique (e.g. centerline versus manual MPR versus axial), and using the most comparable images in terms of contrast phase, slice thickness and gating parameters. Any areas of maximal aortic dimension should be directly compared between the prior and current scans by the same person, using the same software, at as close to the same anatomic location as possible, and ideally in a side-by-side fashion to allow for confirmation of the visual similarity of measurement planes. Additionally, all readers should be instructed to use the same measurement landmarks along the length of the aorta, and diameter measurements should extend from the outer aortic wall to outer aortic wall have been shown to be most reproducible in TAA, although outer aortic wall can be difficult to locate in aortic dissection if the false lumen enhancement is low [3, 15]. Furthermore, it important that if prior CT images/measurements were obtained a different institution, that the measurements on the external prior study be repeated by the current institution, as significant inter-institutional measurement variability has been documented, mostly owing to differences in institutional specific measurement protocols [41]. Lastly, to maximize the interpretability and comparability of documented aortic measurements, it is ideal to utilize a standardized measurement reporting/storage format, and many image analysis programs currently support generation of standardized measurement reports.

Advances and Future Directions

While seemingly a simple task, long-term imaging surveillance of aortic disease struggles with measurement inaccuracies and can be exceedingly time consuming, particularly in the aortic dissection or post-endograft settings where patient-specific considerations, and variations in aortic anatomy, image quality and measurement technique are accentuated. There are two areas in which we believe ongoing advancements in aortic imaging will have a significant impact on the quality of aortic imaging surveillance in the future. First, while MRA is clearly a secondary modality to CTA in majority of institutions due to issues of time, cost and image quality, given MRI's inherent ability to resolve the aortic blood pool and aortic wall without the need for radiation or contrast, and given its ability to provide a dynamic assessment of aortic morphology, distensibility and blood flow, MRI/MRA may be an ideal method to more fully characterize aortic disease. While further advancements are needed to shorten acquisition times for MRI/MRA and to establish the clinical relevance of dynamic aortic parameters in aortic dissection (e.g., distensibility, blood flow, flap motion), active research in these areas has shown promising results [42–44]. Secondly, there is a critical need to advance the speed and accuracy of aortic size and growth assessment in long-term imaging surveillance. Advanced computational methods in the fields of computer vision and machine learning may

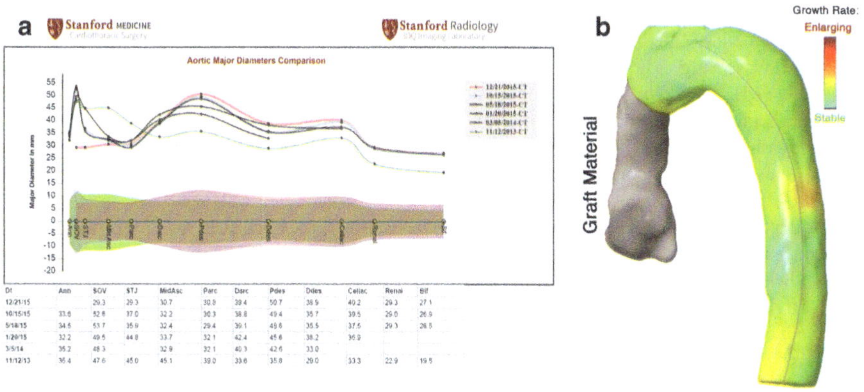

Fig. 6 *Future Directions to Improve Aortic Measurements and Imaging Surveillance:* Software exists that permits tabulation and graphical representation of aortic measurements along the length of the aorta at each surveillance imaging study allowing for improved depiction of long-term growth trends. A sample report is shown from a patient with acute type A aortic dissection treated with ascending aortic repair, with residual dissection involving the arch and descending thoracoabdominal aorta. Five series follow-up studies demonstrate gradual increase in maximum diameter of the proximal descending thoracic aorta over two years. Courtesy of Dominik Fleischman, Stanford 3D/Quantitative Imaging Laboratory (**a**). Image analysis tools are being developed that allow for a three-dimensional analysis of aortic growth in aortic dissection that overcomes many of the limitations of diameter measurements, and an example of such a 3D analysis in a repaired type A dissection patient with stable aortic dimensions is shown (**b**)

be ideal solutions. Preliminary studies have shown that automated segmentation and classification of aortic aneurysms as well as three-dimensional deformation analysis of aortic growth are both possible, and suggest the possibility that the future of aortic imaging surveillance may evolve from the hands of human readers to the servers of medical imaging software companies (Fig. 6) [45, 46].

References

1. Tsai TT, Fattori R, Trimarchi S, Isselbacher E, Myrmel T, Evangelista A, et al. Long-term survival in patients presenting with type B acute aortic dissection insights from the international registry of acute aortic dissection. Circulation. 2006;114(21):2226–31.
2. Durham CA, Cambria RP, Wang LJ, Ergul EA, Aranson NJ, Patel VI, et al. The natural history of medically managed acute type B aortic dissection. J Vasc Surg. 2015;61(5):1192–8.
3. Hiratzka LF, Bakris GL, Beckman JA, Bersin RM, Carr VF, Casey DE Jr, et al. 2010 ACCF/AHA/AATS/ACR/ASA/SCA/SCAI/SIR/STS/SVM guidelines for the diagnosis and management of patients with thoracic aortic disease: a report of the American College of Cardiology Foundation/American Heart Association task force on practice guidelines, American Association for Thoracic Surgery, American College of Radiology, American Stroke Association, Society of Cardiovascular Anesthesiologists, Society for Cardiovascular Angiography and Interventions, Society of Interventional Radiology, Society of Thoracic Surgeons, and Society for Vascular Medicine. Circulation. 2010;121(13):e266–369.

4. Kimura N, Itoh S, Yuri K, Adachi K, Matsumoto H, Yamaguchi A, et al. Reoperation for enlargement of the distal aorta after initial surgery for acute type a aortic dissection. J Thorac Cardiovasc Surg. 2015;149(2 Suppl):S91–8. e1
5. Jonker FH, Trimarchi S, Rampoldi V, Patel HJ, O'Gara P, Peterson MD, et al. Aortic expansion after acute type B aortic dissection. Ann Thorac Surg. 2012;94(4):1223–9.
6. Sueyoshi E, Sakamoto I, Hayashi K, Yamaguchi T, Imada T. Growth rate of aortic diameter in patients with type B aortic dissection during the chronic phase. Circulation. 2004;110(11 suppl 1):II-256–I-61.
7. Sailer AM, Nelemans PJ, Hastie TJ, Chin AS, Huininga M, Chiu P, et al. Prognostic significance of early aortic remodeling in acute uncomplicated type B aortic dissection and intramural hematoma. J Thorac Cardiovasc Surg. 2017;154(4):1192–200.
8. Cho KR, Stanson AW, Potter DD, Cherry KJ, Schaff HV, Sundt TM. Penetrating atherosclerotic ulcer of the descending thoracic aorta and arch. J Thorac Cardiov Sur. 2004;127(5):1393–401.
9. Ganaha F, Miller C, Sugimoto K, Do YS, Minamiguchi H, Saito H, et al. Prognosis of aortic intramural hematoma with and without penetrating atherosclerotic ulcer–a clinical and radiological analysis. Circulation. 2002;106(3):342–8.
10. Nathan DP, Boonn W, Lai E, Wang GJ, Desai N, Woo EY, et al. Presentation, complications, and natural history of penetrating atherosclerotic ulcer disease. J Vasc Surg. 2012;55(1):10–5.
11. Kitai T, Kaji S, Yamamuro A, Tani T, Kinoshita M, Ehara N, et al. Impact of new development of ulcer-like projection on clinical outcomes in patients with type B aortic dissection with closed and thrombosed false lumen. Circulation. 2010;122(11 Suppl):S74–80.
12. Evangelista A, Flachskampf FA, Erbel R, Antonini-Canterin F, Vlachopoulos C, Rocchi G, et al. Echocardiography in aortic diseases: EAE recommendations for clinical practice. Eur J Echocardiogr. 2010;11(8):645–58.
13. Goldstein SA, Evangelista A, Abbara S, Arai A, Asch FM, Badano LP, et al. Multimodality imaging of diseases of the thoracic aorta in adults: from the American Society of Echocardiography and the European Association of Cardiovascular Imaging: endorsed by the Society of Cardiovascular Computed Tomography and Society for cardiovascular magnetic resonance. J Am Soc Echocardiogr. 2015;28(2):119–82.
14. Plonek T, Berezowski M, Bochenek M, Filip G, Rylski B, Golesworthy T, et al. A comparison of aortic root measurements by echocardiography and computed tomography. J Thorac Cardiovasc Surg. 2019;157(2):479–86.
15. Blondheim DS, Vassilenko L, Glick Y, Asif A, Nachtigal A, Meisel SR, et al. Aortic dimensions by multi-detector computed tomography vs. echocardiography. J Cardiol. 2016;67(4):365–70.
16. Chaturvedi A, Oppenheimer D, Rajiah P, Kaproth-Joslin KA, Chaturvedi A. Contrast opacification on thoracic CT angiography: challenges and solutions. Insights Imaging. 2017;8(1):127–40.
17. Litmanovich D, Bankier AA, Cantin L, Raptopoulos V, Boiselle PM. CT and MRI in diseases of the aorta. AJR Am J Roentgenol. 2009;193(4):928–40.
18. Krishnam MS, Tomasian A, Malik S, Desphande V, Laub G, Ruehm SG. Image quality and diagnostic accuracy of unenhanced SSFP MR angiography compared with conventional contrast-enhanced MR angiography for the assessment of thoracic aortic diseases. Eur Radiol. 2010;20(6):1311–20.
19. von Knobelsdorff-Brenkenhoff F, Gruettner H, Trauzeddel RF, Greiser A, Schulz-Menger J. Comparison of native high-resolution 3D and contrast-enhanced MR angiography for assessing the thoracic aorta. Eur Heart J Cardiovasc Imaging. 2014;15(6):651–8.
20. Stankovic Z, Allen BD, Garcia J, Jarvis KB, Markl M. 4D flow imaging with MRI. Cardiovasc Diagn Ther. 2014;4(2):173–92.
21. Barrett JF, Keat N. Artifacts in CT: recognition and avoidance. Radiographics: a review publication of the Radiological Society of North America, Inc. 2004;24(6):1679–91.
22. Katsura M, Sato J, Akahane M, Kunimatsu A, Abe O. Current and novel techniques for metal artifact reduction at CT: practical guide for radiologists. Radiographics: a review publication of the Radiological Society of North America, Inc. 2018;38(2):450–61.

23. Kalisz K, Buethe J, Saboo SS, Abbara S, Halliburton S, Rajiah P. Artifacts at cardiac CT: physics and solutions. Radiographics: a review publication of the Radiological Society of North America, Inc. 2016;36(7):2064–83.
24. Habets J, Zandvoort HJ, Reitsma JB, Bartels LW, Moll FL, Leiner T, et al. Magnetic resonance imaging is more sensitive than computed tomography angiography for the detection of endoleaks after endovascular abdominal aortic aneurysm repair: a systematic review. Eur J Vasc Endovasc Surg. 2013;45(4):340–50.
25. Hendee WR, O'Connor MK. Radiation risks of medical imaging: separating fact from fantasy. Radiology. 2012;264(2):312–21.
26. Shuryak I, Sachs RK, Brenner DJ. A new view of radiation-induced cancer. Radiat Prot Dosim. 2011;143(2–4):358–64.
27. Pearce MS, Salotti JA, Little MP, McHugh K, Lee C, Kim KP, et al. Radiation exposure from CT scans in childhood and subsequent risk of leukaemia and brain tumours: a retrospective cohort study. Lancet. 2012;380(9840):499–505.
28. Lopez-Ruiz A, Chandrashekar K, Juncos LA. Changing paradigms in contrast nephropathy. J Am Soc Nephrol. 2017;28(2):397–9.
29. Beckett KR, Moriarity AK, Langer JM. Safe use of contrast media: what the radiologist needs to know. Radiographics: a review publication of the Radiological Society of North America, Inc. 2015;35(6):1738–50.
30. Gulani V, Calamante F, Shellock FG, Kanal E, Reeder SB. International Society for Magnetic Resonance in M. gadolinium deposition in the brain: summary of evidence and recommendations. Lancet Neurol. 2017;16(7):564–70.
31. Expert Panels on Vascular I, Interventional R, Bonci G, Steigner ML, Hanley M, Braun AR, et al. ACR appropriateness criteria((R)) thoracic aorta Interventional planning and follow-up. J Am Coll Radiol. 2017;14(11S):S570–S83.
32. Patterson BO, Cobb RJ, Karthikesalingam A, Holt PJ, Hinchliffe RJ, Loftus IM, et al. A systematic review of aortic remodeling after endovascular repair of type B aortic dissection: methods and outcomes. Ann Thorac Surg. 2014;97(2):588–95.
33. Kret MR, Azarbal AF, Mitchell EL, Liem TK, Landry GJ, Moneta GL. Compliance with long-term surveillance recommendations following endovascular aneurysm repair or type B aortic dissection. J Vasc Surg. 2013;58(1):25–31.
34. Golzarian J, Dussaussois L, Abada HT, Gevenois PA, Van Gansbeke D, Ferreira J, et al. Helical CT of aorta after endoluminal stent-graft therapy: value of biphasic acquisition. AJR Am J Roentgenol. 1998;171(2):329–31.
35. Zoli S, Trabattoni P, Dainese L, Annoni A, Saccu C, Fumagalli M, et al. Cumulative radiation exposure during thoracic endovascular aneurysm repair and subsequent follow-up. Eur J Cardiothorac Surg. 2012;42(2):254–9. Discussion 9–60
36. Rasche V, Oberhuber A, Trumpp S, Bornstedt A, Orend KH, Merkle N, et al. MRI assessment of thoracic stent grafts after emergency implantation in multi trauma patients: a feasibility study. Eur Radiol. 2011;21(7):1397–405.
37. Davies RR, Goldstein LJ, Coady MA, Tittle SL, Rizzo JA, Kopf GS, et al. Yearly rupture or dissection rates for thoracic aortic aneurysms: simple prediction based on size. Ann Thorac Surg. 2002;73(1):17–27. Discussion-8
38. Elefteriades JA, Farkas EA. Thoracic aortic aneurysm clinically pertinent controversies and uncertainties. J Am Coll Cardiol. 2010;55(9):841–57.
39. Quint LE, Liu PS, Booher AM, Watcharotone K, Myles JD. Proximal thoracic aortic diameter measurements at CT: repeatability and reproducibility according to measurement method. Int J Cardiovasc Imaging. 2013;29(2):479–88.
40. Lu TLC, Rizzo E, Marques-Vidal PM, von Segesser LK, Dehmeshki J, Qanadli SD. Variability of ascending aorta diameter measurements as assessed with electrocardiography-gated multidetector computerized tomography and computer assisted diagnosis software. Interact Cardiovasc Thorac Surg. 2010;10(2):217–21.

41. Asch FM, Yuriditsky E, Prakash SK, Roman MJ, Weinsaft JW, Weissman G, et al. The need for standardized methods for measuring the aorta: multimodality Core lab experience from the GenTAC registry. JACC Cardiovasc Imaging. 2016;9(3):219–26.
42. Burris NS, Patel HJ, Hope MD. Retrograde flow in the false lumen: marker of a false lumen under stress? J Thorac Cardiovasc Surg. 2019;157(2):488–91.
43. Bollache E, Barker AJ, Dolan RS, Carr JC, van Ooij P, Ahmadian R, et al. K-t accelerated aortic 4D flow MRI in under two minutes: feasibility and impact of resolution, k-space sampling patterns, and respiratory navigator gating on hemodynamic measurements. Magn Reson Med. 2018;79(1):195–207.
44. Lim RP, Winchester PA, Bruno MT, Xu J, Storey P, McGorty K, et al. Highly accelerated single breath-hold noncontrast thoracic MRA: evaluation in a clinical population. Investig Radiol. 2013;48(3):145–51.
45. Burris NS, Hoff BA, Kazerooni EA, Ross BD. Vascular deformation mapping (VDM) of thoracic aortic enlargement in aneurysmal disease and dissection. Tomography. 2017;3(3):163–73.
46. Kovacs T, Cattin P, Alkadhi H, Wildermuth S, Szekely G. Automatic segmentation of the aortic dissection membrane from 3D CTA images. Lect Notes Comput Sc. 2006;4091:317–24.

Part III
Treatment of Acute Thoracic Aortic Syndromes

Blunt Traumatic Aortic Injury: Etiology, Diagnosis, and Management

Bruce L. Tjaden and Anthony L. Estrera

History

The first report of a BTAI is widely attributed to Andreas Vesalius in 1557. However, this is factually incorrect. The case was first brought to Vesalius' attention in 1555, and it was not until 1609 when a report by Dr. Adolph Occo III (a friend and colleague of Vesalius) was posthumously published describing the situation in detail.

While references to this famous injury abound, finding the actual text of the case report can be challenging, due to its age. Thankfully, Drs. Suy and Fourneau of the University of Leuven in Belgium recently provided an excellent English translation of Dr. Occo III's "Famous Case of an Aneurysm," which is reproduced here with permission:

> Leonard Welser, a gentleman of Augsburg, [had] sustained a violent concussion when handling an agitated horse. He became ill with pertinent sickness, whose principal symptom was excruciating pain in the dorsal region. He failed to respond to any of the medicines proposed by his physicians, and so the advice of Vesalius from Belgium, who then taught anatomy, was sought. This illustrious man instantly recognised the symptoms of an aortic aneurysm, which he predicted would be fatal. Immediately on discovering a small pulsating tumour under the dorsal spine, he declared it to be an aneurysm caused by dilation of the aorta.
>
> Given that this resulted from a concussion, it was incurable. He also stated that he had seen such a disease in the neck, the chest, the popliteal space, and the arm, and that it always was associated with excruciating pain, and at the end, sideration [gangrene]. [Vesalius stated that] this condition is incurable unless it is possible to remove it, and that these aneurysms frequently contain a concrete fluid resembling ice or the crystalline humour, sometimes coagulated blood, or a polypous substance. [He also stated that] while alive, the aneurysmal blood remains fluid, but that is black and sidareted [sic] after death, [and that the] patient dies suffering from exquisite pain, [and that] sometimes these vascular

B. L. Tjaden · A. L. Estrera (✉)
Department of Cardiothoracic and Vascular Surgery, McGovern Medical School at The University of Texas Health Science Center at Houston (UTHealth), Houston, TX, USA
e-mail: Anthony.L.Estrera@uth.tmc.edu

J. S. Coselli et al. (eds.), *Aortic Dissection and Acute Aortic Syndromes*,
https://doi.org/10.1007/978-3-030-66668-2_14

> dilatations form spontaneously, sometimes they are the results of an external cause, as in the present case. Two years after the consultation, the patient finally ran out of patience in the face of this pain, which had resisted all medical treatment. [The patient] ultimately threw himself into the hands of an empiric [a charlatan], who administered certain catapotia [internal remedies], the use of which was soon followed by expectoration of blood, causing the patient to choke on his own blood, resulting in sudden death on June 25, 1557. From the section of the body we found, as predicted by Vesalius, a very large, cavernous, fleshy, tumour protruding from the aorta, which was the source of the pain and the pulsations in the back. As predicted by Vesalius, the good man died from this incurable disease [1].

While most patients with BTAI injuries now sustain their injury in motor vehicle accidents rather than equestrian misadventures, this famous first account of the pathology sheds light on the timeless features of aortic trauma.

Epidemiology and Terminology

In general, penetrating trauma has accounted for the majority of historic aortic injuries (83% in one large trauma registry [2].) However, due to the predominance of blunt traumatic mechanisms—along with the survivability of BTAI—most traumatic aortic injuries that surgeons encounter will be BTAI.

The vast majority of these BTAI involve the descending thoracic aorta [2]. This has the potential to lead to confusion, as blunt *traumatic* aortic injury (which can also include the abdominal aorta) and blunt *thoracic* aortic injury have both been abbreviated BTAI. Authors have historically used these terms interchangeably in the literature because, again, they are epidemiologically nearly synonymous. In light of that, we will not draw distinctions in our review of the literature between the two concepts. In our text, we will use the abbreviation BTAI to mean blunt *thoracic* aortic injury, exclusive of abdominal injury.

Motor vehicle crashes account for the largest subset of BTAI cases [3]. While BTAI are infrequent overall (incidence <0.5% of trauma patients in our registry [4]), they carry a high mortality risk. They are the second-most common cause of blunt traumatic fatalities [3]. In fact, nearly one-third of blunt trauma-related deaths were associated with BTAI on in an autopsy study [5].

As trauma patients are younger on average than most other patients suffering from acute aortic syndromes, it should come as no surprise that most patients with BTAI are young. One 18-year institutional review found an average age of 38 years [6]. This has implications for device selection and treatment strategies [7], and will be discussed later.

Diagnosis: Physical Exam and Imaging Modality

Physical exam is not reliable in ruling in or ruling out BTAI [8]. For this reason, virtually all patients with BTAI will be diagnosed by virtue of imaging. A widened mediastinum on chest x-ray (CXR) may be present, though in isolation, this finding is not particularly useful. Even when considering multiple radiographic findings in aggregate, CXR is not an adequate test for diagnosing BTAI [9], and has been shown to have a sensitivity as low as 41% [10]. A multicenter study found that the constellation of several CXR findings, *in addition to other organ injury and clinical criteria* ("widened mediastinum, hypotension less than 90 mmHg, long bone fracture, pulmonary contusion, left scapula fracture, hemothorax, and pelvic fracture") could be used to diagnose BTAI with a sensitivity of 92% and specificity of 85% [11].

As early as 1996, contrast-enhanced CT of the chest was found to be 97% sensitive and 99.8% specific for BTAI [12]. Over the ensuing decade, from 1997–2007, there was a fundamental shift in the diagnosis of BTAI [13]. CT has become the new gold standard for identifying this injury, and is the modality according to which most diagnostic and treatment decisions are made [13]. Recent work also supports the adequacy of CT with venous contrast instead of formal CT angiography (CTA) in diagnosing BTAI [14]. CT allows for excellent visualization of the injury in axial, coronal, and parasagittal projections, as well as 3D reconstruction of the injury and accurate measurements of the aortic diameter and lengths along centerline, greater curve, and lesser curve using specialized software. (Fig. 1).

If the diagnosis of BTAI is equivocal, adjunctive tests can be performed to rule aortic injury in or out. When comparing CTA, angiogram, and IVUS, IVUS has been shown to be the least equivocal in cases of BTAI [15]. One observational study suggested that IVUS has a sensitivity of 91.7% and specificity of 100% for BTAI. The same publication found transesophageal echocardiography (TEE) to have a 60% sensitivity and 66.7% specificity [16].

BTAI most often occurs in the proximal descending thoracic aorta at the level of the aortic isthmus, but concomitant injury in other locations, such as the ascending, arch, and distal descending thoracic aorta, may be present as well. The adoption of the Ishimaru zones of the aorta may be used in order to more accurately categorize the location of BTAI [17]. According to this schema, the common locations of BTAI would be classified as zone 2 and 3 [7].

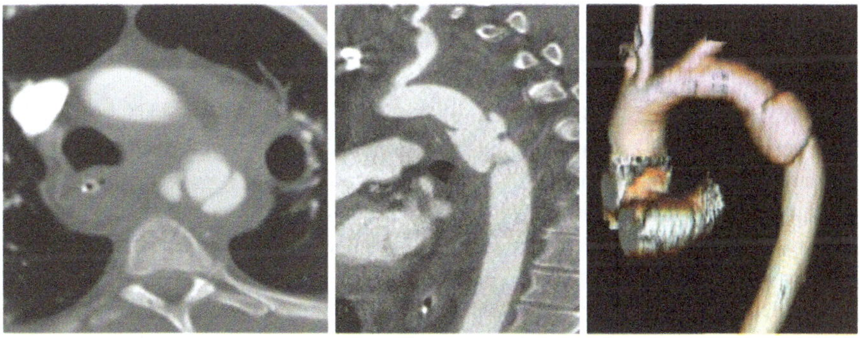

Fig. 1 From left: Axial, parasagittal, and reconstructed images from a computed tomographic angiogram of the chest, demonstrating a severe (Grade IV) blunt thoracic aortic injury

Due to the relative rarity of more proximal aortic injuries, they will not be extensively discussed in this chapter. In the near future, endovascular options for treating these proximal injuries will be available. Currently, however, options are limited to open reconstruction (often using cardiopulmonary bypass) or off-label uses of commercially available endovascular devices.

Diagnosis: Grading

BTAI are commonly classified on a grading scale ranging from I-IV. This grading system was first proposed by Azizzadeh et al. in 2009 [18] and, subsequently, adopted in the 2011 Society for Vascular Surgery (SVS) clinical practice guidelines [19]. Grade I injuries consist of an intimal flap. Grade II injuries are defined as intramural hematoma (IMH), though we also include formal "double-barrel" dissection in this category. Grade III injuries are pseudoaneurysms, identified by a contour abnormality of the outer wall of the aorta. Grade IV injuries include total aortic transections or ruptures. (Fig. 2).

This grading system is not simply a framework for the academic discussion of these injuries—it has been shown to correlate with real-world outcomes. Furthermore, stratification by grades can help to determine when and if intervention is needed [20, 21].

Management: Decision Making

Evaluation and management of a patient with a BTAI almost never occurs in isolation. The traumatic forces required to injure the thoracic aorta are so strong that polytrauma is the rule, rather than the exception. Therefore, the management of each patient with BTAI must be individualized, taking into account the competing priorities of other injuries.

The SVS has issued guidelines for the management of BTAI [19], though it should be noted that the evidence in support of these guidelines is limited and, as such, this document provides only Grade 2 (weak) "suggestions," not "recommendations."

In summary, the SVS suggests that Grade I injuries should be managed nonoperatively with serial imaging. For injuries Grade II-IV, urgent/emergent thoracic endovascular repair (TEVAR) is suggested with several specific technical considerations: general anesthesia, no routine spinal drainage, open femoral exposure, routine low dose heparinization, and selective revascularization of the left subclavian artery (LSA) [19].

Further discussion of the specifics of medical management, as well as endovascular and open surgery, will follow in the subsequent sections.

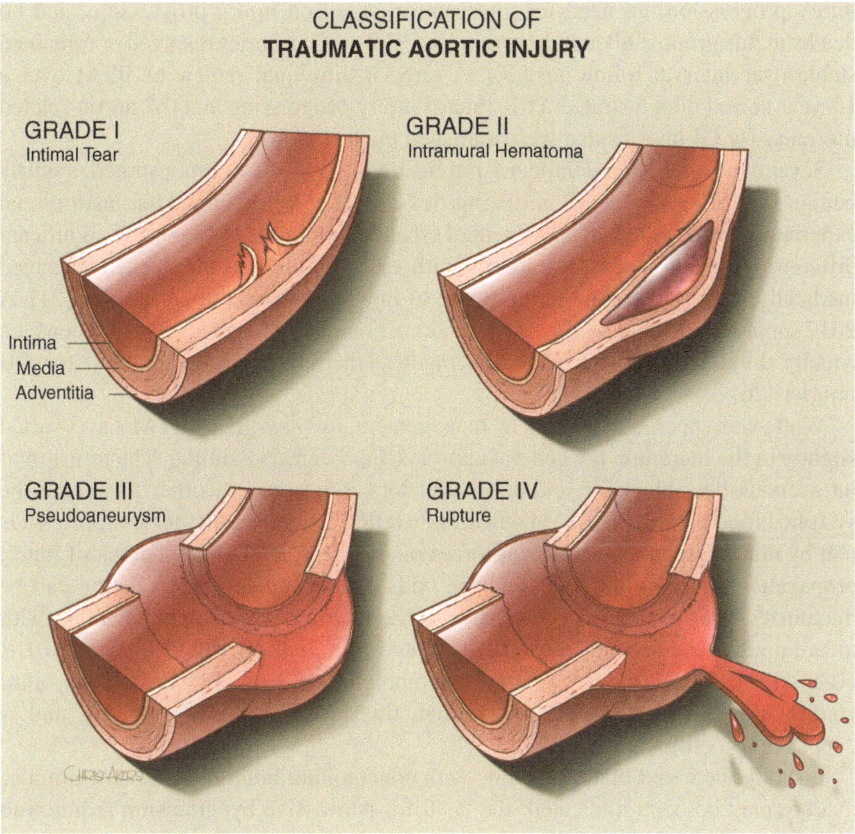

Fig. 2 Grading system for blunt traumatic aortic injuries

Management: Medical

For nearly two decades, nonoperative management of BTAI with intimal disruption alone (GI) has been considered the standard of care. Until recently, however, this principle has been supported by relatively little data. In 2001, Malhotra et al. wrote that that "[GI] injuries heal spontaneously and, hence, may be managed nonoperatively." [22] This conclusion was based on only 6 patients who underwent surveillance scanning after nonoperative management, in which 3 developed small pseudoaneurysms. The series reported by Azizzadeh et al. from Houston demonstrated no deaths in 10 patients with GI injury who were managed medically [18]. In a later publication from the same institution, follow-up CTA performed 4–6 weeks after injury demonstrated complete aortic healing in 5 patients with GI injuries who were managed nonoperatively [15].

Recently, larger series have proven the safety of nonoperative management. Osgood et al. published a series of 46 GI BTAI [23]. They found only a 5% rate of injury progression, no need for intervention based on injury progression, and no deaths in this group. Other authors reported 91% of GI injuries resolved or remained stable over interval follow up [20]. A large institutional review of BTAI over a 15-year period demonstrated a 0% rate of injury progression and 0% aortic-related mortality for GI injuries that were managed medically [24].

Several of these more modern publications have also demonstrated a fairly benign natural history of GII aortic injuries [23–25]. We examined our institutional experience with medical management of GI and GII injuries and found no significant differences in outcomes for patients with either grade of injury when managed medically—other than a more rapid rate of injury resolution in GI injuries [21]. A 2017 survey carried out by the Aortic Trauma Foundation revealed that surgeons are equally divided as to whether or not medical therapy or TEVAR is best for GII injuries [26].

While the specifics of medical management for low-grade BTAI have varied slightly in the literature, the general approach has been very similar. The infusion of intravenous beta blockade and/or vasodilators is initiated in order to reduce the systolic blood pressure (SBP) and heart rate (HR). The rationale for this approach is that by minimizing the mechanical forces on the disrupted intima, the risk of injury propagation can be minimized and the odds of healing/aortic remodeling can be maximized. Our institutional practice is to begin with an infusion of labetalol (with nicardipine as the second-line agent), titrated to a goal of SBP 100–120 and HR 60–90 [21]. In addition, we often recommend 81 mg of aspirin daily until confirmation of injury resolution, though this practice is more variable and is dependent on other injuries.

It should be noted that in patients with concomitant brain injuries, anti-impulse therapy may be contraindicated: the need for permissive hypertension required to optimally perfuse the injured brain may preclude the relative hypotension required for aortic protection. In this case, a joint decision should be made with the trauma and neurosurgical teams in order to agree on acceptable hemodynamic parameters. Rarely, this may require repair of a low-grade aortic injury in order to allow for increased blood pressure.

Interval imaging is needed for patients undergoing medical management of GI or GII aortic injuries, as some injuries can progress to higher grades of injury with time. It is our practice to obtain a repeat CTA after 7–10 days, with further imaging surveillance at 1-, 6-, and 12-month intervals thereafter if the lesion persists [21].

Management: Surgical: Endovascular Rationale, Changing Practice Patterns

Historically, there has been little question that higher grades of aortic injuries (GIII/GIV) benefit from repair to reduce the risk of death. However, in the pre-endovascular era, open repair of BTAI was plagued by high rates of complications and mortalities.

A meta-analysis of open repairs reported paraplegia rates of 9.9% and mortality rates of 21.3% [27]. Even in more modern series, open repair was associated with a 17% mortality rate [28].

TEVAR for BTAI has been associated with significantly decreased morbidity and mortality when compared to open repair, with some centers reporting paraplegia rates and operative mortality rates of 0% [28, 29]. In addition, the overall rate of major complications and length of stay is shorter with TEVAR [30].

In light of these benefits, it should come as no surprise that TEVAR has rapidly supplanted open repair in the treatment of BTAI [30–32]. The utilization of TEVAR in the treatment of BTAI at a large volume center is illustrated in the figure from Fortuna et al.'s 2016 publication (Fig. 3) [24].

Management: Surgical: Endovascular, Technical Considerations

The SVS clinical practice guidelines provide suggestions in regard to technical steps for TEVAR to treat BTAI, as described above. Our institutional practice varies slightly from this document, and is described below.

1. *Timing of Repair*
   (a) For GIII injuries (or particularly large/ominous GII injuries), we generally perform TEVAR within 48 hours.
   (b) For GIV injuries, we generally perform TEVAR within 24 hours.

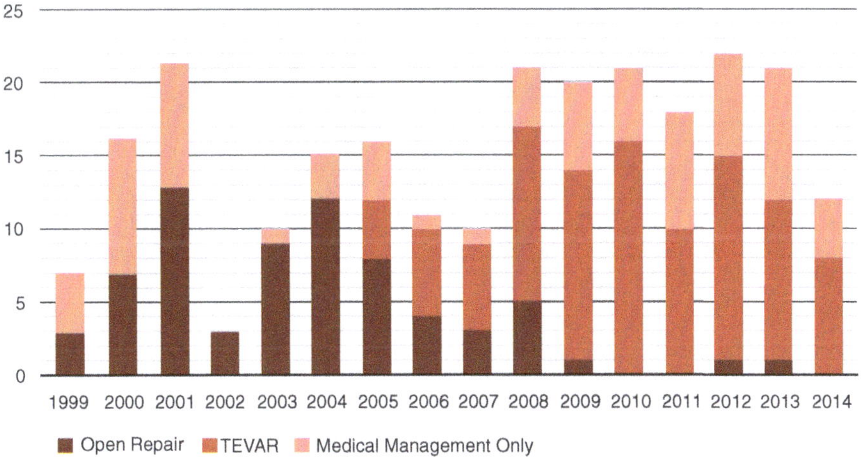

Fig. 3 Utilization of open repair vs. thoracic endovascular aortic repair (TEVAR) at a large-volume center over a 15-year period. This illustrates a dramatic reduction in the number of open repairs with the advent of endovascular options

2. *Preoperative Considerations*

   (a) Preoperative lumbar drains are not placed. This is because only a short segment of aortic coverage is usually required [7], allowing for the use of a single, 10-cm device in most cases—and the risk of spinal paraplegia is very low in historical cohorts of trauma patients treated with TEVAR without drainage [19].
   (b) Decisions regarding intraoperative heparinization are made before the operation in conjunction with our trauma surgery and neurosurgery colleagues.
   (c) Endografts are selected to achieve 5–10% oversizing relative to the native aorta. Trauma patients tend to be young with fairly normal aortas, and the average aortic diameter in BTAI cases is 24 mm [7].
   (d) When considering a BTAI patient for TEVAR, we are willing to accept shorter proximal seal zones. Ideally, we would still like at least 1 cm of healthy aorta proximal to the tear to achieve endograft wall apposition. This is possible in the majority of cases (Fig. 4), as the tear is, on average, 1.6 cm distal to the LSA [7]. However, we usually approach these cases with the philosophy that *any* proximal seal zone is adequate—i.e., we will be satisfied if the entry tear can be covered without the endograft slipping into the tear itself. This is because, unlike aneurysmal disease, there is little concern for impending aortic degeneration and loss of seal or fixation.
   (e) If the tear encroaches on the LSA and the ability to achieve seal distal to it is questionable, care should be taken to preoperatively identify the absolute

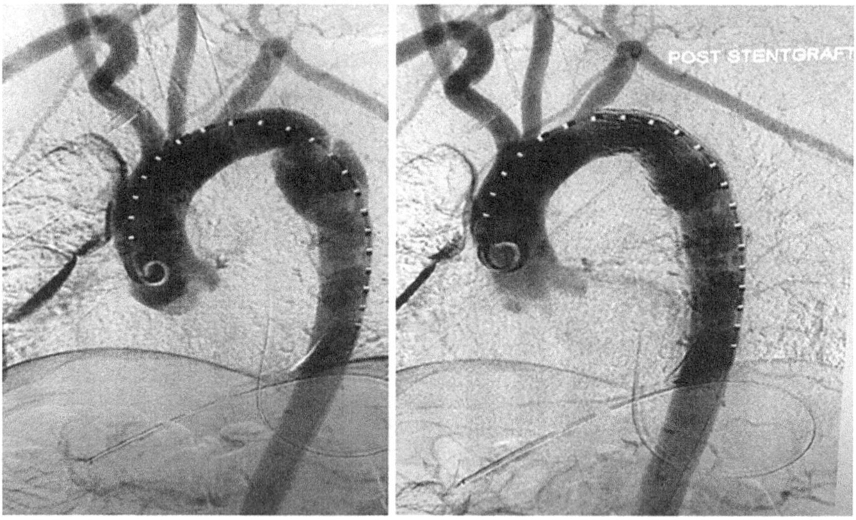

Fig. 4 Left: Initial angiogram of a Grade IV blunt thoracic injury (the same injury as pictured in Fig. 1) demonstrating typical anatomy, with a generous potential seal-zone distal to the left subclavian artery. Right: Completion angiogram showing exclusion of the injury without evidence of endoleak

contraindications to LSA coverage without revascularization. These include: a left vertebral artery that terminates in a posterior inferior cerebellar artery (PICA); a previous coronary artery bypass using a left internal mammary artery; an absent, atretic, or occluded right vertebral artery; or a functional left arm hemodialysis access.

3. *Intraoperative Specifics*

(a) A unilateral percutaneous approach is usually employed, with contralateral access obtained, if needed. Percutaneous TEVAR for BTAI has been shown to be feasible with very low rates of complications [33]. In our experience, we found that the lack of calcific femoral disease in most young trauma patients renders percutaneous access straightforward and safe in almost all cases of BTAI.

- Ultrasound guidance is mandatory [34].
- After securing access with a 5 French (Fr) sheath, the arteriotomy is "pre-closed" using two ProGlide® devices (Abbott, Abbott Park, IL). The femoral artery is then plugged with an 8Fr sheath, which will facilitate diagnostic angiography and/or IVUS.
- If heparinization is planned, it is initiated at the time of 8Fr sheath placement.

(b) A floppy guidewire and marker flush catheter are used for initial angiography. A wire exchange for a stiff wire (e.g. a Lunderquist® wire [Cook Medical, Bloomington, IN]) is performed.
(c) IVUS is used selectively. If adequate CT imaging is available to size the endograft, then IVUS is not usually employed. However, if the aortic diameter or the area requiring coverage is questionable, then IVUS is performed.
(d) The endograft is delivered and positioned over the stiff wire. If the stiff wire and/or device appear to displace the aorta relative to its initial angiographic position, an additional angiogram should be obtained with the device in place in order to ensure appropriate positioning. This can be performed either via a "buddy" catheter through the ipsilateral groin, or through contralateral femoral access.
(e) In the absence of absolute contraindications, coverage of the LSA will be performed, if necessary, to exclude the injury. This has been shown to be associated with low rates of complications in cases of BTAI [19, 35–37].
(f) After device deployment, completion angiography is performed. Percutaneous hemostasis is achieved via the previously placed ProGlide® devices and protamine administration. Rarely, adjunctive techniques for hemostasis may be needed, such as creation of a Rummel-type tourniquet, with or without topical thrombin [38]. (Fig. 5)

4. *Postoperative Management*

(a) Patients are cared for postoperatively in a critical care unit to be monitored for extremity ischemia or neurologic deficits.

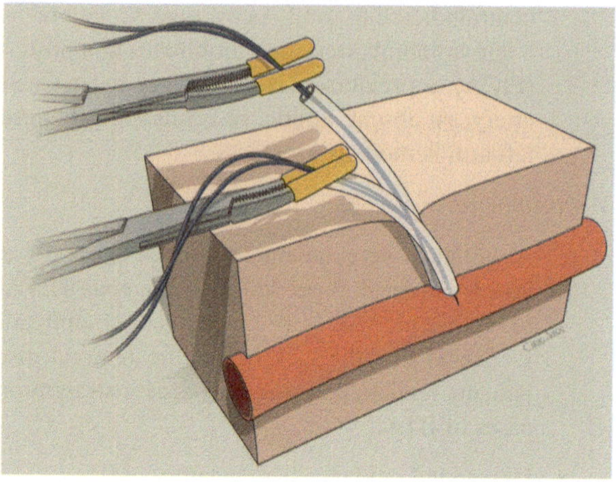

Fig. 5 Illustration of the ProGlide® Rumel tourniquet technique, an effective adjunct for achieving hemostasis after percutaneous TEVAR

(b) Anti-impulse therapy is discontinued after TEVAR.
(c) In the event of symptomatic and ongoing ischemia after LSA coverage (ischemic rest pain, claudication, spinal ischemia), left subclavian revascularization is performed via subclavian-to-carotid transposition or carotid-subclavian bypass [19].

In the near future, branched thoracic endografts will be commercially available, providing options for treatment of more proximal injuries (Fig. 6) while still preserving flow into the arch vessels. The Gore Thoracic Branched Endograft (TBE) (W.L. Gore & Associates, Flagstaff, AZ) is a single-branch thoracic endograft currently in clinical trials. It is based on the Conformable Thoracic Aortic Graft (CTAG), and contains a single internal portal oriented in a caudal direction. We have found that implantation of the TBE is expedited and simplified by first obtaining through-and-through (body floss) wire access through the groin and the left arm (Fig. 7). Prior to transfemoral delivery of the device, it is pre-cannulated with the main body device loaded on a stiff aortic wire and the second through-and-through wire through the portal. The main body device is delivered into the thoracic aorta (with care taken to ensure no wire-wrap). (Fig. 8) The main body is deployed, and a purpose-built side branch endograft is then delivered transfemorally over this second wire and positioned to bridge from the portal into the desired branch vessel (Figs. 9 and 10). At our institution, we have used this device on trial many times to treat a variety of pathologies, and find it well-suited to some trauma cases.

Management: Surgical—Open

Since the introduction of TEVAR, open surgical repair of BTAI has been supplanted by endovascular repair. However, in rare circumstances, open repair might be necessary. For example, a natural disaster or mass casualty incident could make it

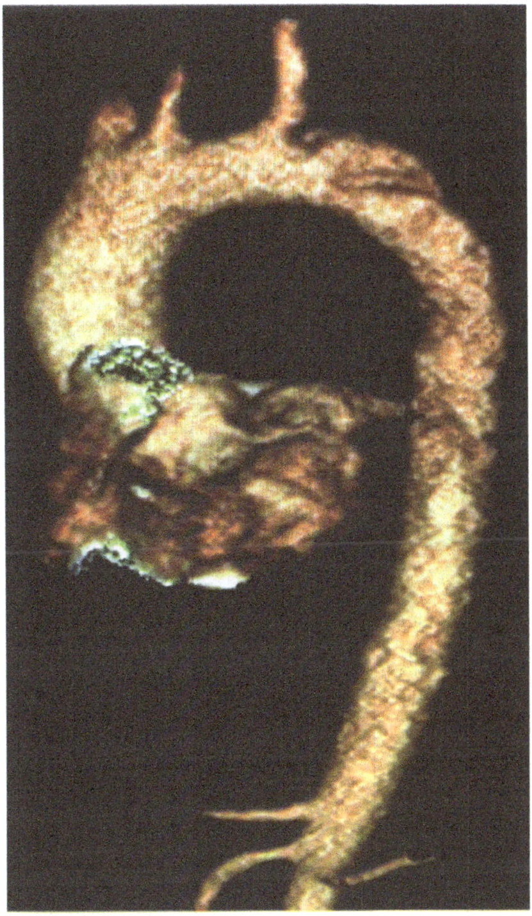

Fig. 6 A reconstructed parasagittal view of the thoracic aorta demonstrating a proximal Grade III blunt thoracic aortic injury encroaching on the left subclavian artery

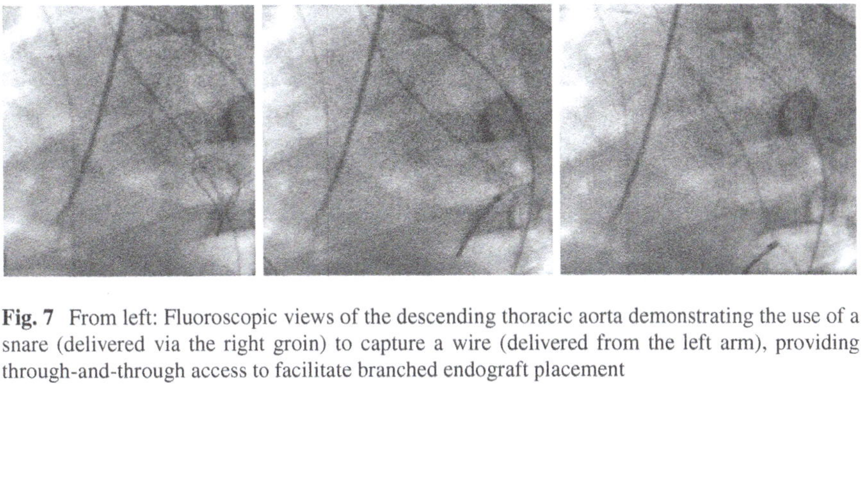

Fig. 7 From left: Fluoroscopic views of the descending thoracic aorta demonstrating the use of a snare (delivered via the right groin) to capture a wire (delivered from the left arm), providing through-and-through access to facilitate branched endograft placement

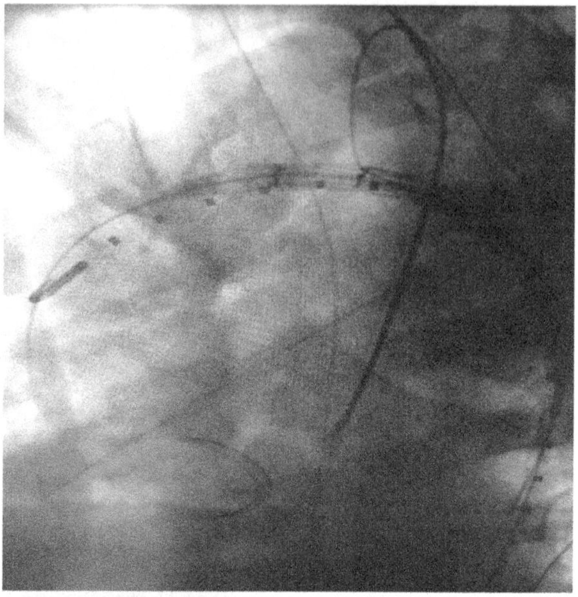

Fig. 8 Fluoroscopic view of the thoracic aorta demonstrating the main body of the thoracic branched device being positioned in the distal arch/proximal descending aorta. The through-and-through wire exits the left arm and right groin, and is used to pre-cannulate the portal of the device prior to inserting it into the body

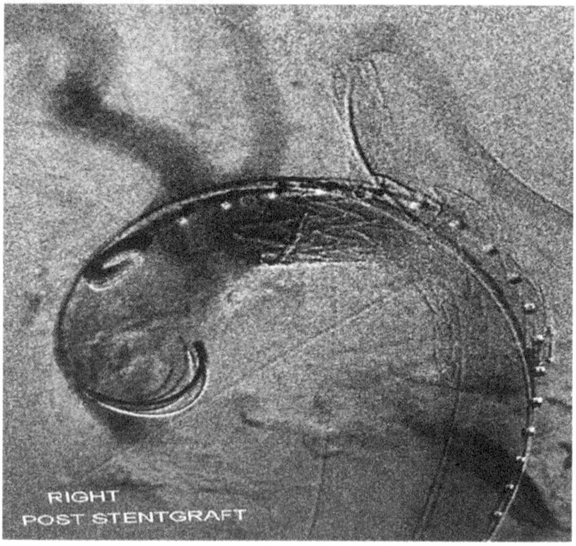

Fig. 9 Completion angiogram after treatment of the blunt thoracic aortic injury using a thoracic branched device

difficult or impossible to obtain an appropriate thoracic endograft for endovascular treatment. Open repair of BTAI is challenging—and should ideally be undertaken by surgeons experienced in open thoracic aortic repair.

Open repair should be performed using a dual-lumen endotracheal tube with single-lung ventilation. The patient should be positioned in the right lateral decubitus position in preparation for a left lateral thoracotomy. Partial left heart bypass is

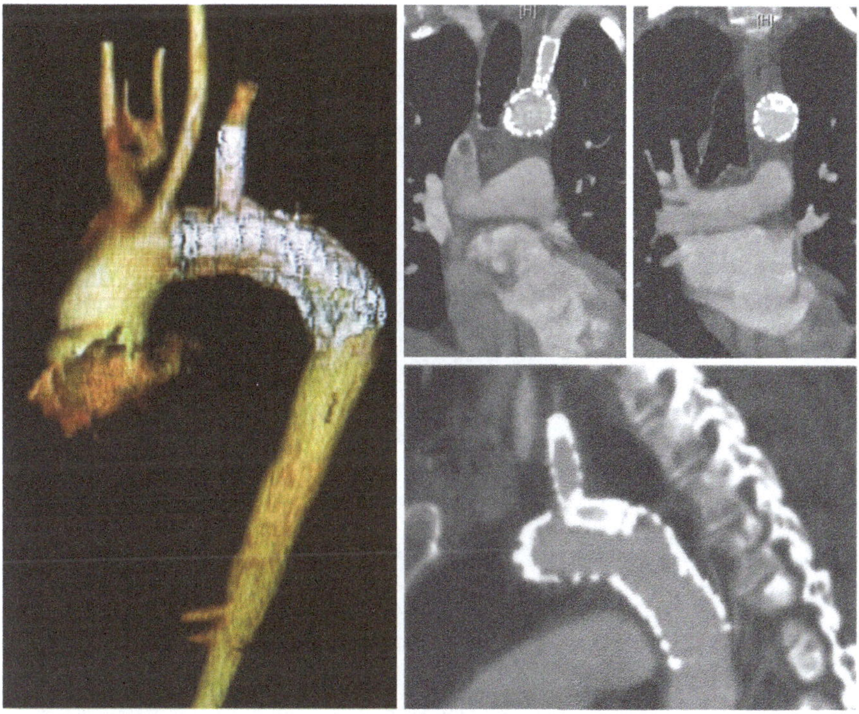

Fig. 10 A selection of images from a CTA of the chest obtained 3 months after treatment of a blunt thoracic aortic injury with a branched endograft. These images demonstrate excellent aortic remodeling and no endoleak

initiated by cannulating the left inferior pulmonary vein for venous drainage and the left common femoral artery or distal thoracic aorta for arterial return. Once the patient is heparinized and partial left heart bypass is initiated, proximal control is obtained by clamping the aorta in zone 2, just proximal to the LSA, and using a separate clamp on the proximal LSA. This is performed because the tear often encroaches on the origin of the LSA. Distal control is easily obtained on the aorta just proximal to the arterial in-flow cannulation site. The aorta is opened (Fig. 11) and the segment involved is replaced using an appropriately sized Dacron graft (Fig. 12). Chest tubes are placed prior to closure [39].

Surveillance

Patients treated for BTAI with open repair may not need dedicated thoracic imaging in the future, unless there is concern for graft contamination or infection due to other associated injuries within the chest. On the other hand, patients treated with TEVAR require surveillance to identify potential endograft complications, such as

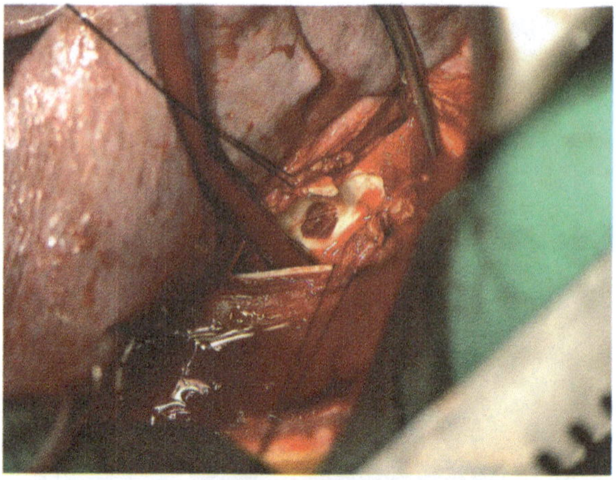

Fig. 11 Intraoperative photograph after the descending thoracic aorta has been clamped and opened, showing a Grade III blunt traumatic aortic injury from inside of the aortic lumen

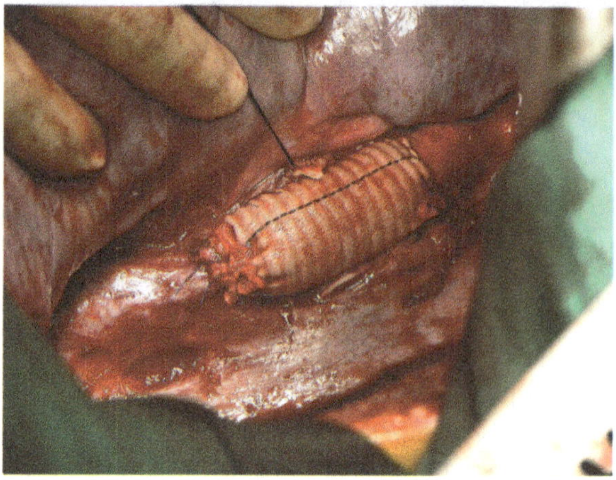

Fig. 12 Dacron replacement of the injured segment of the descending thoracic aorta

migration, kinking, or thrombosis. In general, we obtain a CTA of the chest post-TEVAR at 1 month, 6 months, 12 months, and yearly thereafter. If there are any doubts about the integrity of the aorta outside of the area of endograft coverage (for example, periaortic hematoma or intramural hematoma extending into the distal thoracic aorta beyond the TEVAR), earlier imaging may be indicated.DisclosuresDr. Estrera is a consultant for W.L. Gore. Dr. Tjaden has no disclosures.

References

1. Suy R, Fourneau I. Vesalius' experience with aortic aneurysms. Acta Chir Belg. 2015;115(1):91–5.
2. Mattox KL, Feliciano DV, Burch J, Beall ACJ, Jordan GLJ, DeBakey ME. Five thousand seven hundred sixty cardiovascular injuries in 4459 patients. Epidemiologic evolution 1958 to 1987. Ann Surg. 1989 Jun;209(6):697–8.

3. Karmy-Jones R, Jurkovich GJ. Blunt chest trauma. Curr Probl Surg. 2004 Mar;41(3):211–380.
4. Estrera AL, Miller CC 3rd, Guajardo-Salinas G, Coogan S, Charlton-Ouw K, Safi HJ, et al. Update on blunt thoracic aortic injury: fifteen-year single-institution experience. J Thorac Cardiovasc Surg. 2013 Mar;145(3 Suppl):S154–8.
5. Teixeira PGR, Inaba K, Barmparas G, Georgiou C, Toms C, Noguchi TT, et al. Blunt thoracic aortic injuries: an autopsy study. J Trauma. 2011 Jan;70(1):197–202.
6. Malgor RD, Bilfinger TV, McCormack J, Shapiro MJ, Tassiopoulos AK. Trends in clinical presentation, management, and mortality of blunt aortic traumatic injury over an 18-year period. Vasc Endovasc Surg. 2013 Jan;47(1):19–23.
7. Rajani RR, Johnson LS, Brewer BL, Brewster LP, Duwayri Y, Reeves JG, et al. Anatomic characteristics of aortic transection: centerline analysis to facilitate graft selection. Ann Vasc Surg. 2014 Feb;28(2):433–6.
8. Sinclair DS. Traumatic aortic injury: an imaging review. Emerg Radiol. 2002 Mar;9(1):13–20.
9. Cook AD, Klein JS, Rogers FB, Osler TM, Shackford SR. Chest radiographs of limited utility in the diagnosis of blunt traumatic aortic laceration. J Trauma. 2001 May;50(5):843–7.
10. Gutierrez A, Inaba K, Siboni S, Effron Z, Haltmeier T, Jaffray P, et al. The utility of chest X-ray as a screening tool for blunt thoracic aortic injury. Injury. 2016 Jan;47(1):32–6.
11. Mosquera VX, Marini M, Muniz J, Asorey-Veiga V, Adrio-Nazar B, Boix R, et al. Traumatic aortic injury score (TRAINS): an easy and simple score for early detection of traumatic aortic injuries in major trauma patients with associated blunt chest trauma. Intensive Care Med. 2012 Sep;38(9):1487–96.
12. Mirvis SE, Shanmuganathan K, Miller BH, White CS, Turney SZ. Traumatic aortic injury: diagnosis with contrast-enhanced thoracic CT—five-year experience at a major trauma center. Radiology. 1996 Aug;200(2):413–22.
13. Demetriades D, Velmahos GC, Scalea TM, Jurkovich GJ, Karmy-Jones R, Teixeira PG, et al. Diagnosis and treatment of blunt thoracic aortic injuries: changing perspectives. J Trauma. 2008 Jun;64(6):1415–9.
14. Zaw AA, Stewart D, Murry JS, Hoang DM, Sun B, Ashrafian S, et al. CT chest with IV contrast compared with CT angiography after blunt trauma. Am Surg. 2016 Jan;82(1):41–5.
15. Azizzadeh A, Valdes J, Miller CC 3rd, Nguyen LL, Estrera AL, Charlton-Ouw K, et al. The utility of intravascular ultrasound compared to angiography in the diagnosis of blunt traumatic aortic injury. J Vasc Surg. 2011 Mar;53(3):608–14.
16. Patel NH, Hahn D, Comess KA. Blunt chest trauma victims: role of intravascular ultrasound and transesophageal echocardiography in cases of abnormal thoracic aortogram. J Trauma. 2003 Aug;55(2):330–7.
17. Mitchell RS, Ishimaru S, Ehrlich MP, Iwase T, Lauterjung L, Shimono T, et al. First international summit on thoracic aortic Endografting: roundtable on thoracic aortic dissection as an indication for endografting. J Endovasc Ther. 2002 Jun;9(Suppl 2):II98–105.
18. Azizzadeh A, Keyhani K, Miller CC, Coogan SM, Safi HJ, Estrera AL. Blunt traumatic aortic injury: initial experience with endovascular repair. J Vasc Surg. 2009;49(6):1403–8. https://doi.org/10.1016/j.jvs.2009.02.234.
19. Lee WA, Matsumura JS, Mitchell RS, Farber MA, Greenberg RK, Azizzadeh A, et al. Endovascular repair of traumatic thoracic aortic injury: clinical practice guidelines of the Society for Vascular Surgery. J Vasc Surg. 2011;53(1):187–92. https://doi.org/10.1016/j.jvs.2010.08.027.
20. Rabin J, DuBose J, Sliker CW, O'Connor JV, Scalea TM, Griffith BP. Parameters for successful nonoperative management of traumatic aortic injury. J Thorac Cardiovasc Surg. 2014;147(1):143–50. https://doi.org/10.1016/j.jtcvs.2013.08.053.
21. Sandhu HK, Leonard SD, Perlick A, Saqib NU, Miller CC 3rd, Charlton-Ouw KM, et al. Determinants and outcomes of nonoperative management for blunt traumatic aortic injuries. J Vasc Surg. 2018 Feb;67(2):389–98.
22. Malhotra AK, Fabian TC, Croce MA, Weiman DS, Gavant ML, Pate JW. Minimal aortic injury: a lesion associated with advancing diagnostic techniques. J Trauma. 2001 Dec;51(6):1042–8.
23. Osgood MJ, Heck JM, Rellinger EJ, Doran SL, Garrard CL, Guzman RJ, et al. Natural history of grade I-II blunt traumatic aortic injury. J Vasc Surg. 2014;59(2):334–42. https://doi.org/10.1016/j.jvs.2013.09.007.

24. Fortuna GR, Perlick A, DuBose JJ, Leake SS, Charlton-Ouw KM, Miller CC, et al. Injury grade is a predictor of aortic-related death among patients with blunt thoracic aortic injury. J Vasc Surg. 2016;63(5):1225–31. https://doi.org/10.1016/j.jvs.2015.11.046.
25. Spencer SM, Safcsak K, Smith CP, Cheatham ML, Bhullar IS. Nonoperative management rather than endovascular repair may be safe for grade II blunt traumatic aortic injuries: an 11-year retrospective analysis. J Trauma Acute Care Surg. 2018 Jan;84(1):133–8.
26. DeSoucy E, Loja M, DuBose J, Estrera A, Starnes B, Azizzadeh A. Contemporary Management of Blunt Thoracic Aortic Injury: results of an EAST, AAST and SVS survey by the aortic trauma foundation. J Endovasc Resusc Trauma Manag. 2017;1(1):4–8. Available from: https://www.jevtm.com/journal/index.php/jevtm/article/view/8/6
27. Von Oppell UO, Sa FCS, Dunne TT, De Groot MK, Frcs C, Zilla P. Traumatic aortic rupture: twenty-year Metaanalysis of mortality and risk of paraplegia. Ann Thorac Surg. 1994;58(2):585–93. https://doi.org/10.1016/0003-4975(94)92270-5.
28. Estrera AL, Gochnour DC, Azizzadeh A, Iii CCM, Coogan S, Charlton-ouw K, et al. ORIGINAL ARTICLES: ADULT CARDIAC ADULT CARDIAC SURGERY: Progress in the treatment of blunt thoracic aortic injury: 12-year single-institution experience. ATS. 2010;90(1):64–71. https://doi.org/10.1016/j.athoracsur.2010.03.053.
29. Li S, Cai W, Li X, Qiu J, Li Q, Shu C. Thoracic endovascular aortic repair for traumatic type B aortic dissection: a 5-year experience from a single center. Int Angiol. 2017 Aug;36(4):316–21.
30. Grigorian A, Spencer D, Donayre C, Nahmias J, Schubl S, Gabriel V, et al. National Trends of thoracic endovascular aortic repair versus open repair in blunt thoracic aortic injury. Ann Vasc Surg. 2018 Oct;52:72–8.
31. Scalea TM, Feliciano DV, DuBose JJ, Ottochian M, O'Connor JV, Morrison JJ. Blunt thoracic aortic injury: endovascular repair is now the standard. J Am Coll Surg. 2019 Apr;228(4):605–10.
32. Jonker FHW, Giacovelli JK, Muhs BE, Sosa JA, Indes JE. Trends and outcomes of endovascular and open treatment for traumatic thoracic aortic injury. J Vasc Surg. 2010;51(3):565–71. https://doi.org/10.1016/j.jvs.2009.10.046.
33. Brenner M, Teeter W, Hadud M, Hoehn M, O'Connor J, Stein D, et al. Long-term outcomes of thoracic endovascular aortic repair: a single institution's 11-year experience. J Trauma Acute Care Surg. 2017 Apr;82(4):687–93.
34. Sobolev M, Slovut DP, Lee Chang A, Shiloh AL, Eisen LA. Ultrasound-guided catheterization of the femoral artery: a systematic review and meta-analysis of randomized controlled trials. J Invasive Cardiol. 2015 Jul;27(7):318–23.
35. DuBose JJ, Leake SS, Brenner M, Pasley J, O'Callaghan T, Luo-Owen X, et al. Contemporary management and outcomes of blunt thoracic aortic injury: a multicenter retrospective study. J Trauma Acute Care Surg. 2015 Feb;78(2):360–9.
36. McBride CL, Dubose JJ, Miller CC 3rd, Perlick AP, Charlton-Ouw KM, Estrera AL, et al. Intentional left subclavian artery coverage during thoracic endovascular aortic repair for traumatic aortic injury. J Vasc Surg. 2015 Jan;61(1):73–9.
37. Matsumura JS, Lee WA, Mitchell RS, Farber MA, Murad MH, Lumsden AB, et al. The Society for Vascular Surgery Practice Guidelines: management of the left subclavian artery with thoracic endovascular aortic repair. J Vasc Surg. 2009 Nov;50(5):1155–8.
38. Furlough CL, Desai SS, Azizzadeh A. Adjunctive technique for the use of ProGlide vascular closure device to improve hemostasis. J Vasc Surg. 2014 Dec;60(6):1693–4.
39. Azizzadeh A, Keyhani K, Miller CC 3rd, Coogan SM, Safi HJ, Estrera AL. Blunt traumatic aortic injury: initial experience with endovascular repair. J Vasc Surg. 2009 Jun;49(6):1403–8.

Catheter-Induced Aortic Dissection

Hannah Chaudry, Marwan Saad, and J. Dawn Abbott

Terminology

Aortic dissection occurs when an injury to the intima, or innermost layer of the aorta, results in a tear, allowing blood to accumulate between the intimal and medial layers of the vessel wall. This split between the layers of the vessel wall results in a dissection flap separating a true and false lumen. Aortic dissection often occurs spontaneously in aortas that are dilated or in which the integrity of the media is compromised. They can also, however, occur in the setting of diagnostic or interventional procedures where a catheter or device manipulation results in injury to the intima with resultant bleeding into the vessel wall. Iatrogenic aortic dissection refers to an aortic dissection that results as a consequence or complication of invasive procedures such as a diagnostic cardiac catheterization, percutaneous coronary interventions (PCI), or cardiac surgery. Catheter-induced iatrogenic aortic dissections are those in which a coronary catheter is responsible for inducing the initial injury in the vessel wall and often occurs as an extension or propagation of a coronary artery dissection. In 2002, the International Registry of Aortic Dissection (IRAD) reported 34 cases of iatrogenic aortic dissections among 723 patients with aortic dissections in the registry at the time. Of these, 19 (2.6%) occurred after major surgery and 14 (2%) were catheter-derived following coronary angiography or intervention [1].

H. Chaudry · M. Saad · J. D. Abbott (✉)
Cardiovascular Institute, Warren Alpert Medical School, Brown University, Providence, RI, USA
e-mail: Jabbott@lifespan.org

J. S. Coselli et al. (eds.), *Aortic Dissection and Acute Aortic Syndromes*,
https://doi.org/10.1007/978-3-030-66668-2_15

Incidence

Catheter-induced aortic dissections are rare. The incidence has been reported at around 0.02–0.06% of all invasive cardiac procedures [2–5] with the incidence being higher in PCIs than diagnostic catheterizations (0.06 to 0.07% vs 0.008 to 0.02%, respectively) [6, 7]. One case series noted an even higher incidence of 0.12% following PCI as compared to 0.01% following diagnostic coronary angiography [4]. Iatrogenic aortic dissections also occur more frequently in the setting of urgent PCI for acute myocardial infarction (AMI) with an incidence of 0.19% [2] and following PCI for chronic total occlusions (CTO) with an incidence of as high as 1.9% [8].

Risk Factors

Previous studies have identified risk factors for iatrogenic catheter-induced aortic dissection; however, these are limited to case reports due to the rarity of the event. Clinical risk factors that have been described include older age, diabetes, hypertension, atherosclerotic burden, calcification of the aortic root as well as history of prior coronary artery bypass grafting [1, 4, 6]. Atherosclerosis is thought to predispose vessels to plaque ulceration when manipulated, which then serves as an entry site for blood flow between the layers of the vessel wall. This link between acute plaque rupture and inflammation may be a factor in the apparent increased susceptibility of patients with AMI to coronary dissection with propagation to the aorta [2]. Additionally, any condition resulting in weakness in the media of the vessel wall carries a higher risk of developing an aortic dissection in general, however, these have not necessarily been linked to the development of an iatrogenic aortic dissection in the current literature. This point highlights the differences in the pathophysiology between spontaneous aortic dissections and those that are iatrogenic and is also reflected in the difference in management strategies between these two conditions. The classic risk factors for spontaneous aortic dissections include; history of aortic aneurysm, Marfan syndrome, Ehlers-Danlos syndrome, bicuspid aortic valve, unicuspid valve as well as cystic medial necrosis [2]. The role of cystic medial necrosis is controversial since low grades of degeneration are non-specific and occur with advancing age [2, 9].

Several procedural characteristics have been associated with iatrogenic aortic dissection. These types of dissections have been noted to occur more frequently during coronary artery engagement (specifically the right coronary artery) and balloon dilation, where there is more risk of traumatic damage to the intima [3, 4]. Certain types of catheters (e.g., the Amplatz catheter) have also been reported in a disproportionate number of catheter-induced dissections [2–4]. In addition, over-vigorous hand injection of contrast is a potential contributing factor, and care must be taken to minimize further injection to prevent propagation once a dissection is identified [6]. Engagement of the right coronary artery (RCA), as well as treatment of chronic total occlusion (CTO), poses an increased risk for catheter-induced aortic dissection [2–4, 6]. In an IRAD report of 74 consecutive iatrogenic dissections, 97% occurred during engagement of a vessel with 57% being the RCA. The dissections were catheter induced in 92% of cases. It is unclear whether technical or anatomical differences between the RCA and left main coronary artery (LM) are responsible for this difference but it is proposed that the larger ostium of the LM, as well as the decreased angulation at which it is engaged, may decrease the risk of aortocoronary dissection.

Mechanism

Iatrogenic catheter-induced aortic dissection most often involves the ostium of a coronary artery and may extend variably in an antegrade or retrograde fashion. Few studies have reported isolated aortic dissection without coronary artery involvement [10, 11]. Antegrade aortic dissections usually occur with an entry point inside a coronary artery and extend in the same direction of blood flow in the true lumen. In contrast, retrograde dissections extend in the opposite direction to blood flow in the true lumen. Due to the fact that blood flow is pulsatile in the same direction as an antegrade dissection, these often remain patent for a longer period, while retrograde dissections usually seal off quicker due to the opposite nature of blood flow. Antegrade dissections can also propagate down coronary vessels resulting in acute vessel closure. Retrograde aortic dissections related to coronary injury can result from a traumatic injury of the coronary artery with the catheter itself or during balloon/stent inflation. Most retrograde iatrogenic aortic dissections originating from the coronary ostia remain limited to the coronary sinus or are confined to the ascending aorta (Stanford type A; DeBakey types 1 or 2) [2, 6, 7]. This is predominantly due to the anatomy of the sinus of Valsalva which has a high content of collagenous fibers near the aortic annulus and is bordered by the thickened supravalvular ridge [6]. Figure 1, *panel A* represents a case of right aortocoronary dissection extending to the aortic root and ascending aorta, as evident with contrast staining within the aortic wall; *panel B*: a coronary stent graft was used to seal the entry site with halting of the extension of the dissection in the same patient. Figure 2, *panel A* represents a second case of proximal RCA dissection from guide catheter manipulation; *panel B* demonstrates the dissection extending retrogradely to the aortic root; *panel C:* a drug-eluting stent was used to seal the dissection entry site; *panel D:* Near complete resolution of the contrast staining in the aortic wall with sealing the dissection entry site.

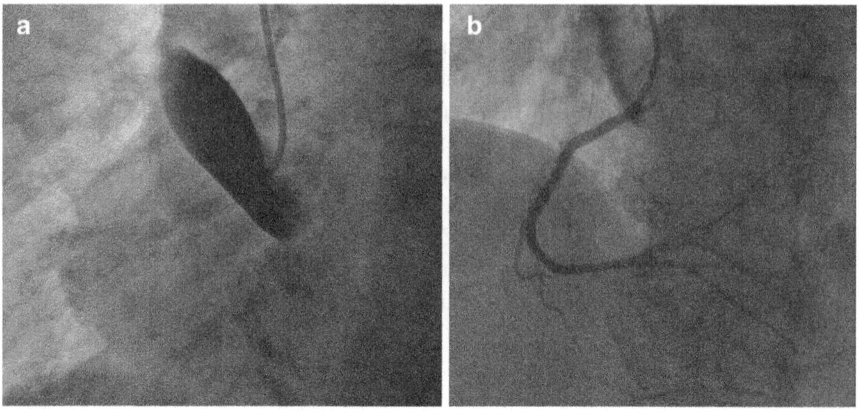

Fig. 1 (**a**) Iatrogenic aortic dissection caused by post-dilatation with non-compliant balloon after stent placement; (**b**) Sealing off the dissection entry using a JOMED® coronary graft stent

Clinical Presentation

The presenting signs and symptoms of iatrogenic aortic dissection vary from that of spontaneous aortic dissection [1]. Patients with iatrogenic aortic dissection are more likely to present with indolent hemodynamic instability, often with hypotension or shock. A review of 723 patients with aortic dissection from the IRAD database showed that patients with iatrogenic aortic dissection are less likely to present with abrupt symptoms (35% vs 87%) and more likely to have no chest or back pain (25% vs 1%) compared with those with spontaneous aortic dissection. Patients with iatrogenic aortic dissection were also more likely to have hypotension (30% vs 9%) and develop cardiac complications such as myocardial ischemia (36% vs 5%) or infarction (15% vs 3%). Aortic regurgitation was less frequent (11% vs 34%) and fewer patients with iatrogenic aortic dissections had a visualized intimal flap (46% vs 60%) or patent false lumen on imaging (48% vs 75%) compared with those with spontaneous aortic dissection.

Diagnosis

Catheter-induced aortic dissection is most often recognized on angiography during the index cardiac procedure, but often subsequently need to be evaluated with non-invasive imaging such as transesophageal echocardiogram (TEE), computed tomography/angiography (CT/CTA) or magnetic resonance imaging/angiography (MRI/MRA).

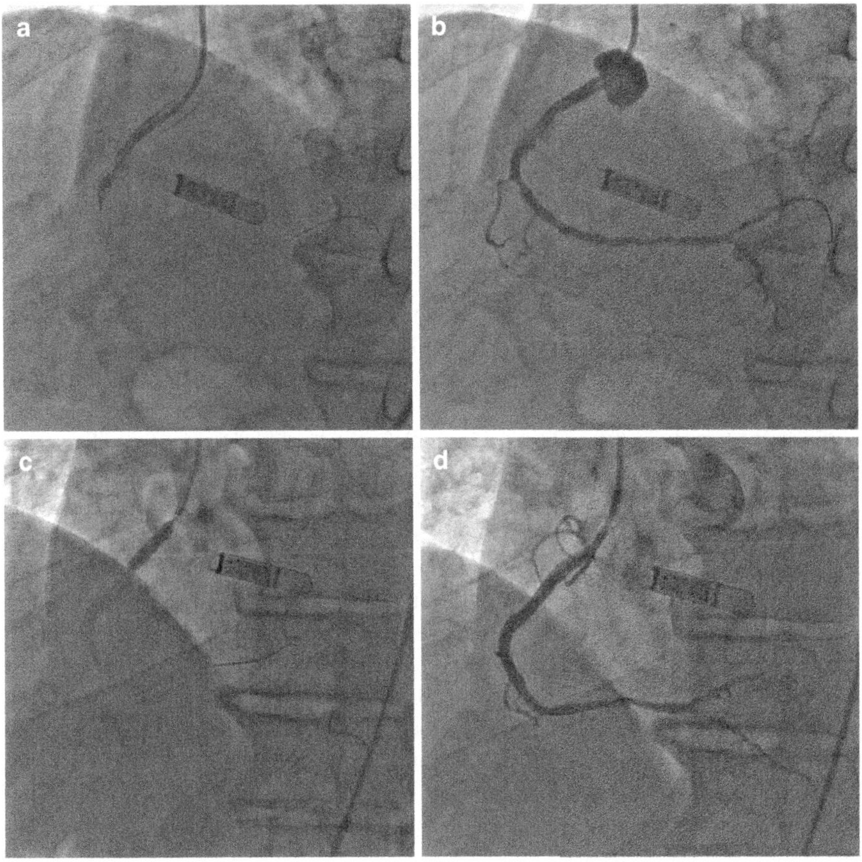

Fig. 2 (**a**) Proximal RCA dissection from guide catheter manipulation; (**b**) demonstrates the dissection extending retrogradely to the aortic root; (**c**) a drug-eluting stent was used to seal the dissection entry site; (**d**) Near complete resolution of the contrast staining in the aortic wall with sealing the dissection entry site

Coronary Angiography

Iatrogenic aortic dissection presents on coronary angiography as persistence of contrast dye staining around the aortic root (Figs. 1a and 2b). In 2000, Dunning et al. proposed a classification system (Table 1) for iatrogenic aortic dissections based on the extent of aortic involvement seen on coronary angiography. Class I includes dissections in which the contrast staining is limited to the ipsilateral coronary cusp; Class II, where contrast extends within 40 mm up the aortic wall; and Class III, where contrast extends to greater than 40 mm up the aortic wall [2]. While Classes I and II are typically medically managed or treated with stenting of the entry point; Class III dissections may necessitate immediate surgical intervention and are associated with higher mortality [2, 3].

Table 1 Dunning Classification

Dunning Class	Aortic Involvement
I	Dissection limited to ipsilateral cusp only
II	Dissection extending <40 mm up the aortic wall
III	Dissection extending >40 mm up the aortic wall

Non-invasive Imaging

Any aortic dissection with evidence of hemodynamic compromise should be evaluated with transthoracic echocardiogram (TTE) to evaluate for extension into the pericardium with pericardial effusion and to rule out cardiac tamponade. In addition, the aortic valve should be evaluated for acute aortic incompetence. TEE can be performed urgently in the catheterization laboratory to identify an aortic dissection flap and evaluate aortic valve function [12]. In most cases, following initial management, urgent imaging with CT or MRI should be performed to determine if there is any residual dissection, evaluate its extent, and for follow-up. There is no consensus as to which imaging technique is preferred. CT has the advantage of rapid, easy acquisition with high sensitivity and specificity, however, it exposes the patient to contrast dye and radiation. MRI, on the other hand, lacks exposure to radiation with high sensitivity and specificity but is time-consuming, and hence may be more suitable for long-term follow-up rather than during the acute situation [13, 14]. Both contrast and non-contrast CT imaging should be obtained in order to differentiate between retained contrast from cardiac catheterization vs contrast from CT scan. Fig. 3: Computed tomography of the chest without contrast in a patient with catheter-induced aortic dissection from RCA percutaneous intervention revealing contrast staining in the aortic wall in relation to RCA (arrows).

Management

Given the rarity of catheter-induced iatrogenic aortic dissection, there are no randomized trials to guide appropriate therapy or inform prognosis. Therefore, most treatment decisions are based on data from previously published care reports and case series of iatrogenic aortic dissections.

Although most spontaneous Stanford type A aortic dissections are treated surgically, several case reports have demonstrated that iatrogenic aortic dissections can be successfully treated by quick sealing of the entry point of the dissection within the coronary vessel [1–4, 7, 15].

Several factors affect management strategies when addressing catheter-induced iatrogenic aortic dissections. These include the hemodynamic stability of the patient, propagation and extent of the aortic injury, presence of aortic valvular incompetence, presence of pericardial effusion or cardiac tamponade,

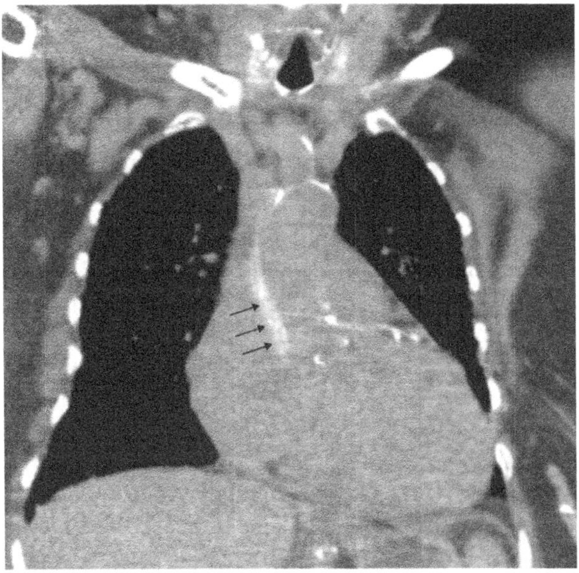

Fig. 3 Computed tomography of the chest without contrast in a patient with catheter-induced aortic dissection from RCA percutaneous intervention revealing contrast staining in the aortic wall in relation to RCA (arrows)

and the condition of the involved coronary artery [16]. Current options for management of catheter-induced aortic dissections include a conservative approach with careful surveillance, percutaneous stenting of the dissection entry point, and surgery.

Medical Management

All patients with identified iatrogenic aortic dissections should have immediate hemodynamic evaluation. As previously mentioned, TTE should be performed to evaluate for the presence of pericardial effusion or valvular dysfunction. Acute hemodynamic optimization should initially take precedence with an attempt at containing and preventing dissection propagation. Further contrast injections should be avoided. Beta-blockers and vasodilators are the mainstays for treatment of spontaneous aortic dissections, and while it may be of limited use in acutely unstable patients, it should be considered in those with stable hemodynamics and small contained dissection, as well as in the follow-up period [16].

Conservative management with watchful waiting has been described with good results for retrograde iatrogenic aortic dissections that are small and contained to the sinus of Valsalva (Dunning class I) and the involved coronary remains with good flow [3, 4]. Additionally, a review of 14 cases with dissection of the descending aorta/arch, without coronary involvement found that if the dissection is small without progression on follow-up imaging, a conservative approach is acceptable and results in good outcomes [3, 11]. In the presence of low-risk dissections with limited damage to the aortic media, medical management with serial hemodynamic monitoring, imaging, and follow-up is appropriate.

Percutaneous Coronary Stenting or Endovascular Repair

When the dissection originates from an entry point within a coronary artery and there is compromise to the flow or extension into the aortic arch, most reports favor management with percutaneous coronary stenting to seal the entry point which is usually located at the coronary ostium (Fig. 1b). One review of 67 cases of iatrogenic aortic dissections, found that 28 (42%) rapidly progressed to the ascending aorta if a stent-based sealing technique was not performed promptly [15]. The authors propose that in all cases where there is dissection into the coronary sinus, the ostium should be sealed immediately to prevent further propagation of the dissection. Moreover, if the ostial stenting failed to halt the dissection progression, it did not compromise the chances of surgical success [15].

Based on historical experience of 9 patients with aortocoronary dissections by Dunning et al., class I and II iatrogenic aortic dissections were all successfully managed with coronary stenting of the entry point whereas more extensive (class III) iatrogenic aortic dissections or patients with hemodynamic instability or ischemia of one of the aortic branches were referred to surgery with poor outcomes [2]. More recently, a retrospective analysis of 74 patients from the Registry on Aortic Iatrogenic Dissection (RAID) found that after a median follow-up of 51.2 months, only 2 deaths were recorded in patients treated conservatively. There were 15 (20%) patients with Dunning class III dissections and only 3 patients were referred for cardiac surgery (2 for aortic surgery and 1 for coronary artery bypass grafting). The remaining 71 cases were treated successfully with either conservative management or PCI [3]. These results suggest that even Dunning class III iatrogenic aortic dissections may be managed with coronary stenting to immediately seal the entry site with favorable outcomes.

Several different stent types have been used to manage iatrogenic aortic dissections. These include bare-metal stents, drug-eluting stents, covered stents, and a covered stent/drug-eluting stent combination [15–19]. A bare-metal stent may be appropriate in cases with extensive aortic dissections that may require early surgical intervention. However, current generation drug eluting stents with biocompatible polymers can also be considered based on studies showing early thromboresistance and higher rates of long-term patency compared to bare metal stents. While covered stents will completely seal the entry point of dissection, their use is not generally required, and drug-eluting stents are likely to be sufficient in most cases. Some authors recommend intravascular ultrasound (IVUS) guided coronary stenting to ensure complete coverage of the dissection and exact placement of the stent to entirely cover the coronary ostium [17]. Optical coherence tomography (OCT) is usually avoided due to the need for contrast injection into the coronary and fear of extension of dissection.

Surgical Repair

Urgent surgical intervention has been necessary in only small minority of previously reported cases of catheter-induced iatrogenic aortic dissections. This is in contrast to spontaneous aortic dissections of the ascending aorta that often require urgent surgical attention due to degeneration of the media that facilitates extensive propagation. High-risk features that should prompt consideration of surgical referral include dissections with significant extension into the aortic arch (Dunning class III), those that involve the aortic branches, or failure of entry sealing with a stent. In addition, patients with significant valvular dysfunction and those in which the coronary artery involved is unsalvageable with stenting or in which coronary artery bypass grafting is indicated should also be considered for surgical management. The goal of surgery is to perform resection of the aortic intimal tear and as much of the dissected aorta as possible, without resulting in excessive operative risk [20]. Surgical resection of the ascending aorta with or without the aortic arch (when involved) is considered the gold standard for patients with spontaneous type A dissection, and this approach has been extended to patients presenting with iatrogenic aortic dissections [20]. Of note, in comparison to spontaneous aortic dissections, the surgical repair of catheter-induced dissection may be riskier, especially in the setting of coronary ischemia and following PCI with full anticoagulation and antiplatelet therapy.

Surveillance

In most cases of catheter-induced iatrogenic aortic dissections where surgical repair is not required, serial imaging with either CT or MRI is needed to monitor the progression of the dissection. The optimal interval between scans has not yet been established. In one series that evaluated the use of multidetector CT (MDCT) in follow-up of catheter-induced aortic dissections, the most common follow-up pattern was MDCT immediately after the occurrence of aortocoronary dissection, followed by repeat imaging at 48 hours and 1 week [14]. The authors proposed repeat follow-up CT after 1–2 months in patients with more extensive class III dissections. In case reports of aortocoronary dissection evaluated with CT, time to resolution of the aortic dissection ranged from 48 hours to 3 months [14].

Prognosis

Historically, iatrogenic aortic dissections have been noted to have a generally poor prognosis similar to that of spontaneous aortic dissections (35% vs 24%, respectively), with type A aortic dissections carrying about a 35% mortality despite regardless of underlying mechanism. It was also noted that the mortality rate was higher (37%) for iatrogenic type B aortic dissections when compared to spontaneous aortic dissection (10%), with the majority of type B dissections (87%) occurring as a consequence of cardiac catheterization procedures [1]. In contrast, Dunning et al. found that patients with limited (Dunning class I and II) dissection had good prognosis with more extensive dissections (Dunning class III) portending a worse outcome.

Based on data from more recent case reports the short- and long-term prognosis of catheter-induced aortic dissections may be more favorable than previously reported [3, 4, 11, 15]. This is likely due to the success of aortocoronary stenting techniques to quickly seal and halt rapid propagation of a dissection. In 5-year follow-up data from the RAID analysis of 74 patients with iatrogenic aortic dissections, there were no long-term complications such as dissection progression, myocardial ischemia, or dissection recurrence in the 72 (97%) patients that survived the acute injury. The authors noted only 2 deaths with a 2.7% mortality in this case series [3]. Similarly, one other series of 18 cases showed a 0% mortality at 1-month follow-up, including cases of extensive dissections requiring urgent surgical intervention [4]. This is in contrast to spontaneous aortic dissections, especially of the ascending aorta (type A) where acute mortality has been reported close to 25%. The authors point out that an acute retrograde type A aortic dissection presents a more favorable prognosis than spontaneous type A dissections that tend to be antegrade in nature with a higher likelihood of propagation.

Conclusion

Iatrogenic aortic dissection is a rare complication of catheter-based procedures, with relatively better outcomes compared with spontaneous aortic dissections. The low event rate had limited our knowledge in regard to the best approach in managing different types of catheter-induced aortic dissections. However, the majority of cases can be adequately managed through conservative or percutaneous approaches, with surgical intervention deemed necessary in a small proportion of these cases.DisclosuresJ Dawn Abbott has received research funding with no personal compensation from AstraZeneca, Bristol Myers Squibb, Abbott, Sinomed, CSL Behring, Biosensors Research USA.

Funding
None.

References

1. Januzzi JL, et al. Iatrogenic aortic dissection. Am J Cardiol. 2002;89(5):623–6.
2. Dunning DW, et al. Iatrogenic coronary artery dissections extending into and involving the aortic root. Catheter Cardiovasc Interv. 2000;51(4):387–93.

3. Nunez-Gil IJ, et al. Incidence, management, and immediate- and long-term outcomes after iatrogenic aortic dissection during diagnostic or interventional coronary procedures. Circulation. 2015;131(24):2114–9.
4. Gómez-Moreno S. Iatrogenic dissection of the ascending aorta following heart catheterisation: incidence, management and outcome. EuroIntervention. 2006;2(2):197. -EOA
5. Vega MR. Aortic dissection—exceedingly rare complication of coronary angioplasty. Catheter Cardiovasc Diagn. 1997;42(4):416.
6. Perez-Castellano N, et al. Dissection of the aortic sinus of Valsalva complicating coronary catheterization: cause, mechanism, evolution, and management. Catheter Cardiovasc Diagn. 1998;43(3):273–9.
7. Carter AJ, Brinker JA. Dissection of the ascending aorta associated with coronary angiography. Am J Cardiol. 1994;73(12):922–3.
8. El Sabbagh A, et al. Angiographic success and procedural complications in patients undergoing retrograde percutaneous coronary chronic total occlusion interventions: a weighted meta-analysis of 3482 patients from 26 studies. Int J Cardiol. 2014;174(2):243–8.
9. Carlson RG, Lillehei CW, Edwards JE. Cystic medial necrosis of the ascending aorta in relation to age and hypertension. Am J Cardiol. 1970;25(4):411–5.
10. El-Haress M, et al. Iatrogenic acute ascending aortic dissection with intramural hematoma during coronary artery stenting: a case report. Front Surg. 2017;4:2.
11. Nunez-Gil IJ, et al. Type a iatrogenic aortic dissection following catheterization without coronary involvement: long-term prognosis. Rev Esp Cardiol (Engl Ed). 2015;68(3):254–5.
12. Alfonso F, et al. Aortic dissection occurring during coronary angioplasty: angiographic and transesophageal echocardiographic findings. Catheter Cardiovasc Diagn. 1997;42(4):412–5.
13. Hartnell GG. Imaging of aortic aneurysms and dissection: CT and MRI. J Thorac Imaging. 2001;16(1):35–46.
14. Tanasie C, et al. Catheter-induced aortic dissection after invasive coronary angiography: evaluation with MDCT. AJR Am J Roentgenol. 2011;197(6):1335–40.
15. Carstensen S, Ward MR. Iatrogenic aortocoronary dissection: the case for immediate aortoostial stenting. Heart Lung Circ. 2008;17(4):325–9.
16. Lindsay A, et al. Complications of percutaneous coronary intervention the survival handbook. London: Springer; 2016. p. XIII, 310 p. 109 illus., 52 illus. in color
17. Abdou SM, Wu CJ. Treatment of aortocoronary dissection complicating anomalous origin right coronary artery and chronic total intervention with intravascular ultrasound guided stenting. Catheter Cardiovasc Interv. 2011;78(6):914–9.
18. Danzi GB, et al. Retrograde dissection during percutaneous coronary intervention: sealing of the entry site by covered stent implantation. BMJ Case Rep. 2012;2012
19. Gorog DA, Watkinson A, Lipkin DP. Treatment of iatrogenic aortic dissection by percutaneous stent placement. J Invasive Cardiol. 2003;15(2):84–5.
20. Leontyev S, et al. Iatrogenic type a aortic dissection during cardiac procedures: early and late outcome in 48 patients. Eur J Cardiothorac Surg. 2012;41(3):641–6.

Aortic Intramural Hematoma

Neel R. Sodha and Frank W. Sellke

Introduction

Acute aortic syndromes (AAS) represent a spectrum of aortic pathologies including aortic dissection, penetrating atherosclerotic ulcer (PAU), and intramural hematoma (IMH). Originally described by Krukenberg in 1920, an aortic intramural hematoma has been defined as "dissection without intimal tear that results from hemorrhage within the aortic wall" [1]. The etiology of, or even the very existence of an aortic intramural hematoma as a distinct pathologic entity from classic aortic dissection, remains controversial. Some physicians believe an acute intramural hematoma results from spontaneous rupture of vasa vasorum within the aortic wall, resulting in bleeding within the tunica media, whereas others believe the imaging and surgical findings associated with an intramural hematoma are the result of a small undetectable intimal tear with subsequent thrombosis, and thus feel an IMH should be referred to as a thrombosed-type aortic dissection [2]. Proponents for the former (IMH as a distinct entity), argue that an intimal defect is often not identified at the time of surgery, and the variability in terms or risk factors and clinical behavior differ significantly from classic aortic dissection, thus supporting IMH as distinct from dissection. Proponents of the latter (IMH as a variant of classic aortic dissection), argue that enhanced imaging and distal inspection of the aorta at the time of surgery may often identify intimal defects which may be missed on initial evaluation [2, 3]. Given the debate as to the existence of IMH as a distinct acute aortic syndrome, it is understandable that management remains controversial as well.

N. R. Sodha (✉)
Division of Cardiothoracic Surgery, Alpert Medical School, Brown University, Providence, Rhode Island, USA
e-mail: nsodha@lifespan.org

F. W. Sellke
Cardiothoracic Surgery, Alpert Medical School, Brown University, Providence, Rhode Island, USA

J. S. Coselli et al. (eds.), *Aortic Dissection and Acute Aortic Syndromes*,
https://doi.org/10.1007/978-3-030-66668-2_16

Classification of acute aortic intramural hematoma is identical that used for aortic dissection. Most commonly, the Stanford classification system as described by Daily and colleagues is used in the clinical setting, with Stanford Type A and B defined as "type A involvement of the ascending aorta, and type B are defined as those limited to the descending aorta with primary intimal tear usually within 2 to 5 cm of the left subclavian artery" [4]. Recent updates from the *Society of Thoracic Surgeons* and *Society for Vascular Surgery* provide for more granular reporting of acute aortic syndromes with Type A lesions described as the primary tear originating in the ascending aorta, Type B lesions with the primary tear originating in the aortic arch or descending aorta, with additional subscripts to describe the extent of pathology depending on zone [5]. Updated classification schemes such as non-A/non-B or Type C are not in widespread clinical use [6, 7] (Fig. 1).

Presentation

Data from the *International Registry of Acute Aortic Dissection (IRAD)* suggest both Type A and Type B acute intramural hematomas are far less common than

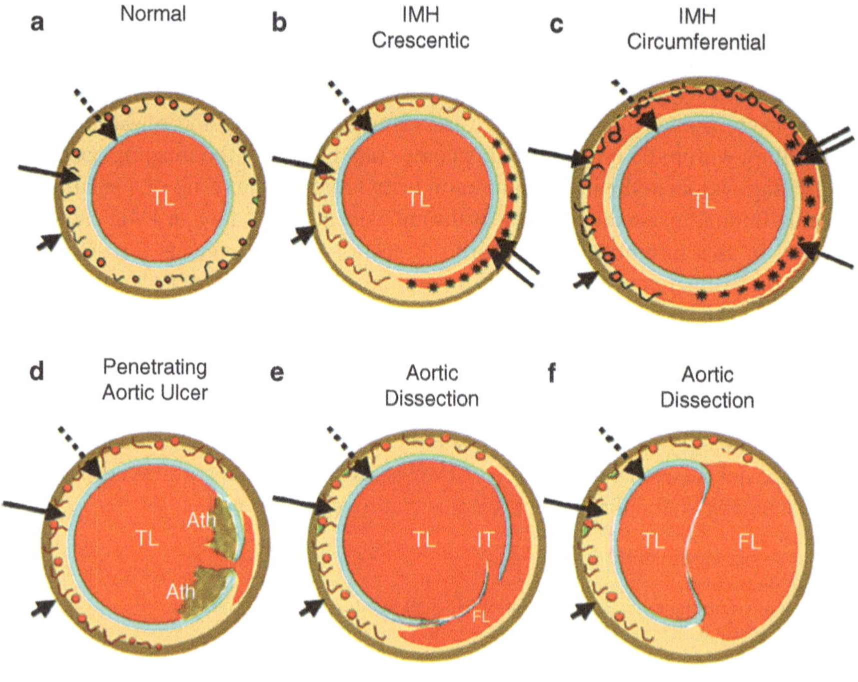

Fig. 1 Schematic representation of acute aortic syndromes. (**a**) Normal, (**b**) Intramural hematoma—Crescenteric, (**c**) Intramural hematoma—Circumferential, (**d**) Penetrating aortic ulcer, (**e**) Aortic dissection, (**f**) Aortic dissection. *TL* True Lumen, *Ath* Atheroma, *IT* Intimal tear, *FL* False lumen. Adapted from Maslow A, Atalay, M, Sodha N. Intramural Hematoma. *J Thorac and Cardiovasc Anesth.* 2018;32:1341–1362

classic aortic dissection, with IMH accounting for less than 10% of acute aortic syndromes [8]. Patients with an acute IMH tend to be about 8 years older than those with acute dissection, averaging near 70 years of age at presentation, and while more common in men than in women, IMH patients trended to a more even distribution between males and females relative to aortic dissection [8]. Arterial hypertension has been more commonly identified as a risk factor for IMH relative to dissection and in contrast with aortic dissection, where Type A is more common than Type B by an approximately 3:1 ratio, Type B IMH is more common than Type A IMH (42% Type A, 58% Type B). Chest pain is the most common presenting symptom for both Type A and B IMH, and is present in approximately 80% of patients, whereas back pain is less common in patients with Type A IMH, but presents with equal frequency to chest pain in patients with Type B IMH. Pain is generally abrupt in onset and severe, but is less commonly described as radiating. Neurologic manifestations, pulse deficits and aortic valve regurgitation are less commonly present relative to aortic dissection [8]. Laboratory analysis is of little value in establishing a diagnosis of intramural hematoma, but may aid in excluding other etiologies of chest pain [9]. Interestingly, aortic intramural hematomas are more likely to present with effusion or pericardial tamponade relative to aortic dissection, possibly related to the location of an IMH relative to the adventitial wall. This finding is thought to be a marker for potential rupture [10]. The above findings highlight the difficulty of diagnosing an intramural hematoma on history or examination alone, as symptoms may be non-specific and mimic other cardiovascular pathology. Rather than elucidate a diagnosis, the presentation findings discussed above and complaints of acute onset chest pain or back pain should raise the suspicion for an acute aortic syndrome and guide the appropriate initial management and diagnostic evaluation (Table 1).

When considering an acute intramural hematoma as a diagnosis based on presentation or imaging, it is essential consider aortitis in the differential diagnosis, as this rare entity may mimic an acute IMH on imaging. On history, aortitis may present with a more chronic or subacute onset of pain relative to an acute IMH. Constitutional symptoms such as fevers, arthralgias and myalgias may be present. A leukocytosis or elevation of inflammatory markers such as erythrocyte sedimentation rate (ESR) of C-reactive protein (CRP) may be present, but are non-specific. CT imaging may be non-specific and unable to differentiate between the two entities, in which case magnetic resonance imaging on weighted T2 sequences or FDG-PET scanning may provide the diagnosis. As surgical intervention for acute aortitis may result in poor outcomes, consideration of this diagnosis in all patients with possible intramural hematoma is essential [11, 12] (Table 2).

The diagnostic imaging for evaluation of acute aortic syndromes, including acute intramural hematoma is discussed in detail elsewhere in the textbook (see Chapter on *Imaging for Acute Aortic Dissection, Intramural Hematoma, and Penetrating Atherosclerotic Ulcer*). Briefly, plain film radiographs/chest x-rays are generally non-diagnostic [8]. Optimal imaging in the stable patient should include computed tomography. Specifically, a non-contrast CT of the chest, abdomen and pelvis should be obtained followed by a contrast-enhanced CT angiogram of the chest,

Table 1 Comparison between acute aortic syndromes

Lesion	Layer affected	Demographics	Presentation	Location	Appearance	Complication
IMH	Medial layer	65–70 y	AAS	Descending > Ascending > Arch	Crescentic thick	
		HTN			Circumferential thick	Rupture
		Males			Varying length	Dissection
		Iatrogenic			No intimal flap	Aneurysm
		Trauma			No false lumen	
AD		58–63 y	AAS	Ascending > Descending		
		HTN				
	Intimal tear	CTD			Intimal flap	Peripheral ischemia
	Intimal flap	Coarctation			Dual lumen: True/false	Embolization
	Medial false lumen	Bicuspid AoV			Low-flow false lumen	Aneurysm
		Pregnancy			False > True lumen	Rupture
		Trauma				
		• Iatrogenic				
AA	Intima		Asymptomatic	Ascending > Descending >>> Arch	Dilation	Rupture
	Media	50–60 y	Compression of proximal structures		No intimal flap	Embolization
	Adventitia	Males	Fistula related		No dual lumen	Fistula
					No false lumen	
PAU	Intimal layer	70 y	AAS	Descending >>> Arch >> Ascending	Irregular surface	IMH
		Males			Crater-like protrusion	Aneurysm
		HTN			No intimal flap	Embolization
		Tobacco			No dual lumen	Dissection
		CAD			No false lumen	Rupture
		COPD				
ULP	Intimal layer		Asymptomatic	Distal Arch Proximal descending >>> Ascending and Distal Descending	Single	
					Contrast-filled	
		65 y			Outpouchings across	Aneurysm
		Males			Intima into medial layer	Regression
					No connections with	
					Aortic branches	

(continued)

Table 1 (continued)

Lesion	Layer affected	Demographics	Presentation	Location	Appearance	Complication
IBP	Medial layer	60–62 y	Asymptomatic	Descending >>> Arch >> Ascending	Multiple pools medial layer	Disappear
		Males			No communication	
					Near branch vessels	

Abbreviations: *AA* aortic aneurysm, *AAS* acute aortic syndrome, *AD* aortic dissection, *AoV* aortic valve, *CAD* coronary artery disease, *COPD*, chronic obstructive pulmonary disease, *CTD* connective tissue disorder, *HTN* hypertension, *IBP* intramural blood pool, *IMH* intramural hematoma, *PAU* penetrating atherosclerotic (aortic) ulcer, *ULP* ulcer-like projection
Adapted from Maslow A, Atalay, M, Sodha N. Intramural Hematoma. *J Thorac and Cardiovasc Anesth.* 2018;32:1341–1362 2018

abdomen, and pelvis. Non-contrast imaging is essential in establishing a diagnosis of an intramural hematoma as a hyperdense area of cresenteric thickening will be visible on these studies. Particular attention should be paid to the location of the IMH, aortic diameter, IMH thickness, presence of a pericardial effusion, and the presence of contrast pools or ulcer-like projections, as each of these findings may play a key role in surgical decision-making. Transesophageal echocardiography can be utilized in the emergent setting for the unstable patient, whereas MRI/MRA may play a role in the stable patient in whom the diagnosis is uncertain [13] (Table 3).

Management

Once the diagnosis of an acute aortic intramural hematoma has been confirmed, immediate medical therapy should be initiated, regardless of whether surgical intervention is planned. Invasive hemodynamic monitoring should be performed with an arterial line and sufficient large-bore intravenous access should be obtained in case of abrupt hemodynamic deterioration. Anti-impulse therapy–systemic arterial blood pressure control combined with reduction in the contractile force of the myocardium, expressed as the change in pressure over time (dP/dt)—should be initiated immediately to reduce the risk of progression to frank dissection or rupture. If the heart rate allows and severe aortic regurgitation is not present, first-line treatment includes the use of beta-adrenergic blockers to reduce systemic blood pressure to less than 120 mmHg systolic and to a heart rate to 60–70 beats per minute. Thereafter, addition of a systemic vasodilator to further reduce arterial blood pressure should be initiated, but should not be used in isolation due to potential reflex tachycardia from the reduction in mean arterial pressure [14].

Table 2 Presentation of intramural hematoma

Sign/Symptom	Type A IMH	Type B IMH
Age (y)	>65	>65
Aortic pain (%)	>90	>90
Chest pain (%)	82.5	77.3
Back pain (%)	41	78.7
Abdominal pain (%)	13.1	36.8
Radiating pain (%)	45.9	35.3
Acute onset pain (%)	86.7	82.6
Hypertension (%)	32.2	58.6
Hypotension (%)	11.9	2.3
Aortic regurgitation (%)	25–35	<10
Pulse deficit (%)	15	<10
Renal complications (%)	<10	<10
Pericardial effusion (%)	≤70	<5
Tamponade (%)	≤50	<5
Coronary ischemia (%)	≤30	≤20
Hemodynamic instability (%)	≤20	<5

Adapted from Maslow A, Atalay, M, Sodha N. Intramural Hematoma. *J Thorac and Cardiovasc Anesth*

Table 3 Adverse outcomes and predictors

		IMH Type A	Intramural Hematoma Type B
Adverse outcomes	Hospital/30-d mortality	10–30%	4–20%
	Long-term mortality	≤40%	4–14%
	Progression, AA, AD, rupture	≤90%	Up to 50%
	Surgery	≤50%	< 10%
Predictors of adverse outcome	Persistent pain	X	X
	Hemodynamic instability	X	X
	Pleural effusion	X	X
	Pericardial effusion	X	X
	Para-aortic hematoma	X	X
	Echolucency	X	X
	Rapid aortic growth	>5 mm/y	> 5 mm/y
	Intimal tear (ULP/FID)	X	X
	PAU-related IMH	Uncommon	> 10 mm depth
	MAD	>45 to >60 mm	> 40 to >60 mm
	Wall thickness	>10 to 15 mm	> 10 to 15 mm

Adapted from Maslow A, Atalay, M, Sodha N. Intramural Hematoma. *J Thorac and Cardiovasc Anesth*. 2018;32:1341–1362

Management: Acute Type A Aortic Intramural Hematoma

Acute Type A aortic intramural hematomas may regress/heal completely with medical therapy alone, progress to a classic aortic dissection, or rupture. Herein lies the difficulty in selecting the optimal management strategy. It is clear the natural history of an acute Type A IMH differs from that of an acute Type A dissection. Reports vary widely on the rates of progression from an IMH to an aortic dissection with Western publications reporting rates of 28%-47%, or rates of progression to rupture ranging from 20%-45% [15, 16]. Given the high-rate of potentially catastrophic complications, guidelines endorsed by the *American Heart Association, Society of Thoracic Surgeons, American Association for Thoracic Surgery,* and the *Society for Vascular Medicine* state "Although the literature gives no compelling guidelines for treatment, the writing committee believes that treatment of IMH corresponding to treatment of aortic dissection in the corresponding segment of the aorta is reasonable", providing a Class IIa/Level of Evidence C recommendation for managing a Type A IMH surgically as would typically be done for a classic dissection [17]. More recent European guidelines from 2014 favor an aggressive approach with urgent surgical intervention for acute Type A IMH as a Class I/Level of Evidence C recommendation for surgery, although specifying "In elderly patients or those with significant comorbidities, initial medical treatment with a 'wait-and-watch strategy' (optimal medical therapy with blood pressure and pain control and repetitive imaging) may be a reasonable option" [18].

In contradistinction to Western management strategies and outcomes, multiple Asian centers have reported excellent outcomes with medical therapy alone for acute Type A IMH in select patients. Reports from Japan and Korea have demonstrated successful resolution of the IMH in up to 40–67% of selected patients [10, 19–22]. The etiology of this difference in outcomes between Eastern and Western populations is unclear, but may be related to differences in hospital referral patterns of genetic differences between populations [23].

While management may vary depending upon region, there are clear risk factors for acute complication which would strongly support a role for early surgical intervention. Hemodynamic compromise or pericardial tamponade are generally indications for emergent surgery. In the hemodynamically stable patient, the following clinical and radiographic findings have been associated with poor outcomes and should prompt consideration for surgical intervention: persistent or recurrent pain, maximal aortic diameter $\geq$ 50 mm, IMH thickness of $\geq$11 mm, or presence of ulcer-like projections. In patients whom are hemodynamically stable without the above findings, if medical management is selected, close monitoring with serial imaging at 48–72 h and 1 week is warranted and surgical intervention is indicated for persistent pain, recurrent effusions, or enlarging aortic diameter [18, 24]. Given the above, the decision to operate on the stable patient with an acute Type A intramural hematoma may be difficult. Upfront surgical therapy provides a rapid and definitive treatment, but is invasive and may result in potential perioperative complications. Conversely, medical therapy alone may subject the patient to the risk of acute deterioration and a prolonged hospitalization due to the need for close surveillance with serial imaging for up to two weeks. We favor an upfront surgical management strategy for most patients, reserving medical therapy for patients who may be of elevated perioperative risk due to age or comorbidities, providing they have low-risk imaging features.

Once a decision has been made to proceed with surgical intervention, the next question which arises is timing of surgery. Immediate surgery is always reasonable, but there are data to suggest that in the stable patient, semi-urgent surgery is acceptable. Estrera and colleagues [25] have demonstrated that in the clinically stable patient, surgery 72 h after symptom onset was safe (no progression to dissection or acute complication) and provided for an easier technical repair [25, 26].

There are limited data specifically addressing the technical aspects of surgical intervention for an acute Type A intramural hematoma, and surgical approaches largely reflect those utilized for acute dissection [27–30]. As with optimal management of acute Type A IMH, there exists wide variability in operative approaches. Most centers favor a peripheral arterial cannulation strategy utilizing either the right or left common femoral artery or the right axillary artery. Advantages of femoral cannulation are primarily technical ease of vascular access, speed of cannulation, and avoidance of aortic manipulation. The primary advantage of right axillary cannulation is the ability to provide antegrade cerebral perfusion to the brain during deep hypothermic circulatory arrest, whereas the primary disadvantage relates to the increased time needed for vessel exposure and placement of a graft. While many prefer to avoid central aortic cannulation over concerns relating to inducing a frank dissection, certain centers have reported good success utilizing a Seldinger technique with transesophageal guidance, preferring this approach as it avoids the added time needed for peripheral access, and may theoretically pose a lower stroke rate based on experience with this technique in acute aortic dissection [27, 29]. We generally employ central venous cannulation unless there is concern for rupture, at which time we utilize a femoral venous approach. While a limited replacement of the ascending aorta with the aortic cross-clamp in place (closed distal anastomosis) can be performed, most centers utilize deep hypothermic circulatory arrest to allow for an open distal anastomosis and replacement of the distal ascending aorta through the hemiarch. Given this, we initiate cooling upon initiation of cardiopulmonary bypass. There is no consensus on the safety or danger of placing a cross-clamp on the ascending aorta in the setting of an acute IMH. Some surgeons prefer to avoid clamping the aorta over concerns for inducing further injury to the aorta or creating a true dissection, and thus they allow the patient to cool to a point where circulatory arrest can be initiated, starting thereafter with distal reconstruction and performing proximal reconstruction during rewarming. Our group and others routinely clamp the ascending aorta during cooling to perform the proximal reconstruction [31], which in the absence of significant root dilation or pathology consists of placement of a supra-coronary tube graft. The distal extent of aortic replacement is largely determined by the size of the distal aorta, evidence of an entry tear in the arch, or evidence of distal visceral compromise which is uncommon in IMH. Generally, in the absence of an aneurysmal aortic arch or intimal tear identified in the arch, an open distal anastomosis is sufficient. Post-operative management is routine with continued strict attention to blood pressure management. We generally obtain a postoperative imaging study prior to discharge and at 3 months if the distal extent of the IMH extends beyond the replaced aorta. If there is extensive residual IMH in the distal aorta, closer surveillance imaging at 1 months, 3 months and 6 months is reasonable. Outcomes of surgical management are relatively favorable with respect to acute aortic dissection, with perioperative mortality rates ranging from 0.9% to 12% in most series [10, 30, 32, 33].

Management: Acute Type B Aortic Intramural Hematoma

The management of acute Type B aortic intramural hematoma is less controversial than that of Type A. Acute Type B IMH is significantly more common than Type A, yet accounts for only about 15% of Type B acute aortic syndromes [8]. Given the absence of an intimal flap or false lumen, Type B intramural hematomas present less frequently with complications such as visceral malperfusion or true luminal compression, thus they are less likely to need emergent intervention. Rates of progression to true aortic dissection are relatively low, ranging from 4–11% [34, 35]. The natural history of acute Type B IMH remains poorly understood as studies have often demonstrated conflicting results. Some studies have raised concern regarding an increased incidence of rupture or sudden death relative to a Type B dissection [16], whereas others have demonstrated the opposite, with high rates of complete regression [35, 36]. Given the conflicting data, there is some increasing interest in early endovascular intervention for acute Type B IMH.

As noted above, current guidelines endorsed by the *American Heart Association, Society of Thoracic Surgeons, American Association for Thoracic Surgery,* and the *Society for Vascular Medicine* state "Although the literature gives no compelling guidelines for treatment, the writing committee believes that treatment of IMH corresponding to treatment of aortic dissection in the corresponding segment of the aorta is reasonable", providing a Class IIa / Level of Evidence C recommendation for managing a Type B IMH medically as would typically be done for a classic uncomplicated dissection [17]. More recent guidelines from the *European Society of Cardiology* in 2014 favor medical treatment as the initial approach for uncomplicated acute Type B IMH (Class I/Level of Evidence C), reserving endovascular therapy or surgery for the same indications as for Type B aortic dissection. They do note the subgroup of patients with aortic dilation or ulcer-like projection (ULP) should be followed up closely and treated more aggressively if symptoms persist or reappear, or if progressive aortic dilation is observed. Indications for intervention (TEVAR rather than surgery) in the acute phase include an expansion of the IMH despite medical therapy, and the disruption of intimal tear on CT with contrast enhancement, with TEVAR given a Class IIa/ Level C recommendation and open surgical repair a Class IIb/Level C recommendation [18].

Open surgical intervention for complicated acute Type B IMH is uncommon, and generally occurs in the emergent setting for rupture when endovascular approaches are not feasible. The technical aspects of open surgical management are described in further detail elsewhere in this text (see Chapter on *Management of Type B Aortic Dissection*). The current preferred approach for complicated acute Type B IMH is via TEVAR. Timing of intervention is dependent upon the patient's clinical status, with emergent intervention required for evidence of rupture or impending rupture, whereas delayed intervention (>14 days) may be preferred to decrease the risk of inducing a retrograde dissection [37]. The need for perioperative spinal drainage and left subclavian arterial revascularization is dependent upon the proximal and distal extent of the planned endograft placement. Ideally, a 20 mm proximal landing zone of healthy aorta should be obtained, with debate as to whether the distal extent of the stent graft should cover the entire IMH or be limited to a segment of the thoracic aorta to decrease the risk of spinal complications [38–40]. Optimal sizing of the stent graft may pose a challenge in the acute setting. Early on, the intramural hematoma can expand resulting in in some degree of compromise of the aortic lumen. As time from the initial injury progresses, the intramural hematoma can thrombose or resolve, resulting in an increase in aortic lumen diameter. Thus, in the early period after development of an IMH, an endograft may potentially be undersized, increasing the risk of endograft migration or type I endoleak. Conversely, sizing based the total aortic diameter, including the hematoma, may predispose to excessive oversizing. A maximal oversize of the stent graft by 10% allows for adequate graft fixation to the diseased aortic wall while avoiding excess wall stress [41]. Outcomes after TEVAR for acute type B IMH are generally favorable with a recent meta-analysis of nine studies comparing 161 patients who underwent TEVAR versus 166 who were medically managed reporting an in-hospital mortality rate of 0–5.9% for patients undergoing TEVAR, and paraparesis/paraplegia rates of 0–5%. While the primary end-points of aortic-related death or IMH regression did not reach statistical differences between medical management and TEVAR, patients undergoing TEVAR did demonstrate a lower rate of progression to dissection or rupture [39].

Conclusions

Aortic intramural hematoma is an acute aortic syndrome characterized by hemorrhage within the medial layer of the aortic wall without evidence of flow or clear luminal communication on imaging or at the time of surgery. Timely diagnosis is essential, and relies on a high index of clinical suspicion, and appropriate imaging. Contrast and non-contrast enhanced CT imaging is the preferred study for stable patients. Echocardiography may be used to assess cardiac and valve function, and can be useful in unstable patients. MRI is typically reserved for stable patients in whom a diagnosis remains unclear. Initial management should include aggressive heart rate and blood pressure control, as done for other acute aortic syndromes. The subsequent management of IMH depends on the location, radiographic appearance, aortic dimensions, and associated pathology. The sum total of these features can allow for some assessment of risk for progression to frank dissection/rupture or potential for regression. Hemodynamically unstable cases warrant emergent surgical management, but factors affecting the decision to operate are evolving. For acute Type A IMH, Western centers have generally favored a more aggressive surgical approach, with urgent/emergent surgical intervention, whereas Asian centers have reported favorable outcomes with medical therapy in select patients. In contrast, the majority of acute Type B IMH are managed medically, with endovascular intervention limited to those experiencing complications or at heightened risk. Outcomes for appropriately managed patients are favorable.

References

1. Krukenberg E. Beitrage zur frage des aneurysma dissecans. Beitr Pathol Anat Allg Pathol. 1920;67:329–51.
2. Uchida K, Imoto K, Karube N, et al. Intramural hematoma should be referred to as thrombosed-type aortic dissection. Eur J Cardiothorac Surg. 2013;44:366–9.
3. Song JK. Update in acute aortic syndrome: intramural hematoma and incomplete dissection as new disease entities. J Cardiol. 2014;64:153–61.
4. Daily PO, Trueblood HW, Stinson EB, et al. Management of acute aortic dissections. Ann Thorac Surg. 1970;10:237–47.
5. Lombardi JV, Hughes GC, Appoo JJ, et al. Society of Thoracic Surgeons and Society for Vascular Surgery reporting standards for aortic dissections. J Vasc Surg. 2020;71:723–47.
6. Von Segesser LK, Killer I, Ziswiler M, et al. Dissection of the descending thoracic aorta extending in to the ascending aorta: a therapeutic challenge. J Thorac Cardiovasc Surg. 1994;108:755–61.
7. Quanadli SD, Malkzadeh S, Villard N, et al. A new clinically driven classification for aortic dissection. Front Surg. 2020;7:37–44.
8. Harris KM, Braverman AC, Eagle KA. Acute aortic intramural hematoma: an analysis from the International Registry for Acute Aortic Dissection. Circulation. 2012;126:S91–6.
9. Suzuki T, Eagle KA. Biomarker-assisted diagnosis of acute aortic dissection. Circulation. 2018;137:270–2.
10. Song JK, Yim JH, Ahn JM, et al. Outcomes of patients with acute type A aortic intramural hematoma. Circulation. 2009;120:2046–52.
11. Nemer DM, Gentryll JL, Jaber WA, et al. Differentiation of aortitis from type A intramural hematoma. Circ Cardiovasc Imaging. 2019;12:834–5.
12. Velez AK, Etchill E, Halushka MK, et al. Aortitis masquerading as intramural hematoma: when to observe, when to operate. J Card Surg. 2020;26:1554–6.
13. Maslow A, Atalay M, Sodha N. Intramural Hematoma. J Thorac Cardiovasc Anesth. 2018;32:1341–62.
14. Sodha NR, Sellke FW. Chapter 161: aortic dissection. In: Vincent JL, Abraham E, Moore FA, et al., editors. Textbook of critical care. 7th ed; 2017.
15. Bossone E, LaBounty TM, Eagle KA. Acute aortic syndromes: diagnosis and management, an update. Eur Heart J. 2018;39:739–49.
16. Tittle SL, Lynch RJ, Cole PE, et al. Midterm follow-up of penetrating ulcer and intramural hematoma of the aorta. J Thorac Cardiovasc Surg. 2002;123:1051–9.
17. Hiratzka LF, Bakris GL, Beckman JA, et al. ACCF/AHA/AATS/ACR/ASA/SCA/SIR/STS/SVM guidelines for the diagnosis and management of patients with thoracic aortic disease. Circulation. 2010;2010:121.
18. Erbel R, Aboyans V, Boileau C, et al. 2014 ESC guidelines on the diagnosis and treatment of aortic diseases: document covering acute and chronic aortic diseases of the thoracic and

abdominal aorta of the adult. The task force for the diagnosis and treatment of aortic diseases of the European Society of Cardiology (ESC). Eur Heart J. 2014;35:2873–926.
19. Moizumi Y, Komatsu T, Motoyoshi N, et al. Clinical features and long-term outcome of type A and type B intramural hematoma of the aorta. J Thorac Cardiovasc Surg. 2004;127:421–7.
20. Song JK, Kim HS, Song JM, et al. Outcomes of medically treated patients with aortic intramural hematoma. Am J Med. 2002;113:181–7.
21. Kaji S, Akasaka T, Horibata Y, et al. Long-term prognosis of patients with type A aortic intramural hematoma. Circulation. 2002;106:I-248–52.
22. Choi YJ, Son JW, Lee SH, et al. Treatment patterns and their outcomes of acute aortic intramural hematoma in real world: multicenter registry for aortic intramural hematoma. BMC Cardiovasc Disord. 2014;14:103.
23. Chow SCY, Wong RHL, Lakhani I, et al. Management of acute Type A intramural hematoma: upfront surgery or individualized approach? A retrospective analysis and meta-analysis. J Thor Dis. 2020;12:680–92.
24. Kitai T, Kaji S, Yamamuro A, et al. Clinical outcomes of medical therapy and timely operation in initially diagnosed type A aortic intramural hematoma: a 20-year experience. Circulation. 2009;120:292–8.
25. Estrera A, Miller C, Lee TY, et al. Acute type A intramural hematoma: analysis of current management strategy. Circulation. 2009;120:287–91.
26. Al Rstum Z, Tanaka A, Eisenberg SB, et al. Optimal timing of type A intramural hematoma repair. Ann Cardiothorac Surg. 2019;8:524–30.
27. Leshnower BG. Cannulation strategies, circulation management and neuroprotection for type A intramural hematoma: tips and tricks. Ann Cardiothorac Surg. 2019;8:561–6.
28. Norton EL, Williams DM, Kim KM, et al. Management of malperfusion syndrome in acute Type A intramural hematoma. Ann Cardiothorac Surg. 2019;8:540–50.
29. Assi R, Siki MA, Desai ND, et al. Repair of type A aortic intramural hematoma. Ann Cardiothorac Surg. 2019;8:567–9.
30. Sandhu HK, Tanaka A, Charlton-Ouw KM, et al. Outcomes and management of type A intramural hematoma. Ann Cardiothorac Surg. 2016;5:317–27.
31. Brown JA, Arnaoutakis GJ, Kilic A, et al. Current trends in the management of acute Type A aortic intramural hematoma. J Card Surg. 2020;35:2331–7.
32. Matsushita A, Fukui T, Tabata M, et al. Preoperative characteristics and surgical outcomes of acute intramural hematoma involving the ascending aorta. J Thorac Cardiovasc Surg. 2016;151:351–8.
33. Hata M, Hata H, Sezai A, et al. Optimal treatment strategy for type A acute aortic dissection with intramural hematoma. J Thorac Cardiovasc Surg. 2014;147:307–11.
34. Kaji S, Akasak T, Katayama M, et al. Long-term prognosis of patients with type B aortic intramural hematoma. Circulation. 2003;18:108–20.
35. Sueyoshi E, Imada T, Sakamoto I, et al. Analysis of predictive factors for progression of Type B aortic intramural hematoma with computed tomography. J Vasc Surg. 2002;35:1179–83.
36. Tolenaar JL, Harris KM, Upchurch GR, et al. The differences and similarities between intramural hematoma of the descending aorta and acute type B dissection. J Vasc Surg. 2013;58:1498–504.
37. Desai ND, Gottret JP, Szeto WY, et al. Impact of timing on major complications after TEVAR for acute type B aortic dissection. J Thorac Cardiovasc Surg. 2015;149:151–6.
38. Ye K, Qin J, Yin M, et al. Acute intramural hematoma of the descending aorta treated with stent graft repair is associated with a better prognosis. J Vasc Interv Radiol. 2017;28:1446–53.
39. Chakos A, Twindyawardhani T, Evangelista A, et al. Endovascular versus medical management of type B intramural hematoma: a meta-analysis. Ann Cardiothorac Surg. 2019;8:447–55.
40. Bischoff MS, Meisenbacher K, Wehrmeister M, et al. Treatment indications for and outcome of endovascular repair of type B intramural aortic hematoma. J Vasc Surg. 2016;64:1569–79.
41. Houben IB, van Bakel TMJ, Patel HJ. Type B intramural hematoma: TEVAR or conservative approach? Ann Cardiothorac Surg. 2019;8:483–7.

Penetrating Atherosclerotic Ulcer: Presentation and Management

Ignas B. Houben, Pieter Van Bakel, and Himanshu J. Patel

Definition and Presentation

Penetrating atherosclerotic ulcer (PAU) was originally defined by Stanson and colleagues as a pathologic diagnosis consistent with localized excavation of the intima and media [1]. In this seminal report, PAU was thought to be a malignant pathology, often associated with intramural hematoma, and required aggressive surgical management. Villacosta and Roman introduced the term "acute aortic syndrome" (AAS) to describe the aortic causes of acute chest pain including aortic dissection (AD), intramural hematoma (IMH) and penetrating aortic ulcer (PAU) [1]. These three aortic pathologies are considered to have similar pathogenesis, clinical presentation and treatment, which depends on the location of the disease, time since onset of symptoms and the presence of accompanying complications.

PAU can be defined as a primary disruption in the arterial intima and elastic lamina extending into the media of the aortic wall [2] (Figs. 1 and 2). The most likely etiology is progression due to an atherosclerotic plaque which causes erosion and inflammatory changes in the aortic wall [1, 3, 4]. Since PAU is now most frequently defined on radiographic imaging rather than in pathologic specimens, it is most important to understand there are three entities that can appear similar on radiographic examination (Fig. 1). These entities can best be distinguished in the context of the overall clinical picture, but in addition, with the description of the entity's natural history. In Fig. 1a, b, ulcerlike projections can present as temporal

This work was generously supported by the Joe D. Morris Professorship, the David Hamilton Fund in Cardiac Surgery, and the Phil Jenkins Breakthrough Fund in Cardiac Surgery

I. B. Houben · P. Van Bakel · H. J. Patel (✉)
Section Head, Adult Cardiac Surgery, University of Michigan Frankel Cardiovascular Center, Ann Arbor, MI, USA
e-mail: hjpatel@med.umich.edu

J. S. Coselli et al. (eds.), *Aortic Dissection and Acute Aortic Syndromes*,
https://doi.org/10.1007/978-3-030-66668-2_17

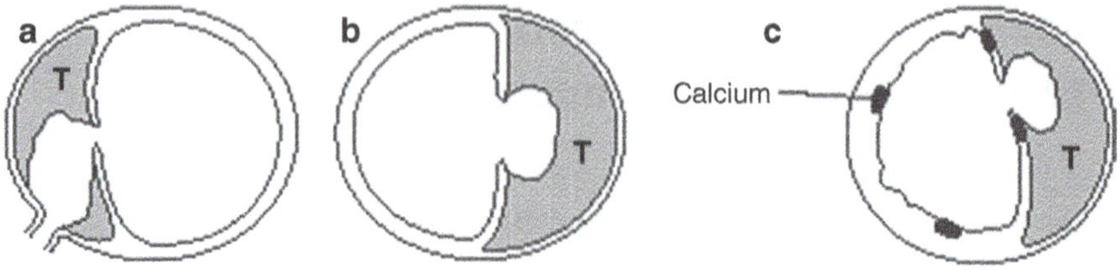

Fig. 1 Schematic representation of aortic cross section in different pathology. The radiographic diagnosis of PAU can encompass three potential pathologic entities. (**a**) A typical branch artery pseudoaneurysm (T = thrombus). (**b**) Reentry tear developing in IMH, and this diagnosis would only be possible if the original scan with the 'fresh' entry tear was available to describe the evolving lesion. (**c**) The original PAU as described by in pathologic specimens by Stanson [2]

Fig. 2 Example of longitudinal aortic tear. This is an ulcerative lesion running along the long axis of the aorta. (**a**) suction device on the medial aspect of the longitudinal tear. (**b**) transverse line across the aorta

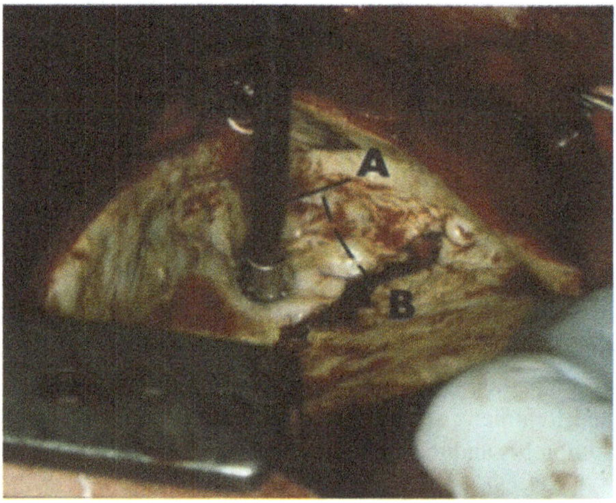

evolution of intramural hematoma either by development of localized perfusion of the false lumen from branch vessels (Fig. 1a) or by development of localized entry tears (Fig. 1b). In contrast, PAU can occur independently of IMH as is shown in Fig. 1c. Given the lack of true pathologic diagnosis, unless the entire historical evolution of the lesion is known, it may be more appropriate to refer to the radiographic anomalies as "ulcer-like projections".

The typical patient presenting with PAU is older and has extensive atherosclerotic disease [4] Risk factors associated with PAU are those of atherosclerosis and include hypertension, hyperlipidemia, and tobacco use. When patients present with PAU, the location of the ulcerlike projection is critical to defining the treatment algorithm. The radiographic classification scheme is according to according to the Stanford classification, and secondly whether there is associated IMH. PAU are most common in the descending thoracic aorta, however they can be found throughout the entire aorta [5]. Type A PAU is found in 6–10% of cases [4, 5]. Nathan et al. found in their study that 62% of all PAU disease originated in the descending thoracic aorta, 31% in the abdominal aorta and 7% in the aortic arch. Isolated PAU can be a stable disease [6], however some PAUs progress over time [5, 7]. It is likely that these progressive PAUs are often associated with other aortic pathologies such as saccular aneurysms. Associated IMH can develop due to erosion of aortic vasa vasorum by the ulcer, and are associated with worse outcomes than isolated IMHs [7]. PAUs vary in size with diameters ranging from 2 to 25 mm and depths ranging from 4 to 30 mm [5]. The increase in diameter and depth of the ulcer is associated with progressive disease [7], and can be associated with the rupture rate of PAUs, which can be as high as 38% [8]. Treatment options depend on the clinical condition of the patient, the location of the PAU and the presence of symptoms.

Clinical Presentation

The clinical presentation of PAU is varied, but often is considered within the spectrum of acute aortic syndromes in many cases. Those PAUs that are found incidentally and in asymptomatic patients may have a different natural history than those identified as part of an acute syndrome [6]. It is not clear whether this is due to the actual natural history, or secondary to the lack of differentiation of the three radiographic entities that manifest as ulcerlike projections on cross sectional imaging studies (Fig. 1). Thoracic PAUs are more likely to develop symptoms [5]. Nathan et al. showed that 18% of patients presented with chest or abdominal pain [5]. The pain associated with symptomatic PAUs is thought to be due to rapid stretching of the aortic adventitia resulting in stimulating of the aortic nerve plexus [9, 10]. In some cases, the tear is oriented in a linear longitudinal manner, and simulates an "unzipping" of the aorta as shown in Fig. 2. In these circumstances, growth rates are robust and the risk of rupture higher than with conventional appearing PAU.

Natural History of Type A PAU

Since the prevalence of Type A PAU is much lower than Type B PAU, literature is more sparse for this disease. Frequently they will be described as part of an entire cohort. Type A PAU is more likely to lead to complications than Type B PAU [8]. In a study by Tittle et al., 10 out of 12 (83%) patients with ascending PAUs received open surgery and 4 out of 12 (33%) presented with rupture [8]. Several studies report malignant natural history in isolated asymptomatic PAU of the ascending aorta, compared to rather benign isolated descending PAU [5, 7, 8]. In these studies, ulcerlike projections in the ascending aorta, often are associated with intramural hematoma, and progress to rupture, IMH expansion or even true double barrel dissection.

Natural History of Type B PAU

The natural history of type B PAU is also poorly understood. The majority of patients with type B PAU are asymptomatic at the time of diagnosis, and display stable natural history [6, 11]. Symptomatic patients have pain, which could be self-limiting and well controlled with antihypertensive medications. Indications for primary repair include: acute recurrent or refractory pain; progression to saccular aneurysm; contained rupture of the aortic wall; IMH expansion; fusiform aortic growth >1 mm per year; or a ulcer like projection with >20 mm in diameter and >10 mm in depth [12, 13]. These patients will need a surgical intervention and the timing dependent on the acuity of presentation (Fig. 3). Asymptomatic patients with PAU without any pain or aortic growth can be medically managed with close CTA surveillance, particularly given the relatively benign natural history seen in some studies.

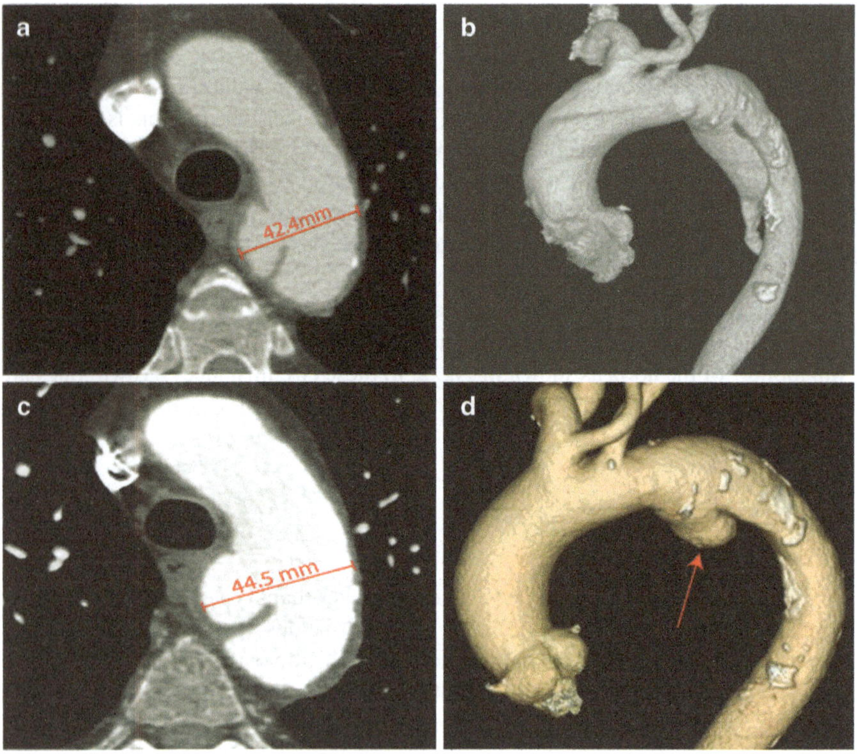

Fig. 3 Example of patient with evolving ulcer-like projection. In (**a**), the patient presented with symptoms and had an ulcer-like projection in the distal arch aorta with the remaining descending aorta with evidence of intramural hematoma. The 3-dimensional reconstruction suggests there is limited flow in the false lumen (**b**). By 2 years (**c**), the aortic dimension was bigger with the 3-dimensional measurement (**d**) suggesting the maximum diameter was 5.8 cm. This patient underwent a successful left carotid to left subclavian artery bypass with associated thoracic endovascular aortic repair from Ishimaru zone 2 to zone 4

Early Management of PAU

Initial management is directed at reducing radial, longitudinal and shear stresses on the aortic wall with medical therapy aimed at lowering systolic blood pressures and pulse pressures. In acute cases, with progression of a PAU towards intramural hematoma (IMH) or aortic dissection, the patient may present with unstable hemodynamics and urgent management is required. Medical management consists of using intravenous beta-blockers to target a heart rate of 60–80 beats per minute, a systolic pressure of 100–120 mmHg and attempts to preserve end-organ perfusion [14, 15]. The main intravenous beta-blocking agents used in this setting are labetalol and esmolol. Esmolol is preferred by many physicians, because of its short duration of action. Additionally, effective pain control should be instituted to aid blood pressure management. In hemodynamically unstable patients, or patients with radiographic evidence of (contained) rupture, emergent surgical repair should be performed.

Treatment Options for Type A PAU

Since there is a higher risk of complications of PAU in the ascending thoracic aorta, and it is often associated with IMH, the management usually consists of surgical intervention (Fig. 3). Open surgical repair is the mainstay of therapy [15, 16], similar to that seen in typical double barrel Type A dissection treatment.

Recently, there is an increasing interest in using thoracic endovascular aortic repair (TEVAR) as an alternative treatment paradigm. Several centers have reported successful endovascular treatment of aortic pathology, such as aneurysm and dissection, in the ascending aorta and transverse arch [17, 18]. Tsilimparis et al. reported on 10 patients undergoing ascending endograft placement. Four underwent cervical debranching, one received a fenestrated and one a branched endograft [17]. The technical success was 100%, the 30-day mortality was 10% and the stroke rate was 10%. Roselli et al. reported on 39 endovascular procedures with 35 stents having proximal and distal landing in Ishimaru zone 0, three occluder devices placed for pseudoaneurysms and one total arch endovascular procedure with an innominate side branch after cervical debranching [18]. Conversion to open surgery was performed in 10%, with the survival at 30 days of 81% and the observed stroke rate of 10%. All patients had significant associated comorbidities and were too high-risk for open surgery. This likely led to the relatively poor reported outcomes when compared to reports of open surgical repair. As only small cohorts of patients have been treated with this approach, and significant complications are reported, endovascular treatment of the ascending aorta should be restricted to high risk patients who are deemed unsuitable for open surgical repair.

After successful repair of the aorta, imaging surveillance is mandatory to ensure there are no further aortic complications in either the treated, adjacent or remote aortic segments, particularly if endovascular therapy has been performed. Regular CT surveillance for endovascular procedures is performed at 1 month, 3 months, 6 months, 12 months and annually after. Medical therapy is also required and typically consists of blood pressure management and control of lipids.

Treatment Options for Type B PAU

In patients with Type B PAU there are several options for management of the PAU (Fig. 1). If a patient is hemodynamically stable, but symptomatic, medical therapy with intravenous beta-blocker and pain management is indicated. If the pain is recurrent or refractory, or there are other signs of impending rupture, repair should be performed urgently. If the patient can be stabilized and transitioned to oral anti-hypertensive medication and becomes asymptomatic, pre-operative planning can take place and the patient should be planned for early repair within 3 months in select circumstances such as development of saccular aneurysms, or rapid expansion of aortic dimension.

TEVAR is an effective therapy for type B PAU and has evolved into the first line strategy. The rate of endoleak and re-interventions are similar to those reported for TEVAR for other indications, and range from 0 to 13% and 0 to 20% respectively [14]. PAUs in patients with progressive disease are usually in more proximal aortic segments with the proximal descending thoracic aorta being the most common site [7]. In many cases, TEVAR needs to be performed in proximal landing is zone 2, and adjunctive left subclavian artery (LSA) management performed as per local practices.

Long-term follow-up on PAU post TEVAR is sparse. The current two longest reported clinical series had a mean follow-up of 51 and 53 months. Demers et al. included 26 descending TEVARs and showed relatively low aortic event related mortality of 4% and an equally low aortic reintervention rate of 4% [19]. Mestres et al. included 22 PAUs and showed a similar aortic event related mortality rate 5% and a higher aortic reintervention rate of 14% [20]. The overall range of follow-up, mortality and reintervention rate ranged from 9–53 months, 0–13% and 0–20% respectively (Table 1). These numbers suggest that at least in the first 2 years after repair, TEVAR compares well to open repair mortality and that attention is needed on the durability of TEVAR. Patel et al. performed a comparison between descending thoracic open repair and TEVAR and found excellent results with the endovascular approach [35]. Early outcomes from descending TEVAR case series over the last two decades can be found in Table 2. Similar to those patients who presented with type A PAU, statin therapy, in addition to blood pressure control and long term imaging surveillance is indicated for the long-term management of these patients (Fig. 4).

Table 1 Late outcomes of contemporary clinical series (n > 5) of descending endovascular repair of penetrating aortic ulcers

References	Year	N	Endoleak	Reintervention	Related mortality	Follow-up (months)
Schoder et al. [21]	2002	8	13%	0	13%	14
Kos et al. [22]	2002	10	20%	–	10%	9
Eggebrecht et al. [23]	2003	10	10%	20%	0	24
Demers et al. [19]	2004	26	14%	4%	4%	51
Brinster et al. [24]	2005	21	0	0	0	14
Eggebrecht et al. [25]	2006	22	5%	9%	0	27
Dalainas et al. [26]	2007	18	6%	0	0	41
Pauls et al. [27]	2007	12	8%	0	0	28
Geisbüsch et al. [28]	2008	48	23%	8%	–	31
Botta et al. [29]	2008	18	17%	11%	0	22
Girn et al. [30]	2009	11	9%	–	18%	32
D'Souza et al. [31]	2009	20	15%	5%	0	24
Patel et al. [13]	2010	37	11%	16%	8%	33
Czerny et al. [32]	2011	72	4%	1%	1%	42
Palombo et al. [33]	2012	16	6%	0	13%	16
Mestres et al. [20]	2012	22	14%	14%	5%	53
Jánosi et al. [34]	2016	63	6%	19%	0	45

Follow Up

Patients with a history of PAU and atherosclerotic aorta should be kept under lifelong CT-surveillance. The guidelines for the first period after surgery or diagnosis are CT angiography at 1, 3, 6 and 12 months and hereafter annually [12, 15, 16]. If the patient remains asymptomatic and the aorta does not grow more than 5 millimeters per year the interval can be increased. It should be noted that aggressive blood pressure control and lifestyle management are critically important to prevent complications during follow-up. PAU should be considered a chronic disease that necessitates lifelong treatment and surveillance.

Conclusion

PAU is a disease of the arterial wall and is mostly asymptomatic. If a patient develops symptoms, they largely overlap with the other causes of AAS (AD and IMH). The management of PAU closely resembles the two other pathologies in acute aortic syndrome. Initial control consists of blood pressure management and pain

Table 2 Early outcomes of contemporary clinical series (n > 5) of descending thoracic endovascular repair of penetrating aortic ulcers

References	Year	N	PAU location			Adjunctive debranching	Early mortality[a]	Stroke	SCI
			Thoracic	Abdominal	Both				
Schoder et al. [21]	2002	8	100%	0	0	0	0	0	13%
Kos et al. [22]	2002	10	100%	0	0	–	0	0	10%
Eggebrecht et al. [23]	2003	10	80%	20%	0	0	0	0	0
Demers et al. [19]	2004	26	100%	0	0	4%	12%	4%	0
Brinster et al. [24]	2005	21	100%	0	0	0	0	0	0
Eggebrecht et al. [25]	2006	22	73%	9%	18%	0	0	5%	0
Dalainas et al. [26]	2007	18	89%	11%	0	0	0	0	0
Pauls et al. [27]	2007	12	100%	0	0	0	0	0	0
Geisbüsch et al. [28]	2008	48	71%	25%	4%	–	6%	4%	0
Botta et al. [29]	2008	18	100%	0	0	5%	11%	0	0
Girn et al. [30]	2009	11	100%	0	0	0	18%	0	9%
D'Souza et al. [31]	2009	20	100%	0	0	5%	0	0	0
Patel et al. [13]	2010	37	100%	0	0	27%	5%	5%	5%
Czerny et al. [32]	2011	72	96%	1%	3%	35%	4%	3%	1%
Palombo et al. [33]	2012	16	81%	19%	0	25%	6%	0	6%
Mestres et al. [20]	2012	22	100%	0	0	27%	5%	0	5%
Jánosi et al. [34]	2016	63	86%	0	14%	5%	8%	0	0

PAU penetrating atherosclerotic ulcer, *SCI* spinal cord ischemia
[a]In-hospital or 30-day mortality

management. Type A PAU necessitates urgent or early elective repair, depending on the hemodynamic stability and symptoms of the patient. Type B lesions are preferably medically managed when asymptomatic and are managed by endovascular repair when symptoms or complications are present. Future advances in endovascular technology may extend the patient population who benefits from the less invasive approach.

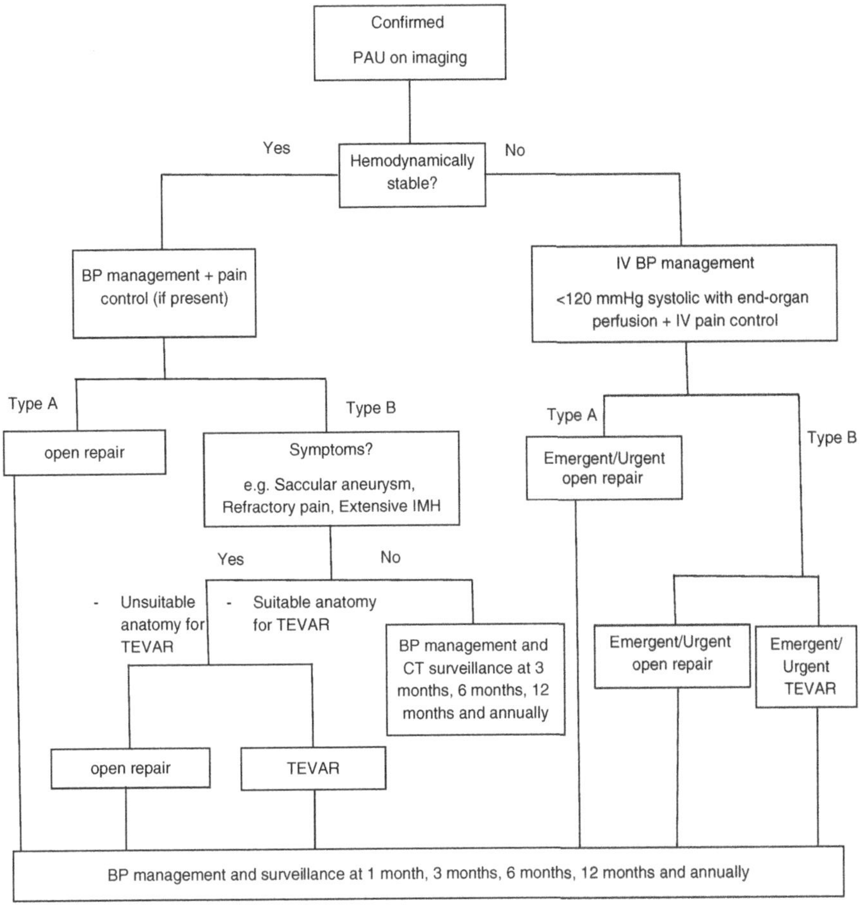

Fig. 4 Flowchart for treatment decision-making in a patient with penetrating aortic ulcer

References

1. Vilacosta I, San Roman JA. Acute aortic syndrome. Heart. 2001;85(4):365–8.
2. Stanson AW, Kazmier FJ, Hollier LH, Edwards WD, Pairolero PC, Sheedy FC, et. al. Penetrating atherosclerotic ulcers of the thoracic aorta: natural history and clinicopathologic correlations. Ann Vasc. Surg. 1986;1:15–23.
3. Coady MA, Rizzo JA, Hammond GL, Pierce JG, Kopf GS, Elefteriades JA. Penetrating ulcer of the thoracic aorta: What is it? How do we recognize it? How do we manage it? J Vasc Surg. 1998;27(6):1006–16.
4. Cho KR, Stanson AW, Donald Potter D, Cherry KJ, Schaff HV, Sundt TM III. Penetrating atherosclerotic ulcer of the descending thoracic aorta and arch. J Thorac Cardiovasc Surg. 2004;127(5):1393–9.
5. Nathan DP, Boonn W, Lai E, Wang GJ, Desai N, Woo EY, et al. Presentation, complications, and natural history of penetrating atherosclerotic ulcer disease. J Vasc Surg. 2012;55(1):10–5.

6. Quint LE, Williams DM, Francis IR, Monaghan HM, Sonnad SS, Patel S, et al. Ulcerlike lesions of the aorta: Imaging features and natural history. Radiology. 2001;218(3):719–23.
7. Ganaha F, Craig Miller D, Sugimoto K, Do YS, Minamiguchi H, Saito H, et al. Prognosis of aortic intramural hematoma with and without penetrating atherosclerotic ulcer: a clinical and radiological analysis. Circulation. 2002;106(3):342–8.
8. Tittle SL, Lynch RJ, Cole PE, Singh HS, Rizzo JA, Kopf GS, et al. Midterm follow-up of penetrating ulcer and intramural hematoma of the aorta. J Thorac Cardiovasc Surg. 2002;123(6):1051–9.
9. Wooley CF, Sparks EH, Boudoulas H. Aortic pain. Prog Cardiovasc Dis. 1998;40(6):563–89.
10. Toda R, Moriyama Y, Iguro Y, Matsumoto H, Masuda H, Ueno T. Penetrating atherosclerotic ulcer. Surg Today. 2001;31(1):32–5. https://doi.org/10.1007/s005950170216.
11. Gifford SM, Duncan AA, Greiten LE, Gloviczki P, Oderich GS, Kalra M, et al. The natural history and outcomes for thoracic and abdominal penetrating aortic ulcers. J Vasc Surg. 2016;63(5):1182–8.
12. Writing Committee, Riambau V, Böckler D, Brunkwall J, Cao P, Chiesa R, et al. Editor's choice – management of descending thoracic aorta diseases: clinical practice guidelines of the European Society for Vascular Surgery (ESVS). Eur J Vasc Endovasc Surg. 2017;53(1):4–52.
13. Patel HJ, Williams DM, Upchurch GR, Dasika NL, Deeb GM. The challenge of associated intramural hematoma with endovascular repair for penetrating ulcers of the descending thoracic aorta. J Vasc Surg. 2010;51(4):829–35.
14. Oderich GS, Kärkkäinen JM, Reed NR, Tenorio ER, Sandri GA. Penetrating aortic ulcer and intramural hematoma. Cardiovasc Intervent Radiol. 2019;42(3):321–34.
15. Erbel R, Aboyans V, Boileau C, Bossone E, Di Bartolomeo R, Eggebrecht H, et al. 2014 ESC guidelines on the diagnosis and treatment of aortic diseases. Russ J Cardiol. 2015;123(7):7–72.
16. Hiratzka LF, Bakris GL, Beckman JA, Bersin RM, Carr VF, Casey DE, et al. 2010 ACCF/AHA/AATS/ACR/ASA/SCA/SCAI/SIR/STS/SVM guidelines for the diagnosis and management of patients with Thoracic Aortic Disease: a report of the American College of Cardiology Foundation/American Heart Association Task Force on Practice Guidelines. A Circulation. 2010;121(13):e266–369.
17. Tsilimparis N, Debus ES, Oderich GS, Haulon S, Terp KA, Roeder B, et al. International experience with endovascular therapy of the ascending aorta with a dedicated endograft. J Vasc Surg. 2016;63(6):1476–82.
18. Roselli EE, Idrees JJ, Johnston DR, Eagleton MJ, Desai MY, Svensson LG. Zone zero thoracic endovascular aortic repair: a proposed modification to the classification of landing zones. J Thorac Cardiovasc Surg. 2018;155(4):1381–9.
19. Demers P, Miller DC, Mitchell RS, Kee ST, Chagonjian L, Dake MD. Stent-graft repair of penetrating atherosclerotic ulcers in the descending thoracic aorta: mid-term results. Ann Thorac Surg. 2004;77(1):81–6.
20. Mestres G, Rodríguez R, García-Madrid C, Montañà X, Burrel M, Cruz LF, et al. Endovascular treatment of penetrating aortic ulcers: mid-term follow-up. Rev Española Cardiol (Engl Ed). 2012;65(1):54–9.
21. Schoder M, Grabenwöger M, Hölzenbein T, Domanovits H, Fleischmann D, Wolf F, et al. Endovascular stent-graft repair of complicated penetrating atherosclerotic ulcers of the descending thoracic aorta. J Vasc Surg. 2002;36(4):720–6.
22. Kos X, Bouchard L, Otal P, Chabbert V, Chemla P, Soula P, et al. Stent-graft treatment of penetrating thoracic aortic ulcers. J Endovasc Therapy. 2002;9(Suppl 2):II25–31.
23. Eggebrecht H, Baumgart D, Schermund A, von Birgelen C, Herold U, Wiesemes R, et al. Endovascular stent-graft repair for penetrating atherosclerotic ulcer of the descending aorta. Am J Cardiol. 2003;91(9):1150–3.
24. Brinster DR, Wheatley GH, Williams J, Ramaiah VG, Diethrich EB, Rodriguez-Lopez JA. Are penetrating aortic ulcers best treated using an endovascular approach? Ann Thorac Surg. 2006;82(5):1688–91.

25. Eggebrecht H, Herold U, Schmermund A, Lind AY, Kuhnt O, Martini S, et al. Endovascular stent-graft treatment of penetrating aortic ulcer: results over a median follow-up of 27 months. Am Heart J. 2006;151(2):530–6.
26. Dalainas I, Nano G, Medda M, Bianchi P, Casana R, Ramponi F, et al. Endovascular treatment of penetrating aortic ulcers: mid-term results. Eur J Vasc Endovasc Surg. 2007;34(1):74–8.
27. Pauls S, Orend KH, Sunder-Plassmann L, Kick J, Schelzig H. Endovascular repair of symptomatic penetrating atherosclerotic ulcer of the thoracic aorta. Eur J Vasc Endovasc Surg. 2007;34(1):66–73.
28. Geisbüsch P, Kotelis D, Weber TF, Hyhlik-Dürr A, Kauczor HU, Böckler D. Early and mid-term results after endovascular stent graft repair of penetrating aortic ulcers. J Vasc Surg. 2008;48(6):1361–8.
29. Botta L, Buttazzi K, Russo V, Parlapiano M, Gostoli V, Di Bartolomeo R, et al. Endovascular repair for penetrating atherosclerotic ulcers of the descending thoracic aorta: early and mid-term results. Ann Thorac Surg. 2008;85(3):987–92.
30. Girn HRS, McPherson S, Nicholson T, Mavor AID, Homer-Vanniasinkam S, Gough MJ. Short series of emergency stent-graft repair of symptomatic penetrating thoracic aortic ulcers (PTAU). Vasc Med. 2009;14(2):123–8.
31. D'Souza S, Duncan A, Aguila F, Oderich G, Ricotta J, Kalra M, et al. TEVAR for non-aneurysmal thoracic aortic pathology. Catheter Cardiovasc Interv. 2009;74(5):783–6.
32. Czerny M, Funovics M, Sodeck G, Dumfarth J, Schoder M, Juraszek A, et al. Results after thoracic endovascular aortic repair in penetrating atherosclerotic ulcers. Ann Thorac Surg. 2011;92(2):562–7.
33. Palombo D, Lucertini G, Robaldo A, Pane B, Spinella G. Treatment of penetrating aortic ulcer by endoprosthesis: A single center experience. Int Angiol. 2012 Feb;31(1):54–61.
34. Jánosi RA, Gorla R, Tsagakis K, Kahlert P, Horacek M, Bruckschen F, et al. Thoracic endovascular repair of complicated penetrating aortic ulcer: an 11-year single-center experience. J Endovasc Ther. 2016;23(1):150–9.
35. Patel HJ, Sood V, Williams DM, Dasika NL, Diener AC, Deeb GM. Late outcomes with repair of penetrating thoracic aortic ulcers: the merits of an endovascular approach. Ann Thorac Surg. 2012;94(2):516–23.

Endovascular Treatment of Type A Aortic Dissections

Maximilian Kreibich and Friedhelm Beyersdorf

Abbreviation

TEVAR Thoracic endovascular aortic repair

Introduction

Patients with acute type A aortic dissection require an immediate surgical intervention to survive [1, 2]. Yet survival after such surgery remains unacceptably low in patients with severe organ malperfusion and/or shock [2, 3], despite considerably improved surgical techniques [3], individualized organ protection and cannulation strategies [4] and integrated, standardized surgical management strategies [5]. In fact, while the predicted mortality of patients with acute type A aortic dissection without shock or malperfusion remains well below 10% even in the elderly, outcomes in older patients presenting shock and malperfusion are dismal, with predicted mortality rates exceeding 50% [2]. Moreover, even in specialized high-volume centers, up to 8% of all patients with an acute type A aortic dissection are deemed inoperable [6].

Thoracic endovascular aortic repair (TEVAR) has significantly improved the perioperative results in the treatment of acute complicated dissections of the descending aorta compared to conventional open surgery [7]. Yet TEVAR's use in the more proximal aortic segments, specifically the ascending aorta, remains experimental and is limited to high-volume aortic centers with specialized aortic teams. In fact, although TEVAR in the ascending aorta remains the subject of only case reports and small case series [8], the rising numbers of successful TEVARs in the ascending aorta highlight this therapy's feasibility. In patients with acute type A aortic dissection and a dismal perioperative risk, TEVAR may help to significantly improve peri- und postoperative outcomes [2, 8, 9]. Nevertheless, four frontiers

M. Kreibich (✉) · F. Beyersdorf
Department of Cardiovascular Surgery, Heart Centre Freiburg University, Freiburg, Germany

Faculty of Medicine, University of Freiburg, Freiburg, Germany
e-mail: maximilian.kreibich@universitaets-herzzentrum.de

J. S. Coselli et al. (eds.), *Aortic Dissection and Acute Aortic Syndromes*,
https://doi.org/10.1007/978-3-030-66668-2_18

currently restrict the routine application of ascending aortic TEVAR to treat acute type A aortic dissection, namely, a physiologic, anatomic, medical, and technical frontier.

Physiologic Frontier

The ascending aorta's motion pattern is uniquely different from the more distal aortic segments such as the tubular, straight descending aorta. In fact, the ascending aorta's flow and motion are significantly influenced by its non-planar curvature, specific inlet flow conditions from the aortic valve, radial expansion-contraction, and transational movement secondary to being attached to the beating heart [10]—effects that result in its substantial deformation, rotation, and craniocaudal movement [11]. The precise implantation of the stent-graft may be perioperatively feasible through rapid over-pacing, halting the heart's ejection and the movement within the ascending aorta. However, when returning to a normal cardiac cycle, the interaction between a dissected, flexible, and highly mobile ascending aorta and stiff tubular stent-graft remains unclear and the potential risk for stent-graft dislocation and other stent-graft induced complications is very high.

Stable fixation to prevent stent-graft dislocation or migration can be ensured by oversizing the stent-graft in comparison to the native aorta. However, particularly in a dissected aorta, oversizing also significantly increases the risk for stent-graft induced new entries and aortic rupture [12]. If we consider a stent-graft's potentially unequal pressure distribution in the ascending aorta's small and large curvature, the risk for stent-graft-induced complications may even be higher in the ascending aorta than in the straight, tubular aortic segments.

Lastly, two small studies, have recently suggested negative aortic remodeling entailing reduced biventricular function following the use of TEVAR in the descending aorta [13, 14]. The impact of stiff endovascular grafts in more proximal aortic segments, particularly the ascending aorta compared with the native flexible aortic wall, and elimination of the Windkessel effect need to be considered when performing ascending aortic TEVAR.

Anatomic Frontier

The length of any stent-graft is defined as the distance between the proximal and distal landing zone. When using short stent-grafts, the landing zone should at least comprise 20 mm to ensure the stent-graft's durable fixation and stabilization [15]. In addition, there must be no entry tear in either of the two landing zones [15]. In this respect, the length of an ascending aortic stent-graft is very limited by the need for proximal and distal landing zons, each measuring at least 20 mm, as well as by the short distance between the aortic sinus with the coronary arteries' offspring and the brachiocephalic trunk with the cerebral arteries'offspring. Because of these preconditions, high quality feasibility studies addressing the application of ascending aortic TEVAR with a straight stent-graft in patients with type A aortic dissection have identified just 32–46% of all patients as being potential candidates suitable for a conventional straight endovascular tube graft because the entry tear would need to be average length of 30–40 mm in the mid ascending aorta for a straight stent-graft to adequately cover it [9, 16, 17]. Therefore, to treat more patients with ascending aortic TEVAR, shorter stent-graft landing zones seem inevitable, yet without additional stent-graft anchorage, the risk for stent-graft-induced complications such as its migration would increase considerably. In addition, a perpendicular angle between the sinotubular junction and distal ascending aorta can further compromise the precise implantation of a straight stent-graft [18].

Medical Frontier

A substantial number of patients with type A aortic dissection develop cardiac tamponade and/or moderate to severe aortic regurgitation [19]. The latter can be a major limitation for isolated ascending aortic TEVAR, while cardiac tamponade may be alleviated by simultaneous pericardial drainage or by transapical, antegrade stent-graft implantation. Antegrade implantation would both remove any pericardial effusion and simplify stent-graft implantation: true lumen wire placement would be simpler, the aortic arch's steep curvature would be avoided, the risk for dissection membrane perforation would be reduced, and accurate and precise stent-graft deployment would be easier because of the shorter distance to the ascending aorta.

Technical Frontier

Currently and commercially available stent-grafts may not be ideal for deployment within a dissected ascending aorta, because most patients presenting an acute type A aortic dissection would require tapered stent-grafts because of significantly different sizes between the proximal and distal landing zones [9]. Moreover, stent-graft dislocation due to the jump phenomenon remains an issue during TEVAR deployment, and even slight displacements of the stent-graft in the short ascending aorta can have devastating consequences because of the high risk for coronary or cerebral malperfusion [20]. The stent-graft's wedge apposition in the ascending aorta is another potential factor limiting durable stent-graft deployment within the ascending aorta as it can also raise the risk for stent-graft-induced complications.

The Endovascular Valve-Carrying Conduit

The concept of a transapically-implantable, endovascular, valve–carrying conduit for treating aortic valve and ascending aortic pathologies was first introduced by Rylski et al. [21]. The endo-conduit consists of a proximal transcatheter aortic valve connected to an uncovered portion of a covered stent-graft. This device is capable of

1. closing a primary entry tear in the ascending aorta,
2. ensuring coronary and cerebral perfusion,
3. stabilizing the distal aorta, initiating true lumen expansion and ensuring distal malperfusion,
4. treating aortic regurgitation, and
5. draining any pericardial effusion via a transapical approach

While conventional TEVAR with a straight tube graft requires two landing zones to affix and seal the graft durably, the valve-carrying conduit would encompass a third, proximal landing zone within the aortic annulus ensuring durable and stable anchorage of the entire device (Fig. 1). Hence, the proximal and distal stent-graft landing zones need not sustain the stent-graft itself, it merely needs to seal it off. Thus, oversizing of the conventional stent-graft landing zones proximally and distally becomes unnecessary, and the landing zones can potentially be even shorter. The latter would enlarge the pool of patients even more.

Individualization is a cornerstone of the conduit because the size of the catheter valve and stent-graft portion can be specifically selected to ideally accommodate the patient's unique anatomy and their specific entry-tear location within the ascending aorta. In a large feasibility study [9], our group was recently able to demonstrate that over two-thirds of all patients suffering an acute type A aortic dissection are potential candidates for the endovascular valve-carrying conduit to stabilize the proximal aorta and close any entry tear within the ascending aorta. Our investigation also showed that just eight different stent-graft lengths would suffice to treat these patients, but also that most of these patients would require short, tapered stent-grafts. Also, 7% of patients would require broader transcatheter aortic valve sizes [9].

A one-stage and a two-stage clinical scenario for implanting the endovascular valve-carrying conduit seem feasible. In the one-stage scenario, the conduit could be used to stabilize the ascending aorta in patients without malperfusion but carrying a high perioperative risk. Frail patients are potential candidates for this one-stage treatment. In the two-stage scenario, the conduit could be the first-step treatment to resolve distal malperfusion by re-expanding the true lumen and proximally stabilizing the dissected ascending aorta. Once the patient has stabilized and both shock and malperfusion have resolved, a stable patient could undergo conventional surgery in the second step with significantly better postoperative outcome prospects. This scenario is comparable to the Emory group's TEVAR first strategy, but would offer these patients the substantial benefit of proximal stabilization [22, 23] (Figs. 2 and 3).

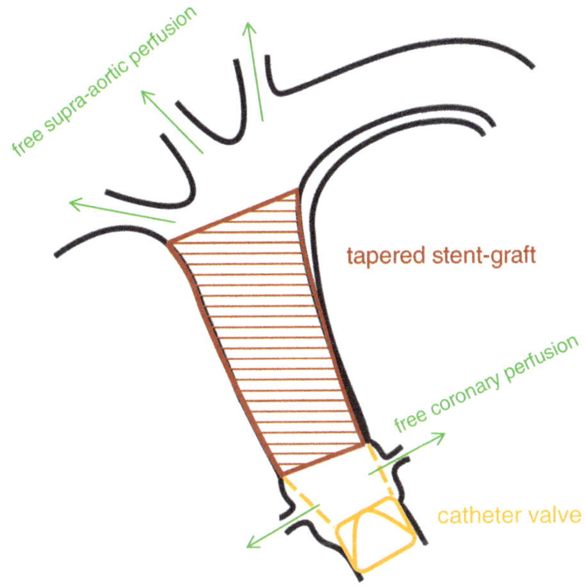

Fig. 1 The endovascular valve-carrying conduit consists of a transcatheter aortic valve connected to an uncovered portion of a covered stent-graft. Three landing zones can be generated by the device: (1) the aortic valve annulus for stable anchorage of the device, (2) a proximal sealing zone at the level of the sinotubular junction, and (3) a distal sealing zone at the level of the distal ascending aorta before the brachiocephalic trunk's takeoff. Individualization is the conduit's fundamental advantage, since the catheter valve size and stent-graft portion can be selected individually to accommodate the patient's unique anatomy, and the two components can be connected shortly before implantation by a suture. Free coronary and supra-aortic perfusion is thus ensured

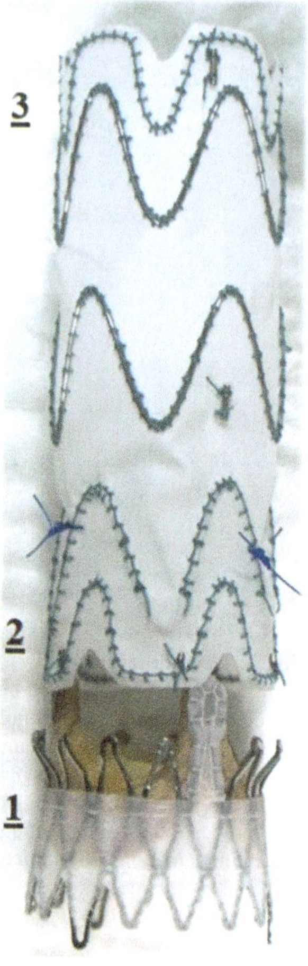

Fig. 2 The endovascular valve-carrying conduit before implantation. The proximal transcatheter aortic valve with proximal landing zone 1 for anchorage is connected to the covered stent-graft with the two sealing zones (2 and 3)

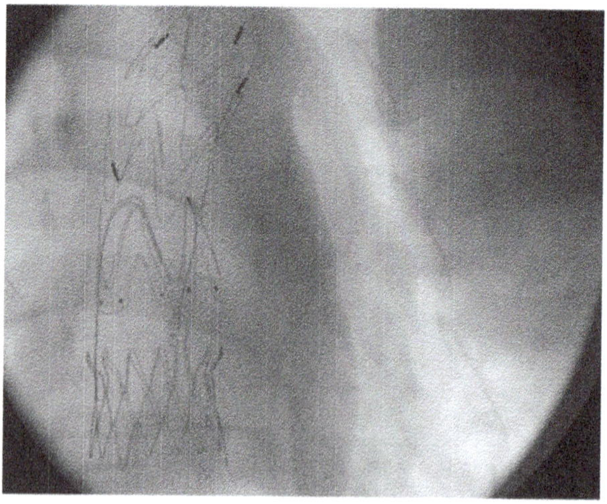

Fig. 3 Representative radiographic image of *in vivo* implantation of the endovascular valve-carrying conduits in a pig model

Conclusion

Ascending aortic TEVAR currently remains confined to the purview of specialized aortic centers treating carefully-selected patients with favorable anatomy and/or a localized pathology. Physiologic, anatomic, medical, and technical problems limit the routine application of TEVAR in the ascending aorta, particularly in patients suffering from type A aortic dissection. The provision of an endovascular valve-carrying conduit raises the potential number of patients eligible for endovascular treatment considerably, and may help to significantly reduce the morbidity and mortality of patients with type A aortic dissections.

Disclosures/conflict of interest No disclosures/conflict of interest for any author.

Funding Institutional funding.

References

1. Dumfarth J, Peterss S, Luehr M, Etz CD, Schachner T, Kofler M, et al. Acute type A dissection in octogenarians: does emergency surgery impact in-hospital outcome or long-term survival? Eur J Cardiothorac Surg. 2017;51:472–7.
2. Kreibich M, Rylski B, Czerny M, Siepe M, Beyersdorf F, Chen Z, et al. Influence of age and the burden of ischemic injury on the outcome of type A aortic dissection repair. Ann Thorac Surg. 2019;108:1391–7.
3. Kreibich M, Bavaria JE, Branchetti E, Brown CR, Chen Z, Khurshan F, et al. Management of patients with coronary artery malperfusion secondary to type A aortic dissection. Ann Thorac Surg. 2019;107:1174–80.
4. Kreibich M, Chen Z, Rylski B, Bavaria JE, Brown CR, Branchetti E, et al. Outcome after aortic, axillary, or femoral cannulation for acute type A aortic dissection. J Thorac Cardiovasc Surg. 2019;158:27–34. e9
5. Bavaria JE, Pochettino A, Brinster DR, Gorman RC, McGarvey ML, Gorman JH, et al. New paradigms and improved results for the surgical treatment of acute type A dissection. Ann Surg. 2001;234:336–42. discussion 42–3
6. Roselli EE, Hasan SM, Idrees JJ, Aftab M, Eagleton MJ, Menon V, et al. Inoperable patients with acute type A dissection: are they candidates for endovascular repair? Interact Cardiovasc Thorac Surg. 2017;25:582–8.
7. Brown CR, Chen Z, Khurshan F, Kreibich M, Bavaria J, Groeneveld P, et al. Outcomes after thoracic endovascular aortic repair in patients with chronic kidney disease in the Medicare population. J Thorac Cardiovasc Surg. 2020;159(2):402–13. https://doi.org/10.1016/j.jtcvs.2019.01.118.
8. Kreibich M, Rylski B, Kondov S, Morlock J, Scheumann J, Kari F, et al. Endovascular treatment of acute Type A aortic dissection—the Endo Bentall approach. J Vis Surg. 2018;4:69.
9. Kreibich M, Soekeland T, Beyersdorf F, Bavaria JE, Schrofel H, Czerny M, et al. Anatomic feasibility of an endovascular valve-carrying conduit for the treatment of type A aortic dissection. J Thorac Cardiovasc Surg. 2019;157:26–34 e1.
10. Jin S, Oshinski J, Giddens DP. Effects of wall motion and compliance on flow patterns in the ascending aorta. J Biomech Eng. 2003;125:347–54.

11. Beller CJ, Labrosse MR, Thubrikar MJ, Robicsek F. Role of aortic root motion in the pathogenesis of aortic dissection. Circulation. 2004;109:763–9.
12. Kreibich M, Bunte D, Berger T, Votsch A, Rylski B, Krombholz-Reindl P, et al. Distal stent-graft-induced new entries following the frozen elephant trunk procedure. Ann Thorac Surg. 2020;110(4):1271–9. https://doi.org/10.1016/j.athoracsur.2020.02.017.
13. van Bakel TMJ, Arthurs CJ, Nauta FJH, Eagle KA, van Herwaarden JA, Moll FL, et al. Cardiac remodelling following thoracic endovascular aortic repair for descending aortic aneurysms. Eur J Cardiothorac Surg. 2019;55:1061–70.
14. Kreibich M, Morlock J, Beyersdorf F, Berger T, Allweier S, Kondov S, et al. Decreased biventricular function following thoracic endovascular aortic repair. Interact Cardiovasc Thorac Surg. 2020;1(30):600–4.
15. Grabenwoger M, Alfonso F, Bachet J, Bonser R, Czerny M, Eggebrecht H, et al. Thoracic Endovascular Aortic Repair (TEVAR) for the treatment of aortic diseases: a position statement from the European Association for Cardio-Thoracic Surgery (EACTS) and the European Society of Cardiology (ESC), in collaboration with the European Association of Percutaneous Cardiovascular Interventions (EAPCI). Eur Heart J. 2012;33:1558–63.
16. Huang C, Zhou M, Liu Z, Huang D, Ran F, Wang W, et al. Computed tomography-based study exploring the feasibility of endovascular treatment of type A aortic dissection in the Chinese population. J Endovasc Ther. 2014;21:707–13.
17. Moon MC, Greenberg RK, Morales JP, Martin Z, Lu Q, Dowdall JF, et al. Computed tomography-based anatomic characterization of proximal aortic dissection with consideration for endovascular candidacy. J Vasc Surg. 2011;53:942–9.
18. Rylski B, Desjardins B, Moser W, Bavaria JE, Milewski RK. Gender-related changes in aortic geometry throughout life. Eur J Cardiothorac Surg. 2014;45:805–11.
19. Kreibich M, Rylski B, Czerny M, Pingpoh C, Siepe M, Beyersdorf F, et al. Type A aortic dissection in patients with bicuspid aortic valve aortopathy. Ann Thorac Surg. 2020;109(1):94–100.
20. Berezowski M, Morlock J, Beyersdorf F, Jasinski M, Plonek T, Siepe M, et al. Inaccurate aortic stent graft deployment in the distal landing zone: incidence, reasons and consequences. Eur J Cardiothorac Surg. 2018;53:1158–64.
21. Rylski B, Szeto WY, Bavaria JE, Branchetti E, Moser W, Milewski RK. Development of a single endovascular device for aortic valve replacement and ascending aortic repair. J Card Surg. 2014;29:371–6.
22. Leshnower BG, Keeling WB, Duwayri YM, Jordan WD Jr, Chen EP. The "thoracic endovascular aortic repair-first" strategy for acute type A dissection with mesenteric malperfusion: Initial results compared with conventional algorithms. J Thorac Cardiovasc Surg. 2019;158:1516–24.
23. Leshnower BG, Veeraswamy RK, Duwayri YM, Chen EP. The "TEVAR-first" approach to DeBakey I aortic dissection with mesenteric malperfusion. Ann Thorac Surg. 2014;97:693–6.

Valve Sparing Aortic Root Replacement for Aortic Valve Insufficiency in Type A Aortic Dissection

Eltayeb Mohamed Ahmed and Edward P. Chen

Introduction

Type A acute aortic dissection (TAAAD) is a surgical emergency that is rapidly fatal if left untreated. The international registry of acute aortic dissection (IRAD) reported an improvement in surgical outcome, as mortality decreased from 25 to 18% over 17 years since its inception. Furthermore, contemporary series reported a mortality as low as 5% [1–3].

The mortality of TAAAD is determined by preoperative risk factors, such as malperfusion syndrome, renal impairment, or preoperative rupture [4, 5]. Therefore, an operation that avoids a high-risk reintervention, and that is not associated with an increase in immediate risk is optimal. Aortic root replacement, when required to completely resect the proximal extent of the dissection, is associated with excellent event-free survival and reoperation rates [6–8]. In fact, several series reported that replacement of the aortic root in patients with TAAAD is not associated with an increase in perioperative morbidity or mortality [5, 9, 10]. Furthermore, there is evidence to show that root replacement decreases the need for reintervention, as shown in a propensity matched cohort where the freedom from reintervention was significantly higher in the root replacement group 98 vs. 86% at 7 years [11]. Surgical options for aortic root replacement can be performed using a composite valve conduit or a valve sparing technique (VSRR).

In this chapter we will discuss the indications for aortic root replacement in TAAAD, valve sparing aortic root replacement (VSRR) in TAAAD, the technical details of VSRR in TAAAD, and the result of valve conserving root surgery.

E. M. Ahmed
Bristol Royal Infirmary, Bristol, UK

E. P. Chen (✉)
Section of Surgical Disciplines, Division of Cardiovascular and Thoracic Surgery, Duke University Medical Center, Durham, NC, USA
e-mail: edward.p.chen@duke.edu

J. S. Coselli et al. (eds.), *Aortic Dissection and Acute Aortic Syndromes*,
https://doi.org/10.1007/978-3-030-66668-2_19

Indications for Aortic Root Replacement in TAAAD

Replacement of the aortic root is indicated in patients with an aortic root diameter ≥5.5 cm, a diameter of 4.0–5.0 cm in patients with concomitant risk factors for rupture or dissection, or a simultaneously indicated valve or ascending aortic surgery [12, 13]. While these indications are well established in the elective setting, they are also applied to patients with TAAAD. In patients with aortic dissection the American Heart Association (AHA) recommended root replacement in patients with extensive destruction of the aortic root or root dilatation [12, 14]. However, the degree of destruction or dilatation is not quantified and is an area of debate over whether root replacement is required in TAAAD. Therefore, the decision to replace the root is often based on an assessment of the risk of extensive repair against the possibility of a complicated redo surgery in the future (Fig. 1) [15].

Following supracomissural repair of TAAAD, the aortic root continues to enlarge at a rate 0.50–0.60 mm/year [16]. Furthermore, a substantial proportion of patients operated for TAAAD will require a reintervention, the freedom from reintervention is in the range 80–30% at 10 years [5, 17]. Conversely, adding a root replacement to an already high-risk operation does increase the risk of the operation as shown in the University of Pennsylvania study, the mortality of aortic root replacement was almost three times higher than supracomissural repair in patients with TAAAD [18, 19]. Therefore, it is important to identify risk factors for reoperation to enable the surgeon to balance the risk of a complex redo procedure against an aggressive index operation in TAAAD.

Several authors investigated the risk factors for reoperation following TAAAD repair. Young-age has been identified as a risk factor for reoperation by several groups [19, 20]. In a study of young patients, under the age of 50, the reoperation rate following TAAAD was 24%. In the same cohort 44% of patients who had a supracomissural replacement required a root procedure [19, 21, 22]. Kirsch et al. studied 160 patients who underwent repair of TAAAD; the freedom from

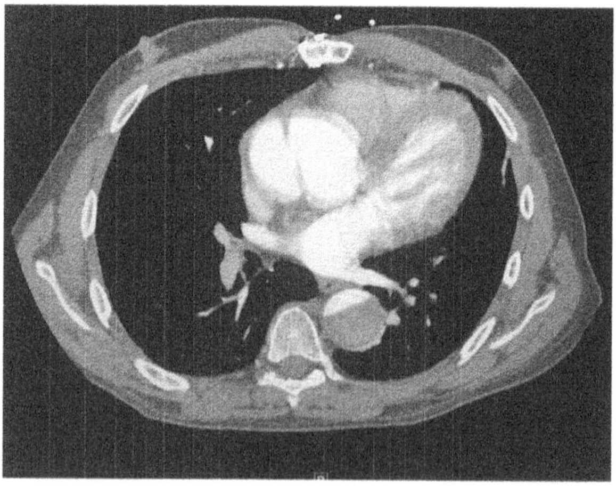

Fig. 1 A 61-year-old male patient who had supracomissural repair of TAAAD presenting with a pseudoaneurysm 1 year following initial repair

reoperation at 10 years was 60%, and they identified severe preoperative AI as a predictor for proximal reoperation, RR 3.6 (95% CI 1.44–9.77) [7]. Certainly, severe AI and root aneurysm are among the commonest indications for reoperation following TAAD repair [23].

Patients with connective tissue disease are at a great risk of requiring a reintervention. In the Nordic Consortium for Acute Aortic Dissection Type A (NORCAAD) study, the risk of reoperation was five times higher in patients with connective tissue disease [24]. A cohort study of over 500 patients, identified Marfan syndrome as a risk factor for reintervention (OR 4.68 95% CI 1.6–13.7) [25]. We believe, among other groups, that limited ascending repair without root replacement will almost certainly result in the need for a root reintervention in this cohort of patients [26]. It must be emphasized that often the diagnosis of Marfan syndrome is made after presentation with TAAAD. Therefore, a high index of suspicion is needed particularly in the young [19].

In addition to hemodynamic characteristics of the aortic valve and the patients' genetic risk profile, certain anatomical features of the dissection flap and the aortic root are associated with a pronounced increase in the risk of a reintervention. The preoperative root diameter, number of commissural detachment, and dissection flap extension into the root are anatomical features that should be recognized and persuade the surgeon to take an aggressive approach to the aortic root in patients with TAAAD (Fig. 2) [27, 28].

The controversy, whether the root should be replaced or not, stems from the fact that high rates of reintervention and the risk factors for reintervention have not been universally identified and agreed upon among investigators. The NORCAAD, for example, reported a reoperation rate of 5% at 8 years, most of the reoperations were in the form of a root replacement; however, the mean follow-up was 3.3 years, and 25% of patients in the cohort had a root replacement [24]. Mayo clinic series had a freedom from reoperation at 91% and 79% at 10 and 20 years respectively. While no predictive factors for reoperation were identified; yet 70% of reoperations were for aortic root dilatation or aortic insufficiency [5]. Low reoperation rates have been reported by other groups in smaller studies [8, 18, 19, 29].

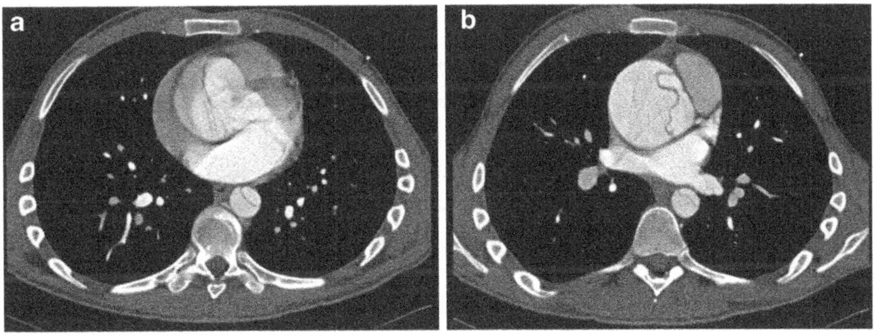

Fig. 2 Preoperative CTA demonstrating a dilated aortic root with the dissection flap extending into the aortic root (**a**) and the ascending aorta (**b**)

The limitations of the evidence available are related to the fact that most studies evaluating long term outcomes of TAAAD patients have a small number of patients, retrospective in nature, single centre, and have a short follow-up. Therefore, a large cohort of TAAAD patients with standardised follow-up is needed to enable the surgical community and patients make an informed decision of the choice of surgery in this fatal disease.

At our institution, we perform root replacement if the tear is in the aortic root, the root is dilated >4.5 cm in diameter, and in patients with suspected connective tissue disease. The IRAD reported a similar strategy of selective root with no difference in outcome between the supracomissural repair group and the root replacement group. In our experience, the outcome of VSRR in the hemodynamically unstable patients and patients with malperfusion syndrome is unfavourable. However, other groups did not preclude patients from a VSRR approach because of haemodynamic instability [9]. Halstead reported excellent results with a similar aggressive strategy towards the root [8]. We also believe that the surgeon's experience should be considered before recommending a liberal root replacement strategy in patients with TAAAD [9, 30, 31].

VSRR in TAAAD

Bentall and De Bono used a Starr valve and a Teflon graft in their technique of composite valve conduit aortic root replacement with reimplantation of the coronary arteries [32]. The technique was modified by Cabrol, as the two ends of an 8 mm Dacron graft were anastomosed to the coronary ostia, the graft is subsequently anastomosed sided-to-side to the aortic prosthesis [33]. The early mortality in Cabrol series, a third of which had aortic dissection, was an outstanding 4% [34].

The prosthetic valve component is the main limitation of the Bentall procedure. Mechanical valves offer better durability, particularly in young patients, in comparison with bioprosthesis. The durability of mechanical prosthesis is offset by the risk of anticoagulation, thromboembolic events and valve thrombosis. Bouhout and associates reported survival, freedom from reoperation, and freedom from significant bleeding of 87%, 82%, and 90% respectively at 10 years in young patients. A meta-analysis of the Bentall procedure, 7629 patients included, reported an annual linearized risk of 2% for mortality, 0.77% thromboembolic events, and 2.66% of valve related adverse events [35].

The risk of structural valve degeneration of bioprosthesis is of a considerable importance when a bio-Bentall is contemplated. Reports of freedom from structural valve degeneration of modern bioprosthesis are limited by short follow-up [36]. In a UK-based registry, the results of biological AVR were not encouraging with a freedom from reintervention or death of 47% at 10 years [37]. The AVR data is pertinent to aortic root replacement using the Bentall technique, and clearly the long-term results of prosthetic valve replacement are suboptimal. It is logical that avoiding the adverse implications of a prosthetic valve, if possible, may result in an improved survival and quality of life in patients undergoing aortic root replacement [38, 39].

Sir Magdi Yacoub recognized in a cohort of patients with aortic insufficiency and aortic root aneurysm with normal cusps morphology that it was feasible to repair the aortic root, restore the aortic valve hemodynamics, and preserve native valve function. In Yacoub's remodelling technique, the aortic sinuses are excised, leaving a rim of 3 mm, the coronary ostia are isolated with a small aortic rim surrounding them (coronary button), and a tube graft, fashioned into three tongues, is sutured to the residual wall of the aortic root; subsequently, the coronary buttons are attached to the tube graft [40, 41]. The remodelling method proved to deliver durable aortic valve repair in selected patients [42]. A comparison between the results of remodelling in patients with type A aortic dissection and those with aneurysm revealed a longer bypass time, longer ICU stay, and a mortality of 19% in line with the average mortality in the IRAD with no difference in the reoperation rate or incidence of AI [43].

Tirone David and Chris Feindel, in 1992, introduced the reimplantation procedure, and reported their experience of ten patients with annuloaortic ectasia; four patients had aortic dissection in the series. In the reimplantation technique, the aortic valve is implanted within a tube graft that is anchored to the VAJ. In their series, there were no deaths, and one patient required reoperation for aortic insufficiency [44].

The advantage of the remodelling is that it preserves the inter-leaflet triangles, which may facilitate the dynamic nature of the native aortic root. Indeed, in-vivo studies demonstrated superior hemodynamics with remodelling in comparison with reimplantation [45]. However, a major limitation of the remodelling procedure is that it doesn't provide external stabilization of the VAJ, which is a potential cause for recurrence of AI and a source for a higher failure rate in patients with TAAAD [46–48]. However, the reimplantation requires more extensive dissection of the aortic root, takes longer, and potentially technically more demanding [42, 46]. Emanuel Lansac addressed stabilisation of the VAJ by adding an expansible ring in the subvalvular plane [49, 50]. The early results of remodelling in addition to subvalvular ring implantation demonstrated a reduction in the rate of reoperations and intraoperative conversion to prosthetic valve replacement [50]. Several modifications of the remodelling were developed, but most remain single-centre and reported in a small number of patients. Dr. C Miller group advocate a conservative partial root replacement, Uni-Yacoub or Bi-Yacoub repair, in selected patients [51].

Technical Aspects of Valve Sparing Root Replacement in TAAAD

The aim of VSRR is to provide durable repair with a low reintervention rate on the aortic valve. At the authors' institution, our procedure of choice is the reimplantation technique. Stabilization of the VAJ with a ring in combination with remodelling of the aortic root is a viable option [52]. Regardless to whether reimplantation or remodelling with ring stabilization is used, the technical aspects pertinent in the setting of TAAAD are shared.

The technical aspects of cardiopulmonary bypass in TAAAD repair are discussed elsewhere in this book. At Emory, we use the right axillary artery or the ascending aorta for arterial return, and the right atrium is used for drainage through a three-stage venous cannula inserted through the right atrial appendage. At a bladder temperature of 24–28 °C, the innominate artery is clamped and unilateral antegrade cerebral perfusion initiated. The aortic arch is reconstructed, using the neo-intima technique, and repaired as indicated. Following completion of distal reconstruction, the distal tube graft is clamped and total body perfusion is resumed through the right axillary artery.

At this stage the aortic root and valve are assessed for indication for root intervention and suitability of the aortic valve for preservation. With regard to the aortic valve, particular attention is paid to leaflets tissue quality, thickening, calcification, leaflet fenestration, leaflet prolapse and valve configuration. If the valve is suitable for preservation, the aortic root tissue is excised, leaving a 4–5 mm rim of aortic tissue, and the coronary buttons created. Subsequently, the aortic root is dissected free from surrounding structures 2 mm below the nadir of each cusp; the dissection is limited in the non-coronary/right coronary commissure because of the natural limitation imposed by the membranous septum and the muscular septum; the left atrium forms the lower limit of left coronary sinus dissection.

It is important to note that in cases of TAAAD tissue planes are more challenging to identify because of the haematoma and the swelling induced by the dissection (Fig. 3). It is worthwhile to invest in careful dissection to avoid inadvertent injury to the right ventricular outflow tract (RVOT), pulmonary artery (PA), and coronary vessels. Should an injury be identified, it should be repaired immediately.

Once the dissection is carried to the lowest point desired, 2-0 Polyester sutures are placed from within the LVOT and used to anchor the aortic prosthesis. We do not use pledgeted subannular sutures, as we believe pledgets can potentially interfere with

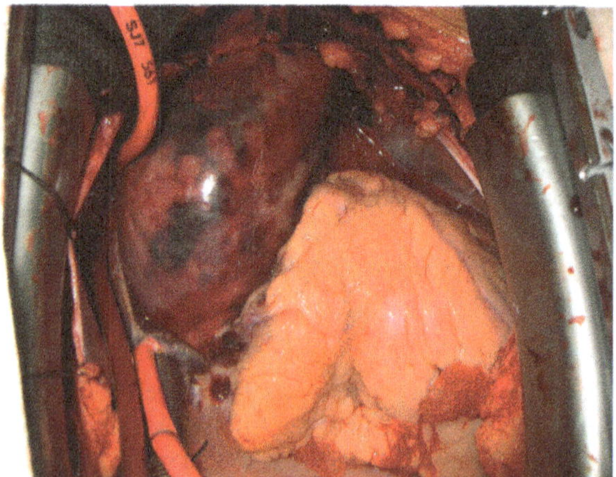

Fig. 3 TAAAD with haematoma extension into the pulmonary artery, dissection of tissue planes for VSRR can be challenging

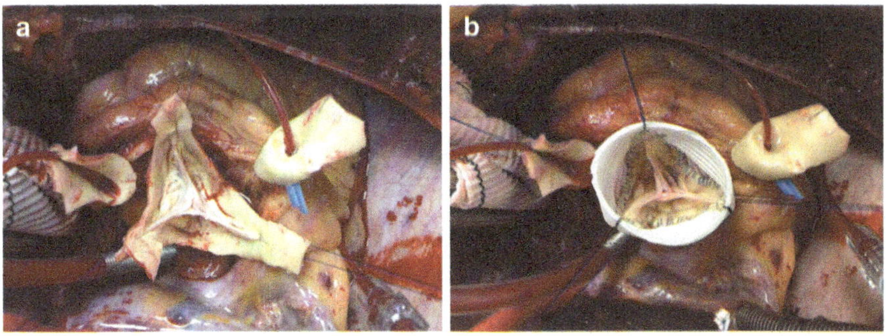

Fig. 4 (**a**) The aortic root is dissected leaving a 3–4 mm of tissue. (**b**) The valve is telescoped within the graft and sutured with 5-0 Polypropylene to the prosthesis prior to implantation of the coronary buttons

the undersurface of the leaflet. The proximal end of the graft is anchored to the subannular sutures with the valve and remnants of the aortic root telescoped within the graft. Subsequently, we assess the height of the commissures and suspend them to the graft with 5/0 Polypropylene under tension. It is important to maintain tension on the commissures at this stage. The aortic root rim is sutured to the graft with 5/0 Polypropylene sutures (Fig. 4); we assess leaflet coaptation, and should leaflet repair be required, it is performed at this stage. The coronary buttons are then anastomosed to the graft, starting with the left coronary artery. If the there is doubt regarding the integrity of the tissue of the coronary button, Cabrol modification of the original Bentall procedure, using a conduit to anastomose the coronary arteries to the graft is a sound strategy that we occasionally employ, as it helps avoid disappointment caused by a bleeding coronary button at the end of a long operation [6, 53]. We administer cardioplegia into the root and assess its' competency prior to releasing the cross clamp.

It is of paramount importance to carefully assess the TEE images after discontinuing CPB for evidence of AI. Should AI be identified, it is helpful to identify the aetiology and mechanism from TEE, as that would shorten the second clamp time required to address AI. It is our strategy to reclamp should AI > +1 be detected on TEE.

Regarding the sizing of the graft, we used David's formula of a graft size = $[2*(C_{usp}*2/3)] + 6$ to 10 mm to select a prosthesis appropriately. The height of the NC/RC commissure as proposed by El Khoury, or a Hegar dilator can also be used as guide prosthesis size [54]. We do not perform complex cusp repair in patients with TAAAD, as a second clamp may prove to be costly in this critically ill cohort of patients.

Results of VSRR in TAAAD

Sir Magdi Yacoub reported the results of remodelling in 158 patients, 31% had acute aortic dissection, with a mortality of 4.6% for the whole cohort; the mortality of patients with acute type A aortic dissection was 18%. However, a third of patients developed moderate aortic insufficiency, during a mean follow-up of 5 years [55].

The partial root replacement, including Uni-Yacoub and Bi-Yacoub, technique has been adopted by other groups, with a reported freedom from reintervention of 100–90% at 10 years or more [3, 56, 57]. Urbanski used a similar strategy in 46 patients with TAAAD with no valve related reintervention at mean follow-up of 4.5 years [58]. However, the selective sinus repair excellent results have not bee replicated by other group; in Chiu series 11% of patients who had unisinus or bisinus repair had a reintervention, while 0% of the Bentall group [27]. A study from Japan reported repair of AAAD in 19 patients, using the remodelling technique with VAJ ring stabilisation; the perioperative mortality was 5.6% and one patient needed reoperation for AI during a follow-up of 56 months [52]. The experience with this strategy in TAAAD is still its infancy, and we would be curious for long-term results and larger series to be reported.

The largest series to date of VSRR in TAAAD is from Hannover; Beckmann et al. reported their results of 109 patients who underwent David procedure for TAAAD. The in-hospital mortality was 11%, despite 40% of patients undergoing concomitant total arch replacement, which is below the mortality reported by IRAD, with a 10-year freedom from reoperation of 85%. Freedom from AI < +1 was 96%. Interestingly, when adjusted for perioperative mortality, the long-term survival of patients treated with VSRR for TAAAD is no different from elective patients [59]. These excellent results should be evaluated bearing in mind that in Hannover, on average, 22 VSRRR are performed electively every year; while in the USA the median number of aortic root surgeries performed by a centre is 2, and only 5% of centres performed more than 16 aortic root operations annually [60].

At Emory we published our experience in VSRR in TAAAD patients over 13 years. Of the 132 patients, 52 had VSRR. The 30-day mortality was 3.4% and 14.3 in the VSRR and root replacement groups respectively. The freedom from AI +2 was 94% at midterm follow-up and no patient required AVR. Furthermore, long-term survival benefit has been demonstrated following VSRR [31, 38, 61].

A comparative study of Bentall and David procedure in 135 TAAAD patients, reported similar adjusted perioperative mortality, no reoperations in the David group, and a better 10 year survival in favour of VSRR, 98% vs. 57% at 10 years. The Leipzig group reported the results of 208 root replacement in TAAAD, 130 Bentall, 51 modified Yacoub, 21 David, with similar perioperative results, despite the longer bypass time in the reimplantation group; the freedom from reoperation was also similar and in excess of 80% in all groups at 5 years [62]. Higher freedom from reoperation rates were reported in smaller series [63]. It is likely that in self-selected institutions good results are obtainable [64]. However, the encouraging results of VSRR in TAAAD are not consistent. Tanka et al. reported 24 VSRR, from a total cohort of 328 TAAAD patients, with a freedom from reoperation and freedom from moderate AI of 65% [65]. Tanaka's series is over a 16 years period, which may reflect a small volume of VSRR, and may explain the discouraging results. On the other hand, an element of publication bias is likely, as centres with good results are more likely to publish them.

A meta-analysis of valve sparing root replacement, 10% had TAAAD, reported a linearized mortality rate of 1.5%, 0.4% thromboembolic events, and a rate of 1.7% of major adverse valve related events [66]. Furthermore, a meta-analysis comparing Bentall and VSRR, including 9 studies and 706 patients, reported an improvement in early mortality and late mortality in the pooled VSRR group with an OR 0.77 (0.21–0.57 95% CI) for early mortality. The linearized late mortality was 4.1% and 19.8% for VSRR and Bentall respectively, OR 0.34 (95% CI 0.21–0.57) for later mortality. However, reintervention rate was higher in the VSRR group. The number of patients included in each study ranged from 52 to 295 patients, and all the studies were cohort studies. It is likely that there is an element of selection bias in all the reported studies based on surgeons' experience and patents' characteristic. Yet it is safe to conclude that in the appropriately selected patient VSRR provides long term benefit, these findings resonate with meta-analysis findings in aneurysmal aortic root disease [67, 68].

Aubin et al. reported a single surgeon experience of liberally employing the reimplantation in 45 patients with TAAAD. All patients with root involvement, in the absence of haemodynamic instability or serious organ dysfunction had reimplantation repair. Despite an increase in ischaemic time, cardiopulmonary bypass time by an approximately 50 min, the 30-day mortality of the reimplantation and non-reimplantation groups was 17% and 23% respectively. No reoperations were required for proximal disease, and the mean AI grade was 0.6 at 5 years follow-up. While Aubin's series is relatively small, it is among the most recently published data reflecting an increase in experience with reimplantation, a trend of a more aggressive approach to the root. It highlights importance of the surgeon's experience in achieving a good outcome in this challenging condition [69].

Others have demonstrated the association between surgeons with aortic interest and an aggressive approach towards the root, with a potential survival benefit [70]. The trend towards a more radical root strategy is particularly evident in the light that the University of Pennsylvania group published a series, just under a decade ago, of "new paradigms" in TAAD in which under a quarter of patients had aortic root replacement [71]. We have seen time and time again in cardiac surgery "the pendulum swing" and only more data would enable us to assess if swing in the other direction is needed.

Conclusion

In experienced centres VSRR should be considered if the valve morphology is favourable and in the absence of increased perioperative mortality risk factors. Young patients and patients with dilated aortic root or genetic aortic syndromes would probably benefit the most from valve conservation and preservation of native valve function.

References

1. Malvindi PG, Modi A, Miskolczi S, Kaarne M, Velissaris T, Barlow C, et al. Open and closed distal anastomosis for acute type A aortic dissection repair. Interact Cardiovasc Thorac Surg. 2016;22(6):776–83.
2. Pape LA, Awais M, Woznicki EM, Suzuki T, Trimarchi S, Evangelista A, et al. Presentation, diagnosis, and outcomes of acute aortic dissection: 17-year trends from the international registry of acute aortic dissection. J Am Coll Cardiol. 2015;66(4):350–8.
3. Huang F, Li L, Qin W, Su C, Wang L, Xiao L, et al. Partial aortic root remodeling for root reconstruction in patients with acute type A dissection. J Biomed Res. 2016;30(5):411–8.
4. Apaydin AZ, Buket S, Posacioglu H, Islamoglu F, Calkavur T, Yagdi T, et al. Perioperative risk factors for mortality in patients with acute type A aortic dissection. Ann Thorac Surg. 2002;74(6):2034–9. discussion 9
5. Wang Z, Greason KL, Pochettino A, Schaff HV, Suri RM, Stulak JM, et al. Long-term outcomes of survival and freedom from reoperation on the aortic root or valve after surgery for acute ascending aorta dissection. J Thorac Cardiovasc Surg. 2014;148(5):2117–22.
6. Ergin MA, McCullough J, Galla JD, Lansman SL, Griepp RB. Radical replacement of the aortic root in acute type A dissection: indications and outcome. Eur J Cardiothorac Surg. 1996;10(10):840–4. discussion 5
7. Kirsch M, Soustelle C, Houel R, Hillion ML, Loisance D. Risk factor analysis for proximal and distal reoperations after surgery for acute type A aortic dissection. J Thorac Cardiovasc Surg. 2002;123(2):318–25.
8. Halstead JC, Spielvogel D, Meier DM, Rinke S, Bodian C, Malekan R, et al. Composite aortic root replacement in acute type A dissection: time to rethink the indications? Eur J Cardiothorac Surg. 2005;27(4):626–32. discussion 32-3
9. Di Eusanio M, Trimarchi S, Peterson MD, Myrmel T, Hughes GC, Korach A, et al. Root replacement surgery versus more conservative management during type A acute aortic dissection repair. Ann Thorac Surg. 2014;98(6):2078–84.
10. Montalvo J, Razzouk A, Wang N, Bansal R, Rasi A, Hasaniya N, et al. Aortic root surgery does not increase the operative risk of acute type A aortic dissection. Am Surg. 2011;77(1):88–92.
11. Castrovinci S, Pacini D, Di Marco L, Berretta P, Cefarelli M, Murana G, et al. Surgical management of aortic root in type A acute aortic dissection: a propensity-score analysis. Eur J Cardiothorac Surg. 2016;50(2):223–9.
12. Hiratzka LF, Bakris GL, Beckman JA, Bersin RM, Carr VF, Casey DE Jr, et al. 2010 ACCF/AHA/AATS/ACR/ASA/SCA/SCAI/SIR/STS/SVM guidelines for the diagnosis and management of patients with thoracic aortic disease: executive summary. A report of the American College of Cardiology Foundation/American Heart Association Task Force on Practice Guidelines, American Association for Thoracic Surgery, American College of Radiology, American Stroke Association, Society of Cardiovascular Anesthesiologists, Society for Cardiovascular Angiography and Interventions, Society of Interventional Radiology, Society of Thoracic Surgeons, and Society for Vascular Medicine. Catheter Cardiovasc Interv. 2010;76(2):E43–86.
13. ACCF/AHA/AATS/ACR/ASA/SCA/SCAI/SIR/STS/SVM Guidelines for the Diagnosis and Management of Patients with Thoracic Aortic Disease Representative Members, Hiratzka LF, Creager MA, Isselbacher EM, Svensson LG, et al. Surgery for aortic dilatation in patients with bicuspid aortic valves: a statement of clarification From the American College of Cardiology/American Heart Association Task Force on Clinical Practice Guidelines. Circulation. 2016;133(7):680–6.
14. Mokashi SA, Svensson LG. Guidelines for the management of thoracic aortic disease in 2017. Gen Thorac Cardiovasc Surg. 2019;67(1):59–65.
15. Fleischman F, Elsayed RS, Cohen RG, Tatum JM, Kumar SR, Kazerouni K, et al. Selective aortic arch and root replacement in repair of acute type A aortic dissection. Ann Thorac Surg. 2018;105(2):505–12.

16. Qiu J, Wu J, Xie E, Luo X, Chen JF, Gao W, et al. Surgical management and outcomes of aortic root in acute type A aortic dissection. Ann Thorac Surg. 2019;110(1):136–43.
17. Pugliese P, Pessotto R, Santini F, Montalbano G, Luciani GB, Mazzucco A. Risk of late reoperations in patients with acute type A aortic dissection: impact of a more radical surgical approach. Eur J Cardiothorac Surg. 1998;13(5):576–80. discussion 80-1
18. Valdis M, Adams C, Chu MWA, Kiaii B, Guo L. Comparison of outcomes of root replacement procedures and supracoronary techniques for surgical repair of acute aortic dissection. Can J Surg. 2017;60(3):198–204.
19. Geirsson A, Bavaria JE, Swarr D, Keane MG, Woo YJ, Szeto WY, et al. Fate of the residual distal and proximal aorta after acute type A dissection repair using a contemporary surgical reconstruction algorithm. Ann Thorac Surg. 2007;84(6):1955–64. discussion 64
20. Fann JI, Smith JA, Miller DC, Mitchell RS, Moore KA, Grunkemeier G, et al. Surgical management of aortic dissection during a 30-year period. Circulation. 1995;92(9 Suppl):II113–21.
21. Niederhauser U, Kaplan Z, Kunzli A, Genoni M, Zund G, Lachat ML, et al. Disadvantages of local repair in acute type A aortic dissection. Ann Thorac Surg. 1998;66(5):1592–9.
22. Piccardo A, Regesta T, Le Guyader A, Di Lorenzo N, Bertin F, Pesteil F, et al. Outcomes after surgery for acute type A aortic dissection in "non-Marfan syndrome" patients with long life expectancy: a 24-year follow-up. Arch Cardiovasc Dis. 2017;110(1):14–25.
23. Concistre G, Casali G, Santaniello E, Montalto A, Fiorani B, Dell'Aquila A, et al. Reoperation after surgical correction of acute type A aortic dissection: risk factor analysis. Ann Thorac Surg. 2012;93(2):450–5.
24. Pan E, Gudbjartsson T, Ahlsson A, Fuglsang S, Geirsson A, Hansson EC, et al. Low rate of reoperations after acute type A aortic dissection repair from The Nordic Consortium Registry. J Thorac Cardiovasc Surg. 2018;156(3):939–48.
25. Dohle DS, El Beyrouti H, Brendel L, Pfeiffer P, El-Mehsen M, Vahl CF. Survival and reinterventions after isolated proximal aortic repair in acute type A aortic dissection. Interact Cardiovasc Thorac Surg. 2019;28(6):981–8.
26. Schoenhoff FS, Carrel TP. Re-interventions on the thoracic and thoracoabdominal aorta in patients with Marfan syndrome. Ann Cardiothorac Surg. 2017;6(6):662–71.
27. Ikeno Y, Yokawa K, Yamanaka K, Inoue T, Tanaka H, Okada K, et al. The fate of aortic root and aortic regurgitation after supracoronary ascending aortic replacement for acute type A aortic dissection. J Thorac Cardiovasc Surg. 2019;161(2):483–493.e1.
28. Malvindi PG, van Putte BP, Sonker U, Heijmen RH, Schepens MA, Morshuis WJ. Reoperation after acute type A aortic dissection repair: a series of 104 patients. Ann Thorac Surg. 2013;95(3):922–7.
29. Kamohara K, Koga S, Takaki J, Yoshida N, Furukawa K, Morita S. Long-term durability of preserved aortic root after repair of acute type A aortic dissection. Gen Thorac Cardiovasc Surg. 2017;65(8):441–8.
30. Yang B, Norton EL, Hobbs R, Farhat L, Wu X, Hornsby WE, et al. Short- and long-term outcomes of aortic root repair and replacement in patients undergoing acute type A aortic dissection repair: twenty-year experience. J Thorac Cardiovasc Surg. 2019;157(6):2125–36.
31. Leshnower BG, Chen EP. When and how to replace the aortic root in type A aortic dissection. Ann Cardiothorac Surg. 2016;5(4):377–82.
32. Bentall H, De Bono A. A technique for complete replacement of the ascending aorta. Thorax. 1968;23(4):338–9.
33. Cabrol C, Pavie A, Gandjbakhch I, Villemot JP, Guiraudon G, Laughlin L, et al. Complete replacement of the ascending aorta with reimplantation of the coronary arteries: new surgical approach. J Thorac Cardiovasc Surg. 1981;81(2):309–15.
34. Cabrol C, Pavie A, Mesnildrey P, Gandjbakhch I, Laughlin L, Bors V, et al. Long-term results with total replacement of the ascending aorta and reimplantation of the coronary arteries. J Thorac Cardiovasc Surg. 1986;91(1):17–25.
35. Mookhoek A, Korteland NM, Arabkhani B, Di Centa I, Lansac E, Bekkers JA, et al. Bentall procedure: a systematic review and meta-analysis. Ann Thorac Surg. 2016;101(5):1684–9.

36. Lam KY, Koene B, Timmermans N, Soliman-Hamad M, van Straten A. Reintervention after aortic valve replacement: comparison of three aortic bioprostheses. Ann Thorac Surg. 2019;110(2):615–21.
37. Hickey GL, Bridgewater B, Grant SW, Deanfield J, Parkinson J, Bryan AJ, et al. National registry data and record linkage to inform postmarket surveillance of prosthetic aortic valve models over 15 years. JAMA Intern Med. 2017;177(1):79–86.
38. Esaki J, Leshnower BG, Binongo JN, Lasanajak Y, McPherson L, Halkos ME, et al. The David V valve-sparing root replacement provides improved survival compared with mechanical valve-conduits in the treatment of young patients with aortic root pathology. Ann Thorac Surg. 2016;102(5):1522–30.
39. Franke UF, Isecke A, Nagib R, Breuer M, Wippermann J, Tigges-Limmer K, et al. Quality of life after aortic root surgery: reimplantation technique versus composite replacement. Ann Thorac Surg. 2010;90(6):1869–75.
40. Sarsam MA, Yacoub M. Remodeling of the aortic valve anulus. J Thorac Cardiovasc Surg. 1993;105(3):435–8.
41. Yacoub M. Valve-conserving operation for aortic root aneurysm or dissection. Oper Tech Card Thorac Surg. 1996;1(1):57–67.
42. Aicher D, Langer F, Lausberg H, Bierbach B, Schafers HJ. Aortic root remodeling: ten-year experience with 274 patients. J Thorac Cardiovasc Surg. 2007;134(4):909–15.
43. Kallenbach K, Leyh RG, Salcher R, Karck M, Hagl C, Haverich A. Acute aortic dissection versus aortic root aneurysm: comparison of indications for valve sparing aortic root reconstruction. Eur J Cardiothorac Surg. 2004;25(5):663–70.
44. David TE, Feindel CM. An aortic valve-sparing operation for patients with aortic incompetence and aneurysm of the ascending aorta. J Thorac Cardiovasc Surg. 1992;103(4):617–21. discussion 22
45. Fries R, Graeter T, Aicher D, Reul H, Schmitz C, Bohm M, et al. In vitro comparison of aortic valve movement after valve-preserving aortic replacement. J Thorac Cardiovasc Surg. 2006;132(1):32–7.
46. Schafers H, Fries R, Langer F, Nikoloudakis N, Graeter T, Grundmann U. Valve-preserving replacement of the ascending aorta: remodeling versus reimplantation. J Thorac Cardiovasc Surg. 1998;116(6):990–6.
47. Leyh RG, Fischer S, Kallenbach K, Kofidis T, Pethig K, Harringer W, et al. High failure rate after valve-sparing aortic root replacement using the "remodeling technique" in acute type A aortic dissection. Circulation. 2002;106(12 Suppl 1):I229–33.
48. Dib B, Seppelt PC, Arif R, Weymann A, Veres G, Schmack B, et al. Extensive aortic surgery in acute aortic dissection type A on outcome—insights from 25 years single center experience. J Cardiothorac Surg. 2019;14(1):187.
49. Lansac E, Di Centa I, Vojacek J, Nijs J, Hlubocky J, Mecozzi G, et al. Valve sparing root replacement: the remodeling technique with external ring annuloplasty. Ann Cardiothorac Surg. 2013;2(1):117–23.
50. Lansac E, Di Centa I, Bonnet N, Leprince P, Rama A, Acar C, et al. Aortic prosthetic ring annuloplasty: a useful adjunct to a standardized aortic valve-sparing procedure? Eur J Cardiothorac Surg. 2006;29(4):537–44.
51. Chiu P, Miller DC. Evolution of surgical therapy for Stanford acute type A aortic dissection. Ann Cardiothorac Surg. 2016;5(4):275–95.
52. Kato Y, Sasaki K, Yamauchi H, Kanno Y, Jinno T, Yamada M, et al. Aortic root remodelling with external ring annuloplasty in acute type A aortic dissection. Interact Cardiovasc Thorac Surg. 2020;30(1):85–90.
53. Moriyama Y, Taira A. Aortic root replacement in type A dissection. Eur J Cardiothorac Surg. 1997;12(2):325–6.
54. de Kerchove L, Mosala Nezhad Z, Boodhwani M, El Khoury G. How to perform valve sparing reimplantation in a tricuspid aortic valve. Ann Cardiothorac Surg. 2013;2(1):105–12.

55. Yacoub MH, Gehle P, Chandrasekaran V, Birks EJ, Child A, Radley-Smith R. Late results of a valve-preserving operation in patients with aneurysms of the ascending aorta and root. J Thorac Cardiovasc Surg. 1998;115(5):1080–90.
56. Irimie V, Atieh A, Kucinoski G, Jankulovski A, Zacher M, Urbanski PP. Long-term outcomes after valve-sparing anatomical aortic root reconstruction in acute dissection involving the root. J Thorac Cardiovasc Surg. 2019;159(4):1176–1184.e1.
57. Sievers HH, Richardt D, Diwoky M, Auer C, Bucsky B, Nasseri B, et al. Survival and reoperation after valve-sparing root replacement and root repair in acute type A dissection. J Thorac Cardiovasc Surg. 2018;156(6):2076–82.e2.
58. Urbanski PP, Hijazi H, Dinstak W, Diegeler A. Valve-sparing aortic root repair in acute type A dissection: how many sinuses have to be repaired for curative surgery? Eur J Cardiothorac Surg. 2013;44(3):439–43. discussion 43-4
59. Beckmann E, Martens A, Pertz J, Kaufeld T, Umminger J, Hanke JS, et al. Valve-sparing David I procedure in acute aortic type A dissection: a 20-year experience with more than 100 patients. Eur J Cardiothorac Surg. 2017;52(2):319–24.
60. Stamou SC, Williams ML, Gunn TM, Hagberg RC, Lobdell KW, Kouchoukos NT. Aortic root surgery in the United States: a report from the Society of Thoracic Surgeons database. J Thorac Cardiovasc Surg. 2015;149(1):116–22.e4.
61. Rosenblum JM, Leshnower BG, Moon RC, Lasanajak Y, Binongo J, McPherson L, et al. Durability and safety of David V valve-sparing root replacement in acute type A aortic dissection. J Thorac Cardiovasc Surg. 2019;157(1):14–23.e1.
62. Subramanian S, Leontyev S, Borger MA, Trommer C, Misfeld M, Mohr FW. Valve-sparing root reconstruction does not compromise survival in acute type A aortic dissection. Ann Thorac Surg. 2012;94(4):1230–4.
63. Graeter TP, Langer F, Nikoloudakis N, Aicher D, Schafers HJ. Valve-preserving operation in acute aortic dissection type A. Ann Thorac Surg. 2000;70(5):1460–5.
64. Monsefi N, Miskovic A, Moritz A, Zierer A. Long-term results of the David Procedure in patients with acute type A aortic dissection. Int J Surg. 2015;22:99–104.
65. Tanaka H, Ikeno Y, Abe N, Takahashi H, Inoue T, Okita Y. Outcomes of valve-sparing root replacement in acute type A aortic dissection. Eur J Cardiothorac Surg. 2018;53(5):1021–6.
66. Arabkhani B, Mookhoek A, Di Centa I, Lansac E, Bekkers JA, De Lind Van Wijngaarden R, et al. Reported outcome after valve-sparing aortic root replacement for aortic root aneurysm: a systematic review and meta-analysis. Ann Thorac Surg. 2015;100(3):1126–31.
67. Wu J, Huang Y, Qiu J, Saeed B, Yu C. Is valve-sparing root replacement a safe option in acute type A aortic dissection? A systematic review and meta-analysis. Interact Cardiovasc Thorac Surg. 2019;29(5):766–75.
68. Salmasi MY, Theodoulou I, Iyer P, Al-Zubaidy M, Naqvi D, Snober M, et al. Comparing outcomes between valve-sparing root replacement and the Bentall procedure in proximal aortic aneurysms: systematic review and meta-analysis. Interact Cardiovasc Thorac Surg. 2019;29(6):911–22.
69. Aubin H, Akhyari P, Rellecke P, Pawlitza C, Petrov G, Lichtenberg A, et al. Valve-sparing aortic root replacement as first-choice strategy in acute type A aortic dissection. Front Surg. 2019;6:46.
70. Bin Mahmood SU, Mori M, Geirsson A, Elefteriades JA, Mangi AA. Acute type A aortic dissection surgery performed by aortic specialists improves 2-year outcomes. Aorta (Stamford). 2019;7(1):1–6.
71. Bavaria JE, Pochettino A, Brinster DR, Gorman RC, McGarvey ML, Gorman JH, et al. New paradigms and improved results for the surgical treatment of acute type A dissection. Ann Surg. 2001;234(3):336–42. discussion 42-3

Basic Approaches for the Surgical Management of Acute Type A Aortic Dissection: Safe Management Strategies for the General Cardiac Surgeon

Tirone E. David

Surgery for acute type A aortic dissection is associated with high operative mortality and morbidity largely because of its heterogeneity in pathology, pathophysiology and clinical presentation. Many patients die before reaching an emergency room whereas others walk in a doctors' office complaining of vague chest discomfort or other symptom and are found to have acute type A aortic dissections. The dissection may involve only the ascending aorta in some cases whereas in most patients the entry tear is in the proximal ascending aorta and the false lumen extends down to the thoracic, abdominal and even femoral arteries causing various degrees of organ malperfusion. The faster the diagnosis is made and the faster the patient can be taken to the operating the better for the patient, and probably for the surgeon too. The mortality of acute type A aortic dissection during the first 24 h is very high and referring these patients to an aortic center may be inappropriate because whatever might be gained in operative mortality if the operation is performed by an experienced aortic surgeon the overall mortality might be higher by delaying surgery. In addition, even experienced aortic surgeons find challenging to operate on certain patients with acute type A aortic dissection. Thus, the general cardiac surgeon working somewhere distant from an "aortic center" is probably the best person to save the patient's life. This is an operation that every cardiac surgeon should be able to perform, and if it is planned and executed well, the mortality and morbidity rates can be reduced.

This chapter was written with the "general cardiac surgeon" in mind, the one who sees only a few patients with acute type A dissection each year. Based on my

The contents of this chapter were largely based on an editorial written by the author and published in the Journal of Thoracic and Cardiovascular Surgery in 2015; volume 150, pages 279–283. Permission from Elsevier was obtained.

T. E. David (✉)
University of Toronto, Toronto, ON, Canada
e-mail: tirone.david@uhn.ca

J. S. Coselli et al. (eds.), *Aortic Dissection and Acute Aortic Syndromes*,
https://doi.org/10.1007/978-3-030-66668-2_20

lifetime experience working in a teaching hospital, I will be describing techniques that I know that are reproducible if only followed correctly and performed with care and attention to the details I will enumerate. Although I already mentioned, I firmly believe that prompt diagnosis and immediate surgery are crucial in this disease, and the sooner you can get the patient on the operating table, the better the operative and long-term outcomes will be.

The Hemodynamically Unstable Patient

Hemodynamic instability after acute type A aortic dissection occurs because acute myocardial ischemia due to the dissection or ruptured of the false lumen into the pericardial cavity with consequent pericardial tamponade or rupture into the chest of abdominal cavities. It is difficult and sometimes impossible to save the patient with acute rupture of the false lumen in the pleural or abdominal cavity. However, it is relatively common to have to operate on patients with myocardial ischemia or pericardial tamponade. Patients with acute type A dissection and myocardial ischemia may have been treated by emergency room doctors with drugs such as ticagrelol which immensely increases the risk of massive postoperative bleeding. I have operated on only two such patients and one died as consequence of massive blood transfusion after a correctly and expeditiously performed operation for acute type A dissection.

An arterial line on the right radial or brachial artery, a central venous line, and a good peripheral IV are indispensable in hemodynamically unstable patients. Although transcutaneous cannulation of the femoral vessels can be performed, I believe you should start the operation by making an incision in the inguinal area and expose the anterior wall of the femoral vein and common femoral artery. If the femoral artery has evidence of a false lumen, mobilize this vessel circumferentially and put tapes around it. If there is no dissection, simply put a purse string suture on the anterior wall of the common femoral artery. A purse string suture should also be place on the femoral vein. Next, go to the chest and do a full median-sternotomy. If the hemodynamic instability is due to tamponade the pericardial cavity will be tense and blue. Don't open it because if you do there is a risk of a hypertensive crisis and the aorta may blow up and make things messy. Give heparin and insert perfusion cannulas in the femoral vessels using the Seldinger technique. If the femoral artery has a false lumen, clamp it and open it transversely and insert a cannular into the true lumen. Both the arterial and venous cardiopulmonary bypass lines should have a second arm of tubing 80–100 cm long in case you need another venous cannula to completely drain the right side of the heart, or another arterial cannula. Go on bypass and start to cool the patient. Make a small incision in the pericardium and begin to drain the fluid slowly. Alert the anesthetist of possible hypertension and reduce the doses of inotropes and vasopressors. The rupture that caused the tamponade is often sealed and there is no active bleeding in most patients. If this is the case, carry on and you may want to insert a cannula in the right atrium for better venous drainage. The heart is not likely to fibrillate very soon if left undisturbed because it is the last organ to receive cold blood when blood is pumped into a femoral artery. However, if the heart is ischemic because of occlusion of the right coronary artery by the dissection and/or if there is severe aortic insufficiency, the heart may fibrillate sooner than you hope. Regardless, it is safer to insert a vent into the right superior pulmonary vein and gently advance it into the left ventricle. In addition, you should do two more things while the patient is being cooled: insert a cardioplegia cannula into the coronary sinus and put a tape around the superior vena cava. If the heart begins to fibrillate but the left ventricle is not distending, wait until the nasopharyngeal temperature reaches 20–22 °C. If the ventricle is distending, apply suction on the ventricular vent and increase the pump flow into the femoral cannula. Uncommonly, the aortic insufficiency is so severe that perfusion pressure cannot be maintained or the heart remains distended and requires more than an occasional manual squeeze to decompress it. In this case, reduce the pump flow to 1 l/min and apply a large clamp on the proximal half of the ascending aorta, as close to the sino-tubular junction as possible without much dissection (you will have to clamp part of the pulmonary artery too), and gently increase the pump flow. When the heart is empty give 1–2 l of cold blood cardioplegia into the coronary sinus. You may also want to use some topical cooling by placing ice over a sponge on top of the right ventricle.

When the target temperature is reached, snare the superior vena cava and wait for 30 s before stopping the pump (venous hypertension prevents air from entering the cerebral circulation). Transect the ascending aorta at its mid-portion and incise its anterior wall (false and true lumens) up to the level of the innominate artery. Visually inspect the intima of the aortic arch for any tear, and if there is none, cut the ascending aorta a few millimeters below the level of the innominate artery.

If you did not have to clamp the aorta because of severe aortic insufficiency, now is the time to give retrograde blood cardioplegia (the perfusionist has to know in advance that cardioplegia will be given during circulatory arrest).

Choose a tubular Dacron graft that fits inside the true lumen of the arch, usually 26–30 mm in diameter, depending of the size of the patient and aorta. Dacron grafts manufacturers make large straight grafts with a side arm (8–10 mm) that can be used for antegrade perfusion. Next, suture the Dacron graft 5–7 mm inside the intima on the posterior wall of the aortic arch with a horizontal mattress suture of 4–0 polypropylene buttressed on a 4–5 mm wide strip of Teflon felt on the adventitia. The needle should be the thinnest you can find. Begin to suture the graft into the posterior wall of the arch by making sure that the graft lies at least 5–7 mm inside the dissected intima of the aortic arch. Every bite should be through the intima first, 3–4 mm apart from each other, and 5–7 mm into the arch and in the graft. Once you reach the innominate artery, take the second arm of the suture and begin to sew the anterior wall of the graft inside the intima with the same precision that you sutured the posterior wall. Never pull the suture against the intima; pull it always against the graft to prevent tears in the intima along the suture line. I do not think you should use French glue or BioGlue® (Cryolife, Kennesaw, GA) but other experienced surgeons believe that it makes the anastomosis more hemostatic. If you are going to use glue, do so sparingly and only in between the dissected layers along the first centimeter where you are going to suture the graft. Fibrin glue can also be used to "glue" the layers together before suturing the graft and it does not cause tissue necrosis like the others do. Next, remove the arterial femoral cannula and insert into the Dacron graft, 1 cm from the distal anastomosis by making a small transverse cut in the graft (smaller than the size of the arterial cannula) and placing two 4-0 polypropylene sutures, one on each end of the cut to secure the cannula, and later to close the hole in the graft. Conversely, if you have large Dacron grafts with a side arm for perfusion, insert the cannula into the perfusion limb of the graft. Start antegrade perfusion with an open graft and carefully de-air the aortic arch. Clamp the Dacron graft close to the new arterial cannula or perfusion limb of the graft and increase perfusion pressure. Release the tape on the superior vena cava and re-establish full cardiopulmonary bypass. The distal anastomosis seldom leaks if performed as described. If it does, place extra stitches but reduce the pump flow to 1 l/min while you are putting the stitches and tying them. When the anastomosis is perfect, begin to re-warm the patient. Figure 1 illustrates the sequence of the technique described above.

I have had a few patients in whom the ascending aorta was bleeding actively when I opened the pericardium and I had to exsanguinate the patient into the venous reservoir, clamp the aorta above the rupture and re-establish full cardiopulmonary bypass before proceeding with the operation as described above. Those patients did not always survive surgery.

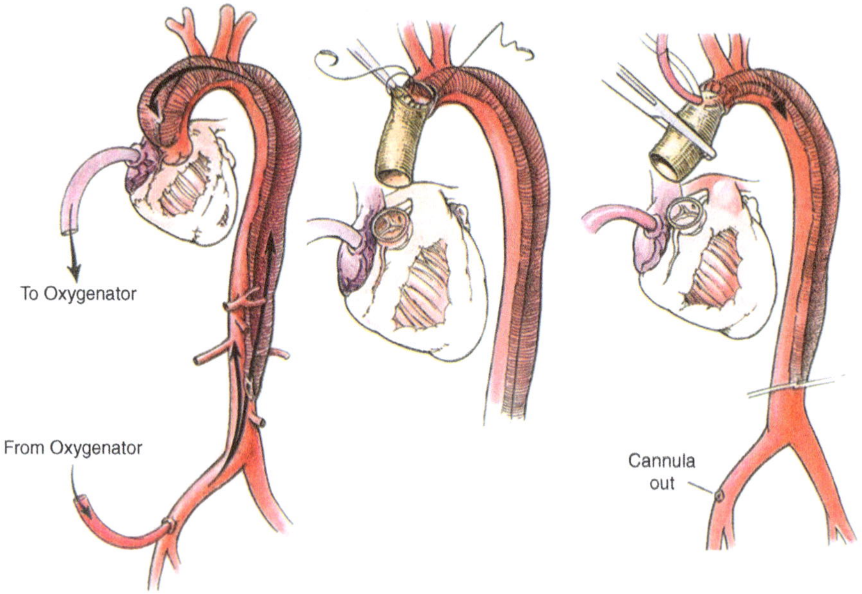

Fig. 1 Femoral artery perfusion reverses the flow in the false lumen and aortic clamping should be avoided to reduce the risk of malperfusion. The distal anastomosis should be performed under circulatory arrest. The femoral cannula should be removed and inserted into the Dacron graft for antegrade perfusion after completion of the distal anastomosis or connected to a perfusion branch already sewn to the Dacron graft

Clamping the aorta just below the takeoff of the innominate artery in acute type A aortic dissection should be avoided when arterial blood is pumped in the femoral artery because it can increase the risk of malperfusion and cause multiple ruptures of the false lumen (Fig. 1).

It is generally believed that it is important to resect the primary tear in type A aortic dissection. Luckily, in most patients the tear starts just above the sinotubular junction in the greater curvature of the ascending aorta. However, the primary tear can be in the aortic arch and resection can be complicated because it may require replacement of the entire aortic arch, and sometimes even replacement of the proximal parts of the brachiocephalic arteries. This is not an operation for a "general cardiac surgeon". I believe that the safest thing for you to do is to replace the ascending aorta as described above and leave the tear in the aortic arch unless you can resect the tear without detaching the brachiocephalic vessels from the aortic arch and descending thoracic aorta. You should do your best to save the patient's life and if further surgery is needed in the future, so be it, and it is certainly much better than death or a devastating stroke if you try to replace the aortic arch and brachiocephalic arteries in this acute setting.

The Hemodynamically Stable Patient

In the hemodynamically stable patient with acute type A aortic dissection you can take a bit more time and do things differently. You should have two monitoring arterial lines, one on each arm, and perhaps even a third one in a femoral artery (all this to control malperfusion during cardiopulmonary bypass). If you know how to expose the right axillary artery, this is the ideal vessel to use as arterial return during cardiopulmonary bypass unless there is a complex arch dissection with tears that extend into the right subclavian artery which his uncommon but when it does you should not use it for arterial return. The right axillary artery should be mobilized for a length of 25–30 mm and elastic vessel loops passed around it proximally and distally or you also can use fine vascular clamps. A tubular graft of 6 or 8 mm (Dacron or Gore-Tex) should be sutured to it in an end-to-side fashion and used for arterial return (Fig. 2). You do not have to give heparin to perform this anastomosis because there are plenty collaterals around the axillary artery. Once the anastomosis is completed, release the distal vessel loop first and let some blood out. Occlude the vessel distally and release the proximal vessel loop for a fraction of second. Clamp the graft a few millimeters from the anastomosis and release both vessel loops. Make sure the anastomosis is intact. The blood pressure in the right radial artery should return to normal after releasing the vessel loops.

Do a full median-sternotomy, open the pericardium and give heparin. Connect the arterial line to the axillary artery graft (Fig. 2). This line should have a second limb of tubing 80–100 cm for another arterial cannula if needed. Use the right atrium for venous drainage. Go on cardiopulmonary bypass and began to cool the patient. If the mean arterial pressure in the right arm is greater than 15–20 mmHg

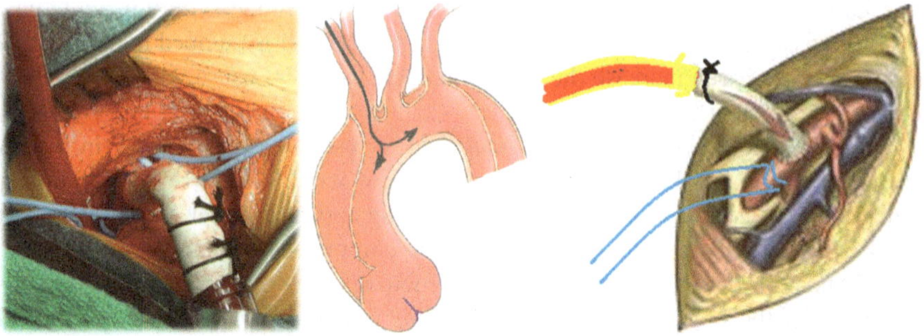

Fig. 2 Axillary artery perfusion may prevent malperfusion because blood is pumped into the true lumen. With this type of arterial return during cardiopulmonary bypass the ascending aorta may be clamped without increasing the risk of malperfusion

than in the left arm, gently snare the distal vessel loop on the axillary artery until the mean pressures are similar. If the arterial resistance in the pump head is too high to deliver the calculated blood flow, you need to insert a second arterial cannula, probably in the femoral artery. Insert a left ventricular vent through the right superior pulmonary vein. You can now clamp the ascending aorta 1–2 cm below the takeoff of the innominate artery and wait for a few seconds to make sure the blood pressure remains the same in both arms. Transect the aorta and give cardioplegia either directly into the coronary arteries or retrograde into the coronary sinus.

Carefully dissect the aortic arch and brachiocephalic arteries. Start by detaching the pericardial reflection around the distal ascending aorta, then the innominate vein, and finally the three brachiocephalic arteries. When the nasopharyngeal temperature is 25 °C and the rectal is below 30 °C (the rectal temperature will not drop as fast as the nasopharyngeal because cold blood is being pumped into the axillary artery) you can reduce the flow to 10 ml/kg/min, clamp all three bachiocephalic vessels, remove the aortic clamp and cut the ascending aorta (true and false lumens) immediately below the level of the innominate artery. Suture a tubular Dacron graft to the aortic arch as described above for the hemodynamically unstable patient. Once this anastomosis is completed you may to use the axillary artery for antegrade perfusion or insert a new arterial cannula into the Dacron graft as described above. If the anastomosis is intact, begin to re-warm the patient.

If you are unfamiliar with axillary artery anatomy or this artery is too small to supply blood to the entire body, you may use the femoral artery for cardiopulmonary bypass and conduct the operation as we described for the hemodynamically unstable patient but avoid clamping the aorta to reduce the risk of malperfusion and further expand the false lumen.

The Patient with Malperfusion

Malperfusion of one or more organs (heart, brain, mesenteric, renal and peripheral arteries) was associated with higher operative mortality in all three large registries on acute type A aortic dissection (International Registry on Acute Aortic Dissection, German Registry for Acute Aortic Dissection Type A, and the Nordic Consortium for Acute Type A Aortic Dissection). Malperfusion of at least one organ occurs in approximately one-third of all patients. The best approach to manage these patients remains controversial and it ranges from immediate surgery and repair of the proximal aorta to force the blood into the true lumen to percutaneous intervention with fenestration and stenting of the descending thoracic aorta and delay repair of the proximal aorta. What should the general cardiac surgeon do when a patient presents with life threatening malperfusion? If the patient has mesenteric ischemia and profound lactic acidosis, surgery may be futile. If resources for percutaneous intervention are available, fenestration and stenting can be considered. If the patient has myocardial, cerebral, renal or peripheral malperfusion and has no serious co-morbidities, I believe immediate surgery with cardiopulmonary bypass with at least two arterial cannulas (axillary and femoral) or one central cannula into the true lumen (if you can do this safely) is probably the safest approach. If malperfusion persists after proximal aortic repair which restored flow into the true lumen, a separate procedure may be necessary and this may involve transcatheter interventions such as fenestration and stenting of large and medium size arteries or an extra-anatomic bypass such as axillary artery to femoral artery bypass for lower limb ischemia. Patients with persistent malperfusion after proximal aortic repair usually succumb postoperatively in spite all available therapies.

The Patient with Aortic Arch Tear

The aortic arch can be the primary site of an aortic tear and the dissection can propagate distally (antegrade false lumen) or proximally (retrograde false lumen) or in both directions. Patients with antegrade aortic arch dissection can be managed medically initially as if they had Type B aortic dissection, however, if the dissection extends proximally the risk of rupture into the pericardial cavity appears to be similar to Type A and surgery with total arch replacement and probably and descending thoracic aortic stent should be done. These types of operations are in the domain of experienced aortic surgeons and referral to an aortic center may be the best for the patient.

The Aortic Root

Once the distal anastomosis is completed attention is turned to the aortic root. Transect the false and true lumens 5–7 mm above the sinotubular junction. Gently suspend the three commissures of the aortic valve and inspect the cusps. If they are normal or near normal, an attempt should be made to save them. Next, inspect the aortic sinuses and the extensiveness of the dissection. If it involves only the non-coronary aortic sinus and part of the right (the most common finding in acute type A dissection), and the sinuses are not aneurysmal, they can be preserved. I don't believe you should use BioGlue® (I prefer to use fibrin glue to seal the intima with the adventitia) but many surgeons disagree with me. If you are going to use glue do so sparingly to minimize tissue necrosis and false aneurysms later on. Suspend the three commissures and approximate them until the three cusps touch each other. Measure the diameter of the imaginary circle that include all three commisures and use a Dacron graft of this size to repair the root. In one end of the graft make three equidistant marks (approximately at 120° from each other), unless the inter-commissural distances are grossly different (the left cusp is usually the smallest of the three and so is its inter-commissural distance). Using three horizontal mattress sutures (4-0 polypropylene with a fine needle) secure the Dacron inside the aortic root immediately above each commissure using the marks made in the end of the graft as reference points. Buttress these sutures on a strip of Teflon felt on the adventitia of the aortic root. As with the distal anastomosis, carefully suture the Dacron graft to the aortic root using the same principles (the bites should be 3–4 mm apart and 5–7 mm into the aortic wall and Dacron graft, and the needle is always passed from the inside to the outside of the aortic root). Once this anastomosis is completed, inject blood cardioplegia under pressure inside graft by clamping its distal part. This maneuver tests the integrity of the proximal anastomosis and aortic valve competence. In my experience, if the ventricle does not distend while cardioplegia is given and the ventricular vent is not on suction there must be none or less than mild aortic insufficiency.

If the aortic sinuses are aneurysmal or extensively dissected but the cusps are normal, an aortic valve-sparing operation can be performed. Reimplantation of the aortic valve in a tubular Dacron graft has been shown to provide excellent long-term results in patients with acute type A aortic dissection that need aortic root repair. Aortic valve sparing operations are complex procedures and usually out of the domain of the general cardiac surgeon and I believe that an aortic root replacement is probably safer in this setting. Depending on the patients' age you may use a mechanical or a tissue valve.

Finally, if the aortic sinuses are relatively normal with minimal dissection but the aortic cusps are diseased, replace the aortic valve, leave the coronary arteries where they are, and suture a graft in the supra-coronary position.

If the dissection involved the orifice of the right coronary artery but the intima of this artery is intact, there is no need to bypass it as elimination of the false lumen alone should re-establish normal flow. If there is an intimal tear around the orifice of the right coronary artery or its intima is damaged, it is safer to tie it off and bypass it with a saphenous vein graft 1 or 2 cm from its origin. Remember that suturing a vein graft into collagen impregnated Dacron can cause ostio-stenosis of the vein due to pannus. Thus, if the vein has a small caliber (<4 mm), it is safer to sew a patch of vein graft on the Dacron graft (a circular patch 1–1.5 cm^2 is adequate) and the saphenous vein graft onto the vein patch.

Trim the distal and proximal Dacron grafts and suture them together. Remember that the total length of the ascending aorta graft should be only 4–5 cm. Thus, both the distal and the proximal grafts should be relatively short to prevent kinking of the graft. De-air the heart and unclamp the distal graft. Reperfuse the heart and when the rectal temperature is around 36 °C discontinue bypass. If things are stable and you have a cannula into the aortic graft, remove it before reversing the heparin and put it into the right atrium in the place of the venous cannula. Tie the sutures that you placed to secure the cannula in the graft and run a fine polypropylene suture for hemostasis. Obviously, this is not necessary if you used a Dacron graft with a perfusing branch. Give protamine and make sure hemostasis is perfect. Transfusion of platelets and other clotting factors are often needed in acute type A aortic dissection because most of these patients develop coagulopathy.

Do this operation as described and your patient will have a 90% chance to go home alive and without neurological deficit. Unfortunately you will lose some patients mostly because of malperfusion, which remains an unresolved problem in surgery for acute type A aortic dissection.

Postoperative Care

Most surgically treated patients with acute type A aortic dissection require more than one day in the intensive care unit. In addition to the routine postoperative care for patients who undergo surgery on cardiopulmonary bypass they need close surveillance for malperfusion and may need further intervention if the malperfusion is life-threatening.

Antihypertensive agents, particularly betablockers, are extremely important to prevent or retard the expansion of the false lumen. A CT angiogram is advisable before discharge from hospital to determine patency, extension and diameter of the false lumen. These patients need lifelong surveillance of the false lumen with periodical images of the entire thoracic and abdominal aorta as well as echocardiography of the aortic root.

Recommended Reading

1. Trimarchi S, de Beaufort HWL, Tolenaar JL, Bavaria JE, Desai ND, Di Eusanio M, Di Bartolomeo R, Peterson MD, Ehrlich M, Evangelista A, Montgomery DG, Myrmel T, Hughes GC, Appoo JJ, De Vincentiis C, Yan TD, Nienaber CA, Isselbacher EM, Deeb GM, Gleason TG, Patel HJ, Sundt TM, Eagle KA. Acute aortic dissections with entry tear in the arch: A report from the International Registry of Acute Aortic Dissection. J Thorac Cardiovasc Surg. 2019;157:66–73.
2. Zindovic I, Gudbjartsson T, Ahlsson A, Fuglsang S, Gunn J, Hansson EC, Hjortdal V, Järvelä K, Jeppsson A, Mennander A, Olsson C, Pan E, Sjögren J, Wickbom A, Geirsson A, Nozohoor S. Malperfusion in acute type A aortic dissection: an update from the Nordic Consortium for Acute Type A Aortic Dissection. J Thorac Cardiovasc Surg. 2019;157:1324–33.
3. Conzelmanna LO, Weigangb E, Mehlhorna U, Abugamehd A, Hoffmanne I, Blettnere M, Etzb DE, Czerny M, Vahld CF on behalf of the GERAADA Investigators. Mortality in patients with acute aortic dissection type A: analysis of pre- and intraoperative risk factors from the German Registry for Acute Aortic Dissection Type A (GERAADA). Eur J Cardio-Thorac Surg. 2016;49:44–52.
4. Pape LA, Awais M, Woznicki EM, Suzuki T, Trimarchi S, Evangelista A, Myrmel T, Larsen M, Harris KM, Greason K, Di Eusanio M, Bossone E, Montgomery DG, Eagle KA, Nienaber CA, Isselbacher EM, O'Gara P. Presentation, diagnosis, and outcomes of acute aortic dissection: 17-year trends from the international registry of acute aortic dissection. J Am Coll Cardio. 2015;66:350–8.
5. Czerny M, Schoenhoff F, Etz C, Englberger L, Khaladj N, Zierer A, Weigang E, Hoffmann I, Blettner M, Carrel TP. The impact of pre-operative malperfusion on outcome in acute type A aortic dissection: results from the GERAADA Registry. J Am Coll Cardiol. 2015;65:2628–35.
6. Di Eusanio M, Trimarchi S, Patel HJ, Hutchison S, Suzuki T, Peterson MD, Di Bartolomeo R, Folesani G, Pyeritz RE, Braverman AC, Montgomery DG, Isselbacher EM, Nienaber CA, Eagle KA, Fattori R. Clinical presentation, management, and short-term outcome of patients with type A acute dissection complicated by mesenteric malperfusion: observations from the International Registry of Acute Aortic Dissection. J Thorac Cardiovasc Surg. 2013;145:385–90.

Valve Repair for Aortic Valve Insufficiency in the Setting of Acute Aortic Dissection

Talal Al-Atassi and Munir Boodhwani

Introduction

Acute Type A aortic dissection is a rare life-threatening condition with an incidence of between 2.9 and 4.7 per 100,000 persons per year [1–6]. Conservative treatment is associated with a high mortality rate approaching 60% within 48 h [7, 8]. Mortality is due to complications associated with type A dissection such as rupture, stroke, myocardial infarction, and acute heart failure from aortic valve insufficiency (AI). Emergency surgery is indicated in acute type A aortic dissection as it significantly improves survival compared to conservative therapy. The primary goal of surgery is to resect the primary entry tear, exclude the false lumen from systemic blood flow, re-establish dominant flow in the true lumen, and in cases with AI, re-establish aortic valve (AV) competence.

Although acute Type A aortic dissection spares the aortic root and AV in many cases, as many as 40–75% of patients present with moderate or severe AI [9–11]. Re-establishing AV competence can be achieved through a variety of surgical options and techniques that include replacement and repair of the AV. Choosing the surgical technique is largely driven by the mechanism of AI. Herein, we explore the different mechanisms of AI in acute type A aortic dissection and associated surgical techniques to repair the AV.

Talal Al-Atassi and Munir Boodhwani contributed equally with all other contributors.

T. Al-Atassi · M. Boodhwani (✉)
Division of Cardiac Surgery, University of Ottawa Heart Institute, Ottawa, ON, Canada
e-mail: mboodhwani@ottawaheart.ca

J. S. Coselli et al. (eds.), *Aortic Dissection and Acute Aortic Syndromes*,
https://doi.org/10.1007/978-3-030-66668-2_21

Aortic Valve Anatomy and Function

A thorough understanding of AV anatomy and function is essential to its successful preservation and repair. The basis of a normally functioning AV is a complex interaction between the annulus and the AV cusps. Although surgeons commonly refer to the annulus as a single entity, in reality, the functional aortic annulus (FAA) is made of three components: the sinotubular junction (STJ), the ventriculo-aortic junction (VAJ), and the anatomic crown-shaped annulus on which the cusps insert. The cusps normally coapt at the center of the AV orifice and midway between the STJ and VAJ. A basic tenet of AV repair is that lesions of the FAA *and* the cusps should both be addressed at the time of valve repair.

Mechanisms of Aortic Valve Insufficiency in Acute Dissection

The optimal management of significant AI in the context of acute Type A aortic dissection remains somewhat controversial. Whereas in the past there was a trend favoring aortic valve replacement [12–15], more recently, there is a growing trend to spare and repair the AV in select patients, which incurs a moderate risk of reoperation but a low risk of thromboembolism, bleeding, and endocarditis [16–22]. A detailed understanding of the possible mechanisms of AI in acute dissections is paramount for the surgeon to decide on a tailored AI management strategy. Preoperative computed tomography (CT) coupled with intraoperative transesophageal echocardiogram (TEE) and visual inspection of the aortic root and AV can help the surgeon describe the mechanism of AI and choose an appropriate surgical technique.

The emergence of a repair-oriented classification of AI (Fig. 1) has allowed AV repair to transition from an art performed by a few skilled surgeons to a systematic and scientific process that can potentially be adopted by most surgeons [23]. First, it provides a framework to understand the mechanisms of AI in a specific patient and choose an appropriately tailored technique or combination of techniques to restore normal valve function. Second, it provides us with a universal vocabulary, which helps with communication in both the clinical and research settings, much like the Carpentier classification did for mitral valve repair [24].

In this classification, type I is aortic insufficiency associated with normal cusp motion. Type I is further divided into type Ia due to dilatation of the ascending aorta and STJ, type Ib due to dilatation of the VAJ and the STJ, type Ic due to dilatation of the VAJ, and type Id due to cusp pathology without involvement of the FAA. Patients presenting with acute type A dissection often have an associated ascending aortic aneurysm leading to dilatation of the STJ (type Ia) and/or an aortic root aneurysm leading to dilatation of the STJ, sinuses of Valsalva, and VAJ (type Ib). In the absence of aneurysms or aortic dilatation, a unique mechanism in acute dissection may be due to a dissection flap prolapsing through the AV and causing valve incompetence (type Id).

AI Class	Type I Normal cusp motion with FAA dilatation or cusp perforation				Type II	Type III
	Ia	Ib	Ic	Id	Cusp Prolapse	Cusp Restriction
Mechanism						
Repair Techniques	STJ Remodeling *Ascending aortic graft*	VSRR *Reimplantation or Remodeling+SCA*	SCA or External Ring	Patch Repair *Autologous or bovine pericardium*	Leaflet Repair *Triangular resection Free margin plication or resuspension Patch repair*	Leaflet Repair *Shaving Decalcification Patch repair*

Fig. 1 Repair-oriented functional classification of aortic insufficiency (AI) with description of disease mechanisms and repair techniques used. Non-shaded columns are the focus of this review. *FAA* functional aortic annulus, *STJ* sinotubular junction, *VSRR* valve sparing root replacement, *SCA* subcommissural annuloplasty

Type II AI is due to cusp prolapse. In patients with acute Type A aortic dissection this may be due to chronic underlying cusp pathology in the form of excessive cusp tissue or due to acute extension of the dissection into the root causing commissural disruption. Prolapse may also be unmasked or induced when a dilated STJ is restored to normal dimensions.

Type III AI is due to cusp restriction from calcification, thickening, or fibrosis of the cusps. In the context of acute Type A aortic dissection, most often these are chronic underlying findings found in a bicuspid, degenerative, or rheumatic valve that are unrelated to the acute dissection. Nevertheless, all lesions found at the time of surgery need to be addressed.

Aortic Valve Repair in Acute Aortic Dissection: Selection

Patient selection for aortic root intervention and AV repair in patients presenting with AI and acute Type A dissection hinges on a combination of factors: the patient's condition, the surgeon's expertise, and anatomic factors.

The first factor in decision-making is the patient's condition upon presentation. The basic principle is that emergency acute type A dissection surgery is a life-saving surgery. Therefore, a hemodynamically unstable patient or one presenting with end organ malperfusion and dysfunction may benefit from a more conservative approach with the shortest ischemic time that saves the patient's life, despite the risk of future re-intervention.

The second factor is surgeon expertise. If limited surgical experience is a factor, then a Bentall procedure may be safer than a valve-sparing root procedure. Furthermore, without a real indication to replace the aortic root such as intimal injury, dissection flap, or dilatation of the aortic root >45 mm, a simple aortic valve replacement (AVR) and a supracoronary ascending aorta replacement may be the safest procedure. In many of these decision-making scenarios, the age of the patient and the risk of re-intervention must be weighed against the increased risk of mortality from a more complex operation.

The third factor relies on understanding the mechanism of AI in terms of anatomy and physiology and deciding whether there is an indication for aortic root and AV intervention and if the conditions are favorable for AV repair. The pre-operative CT scan is the surgeon's first glimpse at anatomy. It shows the extent of the dissection (whether it extends into the aortic root) as well as the dimension of the aorta at various levels (ascending, STJ, sinuses of Valsalva). An underlying aneurysmal ascending aorta sparing the root versus one that involves the aortic root may be the first indication of the extent of surgery required. In most patients, the aortic root and valve can be safely spared and repaired using aortic valve resuspension [22].

Next, an intra-operative TEE corroborates the anatomic factors seen on CT. In addition, it provides physiological information about the mechanism of AI. Key aspects to consider include jet origin and direction, end-diastolic measurements of the VAJ, STJ, and Sinuses of Valsalva, cusp thickness, mobility, and presence of calcification.

Despite gathering essential information from CT and TEE, intra-operative visual inspection remains the final arbiter on the reparability of the AV. Cusp tissue quality is perhaps the most important factor in deciding whether preservation and repair of the AV is feasible. Heavily calcified or fibrotic cusps usually preclude repair. Similarly, severely dilated STJs are associated with stress fenestrations along the commissures, which makes a durable AV repair unlikely. Decreased cusp geometric height (<16 mm) is another marker of cusp restriction that may preclude a good AV repair. Sievers type 1 bicuspid AVs [25] with commissural angles <140° also can be challenging to repair and may require techniques such as tricuspidization. In the context of a root aneurysm and one of the above cusp findings, a valve replacement may be the preferred technique [26]. Finally, visual inspection is essential in cases of a prolapsing ascending intimal flap. Relying on TEE may be difficult as the prolapsing flap interacting with the AV may be the only cause of AI or there may be other underlying mechanisms for AI obscured by the flap.

Aortic Valve Repair in Acute Aortic Dissection: Techniques

Type I AI lesions are most frequently due to dilatation of the various components of the FAA and may occur in isolation or with associated cusp disease.

Repair of Type Ia AI

An acute aortic dissection is associated with a rapid increase in the size of the affected aorta [27]. When this rapid increase is greater than 30% of baseline, STJ dilatation alone may be sufficient to cause AI [28]. Type Ia aortic valve insufficiency

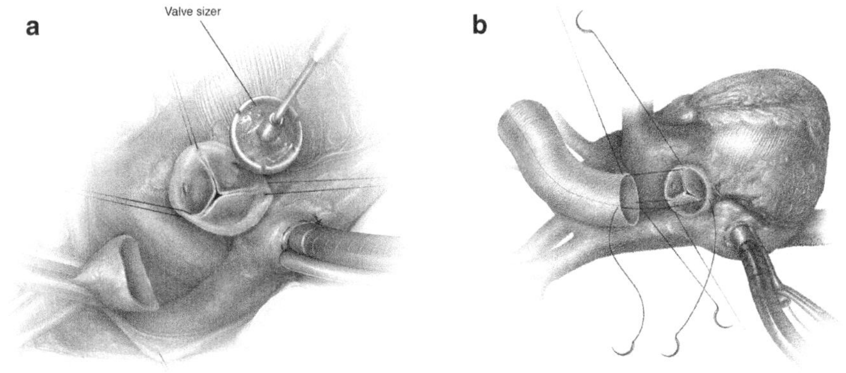

Fig. 2 (**a**) Sizing of aortic prosthesis. Traction is applied to the commissural retraction sutures to place the valve in physiologic closing position with adequate cusp coaptation. The sinotubular junction is sized in this position. Oversizing the prosthesis can lead to central regurgitation, whereas undersizing can induce cusp prolapse. (**b**) Orientation and spacing. The anastomosis is performed at the level of the sinotubular junction starting with three separate sutures, one at each commissure. This ensures correct orientation of the prosthesis and appropriate spacing. Unequal spacing between commissures can induce cusp prolapse. Reprinted with permission from Boodhwani, M and El Khoury, G. Aortic Valve Repair. Operative Techniques in Thoracic and Cardiovascular Surgery. Volume 14, Issue 4, Winter 2009:266–280.

is due to dilatation of the ascending aorta with concomitant STJ dilatation leading to a central cusp coaptation defect and ensuing central regurgitant jet. In milder cases without associated cusp disease, cusp tissue quality remains intact and the valve can easily be repaired. However, a chronic, severely dilated STJ will often be associated with stress fenestrations along the commissures. If large fenestrations exist in multiple cusps and especially if they are within the coaptation zone of the valve, it may be best to replace the valve. The former case can be corrected by replacing the ascending aorta and remodeling the STJ using a Dacron tube graft. Sizing of the aortic prosthesis is performed by placing three commissural retraction sutures and applying traction to place the valve in physiologic closing position. The STJ is sized in that position using a valve sizer (Fig. 2). Accurate sizing is essential as oversizing can lead to central AI and undersizing can lead to cusp prolapse. The anastomosis is performed at the level of the STJ using the three separate commissural sutures, ensuring correct orientation and appropriate spacing between the commissures. Uneven spacing between the commissures can induce cusp prolapse. When the dissection flap extends to the STJ, then either one or two layers of Teflon felt strip can initially be added on the inside and outside of the aorta to bring back together the layers of the aortic wall and the commissural sutures can be pledgeted. In cases of significant AI and widening of the interleaflet triangle, the surgeon may need to add a subcommissural annuloplasty using braided sutures (Fig. 3). The first arm of the pledgeted braided suture is passed from the aortic to the ventricular side, in the interleaflet triangle, and comes back out to the aortic side at the same level. The second arm of the suture is passed in a similar fashion below the first. A free pledget is added and the suture is tied, reducing the width of the interleaflet triangle

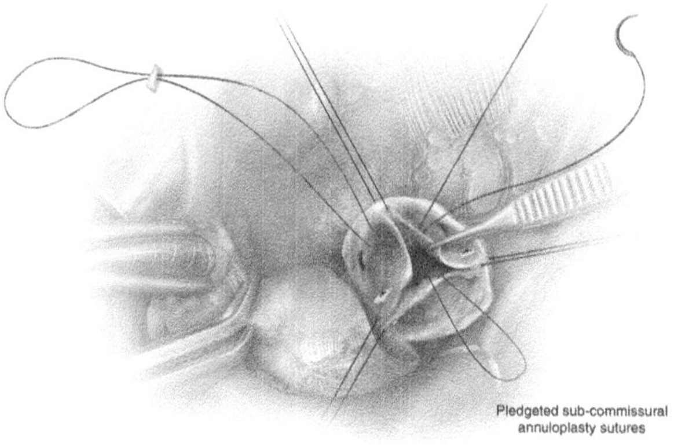

Fig. 3 Reprinted with permission from Boodhwani, M and El Khoury, G. Aortic Valve Repair. Operative Techniques in Thoracic and Cardiovascular Surgery. Volume 14, Issue 4, Winter 2009: 266–280.

and increasing the coaptation surface of the valve leaflets. This is performed at each commissure. These sutures are usually placed at midcommissural height, except at the noncoronary/right coronary commissure, where it should be placed higher to avoid the membranous septum and conduction tissue. A sub-commissural annuloplasty, or Cabrol stitch, should NOT be performed within a dissected aortic root as it will further exacerbate the dissection and potentially cause new tears in an already dissected aorta. This technique should be reserved for roots that are completely intact.

Repair of Type Ib AI

Type Ib lesions are due to dilatation of the VAJ and STJ leading to a central cusp coaptation defect and regurgitant jet. In the context of acute Type A dissection, the surgeon should consider replacing the aortic root when it is >45 mm in diameter, when there is an entry tear or significant dissection involving the root, and in genetic syndromes. If there is only limited dissection of the aortic root and no tears in the root, then it may be preserved in select cases. If the cusps are heavily calcified, fibrotic, or have fenestrations and in Sievers type 1 bicuspid AVs with commissural angles <140°, the surgeon should proceed with a Bentall procedure. Otherwise, a valve-sparing root replacement (VSRR) is reasonable in expert hands. Details of Bentall and VSRR in type A dissection are discussed in other chapters of this book. Briefly, for VSRR, either the reimplantation or remodeling plus annuloplasty technique can be used. However, an important disadvantage of the remodeling technique is the need to sew the graft to a potentially dissected aortic rim and the resulting risk of bleeding complications. In contrast, since the reimplantation technique anchors the graft below the aortic valve, in an area unaffected by the dissection, it can be a safe procedure from a hemostatic perspective. Remodeling of the aortic root is also postulated to better preserve annular dynamics during the cardiac cycle, though the impact on clinical outcome remains uncertain [29]. However, long-term results of the remodeling technique have not been as good as the reimplantation technique, especially in patients with aortic root aneurysms associated with bicuspid AV insufficiency and genetic syndromes [30–33]. Lastly, there is little published data on the use of the remodeling technique in acute aortic dissection. In addition to the root replacement, the cusps need to be assessed after the root is replaced and possible adjunctive cusp repair techniques may be used at that point. These techniques are further discussed under type II and type II lesions.

Type Ic AI Repair

Type Ic lesions are due to dilatation of the VAJ due to dilatation of the left ventricle. This is uncommon in acute type A dissections, unless there was an underlying chronic left ventricular pathology leading to dilatation. Severe VAJ dilation in the context of acute dissection may be best treated with a reimplantation procedure, when indicated.

Type Id AI Repair

This lesion typically includes cusp defects due to large fenestrations or defects from endocarditis. However, in the context of acute Type A dissection there is a more frequent scenario of a prolapsing flap from the ascending aorta that interferes with the functioning of the AV. The valve and root may be completely normal, but the prolapsing flap interacts with the AV and sometimes protrudes into the left ventricular outflow tract, leading to AI [34]. This is easily repaired with a supracoronary ascending aorta replacement. However, the surgeon must be careful in assessing for the presence of other lesions that may be difficult to see on TEE, which are masked by the prolapsing flap.

Type II AI Repair

Type II lesions are due to cusp prolapse and leads to an eccentric regurgitant jet seen on TEE. One or more cusps will coapt lower than the usual midpoint between the STJ and VAJ. It is the most frequent cusp pathology and may be due to underlying intrinsic cusp pathology or in the context of VSRR using the reimplantation technique to reduce the annular dimension. Central free margin plication using a small caliber Prolene suture placed in the center of the free margin can correct slight cusp prolapse [35]. This suture plicates, shortens, and reduces the length and therefore raises the height of the prolapsing cusp. For slightly larger degrees of prolapse, an alternative technique is free margin resuspension performed by passing a PTFE suture over and over the free margin and exteriorizing the suture at the commissures. Pulling on this suture has the effect of performing multiple plications along the free margin thereby shortening and raising it [35]. For severely prolapsing cusps with excess tissue, a larger degree of correction may be needed by resecting a small portion of the cusp with primary reapproximation.

Type III AI Repair

Type III lesions are due to cusp motion restriction. This is usually caused by underlying cusp pathology and is unrelated to the acute type A dissection. Nevertheless, the lesion must be addressed if it is causing significant AI at the time of surgery. This may be due to a calcified or fibrotic cusp in degenerative and rheumatic valves or in type I bicuspid aortic valves with conjoint cusp restriction due to a fibrous or calcified raphe. If the valve pathology is degenerative or rheumatic, then the valve should be replaced. For bicuspid valves, shaving the fibrous raphe may be all that is needed. If shaving is not adequate then resection of the raphe with primary reapproximation can be performed if there is sufficient cusp tissue. Alternatively, resection and cusp restoration with patch material may be required if there is insufficient cusp tissue left for primary reapproximation. Patch material has also been used for tricuspidization of bicuspid valves. However, the use of patch material in AV repair is a predictor or long-term failure [36]. In addition, if the surgeon lacks experience or complex bicuspid valve repair is required, an aortic valve replacement should be performed.

Aortic Valve Repair in Acute Aortic Dissection: Outcomes

The decision to intervene on the aortic root and to repair or replace the aortic valve can be a complex one and requires consideration of numerous factors. The primary objective of the operation is to save the patient's life by eliminating potentially fatal complications. Intervening on the aortic root without a clear indication and attempts at AV repair that significantly prolong myocardial ischemic time, fail and require AV re-exploration are undesirable and can increase the risk of the operation. On the other hand, the risk of prosthetic valve-related events and lifelong anticoagulation may complicate future management of residual aortopathy in these patients. Although aortic valve repair and leaving the native aortic root increase the risk of long-term reintervention, these patients often have competing risks of morbidity and mortality related to their aortopathy, making such risks less relevant. Furthermore, the cases requiring re-intervention can be done in a more elective and controlled setting. Data on mid- and long-term valvular outcomes shows that the risk of proximal re-intervention after a dissection repair is low. All studies around these topics are retrospective and have inherent limitations related to heterogeneity of patient populations, surgeon experience, myriad of surgical techniques and permutations, and biases in surgeons' complex decision-making processes.

When the aortic root is not dilated and does not have an entry tear, then AV repair through an AV resuspension has good immediate outcomes even with severe AI at presentation [37]. Long-term freedom from reoperation rates at 10 years on repaired AVs range from 69% to 95% [38–40]. Sievers et al. found that a valve-sparing root *repair* strategy has similar 30-day mortality and 15-year freedom from reoperation compared to valve sparing root *replacement* using reimplantation or remodeling techniques [41]. In patients without an indication to replace the root, they found a valve-sparing root repair strategy as a less complex and faster technique in this emergent setting. Others have argued that given the similar short- and long-term results of a root replacement strategy compared with a supracoronary ascending replacement and AV resuspension, then one should perform the "curative proximal repair" by replacing the root, whether by a composite valve conduit (Bentall procedure) or a valve sparing root replacement [42, 43].

A contemporary meta-analysis of AV preservation and repair in acute type A dissection evaluated 2402 patients in 19 observational studies [22]. Early pooled mortality was 19% with a late estimated mortality pooled rate of 4.7%/patient-year. From this data the survival estimates at 5 and 10 years were 58% and 34%, respectively. In the 13 studies reporting late AV re-intervention, the pooled rate was 2.1%/patient-year, with a 5- and 10-years freedom from AV reintervention of 89% and 79%, respectively. The composite outcome of thromboembolism and bleeding had a pooled rate of 1.4%/patient-year. This study highlighted the limited long-term survival of acute type A dissection patients, moderate risk of reoperation and low risk of valve-related complications in preserved valves.

Conclusions

Acute type A dissection is a complex, life-threatening disease with multiple considerations for management. Adding to this complexity, decision-making related to the aortic valve in acute type A dissection needs to factor in the perioperative risks of morbidity and mortality, which may be affected by the patient's stability at presentation, procedural complexity, and the surgeon expertise, as well as competing risks of late mortality related to residual aortopathy or other comorbidities. Other important considerations include the incidence of valve-related events and risk of late aortic valve reoperation. In carefully selected patients, aortic valve repair techniques can prove useful with similar outcomes to valve replacement in expert hands.

Acknowledgements None.
Sources of fundingNone.

Conflicts of Interest None declared.

References

1. Bavaria JE, Brinster DR, Gorman RC, Woo YJ, Gleason T, Pochettino A. Advances in the treatment of acute type A dissection: an integrated approach. Ann Thorac Surg. 2002;74(5):S1848–52; discussion S57–63.
2. Hagan PG, Nienaber CA, Isselbacher EM, Bruckman D, Karavite DJ, Russman PL, et al. The International Registry of Acute Aortic Dissection (IRAD): new insights into an old disease. JAMA. 2000;283(7):897–903.
3. Mehta RH, Suzuki T, Hagan PG, Bossone E, Gilon D, Llovet A, et al. Predicting death in patients with acute type a aortic dissection. Circulation. 2002;105(2):200–6.
4. Meszaros I, Morocz J, Szlavi J, Schmidt J, Tornoci L, Nagy L, et al. Epidemiology and clinicopathology of aortic dissection. Chest. 2000;117(5):1271–8.
5. Pacini D, Di Marco L, Fortuna D, Belotti LM, Gabbieri D, Zussa C, et al. Acute aortic dissection: epidemiology and outcomes. Int J Cardiol. 2013;167(6):2806–12.
6. Stamou SC, Kouchoukos NT, Hagberg RC, Smith CR, Nussbaum M, Hooker RL, et al. Differences in clinical characteristics, management, and outcomes of intraoperative versus spontaneous acute type A aortic dissection. Ann Thorac Surg. 2013;95(1):41–5.
7. Erbel R, Alfonso F, Boileau C, Dirsch O, Eber B, Haverich A, et al. Diagnosis and management of aortic dissection. Eur Heart J. 2001;22(18):1642–81.
8. Kruger T, Conzelmann LO, Bonser RS, Borger MA, Czerny M, Wildhirt S, et al. Acute aortic dissection type A. Br J Surg. 2012;99(10):1331–44.
9. Hiratzka LF, Bakris GL, Beckman JA, Bersin RM, Carr VF, Casey DE Jr, et al. 2010 ACCF/AHA/AATS/ACR/ASA/SCA/SCAI/SIR/STS/SVM guidelines for the diagnosis and management of patients with Thoracic Aortic Disease: a report of the American College of Cardiology Foundation/American Heart Association Task Force on Practice Guidelines, American Association for Thoracic Surgery, American College of Radiology, American Stroke Association, Society of Cardiovascular Anesthesiologists, Society for Cardiovascular Angiography and Interventions, Society of Interventional Radiology, Society of Thoracic Surgeons, and Society for Vascular Medicine. Circulation. 2010;121(13):e266–369.
10. Kruger T, Weigang E, Hoffmann I, Blettner M, Aebert H, Investigators G. Cerebral protection during surgery for acute aortic dissection type A: results of the German Registry for Acute Aortic Dissection Type A (GERAADA). Circulation. 2011;124(4):434–43.
11. Movsowitz HD, Levine RA, Hilgenberg AD, Isselbacher EM. Transesophageal echocardiographic description of the mechanisms of aortic regurgitation in acute type A aortic dissection: implications for aortic valve repair. J Am Coll Cardiol. 2000;36(3):884–90.
12. DeBakey ME, McCollum CH, Crawford ES, Morris GC Jr, Howell J, Noon GP, et al. Dissection and dissecting aneurysms of the aorta: twenty-year follow-up of five hundred twenty-seven patients treated surgically. Surgery. 1982;92(6):1118–34.
13. Kouchoukos NT, Karp RB, Blackstone EH, Kirklin JW, Pacifico AD, Zorn GL. Replacement of the ascending aorta and aortic valve with a composite graft. Results in 86 patients. Ann Surg. 1980;192(3):403–13.
14. Kouchoukos NT, Marshall WG Jr, Wedige-Stecher TA. Eleven-year experience with composite graft replacement of the ascending aorta and aortic valve. J Thorac Cardiovasc Surg. 1986;92(4):691–705.
15. Seybold-Epting W, Meyer J, Hallman GL, Cooley DA. Surgical treatment of acute dissecting aneurysm of the ascending aorta. J Cardiovasc Surg. 1977;18(1):43–8.
16. Dell'Aquila AM, Concistre G, Gallo A, Pansini S, Piccardo A, Passerone G, et al. Fate of the preserved aortic root after treatment of acute type A aortic dissection: 23-year follow-up. J Thorac Cardiovasc Surg. 2013;146(6):1456–60.
17. Immer FF, Aeschimann R, Englberger L, Stadler M, Eckstein FS, Tevaearai H, et al. Resuspension of the aortic valve in acute type A dissection: long-term results. J Heart Valve Dis. 2008;17(1):94–7; discussion 7.

18. Piccardo A, Regesta T, Pansini S, Dell'Aquila AM, Concistre G, Martinelli L, et al. Fate of the aortic valve after root reconstruction in type A aortic dissection: a 20-year follow up. J Heart Valve Dis. 2009;18(5):507–13.
19. Ro SK, Kim JB, Hwang SK, Jung SH, Choo SJ, Chung CH, et al. Aortic root conservative repair of acute type A aortic dissection involving the aortic root: fate of the aortic root and aortic valve function. J Thorac Cardiovasc Surg. 2013;146(5):1113–8.
20. Subramanian S, Leontyev S, Borger MA, Trommer C, Misfeld M, Mohr FW. Valve-sparing root reconstruction does not compromise survival in acute type A aortic dissection. Ann Thorac Surg. 2012;94(4):1230–4.
21. Yamanaka K, Hori Y, Ikarashi J, Kusuhara T, Nakatsuka D, Hirose K, et al. Durability of aortic valve preservation with root reconstruction for acute type A aortic dissection. Eur J Cardio-thoracic Surg. 2012;41(4):e32–6.
22. Saczkowski R, Malas T, Mesana T, de Kerchove L, El Khoury G, Boodhwani M. Aortic valve preservation and repair in acute Type A aortic dissection. Eur J Cardio-thoracic Surg. 2014;45(6):e220–6.
23. Boodhwani M, de Kerchove L, Glineur D, Poncelet A, Rubay J, Astarci P, et al. Repair-oriented classification of aortic insufficiency: impact on surgical techniques and clinical outcomes. J Thorac Cardiovasc Surg. 2009;137(2):286–94.
24. Carpentier A. Cardiac valve surgery–the "French correction". J Thorac Cardiovasc Surg. 1983;86(3):323–37.
25. Sievers HH, Schmidtke C. A classification system for the bicuspid aortic valve from 304 surgical specimens. J Thorac Cardiovasc Surg. 2007;133(5):1226–33.
26. McCarthy FH, Bavaria JE, McDermott KM, Moeller P, Spragan D, Hoedt A, et al. At the root of the repair debate: outcomes after elective aortic root replacements for aortic insufficiency with aneurysm. Ann Thorac Surg. 2016;102(4):1199–205.
27. Rylski B, Blanke P, Beyersdorf F, Desai ND, Milewski RK, Siepe M, et al. How does the ascending aorta geometry change when it dissects? J Am Coll Cardiol. 2014;63(13):1311–9.
28. Al-Atassi T, Toeg HD, Jafar R, Sohmer B, Labrosse M, Boodhwani M. Impact of aortic annular geometry on aortic valve insufficiency: insights from a preclinical, ex vivo, porcine model. J Thorac Cardiovasc Surg. 2015;150(3):656–64.e1.
29. Leyh RG, Schmidtke C, Sievers HH, Yacoub MH. Opening and closing characteristics of the aortic valve after different types of valve-preserving surgery. Circulation. 1999;100(21):2153–60.
30. David TE, David CM, Manlhiot C, Colman J, Crean AM, Bradley T. Outcomes of aortic valve-sparing operations in Marfan syndrome. J Am Coll Cardiol. 2015;66(13):1445–53.
31. David TE, Feindel CM, David CM, Manlhiot C. A quarter of a century of experience with aortic valve-sparing operations. J Thorac Cardiovasc Surg. 2014;148(3):872–9; discussion 9-80.
32. de Kerchove L, Boodhwani M, Glineur D, Vandyck M, Vanoverschelde JL, Noirhomme P, et al. Valve sparing-root replacement with the reimplantation technique to increase the durability of bicuspid aortic valve repair. J Thorac Cardiovasc Surg. 2011;142(6):1430–8.
33. Erasmi AW, Sievers HH, Bechtel JF, Hanke T, Stierle U, Misfeld M. Remodeling or reimplantation for valve-sparing aortic root surgery? Ann Thorac Surg. 2007;83(2):S752–6; discussion S85-90.
34. Knio Z, Montealegre-Gallegos M. Aortic regurgitation with a prolapsing aortic dissection flap: is valve replacement necessary? J Cardiothorac Vasc Anesth. 2016;30(6):1750–3.
35. de Kerchove L, Boodhwani M, Glineur D, Poncelet A, Rubay J, Watremez C, et al. Cusp prolapse repair in trileaflet aortic valves: free margin plication and free margin resuspension techniques. Ann Thorac Surg. 2009;88(2):455–61; discussion 61.
36. Boodhwani M, de Kerchove L, Glineur D, Rubay J, Vanoverschelde JL, Noirhomme P, et al. Repair of regurgitant bicuspid aortic valves: a systematic approach. J Thorac Cardiovasc Surg. 2010;140(2):276–84.e1.

37. Tang PC, Badami A, Akhter SA, Osaki S, Lozonschi L, Kohmoto T, et al. Efficacy of aortic valve resuspension in establishing valve competence in acute type A dissections. Ann Thorac Surg. 2017;103(5):1460–6.
38. Fann JI, Glower DD, Miller DC, Yun KL, Rankin JS, White WD, et al. Preservation of aortic valve in type A aortic dissection complicated by aortic regurgitation. J Thorac Cardiovasc Surg. 1991;102(1):62–73; discussion 5.
39. Mazzucotelli JP, Deleuze PH, Baufreton C, Duval AM, Hillion ML, Loisance DY, et al. Preservation of the aortic valve in acute aortic dissection: long-term echocardiographic assessment and clinical outcome. Ann Thorac Surg. 1993;55(6):1513–7.
40. von Segesser LK, Lorenzetti E, Lachat M, Niederhauser U, Schonbeck M, Vogt PR, et al. Aortic valve preservation in acute type A dissection: is it sound? J Thorac Cardiovasc Surg. 1996;111(2):381–90; discussion 90-1.
41. Sievers HH, Richardt D, Diwoky M, Auer C, Bucsky B, Nasseri B, et al. Survival and reoperation after valve-sparing root replacement and root repair in acute type A dissection. J Thorac Cardiovasc Surg. 2018;156(6):2076–82. e2
42. Di Eusanio M, Trimarchi S, Peterson MD, Myrmel T, Hughes GC, Korach A, et al. Root replacement surgery versus more conservative management during type A acute aortic dissection repair. Ann Thorac Surg. 2014;98(6):2078–84.
43. Urbanski PP, Lenos A, Irimie V, Bougioukakis P, Zacher M, Diegeler A. Acute aortic dissection involving the root: operative and long-term outcome after curative proximal repair. Interact Cardiovasc Thorac Surg. 2016;22(5):620–6.

Management of the Aortic Arch in Acute Aortic Dissection Type A

Takashi Kunihara and Hans-Joachim Schäfers

General Considerations

The goal of surgical treatment of acute aortic dissection is the replacement of the ascending aorta in order to eliminate the segment that can and will lead to pericardial tamponade. The seemingly "straightforward" operation is performed under emergency conditions due to the characteristics of acute aortic dissection type A (AADA). The inherent risks or difficulties are related to the disease, i.e. the patient often presenting in shock, the frequent occurrence and dynamic character of malperfusion of vital organs, and the fragility of the aortic wall. The need for surgery is clear. Different opinions exist regarding extent of aortic replacement, handling of the fragile aortic wall, details of cannulation, and cerebral protection. In view of all differing opinions regarding patient management it must not be forgotten the primary goal is to save the patient's life.

In this chapter we review the evidence regarding the controversial issues with a focus on management of the aortic arch and then describe our routine in more detail.

T. Kunihara
Department of Cardiac Surgery, The Jikei University School of Medicine, Tokyo, Japan

H.-J. Schäfers (✉)
Department of Thoracic and Cardiovascular Surgery, Saarland University Medical Center, Homburg/Saar, Germany
e-mail: h-j.schaefers@uks.eu

J. S. Coselli et al. (eds.), *Aortic Dissection and Acute Aortic Syndromes*,
https://doi.org/10.1007/978-3-030-66668-2_22

Extent of Aortic Replacement

The primary goal of the operation is to bring the patient out of the operating room and hospital alive. A second goal is and has been to minimize the probability of later downstream aortic dilatation; this has long been known to be more frequent if arch dissection and a patent false lumen persist.

Traditionally, this operation has been performed as replacement of the tubular ascending aorta with a cross clamp placed just below the brachiocephalic trunk [1]. Later it was proposed to perform the aortic replacement with an open anastomosis, i.e. include the proximal arch in the replaced aortic segment (Fig. 1) [2, 3]. The early mortality for limited replacement of the ascending aorta has been 7–25%, and that for proximal arch replacement 9–22% [2–10]. The mortality has apparently been mostly related to patient-specific risk factors, such as preoperative shock or the existence of relevant malperfusion [7, 11–13]. Smaller studies, even an early meta-analysis, did not find obvious differences in postoperative morbidities and early/late mortality between open (with deep hypothermia) and closed (with cross-clamp) distal anastomosis techniques [4–6]. A large registry study (NORCAAD, n = 1134) showed that patients who were operated by closed technique had worse short- and mid-term survival than those who had been treated by open anastomosis [7].

The rationale for routine partial arch replacement, which has become the standard in most cardiac surgical units, has been that this eliminates entry tears created

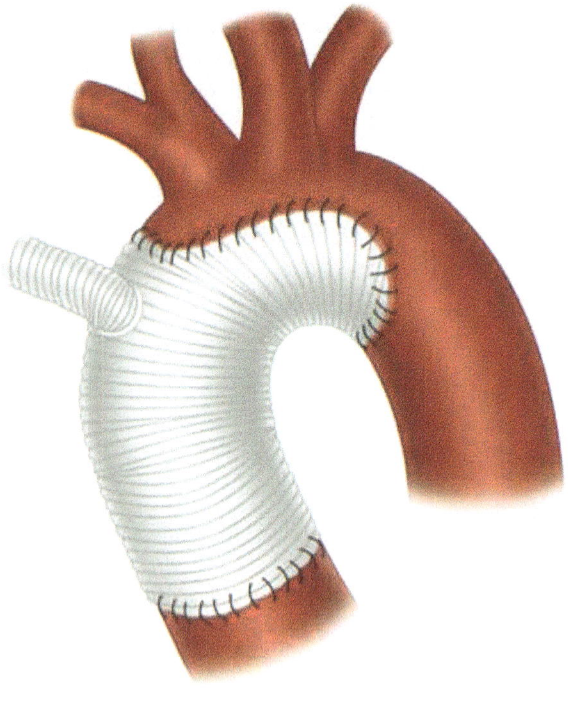

Fig. 1 Partial arch replacement. Depending on the location of an entry or re-entry tear the replacement of the arch may be extended in the convexity of the arch

by the aortic cross clamp [5]. In addition, it allows inspection of the arch for a possible entry site and its resection. Partial arch replacement seems to reduce the prevalence of a persistent false lumen in the downstream aorta. If the dissection is limited to the proximal aorta (DeBakey type II), an open arch anastomosis will lead to complete elimination of dissection by suturing to the non-dissected arch. The positive effects were confirmed in several series [8, 14]. The open distal anastomosis using hypothermic circulatory arrest with or without cerebral perfusion has become a standard part of AADA surgery for the majority of western surgeons. In the German registry circulatory arrest was not used in only 5% of patients, and thus some form of arch replacement in 95% [15]. Freedom from secondary operations for progressive dilatation of the downstream aorta is 87–97% at 5 years after the initial operation [16–21].

Total replacement of the arch has been used rarely in most western series, while it was proposed on an almost routine basis, primarily by Japanese groups [13, 22–24] in order to minimize the probability of distal aortic dilatation. Others have been concerned over an increased risk of mortality and morbidity and employed total arch replacement rarely [25–28]. Over the years total arch replacement has become more popular, in part driven by increasing popularity of the frozen elephant trunk extension [24, 29–32]. In judging the value of the more extensive operation, we need to keep in mind that operative mortality largely depends on patient characteristics. In previous series, partial arch replacement had at an average an early mortality of 10–15%, while total arch replacement was associated with a higher mortality of 20% [11, 12].

Total arch replacement may be performed using different technical variants. The anatomic form of total replacement of the arch with implantation of the aortic island carrying the orifices of the supraaortic vessels (Fig. 2) [19, 20, 28, 29, 32, 33] is feasible also in acute dissection. On the other hand, achieving hemostasis on the

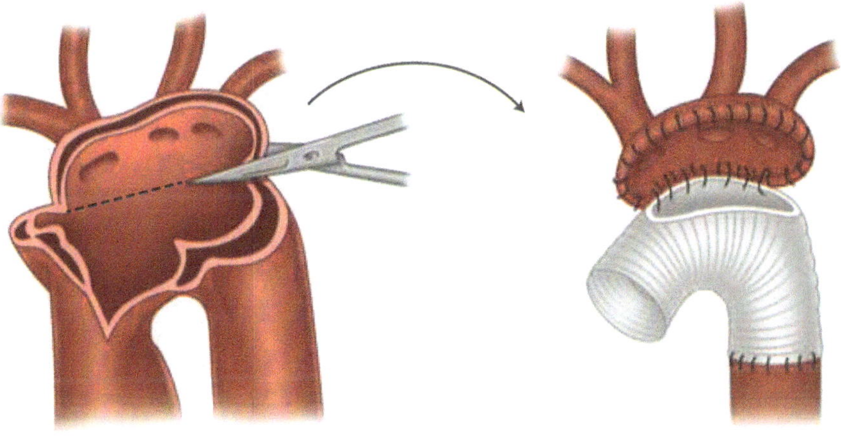

Fig. 2 Total arch replacement in its anatomic form. The island of the aortic arch carrying the orifices of the supraaortic branches is implanted in the arch graft

distal suture line, i.e. between graft and descending aorta, may be challenging in acute dissection. The Japanese variant (Fig. 3) of this operation includes the distal anastomosis and three separate grafts connected to the supraaortic branches. The time required to complete the arch repair is thus longer, but control of the distal anastomosis is facilitated. The Griepp group suggested a modification, which combines advantages of both approaches (Fig. 4). In this technique a smaller graft (e.g. 14 or 16 mm) is anastomosed in end-to-side fashion to the island carrying the supraaortic branches. The aortic graft is connected to the descending aorta while the supraaortic graft is intubated or clamped for antegrade cerebral perfusion. All variants may be combined with a short conventional or frozen elephant trunk [34, 35].

A recent meta-analysis including a large number of Asian patients (42%) revealed that total arch replacement was performed in 32.3% of all procedures [36]. Total arch replacement was performed in almost 50% of all operations for cute type A dissection in 2017 in Japan [37]. In the international registry (IRAD), the German registry (GERAADA), and American database (STS) the frequency of total arch replacement has been only 26.9%, 16.2%, and 14.1%, respectively [11, 12, 38]. It is even less than 10% in Italian and Nordic registry; 6.9% and 5.9%, respectively [39, 40].

One Japanese series demonstrated superior freedom from aortic events after total arch replacement (83%) compared with ascending aortic replacement (51%) at 9 years [41]. A lower rate of reoperation was observed during 10 years after extensive repair than proximal repair (5.4% vs 16.9%, $P < .05$) in another series [42]. Many other studies have not found any significant difference in the incidence of late distal reoperation or major adverse events between aggressive and conservative approach for the aortic arch [11, 16, 36, 40, 43]. One meta-analysis identified increased incidence of aortic reoperation (proximal or distal unknown) after proximal

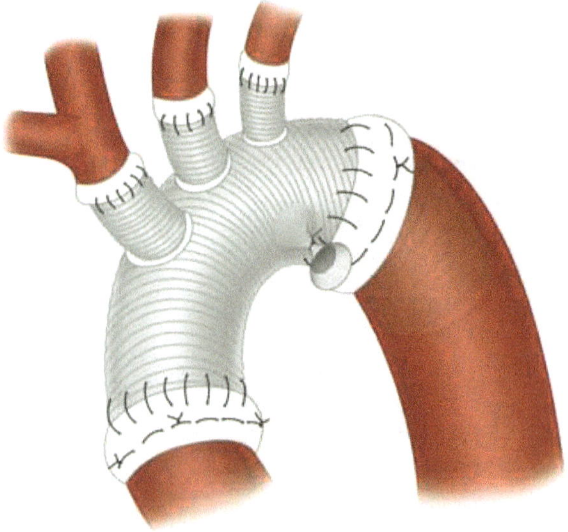

Fig. 3 Total arch replacement with separate anastomoses of the supraaortic vessels. It may or may not be combined with a limited elephant trunk extension into the descending aorta

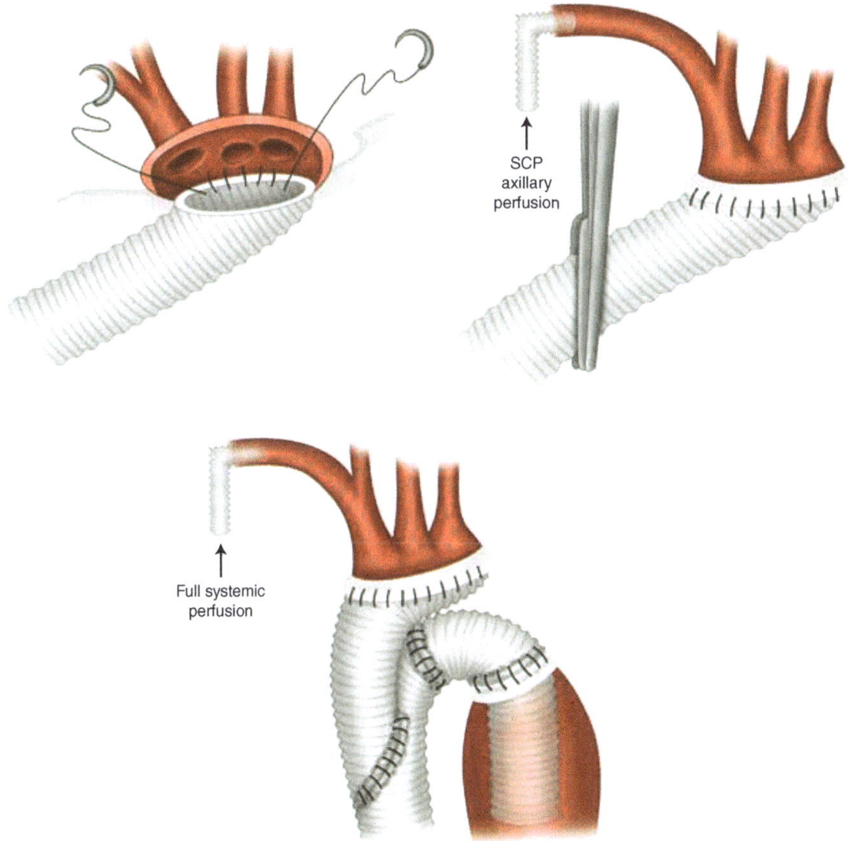

Fig. 4 Modified total arch replacement. A smaller graft is anastomosed to the island carrying the orifices of the supraaortic branches. This graft can then be perfused in antegrade fashion while total arch replacement is performed. The two grafts are then connected. The operation may be combined with a limited elephant trunk extension into the descending aorta

replacement compared with total arch replacement [44]. Failure to exclude the primary entry site was identified as predictor for distal aortic events [45]. On the other hand, one should keep in mind that elective reoperation for progressive enlargement of the distal aorta was not necessary in more than 80% of the patients undergoing proximal arch replacement only; in addition, the complexity of such an elective procedure is far from that of acute dissection.

This increased complexity is confirmed by a higher early mortality after total arch replacement in the majority of registries [11, 12, 36], and it was statistically significant so in a recent meta-analysis (odds ratio = 0.77) [36]. So far, only the Japanese database shows a different result [37]. It is unclear whether this is related to the procedure per se or rather differences in patient selection. Total arch replacement is unquestionably associated with longer procedural time [11, 16, 36, 41–44, 46]. Several registries show a similar incidence of postoperative stroke between replacement of the total arch and the ascending aorta [11, 12, 29, 36], while the STS database and Nordic database report a higher incidence for total arch replacement [38, 40]. The incidence of postoperative acute renal failure was also increased in extended arch replacement according to the IRAD data [11]. So far, total arch replacement has not improved log-term survival [11, 36, 41, 43]; survival seems to be affected mainly by patient-related factors [43, 45, 46].

The addition of a (frozen) elephant trunk (Fig. 5) has been associated with thrombosis of the distal false lumen, at least in the proximal descending aorta [30, 31, 42, 47]. While this technical variant does not prolong cross-clamping time, there is a prolonged lower-body arrest time [29, 30]. In a meta-analysis thrombosis of the distal false lumen was seen in 96.8% of cases who were treated with frozen elephant trunk [29]. Thrombosis rate of the proximal descending aorta was 25–66% after proximal repair and 82–100% after extended repair with frozen elephant trunk in single center experiences [31, 42, 47]. It is yet unclear whether this technique indeed reduces the need for secondary distal aortic replacement sufficiently.

Cannulation for Extracorporeal Circulation

Venous cannulation for these procedures is standard. Single venous drainage from the right atrium using a two-stage cannula is sufficient in essentially all patients. In unusual instances, venous cannulation through a femoral vein may be used alternatively.

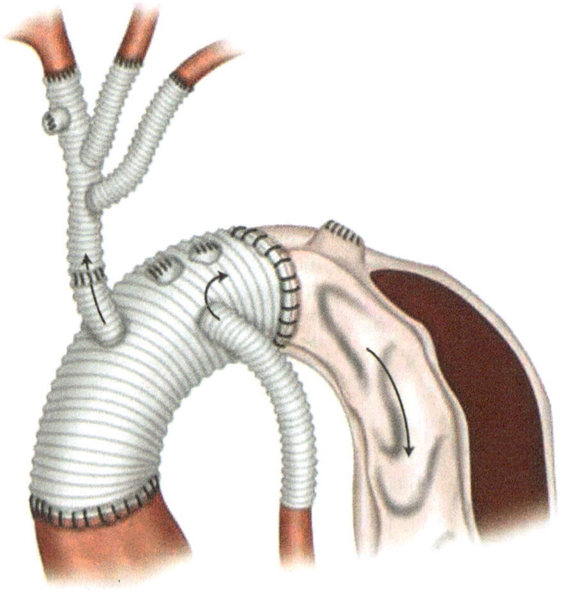

Fig. 5 Total arch replacement combined with a frozen elephant trunk. In this variant separate grafts are connected to the supraaortic vessels

Arterial cannulation has undergone changes over time. The femoral artery has been the traditional cannulation site, and it remains one of the fastest and easiest sites for arterial cannulation. In 2011–2012, the femoral artery was still the first choice of arterial cannulation site for AADA (45.9%), however, the aorta (29.1%) and the axillary artery (31.0%) were used equally as the second choice in STS database [48]. Retrograde perfusion may, however, decrease cerebral perfusion intraoperatively if the false lumen is perfused preferentially. The potential risk of malperfusion of other vital organs is also inherent with this adjunct. In order to minimize these problems, it has been combined with cannulation of the aortic graft once arch repair was finished in order to establish antegrade perfusion into the true lumen [2].

In the 2000s, right axillary artery cannulation became popular as an alternative. Its use in aneurysm surgery has reduced the incidence of embolic cerebral complications [49, 50] by avoiding retrograde flow through an atherosclerotic descending aorta. In acute dissection, its main advantage lies in the fact that there is probably better maintenance of blood flow through the right carotid artery. The axillary artery can be cannulated directly using Seldinger technique [34]. Alternatively, an 8 mm Dacron graft is anastomosed in end-to side fashion to the artery and intubated with the arterial cannula [51]. After termination of cardiopulmonary bypass this Dacron graft can simply be oversewn or ligated, thus avoiding potential repair procedure on the artery itself.

Two meta-analyses published in 2015 found the superiority of axillary artery cannulation over femoral artery cannulation in reducing early mortality and the incidence of permanent neurological dysfunction [52, 53]. However, one of them failed to find clinical benefit of axillary artery cannulation in preventing malperfusion [53]. In 2015, the axillary artery was used as the first choice of arterial cannulation site in more than half of European and Canadian patients with acute setting (54% and 76%, respectively) followed by the femoral artery (28% and 17%, respectively) [33, 54].

Direct cannulation of the proximal aorta has emerged in recent years [55, 56]. This can easily be done by cannulating the non-dissected arch in type II dissections. Different approaches have been proposed for cannulation of the dissected arch [57–59]. The aorta may be cannulated using Seldinger technique guided by epiaortic ultrasonography or transesophageal echocardiography [57]. The position of the cannula within the true lumen can be confirmed by a guidewire, which is in the true lumen both in the ascending and descending aorta as judged by echocardiography. At times the fragility of the aortic tissue may make this form of cannulation difficult. We therefore use it only in selected circumstances.

Some groups cannulate inside the true lumen directly after transection of the ascending aorta [58, 59]. The senior author has a limited personal experience with this approach; it has been difficult to ascertain a stable position in the ascending aorta for controlled perfusion. We therefore do not use this technique. Finally, also the left ventricular apex has been proposed as cannulation site. In the authors' experience, this has been difficult, and left ventricular distension may occur in the presence of aortic regurgitation. Even though there have been small studies showing that the transapical cannulation is safe [60, 61] it should not be one of the preferred approaches.

Cerebral Protection

Any form of arch replacement has to consider the different options of cerebral protection. Deep hypothermia has traditionally been used as the main method of cerebral protection and is probably safe at a nasopharyngeal temperature of 20 °C for up to 20–25 min [62, 63]. Different other temperatures have been stated to be followed, such as rectal, bladder, or tympanic. In interpreting the results of different groups it is important to look at this in detail; tympanic or nasopharyngeal temperature best represent brain temperature [64]. A target brain temperature may already be reached at a bladder temperature of 28 °C.

Retrograde perfusion via the superior vena cava has originally been proposed by a Japanese group [65]. Later studies [66, 67] showed a positive effect in that it reduced the incidence of embolic cerebral complications. Since it probably does not provide nutritive blood flow to the brain [68] it can be used as a way of cooling the head and brain and reducing potential embolic phenomena. Exclusively in patients with acute aortic dissection who underwent isolated proximal aortic repair, retrograde perfusion was associated with shorter procedural time and similar mortality and neurological outcome to antegrade fashion [69]. We use it only for that purpose and commonly employ a flow of 600–1000 ml/min, adjusted to have a central venous pressure of less than 20 mmHg.

More recently, antegrade perfusion of the brain has become a popular means of cerebral protection. This can be achieved by placing perfusion catheters into the supraaortic branches. Alternatively, when the right axillary artery is used for arterial inflow, the brachiocephalic trunk may be clamped and a catheter introduced only into the left carotid artery. Installing such catheters requires a certain time of circulatory arrest [70], so it is commonly used in conjunction with hypothermia. Antegrade perfusion provides nutritive blood flow to the brain and is the only safe means of cerebral protection if the time for arch repair exceeds 30 min [71, 72].

Management of Dissected Tissue

Traditionally, the biggest challenge in surgery for AADA has been handling of the fragile tissue and consecutive hemostasis. This changed dramatically when the so-called "French Glue" became available [73]. The glue is injected between the dissected wall layers, which are then adapted with special clamps or bulldog clamps (Fig. 6a, b). While the adhesive capacity of this glue is limited, it resulted in tanning of the tissue and creation of more normal aortic wall texture. Later Bioglue (CryoLife, Kennesaw, GA, USA) [74] became available with similar effect. Both

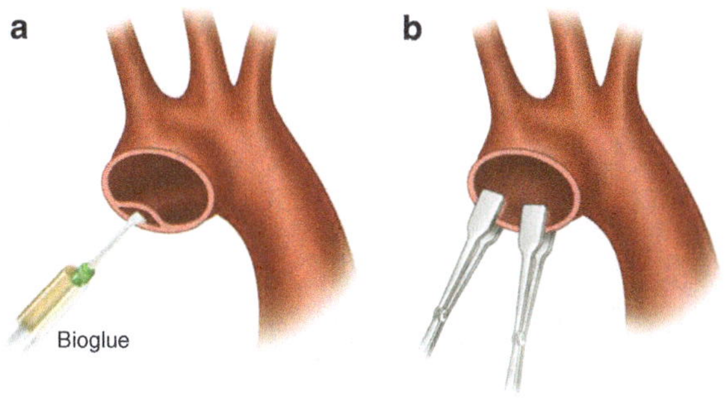

Fig. 6 (**a**) The application of adhesive to the dissected wall layers improves the handling characteristics in acute dissection. Because of possible local toxicity the adhesive should be used sparingly. (**b**) Using clamps the aortic wall layers are adapted until the adhesive has hardened

adhesives have facilitated hemostasis similarly and apparently reduced mortality. Early series reported that the use of GRF glue decreased in-hospital mortality from 23% to 10.5% [75] or 45% to 21% [76, 77]. The use of Bioglue has been associated with reductions in postoperative blood loss and hospital length of stay [78].

Due to the limited adhesive effect, this surgical glue has not affected the patency of the distal false lumen [8, 79]. There have been observations indicating that an excessive amount of glue may negatively influence tissue stability, possibly as a consequence of local tissue necrosis [80, 81]. Therefore, sparing use of such glue seems advisable.

In order to support the suture line and facilitate hemostasis, an intussusception (adventitia inversion) technique has been proposed (Fig. 7) [82]. With this technique, the aorta is transected completely, and the dissected media is shortened by approximately 1 cm compared to the adventitia. The adventitia is then invaginated into the true lumen. In creating the suture line, each bite on the aorta will have adventitia on the outside and inside. We have explored this technique and found it easy to use and very hemostatic.

How We Do It

In view of all knowledge and considerations, we attempt to keep the operations as simple as possible. This involves standard cannulation, hypothermia, and an open anastomosis to the arch. We rarely deviate from this standard approach. If the patient is in shock due to tamponade, the first procedure is the median sternotomy and limited opening of the pericardium to relieve the tamponade. Blood pressure will always increase, and anesthesia carefully monitors blood pressure and—if necessary—administers a vasodilator to avoid sudden rupture due to hypertension. This allows us to rapidly treat hypotension and continue under controlled conditions.

Following a median sternotomy, our standard cannulation involves an 8 mm Dacron graft sutured to the right axillary artery. A standard arterial cannula is ligated into the graft. We always use a two-stage, single venous cannula for optimal venous drainage. Extracorporeal circulation is started, and the core temperature is cooled to

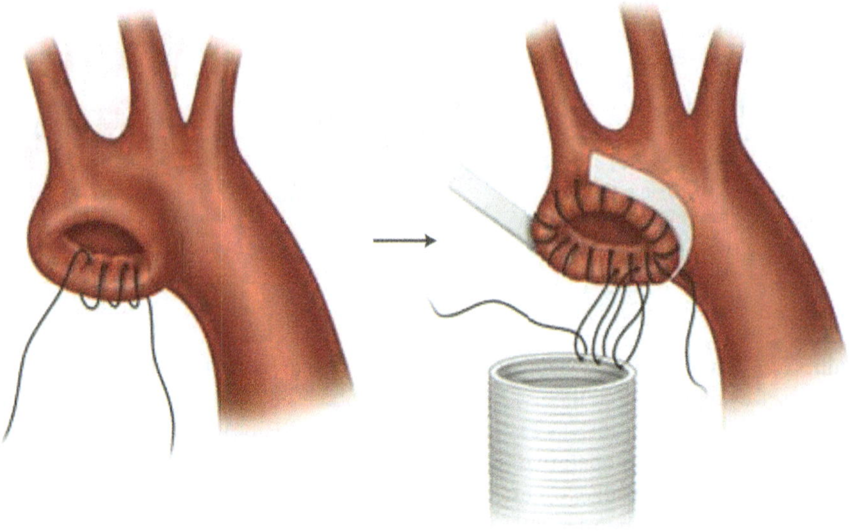

Fig. 7 Invagination technique without tissue adhesive in acute dissection. Following transection of the aorta the adventitia is left longer than the media and folded around the media. The aortic graft is then sutured to the folded aortic edge. A strip of Teflon may or may not be used for the arch suture line

a nasopharyngeal temperature of 20 °C. In cases where the patient's history (back pain as initial presentation) or the CT scan indicate a distal location of the entry, we will cool to a nasopharyngeal temperature of 18 °C. If the degree of aortic regurgitation is limited, we will introduce a left atrial vent catheter through the right superior pulmonary vein when the heart fibrillates and will continue cooling until the desired temperature is reached. If aortic regurgitation is severe and the left ventricle is distending upon fibrillation, we will cross-clamp the aorta and give blood cardioplegia directly into the coronary ostia. At this time the aorta is carefully inspected for the location of the entry tear. If it is found in the ascending aorta the procedure is continued according to plan. If there is no entry in the ascending aorta the patient is cooled to a temperature of 18 °C.

Independent of the type of root procedure, extracorporeal circulation is stopped when the desired nasopharyngeal temperature is reached. With the patient in an anti-Trendelenburg position the cross-clamp is removed. The distal ascending aorta is transected approximately 0.5–1 cm proximal to the brachiocephalic trunk and the arch inspected.

If there is an entry in the concavity of the arch it is resected by extending the aortic transection level to the entry. Similarly, if there is no entry in the arch, the operation is continued as planned, i.e. a hemi-arch replacement is performed. The arch tissue is mobilized for 1 cm, and Bioglue is administered sparingly. The layers of the aortic wall are compressed with special clamps (Fig. 6b) or strong bulldog clamps until the glue has become firm. The chosen Dacron graft is then obliquely anastomosed to the arch using a 4-0 polypropylene suture. In the past years we have explored the use of the intussusception technique (Fig. 7) as alternative to adhesive and found it similarly effective. This type of arch repair can usually be accomplished within a cerebral ischemic time of less than 15 min, and we therefore do not employ antegrade cerebral perfusion.

If the entry is located in the convexity of the arch or in the proximal descending aorta, a decision for total arch replacement is made. Our preferred approach to total arch replacement is the modification proposed by the Griepp group [25, 34, 68], since we feel it gives us best control of the operation and exposure of the distal anastomosis while minimizing operative complexity (Fig. 4).

As a first step most of the aortic tissue is resected around the orifices of the supraaortic branches. A 14 or 16 mm Dacron graft is anastomosed to the island of the origins of the head and neck vessels. Since the duration of hypothermic circulatory arrest is less predictable under these circumstances, we then clamp the graft and resume antegrade perfusion with a blood temperature of 15 °C and a flow rate of 500 ml/min. Alternatively (if the right axillary artery had not been used for arterial cannulation) we place the aortic cannula into this arch graft and snug it with a tourniquet or clamp for antegrade perfusion.

A second graft is then chosen for the aortic arch. If the descending aorta is of normal caliber, end-to-end anastomosis is created. In order to secure hemostasis, either application of adhesive (Bioglue, CryoLife, Kennesaw, GA, USA) or the intussusception technique are employed. We rarely employ Teflon felt to buttress the suture line; for the suture to the descending aorta, however, we always use it. If the diameter of the descending aorta is larger than 3 cm, either a short elephant trunk extension or a frozen trunk are added. This seems particularly helpful if true lumen compression was present on the preoperative CT.

After the distal suture is complete an opening is created on the cephalad circumference of the aortic graft. The smaller graft connected to the head and neck vessels is shortened and implanted into the aortic prosthesis. Full aortic perfusion is restarted, and hemostasis can be checked on the two anastomoses.

If a complex entry is present between the origins of the supraaortic orifices we choose total arch replacement using a branched aortic graft. The distal aortic arch is transected at just distal to the left subclavian artery take-off, taking care not to injure the left recurrent nerve. The false lumen is obliterated by surgical glue, expanding the true lumen with a Foley catheter.

A short tube graft with the same diameter of the distal aorta is inserted into the true lumen as an elephant trunk (Fig. 8). This will not only facilitate distal hemostasis but also improve reverse remodeling of the downstream aorta. The distal end of the prefabricated arch graft with four branches is cut short and anastomosed to the distal aorta using a 4-0 polypropylene suture with the graft inside and felt reinforcement outside. Subsequently the separate arch grafts are connected to the respective arch vessels using 5-0 polypropylene running suture and perfusion is resumed sequentially followed by gradual rewarming. After termination of selective cerebral perfusion, full systemic rewarming becomes feasible. One of the advantages of

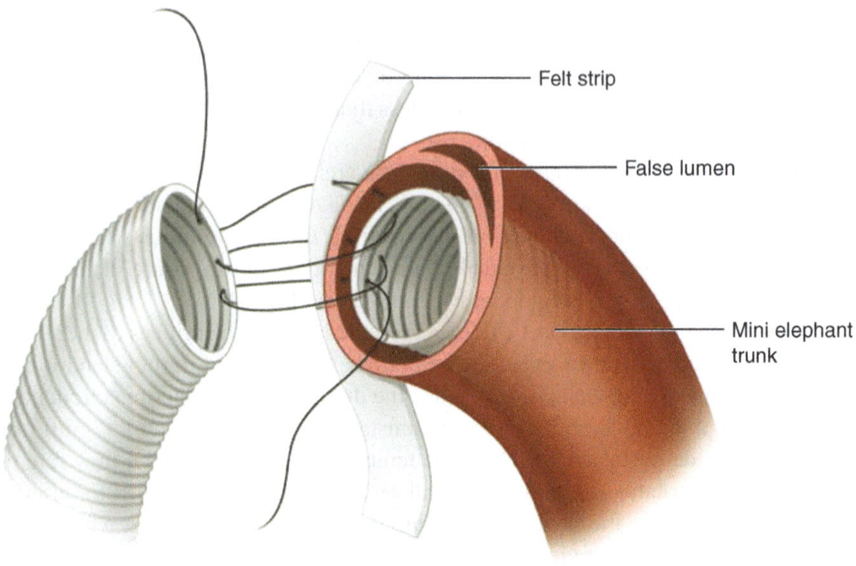

Fig. 8 Creation of the distal anastomosis in total arch replacement for AADA. A short graft (5–8 cm long) is introduced into the true lumen of the descending aorta and a Teflon strip is placed outside the aorta. The aortic graft is connected to the distal aorta, "sandwiching" the aortic wall between the trunk graft and the Teflon strip

individual branch reconstruction is small anastomosis with low tension and good hemostasis.

Antegrade selective cerebral perfusion is performed through an individual circuit and pump other than systemic one. Three balloon catheters (15 Fr for the brachiocephalic artery, 12 Fr for the left common carotid artery and the left subclavian artery) are inserted into the true lumen of the three arch vessels. Total perfusion flow is initially set at 12 ml/kg and adjusted according to the bilateral radial artery pressures and regional cerebral oxygen saturation. When cannulation to the left subclavian artery is complicated, it can be clamped and perfusion flow is reduced. In case of right axillary artery cannulation, all three arch vessels can simply be clamped at their origin and cerebral perfusion can simply be performed through the right axillar artery alone.

In patients with marked true lumen collapse preoperatively, the use of a frozen elephant trunk can be considered aiming at early reverse remodeling of the downstream aorta. In this scenario, one or two arch vessels can be translocated, which will also facilitate anastomosis and hemostasis. An advantage of this technique is that injury of the left recurrent nerve or phrenic nerve can absolutely be avoided. The aortic arch is transected just distal or proximal of the left common carotid artery according to the location of primary intimal tear. The left subclavian artery with or without the left common carotid artery are transected and their proximal ends are closed. Each arch vessel is connected to the respective branch of the prefabricated arch graft which originates from more proximal than natural anatomy (=translocation). A frozen elephant trunk is inserted into the true lumen of the distal aorta. Care must be taken not to injure the intimal flap and not to extend it too far distally to minimize the risk of spinal cord injury [29, 83]. The major drawback is kinking of the branches of the prefabricated arch graft because of unfavorable angles.

References

1. Crawford ES, Kirklin JW, Naftel DC, Svensson LG, Coselli JS, Safi HJ. Surgery for acute dissection of ascending aorta. Should the arch be included? J Thorac Cardiovasc Surg. 1992;104:46–59.
2. David TE, Armstrong S, Ivanov J, Barnard S. Surgery for acute type A aortic dissection. Ann Thorac Surg. 1999;67:1999–2001.
3. Lai DT, Robbins RC, Mitchell RS, Moore KA, Oyer PE, Shumway NE, et al. Does profound hypothermic circulatory arrest improve survival in patients with acute type A aortic dissection? Circulation. 2002;106:I218–28.
4. Stamou SC, Kouchoukos NT, Hagberg RC, Khabbaz KR, Robicsek F, Nussbaum M, et al. Does the technique of distal anastomosis influence clinical outcomes in acute type A aortic dissection? Interact Cardiovasc Thorac Surg. 2011;12:404–8.
5. Malvindi PG, Modi A, Miskolczi S, Kaarne M, Velissaris T, Barlow C, et al. Open and closed distal anastomosis for acute type A aortic dissection repair. Interact Cardiovasc Thorac Surg. 2016;22:776–83.
6. Myrmel T, Lai DT, Miller DC. Can the principles of evidence-based medicine be applied to the treatment of aortic dissections? Eur J Cardiothorac Surg. 2004;25:236–42.
7. Geirsson A, Shioda K, Olsson C, Ahlsson A, Gunn J, Hansson EC, et al. Differential outcomes of open and clamp-on distal anastomosis techniques in acute type A aortic dissection. J Thorac Cardiovasc Surg. 2019;157:1750–8.
8. Nguyen B, Müller M, Kipfer B, Berdat P, Walpoth B, Althaus U, et al. Different techniques of distal aortic repair in acute type A dissection: impact on late aortic morphology and reoperation. Eur J Cardiothorac Surg. 1999;15:496–500.
9. Danner BC, Natour E, Horst M, Dikov V, Ghosh PK, Dapunt OE. Comparison of operative techniques in acute type A aortic dissection performing the distal anastomosis. J Card Surg. 2007;22:105–10.
10. Yamashita C, Okada M, Ataka K, Yoshida M, Yoshimura N, Azami T, et al. Open distal anastomosis in retrograde cerebral perfusion for repair of ascending aortic dissection. Ann Thorac Surg. 1997;64:665–9.
11. Larsen M, Trimarchi S, Patel HJ, Di Eusanio M, Greason KL, Peterson MD, et al. Extended versus limited arch replacement in acute Type A aortic dissection. Eur J Cardiothorac Surg. 2017;52:1104–10.
12. Conzelmann LO, Weigang E, Mehlhorn U, Abugameh A, Hoffmann I, Blettner M, et al., GERAADA Investigators. Mortality in patients with acute aortic dissection type A: analysis of pre- and intraoperative risk factors from the German Registry for Acute Aortic Dissection Type A (GERAADA). Eur J Cardiothorac Surg. 2016;49:e44–52.
13. Inoue Y, Matsuda H, Uchida K, Komiya T, Koyama T, Yoshino H, et al. Analysis of acute type A aortic dissection in Japan registry of aortic dissection (JRAD). Ann Thorac Surg. 2020. pii: S0003-4975(20)30170-3. https://doi.org/10.1016/j.athoracsur.2019.12.051. [Epub ahead of print].
14. Bernard Y, Zimmermann H, Chocron S, Litzler JF, Kastler B, Etievent JP, et al. False lumen patency as a predictor of late outcome in aortic dissection. Am J Cardiol. 2001;87:1378–82.

15. Krüger T, Weigang E, Hoffmann I, Blettner M, Aebert H, GERAADA Investigators. Cerebral protection during surgery for acute aortic dissection type A: results of the German Registry for Acute Aortic Dissection Type A (GERAADA). Circulation. 2011;124:434–43.
16. Rylski B, Beyersdorf F, Kari FA, Schlosser J, Blanke P, Siepe M. Acute type A aortic dissection extending beyond ascending aorta: limited or extensive distal repair. J Thorac Cardiovasc Surg. 2014;148:949–54.
17. Shiono M, Hata M, Sezai A, Iida M, Yagi S, Negishi N. Emergency surgery for acute type A aortic dissection in octogenarians. Ann Thorac Surg. 2006;82:554–9.
18. Omura A, Miyahara S, Yamanaka K, Sakamoto T, Matsumori M, Okada K, et al. Early and late outcomes of repaired acute DeBakey type I aortic dissection after graft replacement. J Thorac Cardiovasc Surg. 2015;151:341–8.
19. Tan ME, Dossche KME, Morshuis WJ, Kelder JC, Waanders FG, Schepens MA. Is extended arch replacement for acute type A aortic dissection an additional risk factor for mortality? Ann Thorac Surg. 2003;76:1209–14.
20. Kim JB, Chung CH, Moon DH, Ha GJ, Lee TY, Jung SH, et al. Total arch repair versus hemiarch repair in the management of acute DeBakey type I aortic dissection. Eur J Cardiothorac Surg. 2011;40:881–7.
21. Lio A, Nicolò F, Bovio E, Serrao A, Zeitani J, Scafuri A, et al. Total arch versus hemiarch replacement for type A acute aortic dissection: a single-center experience. Texas Heart Inst J. 2016;43:488–95.
22. Kazui T, Washiyama N, Bashar AH, Terada H, Suzuki T, Ohkura K, et al. Surgical outcome of acute type A aortic dissection: analysis of risk factors. Ann Thorac Surg. 2002;74:75–81.
23. Ikeno Y, Yokawa K, Koda Y, Gotake Y, Henmi S, Nakai H, et al. The fate of the downstream aorta after open aortic repair for acute DeBakey type I aortic dissection: total arch replacement with elephant trunk technique versus non-total arch replacement†. Eur J Cardiothorac Surg. 2019;55:966–74.
24. Inoue Y, Matsuda H, Omura A, Seike Y, Uehara K, Sasaki H, et al. Comparative study of the frozen elephant trunk and classical elephant trunk techniques to supplement total arch replacement for acute type A aortic dissection. Eur J Cardiothorac Surg. 2019;56:579–86.
25. Halstead JC, Meier M, Etz C, Spielvogel D, Bodian C, Wurm M, et al. The fate of the distal aorta after repair of acute type A aortic dissection. J Thorac Cardiovasc Surg. 2007;133:127–35.
26. Heinemann M, Laas J, Jurmann M, Karck M, Borst HG. Surgery extended into the aortic arch in acute type A dissection. Indications, techniques, and results. Circulation. 1991;84:III25–30.
27. Preventza O, Cervera R, Cooley DA, Bakaeen FG, Mohamed AS, Cheong BY, et al. Acute type I aortic dissection: traditional versus hybrid repair with antegrade stent delivery to the descending thoracic aorta. J Thorac Cardiovasc Surg. 2014;148:119–25.
28. Westaby S, Saito S, Katsumata T. Acute type A dissection: conservative methods provide consistently low mortality. Ann Thorac Surg. 2002;73:707–13.
29. Poon SS, Tian DH, Yan T, Harrington D, Nawaytou O, Kuduvalli M, et al., International Aortic Arch Surgery Study Group. Frozen elephant trunk does not increase incidence of paraplegia in patients with acute type A aortic dissection. J Thorac Cardiovasc Surg. 2020;159:1189–96.e1.
30. Takagi H, Umemoto T, ALICE Group. A meta-analysis of total arch replacement with frozen elephant trunk in acute type A aortic dissection. Vasc Endovascular Surg. 2016;50:33–46.
31. Vallabhajosyula P, Gottret JP, Robb JD, Szeto WY, Desai ND, Pochettino A, et al. Hemiarch replacement with concomitant antegrade stent grafting of the descending thoracic aorta versus total arch replacement for treatment of acute DeBakey I aortic dissection with arch tear. Eur J Cardiothorac Surg. 2016;49:1256–61.
32. Jakob H, Tsagakis K, Tossios P, Massoudy P, Thielmann M, Buck T, et al. Combining classic surgery with descending stent grafting for acute DeBakey type I dissection. Ann Thorac Surg. 2008;86:95–101.
33. Peterson MD, Mazine A, El-Hamamsy I, Manlhiot C, Ouzounian M, MacArthur RG, et al., Canadian Thoracic Aortic Collaborative Investigators. Knowledge, attitudes, and practice preferences of Canadian cardiac surgeons toward the management of acute type A aortic dissection. J Thorac Cardiovasc Surg. 2015;150:824–31.e1–5.

34. Spielvogel D, Etz CD, Silovitz D, Lansman SL, Griepp RB. Aortic arch replacement with a trifurcated graft. Ann Thorac Surg. 2007;83:S791–5.
35. Galla JD, McCullough JN, Ergin MA, Apaydin AZ, Griepp RB. Surgical techniques. Aortic arch and deep hypothermic circulatory arrest: real-life suspended animation. Cardiol Clin. 1999;17:767–78, ix.
36. Hsieh WC, Kan CD, Yu HC, Aboud A, Lindner J, Henry BM, et al. Ascending aorta replacement vs. total aortic arch replacement in the treatment of acute type A dissection: a meta-analysis. Eur Rev Med Pharmacol Sci. 2019;23:9590–611.
37. Committee for Scientific Affairs, The Japanese Association for Thoracic Surgery, Shimizu H, Okada M, Tangoku A, Doki Y, Endo S, Fukuda H, et al. Thoracic and cardiovascular surgeries in Japan during 2017: Annual report by the Japanese Association for Thoracic Surgery. Gen Thorac Cardiovasc Surg. 2020;68:414–49.
38. Ghoreishi M, Sundt TM, Cameron DE, Holmes SD, Roselli EE, Pasrija C, et al. Factors associated with acute stroke after type A aortic dissection repair: an analysis of the Society of Thoracic Surgeons National Adult Cardiac Surgery Database. J Thorac Cardiovasc Surg. 2020;159:2143–54.e3.
39. Russo CF, Mariscalco G, Colli A, Santè P, Nicolini F, Miceli A, et al. Italian multicentre study on type A acute aortic dissection: a 33-year follow-up. Eur J Cardiothorac Surg. 2016;49:125–31.
40. Pan E, Gudbjartsson T, Ahlsson A, Fuglsang S, Geirsson A, Hansson EC, et al. Low rate of reoperations after acute type A aortic dissection repair from The Nordic Consortium Registry. J Thorac Cardiovasc Surg. 2018;156:939–48.
41. Uchida K, Minami T, Cho T, Yasuda S, Kasama K, Suzuki S, et al., Yokohama City University CVS Group. Results of ascending aortic and arch replacement for type A aortic dissection. J Thorac Cardiovasc Surg. 2020. pii: S0022-5223(20)30531-6. https://doi.org/10.1016/j.jtcvs.2020.02.087. [Epub ahead of print].
42. Zhang H, Lang X, Lu F, Song Z, Wang J, Han L, et al. Acute type A dissection without intimal tear in arch: proximal or extensive repair? J Thorac Cardiovasc Surg. 2014;147:1251–5.
43. Di Eusanio M, Berretta P, Cefarelli M, Jacopo A, Murana G, Castrovinci S, et al. Total arch replacement versus more conservative management in type A acute aortic dissection. Ann Thorac Surg. 2015;100:88–94.
44. Yan Y, Xu L, Zhang H, Xu ZY, Ding XY, Wang SW, et al. Proximal aortic repair versus extensive aortic repair in the treatment of acute type A aortic dissection: a meta-analysis. Eur J Cardiothorac Surg. 2016;49:1392–401.
45. Kimura N, Itoh S, Yuri K, Adachi K, Matsumoto H, Yamaguchi A, et al. Reoperation for enlargement of the distal aorta after initial surgery for acute type A aortic dissection. J Thorac Cardiovasc Surg. 2015;149:S91–8.e1.
46. Rice RD, Sandhu HK, Leake SS, Afifi RO, Azizzadeh A, Charlton-Ouw KM, et al. Is total arch replacement associated with worse outcomes during repair of acute type A aortic dissection? Ann Thorac Surg. 2015;100:2159–65.
47. Dai XF, Chen LW, Wu XJ, Dong Y, Wang QM. Total aortic arch reconstruction with triple-branched stent graft or hemiarch replacement for acute Debakey type I aortic dissection: five-years experience with 93 patients. J Card Surg. 2015;30:749–55.
48. Lee TC, Kon Z, Cheema FH, Grau-Sepulveda MV, Englum B, Kim S, et al. Contemporary management and outcomes of acute type A aortic dissection: an analysis of the STS adult cardiac surgery database. J Card Surg. 2018;33:7–18.
49. Etz CD, Plestis KA, Kari FA, Silovitz D, Bodian CA, Spielvogel D, et al. Axillary cannulation significantly improves survival and neurologic outcome after atherosclerotic aneurysm repair of the aortic root and ascending aorta. Ann Thorac Surg. 2008;86:441–6.
50. Svensson LG, Blackstone EH, Rajeswaran J, Sabik JF III, Lytle BW, Gonzalez-Stawinski G, et al. Does the arterial cannulation site for circulatory arrest influence stroke risk? Ann Thorac Surg. 2004;78:1274–84.
51. Pasic M, Schubel J, Bauer M, Yankah C, Kuppe H, Weng YG, et al. Cannulation of the right axillary artery for surgery of acute type A aortic dissection. Eur J Cardiothorac Surg. 2003;24:231–5.

52. Benedetto U, Mohamed H, Vitulli P, Petrou M. Axillary versus femoral arterial cannulation in type A acute aortic dissection: evidence from a meta-analysis of comparative studies and adjusted risk estimates. Eur J Cardiothorac Surg. 2015;48:953–9.
53. Ren Z, Wang Z, Hu R, Wu H, Deng H, Zhou Z, et al. Which cannulation (axillary cannulation or femoral cannulation) is better for acute type A aortic dissection repair? A meta-analysis of nine clinical studies. Eur J Cardiothorac Surg. 2015;47:408–15.
54. De Paulis R, Czerny M, Weltert L, Bavaria J, Borger MA, Carrel TP, et al., EACTS Vascular Domain Group. Current trends in cannulation and neuroprotection during surgery of the aortic arch in Europe. Eur J Cardiothorac Surg. 2015;47:917–23.
55. Reece TB, Tribble CG, Smith RL, Singh RR, Stiles BM, Peeler BB, et al. Central cannulation is safe in acute aortic dissection repair. J Thorac Cardiovasc Surg. 2007;133:428–34.
56. Kamiya H, Kallenbach K, Halmer D, Ozsöz M, Ilg K, Lichtenberg A, et al. Comparison of ascending aorta versus femoral artery cannulation for acute aortic dissection type A. Circulation. 2009;120:S282–6.
57. Shimura S, Odagiri S, Furuya H, Okada K, Ozawa K, Nagase H, et al. Echocardiography-guided aortic cannulation by the Seldinger technique for type A dissection with cerebral malperfusion. J Thorac Cardiovasc Surg. 2020;159:784–93.
58. Conzelmann LO, Kayhan N, Mehlhorn U, Weigang E, Dahm M, Vahl CF. Reevaluation of direct true lumen cannulation in surgery for acute type A aortic dissection. Ann Thorac Surg. 2009;87:1182–6.
59. Kanamori T, Ichihara T, Sakaguchi H, Inoue T. A safe and rapid direct true lumen cannulation for acute type A aortic dissection. Gen Thorac Cardiovasc Surg. 2013;61:336–9.
60. Djukanovic BP, Micovic S, Peric MS, Milojevic PS, Cirkovic MV, Boricic M, et al. The role of transapical cannulation in the operative management of acute aortic dissection. Perfusion. 2015;30:332–6.
61. Wada H, Matsumura H, Minematsu N, Amako M, Nishimi M, Tashiro T. Direct and transapical central cannulation for acute type A aortic dissection. Ann Vasc Dis. 2014;7:286–91.
62. Kunihara T, Grün T, Aicher D, Langer F, Adam O, Wendler O, et al. Hypothermic circulatory arrest is not a risk factor for neurologic morbidity in aortic surgery: a propensity score analysis. J Thorac Cardiovasc Surg. 2005;130:712–8.
63. Damberg A, Carino D, Charilaou P, Peterss S, Tranquilli M, Ziganshin BA, et al. Favorable late survival after aortic surgery under straight deep hypothermic circulatory arrest. J Thorac Cardiovasc Surg. 2017;154:1831–9.e1.
64. Kaukuntla H, Harrington D, Bilkoo I, Clutton-Brock T, Jones T, Bonser RS. Temperature monitoring during cardiopulmonary bypass–do we undercool or overheat the brain? Eur J Cardiothorac Surg. 2004;26:580–5.
65. Ueda Y, Miki S, Kusuhara K, Okita Y, Tahata T, Yamanaka K. Surgical treatment of aneurysm or dissection involving the ascending aorta and aortic arch, utilizing circulatory arrest and retrograde cerebral perfusion. J Cardiovasc Surg (Torino). 1990;31:553–8.
66. Safi HJ, Letsou GV, Iliopoulos DC, Subramaniam MH, Miller CC III, Hassoun H, et al. Impact of retrograde cerebral perfusion on ascending aortic and arch aneurysm repair. Ann Thorac Surg. 1997;63:1601–7.
67. Tian DH, Weller J, Hasmat S, Oo A, Forrest P, Kiat H, et al. Adjunct retrograde cerebral perfusion provides superior outcomes compared with hypothermic circulatory arrest alone: a meta-analysis. J Thorac Cardiovasc Surg. 2018;156:1339–48.e7.
68. Ehrlich MP, Hagl C, McCullough JN, Zhang N, Shiang H, Bodian C, et al. Retrograde cerebral perfusion provides negligible flow through brain capillaries in the pig. J Thorac Cardiovasc Surg. 2001;122:331–8.
69. Tokuda Y, Miyata H, Motomura N, Oshima H, Usui A, Takamoto S, Japan Adult Cardiovascular Database Organization. Brain protection during ascending aortic repair for Stanford type A acute aortic dissection surgery. Nationwide analysis in Japan. Circ J. 2014;78:2431–8.

70. Khaladj N, Shrestha M, Meck S, Peterss S, Kamiya H, Kallenbach K, et al. Hypothermic circulatory arrest with selective antegrade cerebral perfusion in ascending aortic and aortic arch surgery: a risk factor analysis for adverse outcome in 501 patients. J Thorac Cardiovasc Surg. 2008;135:908–14.
71. Fan S, Li H, Wang D, Wu C, Pan Z, Li Y, et al. Effects of four major brain protection strategies during proximal aortic surgery: a systematic review and network meta-analysis. Int J Surg. 2019;63:8–15. https://doi.org/10.1016/j.ijsu.2019.01.009. Epub 2019 Jan 20.
72. Poon SS, Estrera A, Oo A, Field M. Is moderate hypothermic circulatory arrest with selective antegrade cerebral perfusion superior to deep hypothermic circulatory arrest in elective aortic arch surgery? Interact Cardiovasc Thorac Surg. 2016;23:462–8.
73. Guilmet D, Bachet J, Goudot B, Laurian C, Gigou F, Bical O, et al. Use of biological glue in acute aortic dissection. Preliminary clinical results with a new surgical technique. J Thorac Cardiovasc Surg. 1979;77:516–21.
74. Bavaria JE, Brinster DR, Gorman RC, Woo YJ, Gleason T, Pochettino A. Advances in the treatment of acute type A dissection: an integrated approach. Ann Thorac Surg. 2002;74:S1848–52.
75. Kazui T, Washiyama N, Bashar AH, Terada H, Suzuki K, Yamashita K, et al. Role of biologic glue repair of proximal aortic dissection in the development of early and midterm redissection of the aortic root. Ann Thorac Surg. 2001;72:509–14.
76. Bachet J, Goudot B, Teodori G, Brodaty D, Dubois C, De Lentdecker P, et al. Surgery of type A acute aortic dissection with Gelatine-Resorcine-Formol biological glue: a twelve-year experience. J Cardiovasc Surg (Torino). 1990;31:263–73.
77. Bachet J, Goudot B, Dreyfus G, Banfi C, Ayle NA, Aota M, et al. The proper use of glue: a 20-year experience with the GRF glue in acute aortic dissection. J Card Surg. 1997;12:243–53.
78. Chao HH, Torchiana DF. BioGlue: albumin/glutaraldehyde sealant in cardiac surgery. J Card Surg. 2003;18:500–3.
79. Kunihara T, Shiiya N, Matsuzaki K, Murashita T, Matsui Y. Recommendation for appropriate use of GRF glue in the operation for acute aortic dissection. Ann Thorac Cardiovasc Surg. 2008;14:88–95.
80. Witter K, Tonar Z, Matejka VM, Martinca T, Jonák M, Rokosný S, et al. Tissue reaction to three different types of tissue glues in an experimental aorta dissection model: a quantitative approach. Histochem Cell Biol. 2010;133:241–59.
81. Fürst W, Banerjee A. Release of glutaraldehyde from an albumin-glutaraldehyde tissue adhesive causes significant in vitro and in vivo toxicity. Ann Thorac Surg. 2005;79:1522–8.
82. Floten HS, Ravichandran PS, Furnary AP, Gately HL, Starr A. Adventitial inversion technique in repair of aortic dissection. Ann Thorac Surg. 1995;59:771–2.
83. Flores J, Kunihara T, Shiiya N, Yoshimoto K, Matsuzaki K, Yasuda K. Extensive deployment of the stented elephant trunk is associated with an increased risk of spinal cord injury. J Thorac Cardiovasc Surg. 2006;131:336–42.

Frozen Elephant Trunk for Aortic Dissection

Emidio Germano, Kyle Miletic, and Eric E. Roselli

The Problem

Interposition graft replacement of the ascending aorta only is the most commonly performed operation for acute aortic dissection. However, arch and downstream aortic dissection persist in the majority of patients following a limited conventional repair and the patency of the downstream false lumen has been associated with worse survival and risk for reoperation [1, 2]. Simultaneous replacement of the ascending aorta and total arch during the primary procedure may improve outcomes by providing better downstream perfusion and can potentially improve prognosis by promoting earlier reverse remodeling of the aorta [3]. This approach has been criticized, however, for adding complexity to the initial emergency/high-risk procedure [4]. Several modifications to the conventional surgical approach to extend repair to the arch have been described including the elephant trunk technique first described in the 1980s [5, 6]. Soon after the development of stentgrafts, stents were added to surgical graft repairs to extend into the proximal descending aorta. This stent fixation of the elephant trunk graft became the frozen elephant trunk [7–9].

Just as was seen with open arch repair, multiple variations of performing frozen elephant trunk repair have been described. Most frozen elephant trunk operations resemble the conventional operations in that a series of multiple anastomoses are performed including the arch branch vessels. Ischemic times during these operations have been directly correlated with neurological risk and the risk of perioperative death [10–13]. The simple addition of a stented component has not necessarily made the technological challenges of performing arch replacement readily accessible to most surgeons who may rarely perform thoracic aortic operations. There is an unmet need in the treatment of aortic dissection involving the arch to provide a more

E. Germano · K. Miletic · E. E. Roselli (✉)
Aorta Center, Department of Thoracic and Cardiovascular Surgery, Heart Vascular and Thoracic Institute, Cleveland Clinic, Cleveland, OH, USA
e-mail: RosellE@ccf.org

J. S. Coselli et al. (eds.), *Aortic Dissection and Acute Aortic Syndromes*,
https://doi.org/10.1007/978-3-030-66668-2_23

extended repair without adding the increased neurologic and bleeding risk commonly associated with the conventional approaches to more extended repairs.

Room for Improvement

With improvements in patient care such as improved imaging, more frequent use of selective antegrade brain perfusion, and dedicated surgical teams performing cardio-aortic operations, surgical outcomes for aortic dissection continue to improve [14]. It has been demonstrated that there is a volume to outcome relationship for treating aortic dissection, and patients who present with end organ ischemia or malperfusion still represent the greatest challenge in the acute phase [15]. During intermediate follow-up, survival depends upon the patency of the downstream false lumen and for a population of patients with an average age less than 60 years usually without significant coronary disease, the 5 year survival is rather poor [16]. An extended operation at the time of acute dissection that optimizes true lumen flow distally holds promise to improve distal malperfusion and promote the reverse remodeling that may also improve later survival [17].

Novel Approaches

As thoracic endovascular devices have become more available, and cardio-aortic surgeons have become more familiar with the characteristics and unique features including advantages and limitations of these devices, they have been used more commonly during open thoracic aortic operations as part of a hybrid reconstruction strategy [18, 19]. Most commonly, TEVAR devices are used in combination with an open repair to perform the so-called frozen elephant trunk repair for patients with multi-segment disease. What is common to all of the frozen elephant trunks is: 1) the use of a commercially available thoracic stentgraft device delivered in an antegrade fashion through the open aortic arch during a period of at least partial circulatory arrest (i.e. nearly always including selective antegrade brain perfusion); 2) direct suturing of the stentgraft device to the patient's native aorta.

These operations have become common at some larger centers of excellence especially in Europe and Asia, but have not been widely adopted due to the complexity of these operations and the lack of dedicated devices (in the US). Furthermore, there is not a standard for how these operations are performed.

The frozen elephant trunk operation can be performed on any patient with type 1 dissection. However, it is particularly helpful for patients with the retrograde aortic dissection extending from a distal entry tear, those with the aneurysmal distal aorta, distal malperfusion from a smaller true lumen, and those who are young or with suspicion for a genetically triggered cause of aortic disease, placing them at higher risk for later false lumen aneurysmal degeneration [20].

A Better Way

Our surgical technique of frozen elephant trunk repair in acute aortic dissection has evolved over the last 10 years into what we refer to as the Branched Stented Anastamosis Frozen Elephant trunk Repair [21, 22] (Fig. 1). The latest iterations of this procedure will be described later in this chapter.

The cornerstone to achieving successful outcomes for treating complex aortic pathology is the creation of a multi-disciplinary Aortic Team that consists of emergency care transport, cardiology intensive care physicians (cardiology), cardiovascular imaging specialist (radiologists/cardiologists/radiology technicians), cardiothoracic anesthesia, cardiovascular surgery, vascular surgery, hybrid trained operating room nursing and perioperative nursing, and perfusion. The entire team is alerted when a possible acute aortic dissection is en route with the goal to provide comprehensive and expeditious care to patients with acute aortic syndromes using standardized protocols with improved coordination and communication across the various disciplines [23, 24] (Fig. 2).

A careful analysis of contrast enhanced 3D computed tomography (CT) imaging by the operating surgeon is essential to understand the individual patient's anatomy, the dissection morphology and to select the endograft devices used during the repair. The stent graft sizing is done precisely based on the aortic measurements in cross section to the centerline of flow, at the level of suturing in the arch (usually zone 1 or 2, adjacent to the left common carotid artery). Over sizing is avoided to minimize

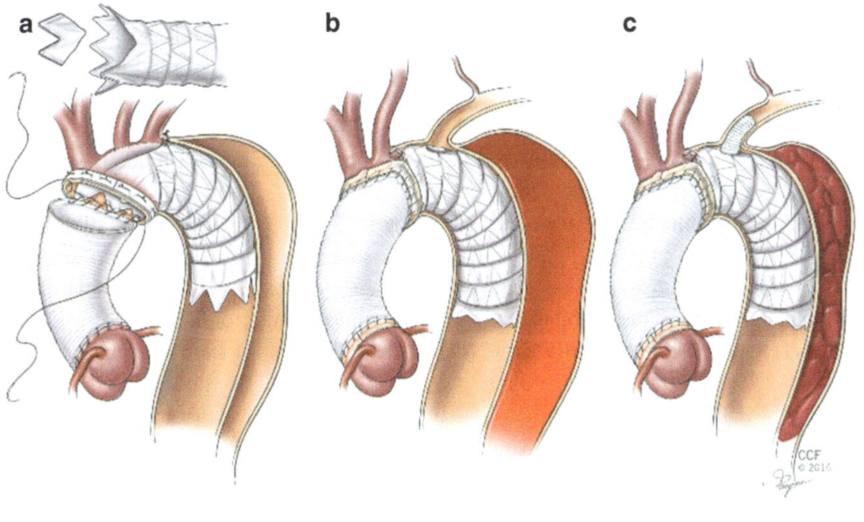

Fig. 1 Chronological evolution of the simplified frozen elephant trunk repair technique for acute aortic dissection. (**a**) Left, 2009 version with a large scallop creation, (**b**) Middle, 2012 version with on table fenestration, and (**c**) Right, latest version with direct bridging arch branch stent grafting—Branched Stented Anastomosis Frozen Elephant trunk Repair (B-SAFER). Image reprint with permission [22]

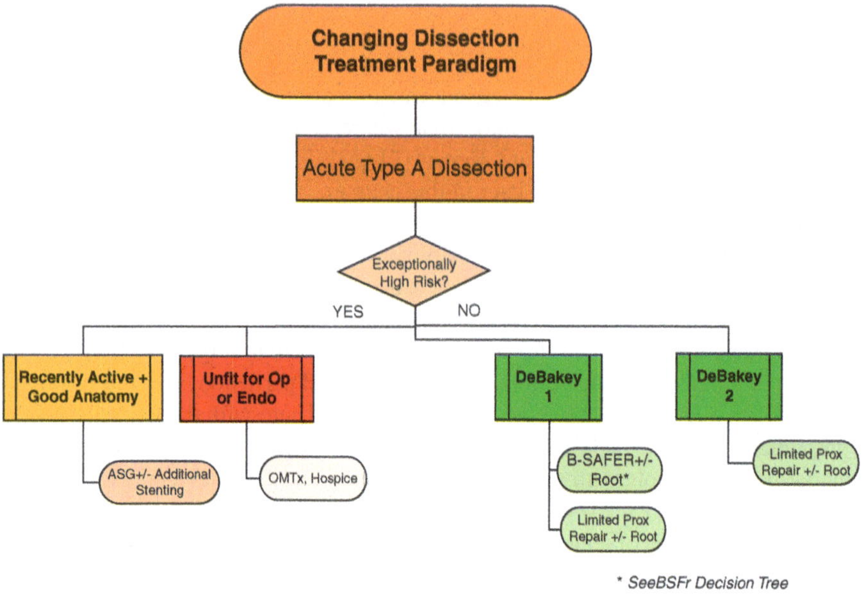

Fig. 2 The current decision-making algorithm for acute ascending aortic dissection at the Cleveland Clinic. *Op* operation, *Endo* endovascular, *ASG* ascending stentgraft, *OMTx* optimal medical treatment, *B-SAFER* branch stented anastomosis frozen elephant trunk repair, *Prox* proximal

graft material infolding at the level of the anastamosis. The frozen elephant trunk device main aortic stent graft is usually 10 or 15 cm long, depending on the shape of the arch so that it can extend beyond the curve of the arch and land parallel into the upper descending aorta. The use of devices longer than 15 cm may increase risk for spinal cord injury and should be avoided. If the arch branch vessel stenting is also planned, these devices are also selected preoperatively based on detailed imaging analysis of target vessels [25].

Our preferred technique for repair in the patient who is hemodynamically stable on presentation begins with cutdown and exposure of the right axillary artery and end-to-side anastomosis of an 8 or 10 mm side graft on the axillary artery [26]. Median sternotomy and standard two-stage venous cannulation are then employed. For patients who undergo this technique, right radial or brachial arterial access is mandatory to monitor brain perfusion pressure during selective antegrade brain perfusion (SABP). A second arterial line in the contralateral arm or either femoral artery is also helpful in determining accurate systemic perfusion pressures. Cardiopulmonary bypass is then initiated via the axillary artery and cooling is begun.

In the hemodynamically unstable patient who presents in extremis, we forego axillary artery cannulation and initiate cardiopulmonary bypass as expeditiously as possible. Our preferred technique in this instance is emergency median sternotomy to relieve tamponade followed by central aortic cannulation utilizing modified

Seldinger technique with echocardiographic guidance to ensure the cannula is in the true lumen of the aorta. As we have gained more experience with this technique, we have increasingly been using it in stable patients as well to save time [27].

Once cardiopulmonary bypass is initiated and as the patient is being cooled, exposure of the distal ascending and aortic arch is obtained. The innominate vein is dissected free and retracted cranially using a self-retaining retractor. The remainder of the arch is dissected via takedown of the pericardial reflection and dissection of the head vessels, which are then encircled with vessel loops. When the patient has been cooled to a goal nasopharyngeal temperature of <24 °C and bladder temperature of <28 °C with electrical silence on bispectral index monitoring, the heart is arrested, the innominate and left common carotid arteries are clamped and selective antegrade brain perfusion (SABP) is initiated. We typically run the SABP perfusate at a rate of ~1 L/min and a perfusate temperature of <18 °C.

The aorta is then transected obliquely from the base of the innominate artery to the underside of the aortic arch. The stent is then brought into the field, precurved, and delivered in an antegrade fashion down the descending aorta. Use of Intravascular Ultrasound (IVUS) to help guide wire placement prior to device delivery can assist with safe access of the stent graft into the true lumen. After deployment, the stent graft is secured to the lesser curve of the aortic arch with a 4-0 polypropylene suture. Fine adjustment to the position of the device can be made before suturing into place. It is usually positioned such that it covers the left subclavian artery ostia and depending upon the location of entry tear, it may also cover the origin of left common carotid artery. Fenestrations in the device are cut with a scalpel at the location of covered arch branch arteries. Short branch stent grafts (typically 2–3 cm in length) are selected so as to minimize branch vessel manipulation. The branch stent grafts are directly positioned through these fenestrations over a wire into the target vessels and deployed. Proper positioning of branch stent is confirmed by direct visualization and the devices are expanded by direct manipulation with a clamp and gently molded with a soft conformable occlusion balloon. The branch devices are aligned with about 5–10 mm of extension into the aortic lumen to assure good overlap and fixation. This first suture line is then run circumferentially to the stentgraft and the aortic wall and typically runs around the distal edge of the left common carotid (zone 2) or innominate artery (zone 1) to optimize fixation and seal in the arch.

The surgical graft to replace the ascending aorta and hemiarch is sized based on the diameter of the sinutubular junction. The graft is beveled distally and then sutured circumferentially to the transected aorta and the stentgraft and along the proximal edge of the innominate artery. In patients with particularly complex branch anatomy, or a large aneurysm of the arch itself, the innominate or left common carotid arteries may be separated from the aorta and reconstructed as separate anastomoses. This multiple anastamotic variation of the B-SAFER operation is typically reserved for chronic dissection cases (Fig. 3).

Following anastomotic completion, the entire graft is deaired and clamped proximally. Full cardiopulmonary bypass is then re-initiated and warming commenced. During re-warming, attention is turned to the aortic root. Next the attention is

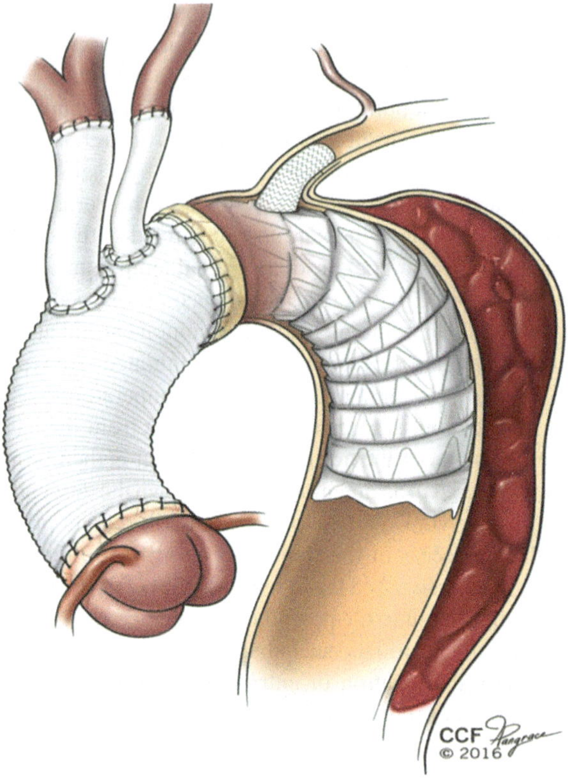

Fig. 3 Illustration of the multiple anastomoses, single stent B-SAFER operation

directed to the proximal aortic reconstruction based on the condition of the aortic root. Mostly, the valve and root can be preserved by re-approximation of the dissected layers at the level just above the coronary ostia. Other options included valve replacement with a bioprosthesis and supracoronary graft anastomosis, total root replacement with reimplantation of the coronaries and valve replacement (modified Bentall), or valve sparing root replacement (modified David's procedure in young stable patients).

In case of concern that the patient may have ongoing distal malperfusion, aortography or intravascular ultrasound may be performed. Based on the findings additional endovascular interventions can be extended distally [28]. This may include the addition of a bare aortic dissections stent (Zenith dissection device, Cook, Indiana, USA) directed at dynamic compression or additional branch vessel stenting directed at treating focal static branch occlusion. These adjunctive procedures can best be performed in a timely manner in the hybrid operating room.

Postoperative care for the patient with the frozen elephant trunk repair is the same as any other patient who presents with acute type A dissection. Patients are imaged with contrast-enhanced CT angiography prior to discharge, 3 months postoperatively, and annually.

Results

Several reports have been published from Europe and Asia where frozen elephant trunk devices have been commercially available for several years. Outcomes for these procedures in most of the experiences have been similar to what is expected with conventional approaches [29, 30]. In a recent combined series from two of the busiest centers in Europe the mortality was 14.9%, stroke rate was 10.8%, and spinal cord injury was 5.5% [31].

One of the biggest concerns with the early reports on the frozen elephant trunk repair has related to the potential for increased risk of spinal cord injury, a complication not typically seen with limited repair of acute dissection [32]. Although results from a recent multi-center analysis of patients undergoing total arch replacement with or without FET demonstrated no increase in risk of spinal cord injury with the addition of FET to a total arch—4% for total arch replacement and 6% for FET [33]. This data suggests that the exact mechanisms of spinal cord injury are yet to be elucidated. The risk is likely related to extent and pattern of disease as much as it is to the techniques used to address it. Improvements in technique and a concerted effort to reduce the circulatory arrest time may help to reduce neurologic risks as the experience improves.

The largest single center series from Beijing have demonstrated excellent results with mortality of 6.5%, stroke 2%, and spinal cord injury of 2.4% [34]. It is important to note that the patient population in the Chinese series was about 10 years younger (mean 46 years old) than their European and American counterparts. Also, the mean time from dissection to operation was 5 days so this likely represents a select population of patients who are less likely to have the severest forms of malperfusion. Malperfusion at presentation has repeatedly been shown to be an important predictor of acute outcomes and the addition of FET to acute repair may prove to be beneficial in these patients as the technique optimizes distal true lumen flow [35, 36].

The primary advantage of the B-SAFER technique is that it allows for repair of the entire ascending, arch, and proximal descending aorta in one relatively efficient operation with a limited period of circulatory arrest. In the early experience with this technique, the results were good with mortality, stroke, and spinal cord injury risk of 4%, respectively. In patients in whose dissection extends only into the arch, this can be the definitive procedure. In those who have residual thoracoabdominal dissection, the residual dissected segment beyond the FET component can be easily addressed with a future endovascular repair [37, 38].

The Future

Next generation frozen elephant trunk devices feature additional branch limbs arising from the surgical graft component and easier to use delivery and deployment systems (Thoraflex, TerumoAortic, Scotland—Fig. 4a; EvitaNeo, Cryolife,

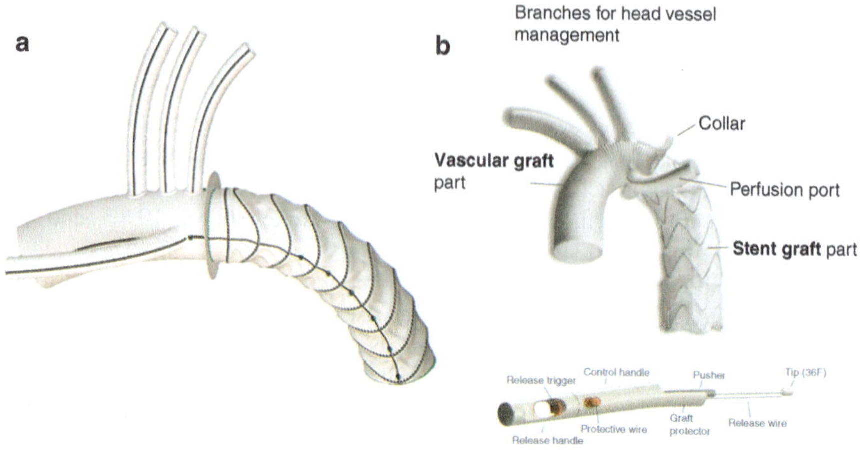

Fig. 4 Commercially available (in Europe; investigational in US) dedicated frozen elephant trunk devices: (**a**) Thoraflex, TerumoAortic and (**b**) EVITA Open Neo, Cryolife. Images provided by manufacturers

Atlanta—Fig. 4b). Additional devices that are currently in trial include a bare stent that extends across the arch with or without and additional descending stentgraft component.

Our experience with the B-SAFER technique has continued and now accounts for the majority of acute DeBakey Type 1 repairs and chronic aortic dissection repairs performed in our center. The operation has been performed by nine of our staff surgeons in over 250 patients. We are currently actively enrolling patients in a physician sponsored investigational device exemption study to allow for prospective assessment of the outcomes for this procedure. Additional advances in the development of frozen elephant trunk repair devices are likely to include built-in branch grafts to accommodate the left subclavian artery and to further simplify extended repair.

Although progress has been slow, it has been steady and we should continue to see improvements in the care of aortic dissection with the use of frozen elephant trunk techniques becoming the new standard of surgical treatment.

References

1. Fattouch K, Sampognaro R, Navarra E, et al. Long-term results after repair of type A acute aortic dissection according to false lumen patency. Ann Thorac Surg. 2009;88(4):1244–50.
2. Yeh C-H, Chen M-C, Wu Y-C, Wang Y-C, Chu J-J, Lin PJ. Risk factors for descending aortic aneurysm formation in medium-term follow-up of patients with type A aortic dissection. Chest. 2003;124(3):989–95.
3. Roselli EE, Loor G, He J, Rafael AE, Rajeswaran J, Houghtaling PL, Svensson LG, Blackstone EH, Lytle BW. Distal aortic interventions after repair of ascending dissection: the argument for a more aggressive approach. J Thorac Cardiovasc Surg. 2015;149(2 Suppl):S117–24.

4. Girardi LN. Total arch for type A dissection? J Thorac Cardiovasc Surg. 2016;151(2):294–5.
5. Borst HG, Walterbusch G, Schaps D. Extensive aortic replacement using "Elephant Trunk" prosthesis. Thorac cardiovasc Surg. 1983;31(1):37–40.
6. Svensson LG. Rationale and technique for replacement of the ascending aorta, arch, and distal aorta using a modified elephant trunk procedure. J Cardiac Surg. 1992;7(4):301–12.
7. Kato M, Ohnishi K, Kaneko M, Ueda T, Kishi D, Mizushima T, et al. New graft-implanting method for thoracic aortic aneurysm or dissection with a stented graft. Circulation. 1996;94(Suppl II):II188–93.
8. Karck M, Chavan A, Hagl C, Friedrich H, Galanski M, Haverich A. The frozen elephant trunk technique: a new treatment for thoracic aortic aneurysms. J Thorac Cardiovasc Surg. 2003;125(6):1550–3.
9. Jakob H, Tsagakis K, Tossios P, Massoudy P, Thielmann M, Buck T, et al. Combining classic surgery with descending stent grafting for acute DeBakey type I dissection. Ann Thorac Surg. 2008;86(1):95–101.
10. Easo J, Weigang E, Hölzl PPF, Horst M, Hoffmann I, Blettner M, et al. Influence of operative strategy for the aortic arch in DeBakey type I aortic dissection: analysis of the German Registry for Acute Aortic Dissection Type A. J Thorac Cardiovasc Surg. 2012;144(3):617–23.
11. Li B, Ma W-G, Liu Y-M, Sun L-Z. Is extended arch replacement justified for acute type A aortic dissection? Interact CardioVasc Thorac Surg. 2015;20(1):120–6.
12. Takagi H, Umemoto T. A meta-analysis of total arch replacement with frozen elephant trunk in acute type A aortic dissection. Vasc Endovascular Surg. 2016;50(1):33–46.
13. Preventza O, Liao JL, Olive JK, Simpson K, Critsinelis AC, Price MD, et al. Neurologic complications after the frozen elephant trunk procedure: a meta-analysis of more than 3000ients. J Thorac Cardiovasc Surg. [Internet]. 2019. https://www.jtcvs.org/article/S0022-5223(19)32242-1/abstract. Accessed 12 May 2020.
14. Pape LA, Awais M, Woznicki EM, Suzuki T, Trimarchi S, Evangelista A, et al. Presentation, diagnosis, and outcomes of acute aortic dissection: 17-year trends from the International Registry of Acute Aortic Dissection. J Am Coll Cardiol. 2015;66(4):350–8.
15. Geirsson A, Szeto WY, Pochettino A, et al. Significance of malperfusion syndromes prior to contemporary surgical repair for acute type A dissection: outcomes and need for additional revascularizations. Eur J Cardiothorac Surg. 2007;32(2):255–62.
16. Omura A, Miyahara S, Yamanaka K, Sakamoto T, Matsumori M, Okada K, et al. Early and late outcomes of repaired acute DeBakey type I aortic dissection after graft replacement. J Thorac Cardiovasc Surg. 2016;151(2):341–8.
17. Roselli EE. Clearing the next hurdles in the treatment of acute ascending aortic syndrome. Eur J Cardiothorac Surg. 2015;47(2):205–8.
18. Roselli EE, Soltesz EG, Mastracci T, Svensson LG, Lytle BW. Antegrade delivery of stent grafts to treat complex thoracic aortic disease. Ann Thorac Surg. 2010;90(2):539–46.
19. Preventza O, Cervera R, Cooley DA, Bakaeen FG, Mohamed AS, Cheong BYC, et al. Acute type I aortic dissection: Traditional versus hybrid repair with antegrade stent delivery to the descending thoracic aorta. J Thorac Cardiovasc Surg. 2014;148(1):119–25.
20. Shrestha M, Bachet J, Bavaria J, Carrel TP, De Paulis R, Di Bartolomeo R, et al. Current status and recommendations for use of the frozen elephant trunk technique: a position paper by the Vascular Domain of EACTS. Eur J Cardiothorac Surg. 2015;47(5):759–69.
21. Roselli EE, Rafael A, Soltesz EG, Canale L, Lytle BW. Simplified frozen elephant trunk repair for acute DeBakey type I dissection. J Thorac Cardiovasc Surg. 2013;145(3 Suppl):S197–201.
22. Roselli EE, Idrees JJ, Bakaeen FG, Tong MZ, Soltesz EG, Mick S, et al. Evolution of simplified frozen elephant trunk repair for acute DeBakey type I dissection: midterm outcomes. Ann Thorac Surg. 2018;105(3):749–55.
23. Aggarwal B, Raymond CE, Randhawa MS, Roselli E, Jacob J, Eagleton M, Kralovic DM, Kormos K, Holloway D, Menon V. Transfer metrics in patients with suspected acute aortic syndrome. Circ Cardiovasc Qual Outcomes. 2014;7(5):780–2.
24. Schoenhagen P, Roselli EE, Harris CM, Eagleton M, Menon V. Online network of subspecialty aortic disease experts: impact of "cloud" technology on management of acute aortic emergencies. J Thorac Cardiovasc Surg. 2016;152(1):39–42.

25. Aftab M, Plichta R, Roselli EE. Acute DeBakey type I dissection repair using frozen elephant trunk: the Cleveland Clinic technique. Semin Cardiothorac Vasc Anesth. 2017;21(3):200–5.
26. Rosinski BF, Idrees JJ, Roselli EE, Germano E, Pasadyn SR, Lowry AM, Blackstone EH, Johnston DR, Soltesz EG, Navia JL, Desai MY, Mick SL, Bakaeen FG, Svensson LG. Cannulation strategies in acute type A dissection repair: a systematic axillary artery approach. J Thorac Cardiovasc Surg. 2019;158(3):647–59.
27. Frederick JR, Yang E, Trubelja A, Desai ND, Szeto WY, Pochettino A, Bavaria JE, Woo YJ. Ascending aortic cannulation in acute type A dissection repair. Ann Thorac Surg. 2013;95(5):1808–11.
28. Huang CY, Hsu HL, Chen PL, Kuo TT, Chen IM, Hsu CP, Shih CC. Aortic remodeling after hybrid provisional extension to induce complete attachment aortic repair of chronic residual type I aortic dissection. J Thorac Cardiovasc Surg. 2019;158(4):1007–16.
29. Di Eusanio M, Borger M, Petridis FD, Leontyev S, Pantaleo A, Moz M, et al. Conventional versus frozen elephant trunk surgery for extensive disease of the thoracic aorta. J Cardiovasc Med. 2014;15(11):803–9.
30. Hanif H, Dubois L, Ouzounian M, Peterson MD, El-Hamamsy I, Dagenais F, et al. Aortic arch reconstructive surgery with conventional techniques vs frozen elephant trunk: a systematic review and meta-analysis. Can J Cardiol. 2018;34(3):262–73.
31. Leone A, Beckmann E, Aandreas M, Di Marco L, Pantaleo A, Reggiani LB, Haverich A, Di Bartolomeo R, Pacini D, Sherestha M. Total aortic arch replacement with frozen elephant trunk technique: results from two European institutes. J Thorac Cardiovasc Surg. 2020;159(4):1201–11.
32. Svensson LG. Commentary: Three reasons for paralysis after elephant trunk procedures. J Thorac Cardiovasc Surg. 2019;158(2):351–2.
33. Poon SS, Tian DH, Yan T, Harrington D, Nawaytou O, Kuduvalli M, Haverich A, Ehrlich M, Ma WG, Sun LZ, Estrera AL, Field M, International Aortic Arch Surgery Study Group. Frozen elephant trunk does not increase incidence of paraplegia in patients with acute type A aortic dissection. J Thorac Cardiovasc Surg. 2020;159(4):1189–96.
34. Ma WG, Zheng J, Zhang W, Sun K, Ziganshin BA, Wang LF, Qi RD, Liu YM, Zhu JM, Chang Q, Elefteriades JA, Sun LZ. Frozen elephant trunk with total arch replacement for type A aortic dissections: does acuity affect operative mortality? J Thorac Cardiovasc Surg. 2014;148(3):963–70; discussion 970-2.
35. Augoustides JG, Geirsson A, Szeto WY, Walsh EK, Cornelius B, Pochettino A, Bavaria JE. Observational study of mortality risk stratification by ischemic presentation in patients with acute type A aortic dissection: the Penn classification. Nat Clin Pract Cardiovasc Med. 2009;6(2):140–6.
36. Olsson C, Hillebrant C-G, Liska J, Lockowandt U, Eriksson P, Franco-Cereceda A. Mortality in acute type A aortic dissection: validation of the Penn classification. Ann Thorac Surg. 2011;92(4):1376–82.
37. Roselli EE, Subramanian S, Sun Z, Idrees J, Nowicki E, Blackstone EH, Greenber RK, Svensson LG, Lytle BW. Endovascular versus open elephant trunk completion for extensive aortic disease. J Thorac Cardiovasc Surg. 2013;146(6):1408–16; discussion 1416-7.
38. Kreibich M, Berger T, Rylski B, Chen Z, Beyersdorf F, Siepe M, Czerny M. Aortic reinterventions after the frozen elephant trunk procedure. J Thorac Cardiovasc Surg. 2019:S0022-5223(19)30516-1.

One-Stage Repair of Extensive Chronic Thoracic Aortic Dissection

Alexander Kulik and Nicholas T. Kouchoukos

Introduction

Following successful repair of acute type A aortic dissection with graft replacement of the ascending aorta and part of the aortic arch, the false lumen frequently remains patent. Progressive dilation of the remaining dissected aorta may thereafter develop [1, 2], occurring most commonly in younger patients and those with connective tissue disease (Marfan syndrome) [3–5]. Ultimately, up to 30% of patients will require operative re-intervention for aneurysmal disease or progressive aortic valve insufficiency 5–10 years after the initial dissection surgery [1–4, 6–10]. Late reoperations for thoracic aortic dilation may also be necessary for patients who develop aortic dissection after coronary or valve operations [11–13], and for those who develop retrograde dissection and enlargement of the aortic arch following type B aortic dissection or endovascular stent-graft repair of the thoracic aorta [14–16]. While several operative techniques exist, the optimal surgical approach for the management of patients who develop substantial enlargement of the remaining dissected thoracic aorta has yet to be determined. Options for management include staged procedures, commonly using conventional [17–19] or frozen elephant trunk techniques [20–23], hybrid procedures using endovascular grafts to exclude the aneurysmal thoracic aortic segments [24–26], and 1-stage procedures [27–29]. Herein, we present our experience with the 1-stage technique which we have used exclusively since 1995 for patients with chronic thoracic aortic dissection who require

A. Kulik (✉)
Lynn Heart and Vascular Institute, Boca Raton Regional Hospital, Boca Raton, FL, USA

Florida Atlantic University, Boca Raton, FL, USA

N. T. Kouchoukos
Division of Cardiovascular and Thoracic Surgery, Missouri Baptist Medical Center, BJC HealthCare, St. Louis, MO, USA

Washington University School of Medicine, St. Louis, MO, USA

J. S. Coselli et al. (eds.), *Aortic Dissection and Acute Aortic Syndromes*,
https://doi.org/10.1007/978-3-030-66668-2_24

extensive resection of the descending thoracic aorta. We have focused on the details of the surgical technique, and have highlighted the early and late clinical outcomes associated with the procedure.

Technique

Previously reported [27, 30–33], our operative technique involves the use of bilateral anterior thoracotomy incisions through the fourth intercostal space and a transverse sternotomy (Fig. 1). Peripheral venous cannulation is performed through the right common femoral vein using a 2-stage cannula with the tip positioned in the superior vena cava, and arterial cannulation is achieved through the right common femoral artery and the right axillary artery. For axillary cannulation, through a right subclavicular incision, an 8- or 10-mm collagen-impregnated polyester graft (Hemashield Platinum straight tube graft; MAQUET Cardiovascular LLC, Wayne, NJ) is sutured to the axillary artery in an end-to-side fashion and the graft is then connected to the cardiopulmonary bypass (CPB) circuit (Fig. 2a, b). Two separate arterial lines from the pump oxygenator are used during aortic arch operations, and the desired ratio of flow through the two arterial lines is achieved

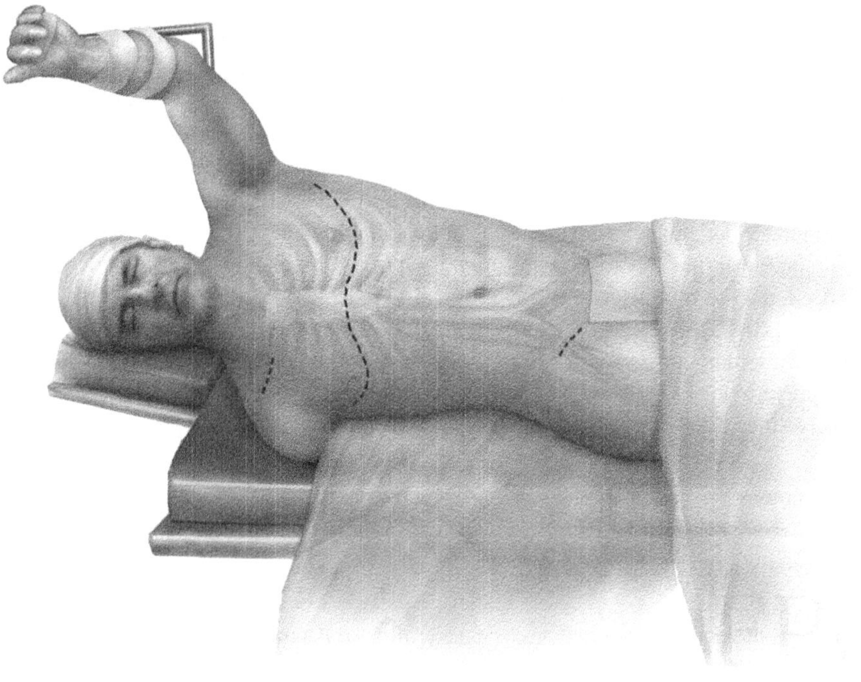

Fig. 1 Patient is positioned in a modified right lateral decubitus position. Dashed lines indicate sites of incision. (From Kouchoukos [33])

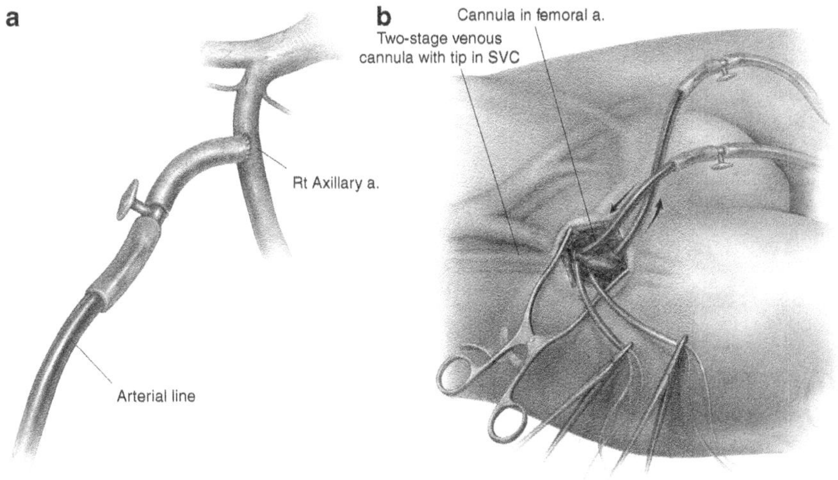

Fig. 2 (**a**) Axillary artery graft. (From Kouchoukos [33]]. (**b**) Right femoral artery and vein cannulation. (From Kouchoukos [33])

during the operation by using occluders and in-line flowmeters. The femoral arterial line is initially clamped, and CPB is established using the axillary perfusion graft. Cooling is then initiated, and a catheter is inserted into the right superior pulmonary vein for venting the left heart. A cannula is also inserted into the coronary sinus for delivery of cold blood cardioplegic solution (Fig. 3). During cooling the head is packed in ice and intravenous methylprednisolone (7–10 mg/kg) and thiopental (10–15 mg/kg) are administered. The pericardium is incised over the distal ascending aorta and aortic arch, and the left phrenic and left vagus nerves are identified and protected without isolation or traction. If the ascending aorta can be safely clamped, additional antegrade cardioplegia is administered (Fig. 4). When the nasopharyngeal temperature reaches 13–18 °C and the electroencephalogram becomes isoelectric, circulatory arrest is established. The axillary perfusion graft is clamped and the ascending aorta and aortic arch are opened with care to prevent dislodgment of atheromatous debris. The brachiocephalic arteries are dissected from the surrounding tissue and transected at their origins from the aorta. In the presence of atheroma or dissection, the arteries may require division more distally (Fig. 5). Perfusion from the axillary artery is then slowly initiated to evacuate trapped air and debris (Fig. 6). The arteries are flushed and individually clamped. Cerebral perfusion is then initiated from the right axillary artery graft (flow 10–15 mL/kg/min; temperature 20–22 °C) to provide perfusion to the right carotid and right vertebral arteries, and, through the circle of Willis and other collateral channels, to the left side of the brain. The flow rate is adjusted to maintain a mixed venous oxygen saturation of 85–95% using bilateral cerebral oximetric monitoring. Perfusion pressure is continuously monitored from the left radial artery. A clamp is placed on the descending thoracic aorta distal to the aneurysmal

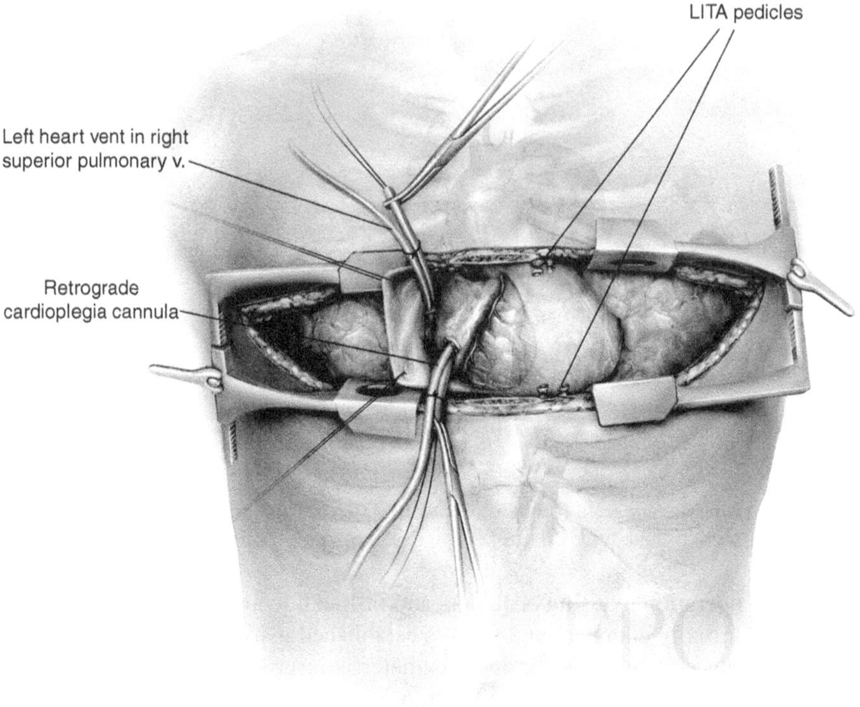

Fig. 3 The left heart is vented through the right superior pulmonary vein. A balloon-tipped cannula is positioned in the coronary sinus through purse-string suture in right atrial wall. (From Kouchoukos [33])

segment and flow to the lower body is initiated through the femoral arterial cannula. An appropriate sized presewn multibranched graft is positioned in the opened aortic arch. The distal limb of the graft is positioned into the descending thoracic aorta beneath the left phrenic and left vagus nerves (Fig. 7). The three adjacent branches of the aortic graft are cut to the appropriate lengths and sutured sequentially to the brachicephalic arteries, beginning with the left subclavian and ending with the innominate artery (Fig. 7). Perfusion from the right axillary artery continues while these anastomoses are performed. When the anastomoses are completed, the aortic graft is clamped distal to the left subclavian artery, the clamps on the three branches are removed, and air is evacuated from the proximal open end of the aortic graft. The aortic graft is then clamped just proximal to the innominate artery and antegrade flow is established through the three arteries, maintaining the same flow rate, pressure, and temperature (Fig. 8). The fourth branch of the aortic graft is ligated. Flow from the femoral artery cannula is discontinued and the site for attachment of the distal end of the graft to the descending thoracic aorta is determined. This is generally where the diameter of the

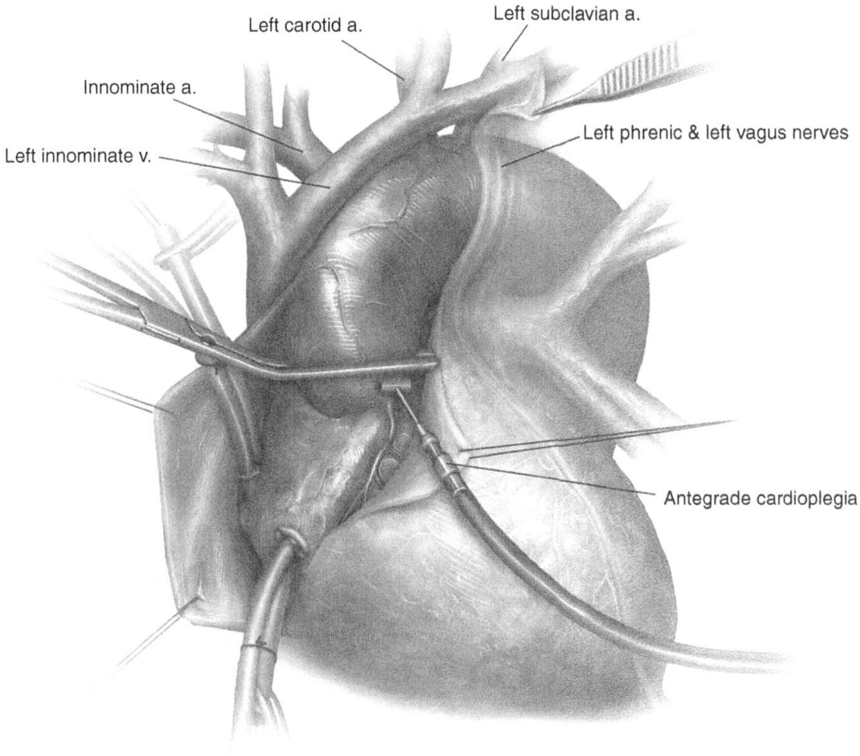

Fig. 4 The ascending aorta is clamped, if feasible, and antegrade cardioplegia is administered. The left inferior pulmonary ligament is divided to mobilize the left lung and the distal limit of excision of the descending aorta is identified. (From Kouchoukos [33])

remaining dissected aorta does not exceed 3.5–4.5 cm. A segment of the septum between the true and false lumens of the distal aorta is excised to permit perfusion of both channels. The graft is stretched tightly to avoid buckling and is anastomosed to the open descending thoracic aorta, reinforcing the suture line with a strip of polytetrafluoroethylene felt (Fig. 8). Intercostal arteries above the seventh intercostal space are ligated. Those below this level, if patent, are preserved by beveling the aorta to preserve the posterior wall. As the distal suture line is being completed, femoral arterial perfusion is initiated slowly to evacuate distal air and debris. Rewarming then commences, using only arterial flow through the right axillary artery. During rewarming, aortic valve or aortic root replacement and coronary artery bypass grafting are performed, if indicated. The proximal end of the aortic graft is sutured to the ascending aorta at the level just above the aortic commissures (Fig. 9), to an existing aortic graft, or to a newly inserted composite graft. CPB is discontinued once rewarming is completed. The axillary artery graft is subsequently ligated close to the artery and divided.

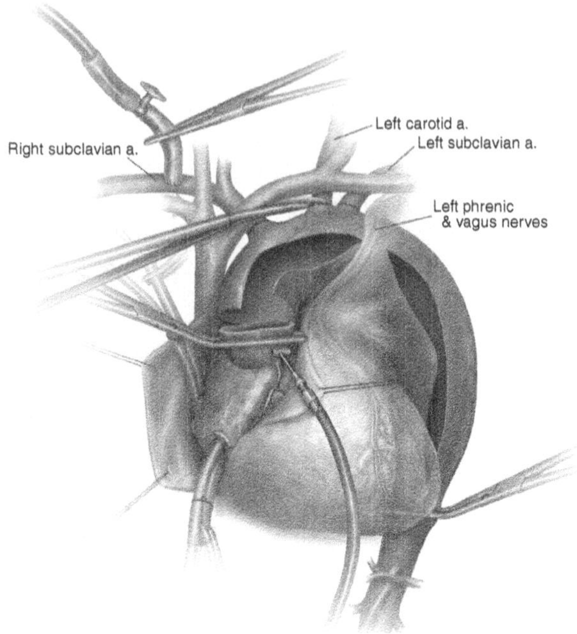

Fig. 5 After circulatory arrest is established, the axillary graft and femoral venous lines are clamped. A clamp is placed on the descending thoracic aorta distal to the aneurysmal segment. The ascending aorta is incised vertically on the anterior surface and the incision is extended across the aortic arch up to the level of the left phrenic nerve. A separate incision is made in the descending thoracic aorta lateral to the left vagus nerve. The three brachiocephalic arteries are transected from their origins or more distally, if necessary. (From Kouchoukos [33])

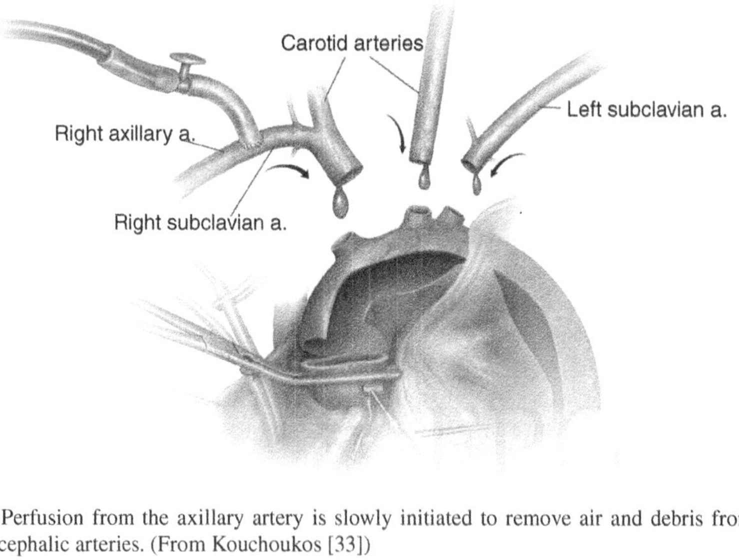

Fig. 6 Perfusion from the axillary artery is slowly initiated to remove air and debris from the brachiocephalic arteries. (From Kouchoukos [33])

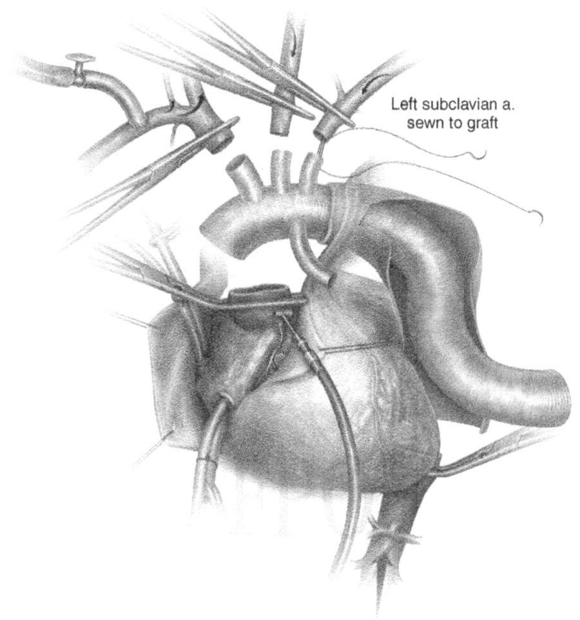

Fig. 7 After brain perfusion is established, a presewn multigraft branch is positioned in the open end of the aortic arch, passing the distal limb into the descending thoracic aorta beneath the phrenic and vagus nerves. The three adjacent branches of the graft are cut to the appropriate lengths and sutured sequentially to the brachial arteries beginning with the left subclavian artery. (From Kouchoukos [33])

Results

During a 21-year interval ending in December, 2015, we employed the technique described above to treat 80 patients with chronic, extensive aortic dissection and aneurysmal enlargement of the thoracic aorta. During the procedure, all aneurysmal aorta was resected and replaced with graft; this included the ascending aorta, the aortic arch, and varying lengths of the descending thoracic aorta. One half or more of the descending thoracic aorta was replaced in 62 of the 80 patients. Seventy-three patients had type A dissection (61 of whom had previously undergone repair of acute type A dissection), and seven patients had type B dissection with proximal extension. The mean patient age was 57 years (range, 22–81 years), and 72% were men. Thirteen patients (16%) had genetically mediated connective tissue disorders. Among the 61 patients undergoing reoperation, the mean interval between the initial and the 1-stage procedures was 62.5 months (range, 1.7–265 months).

In the operating room, the mean transfusion requirements were 8 ± 5.1 units of packed red blood cells, 6.3 ± 3.9 units of fresh-frozen plasma, 4.6 ± 3 units of platelets, and 10.8 ± 18 units of cryoprecipitate. The average hospital length of stay after surgery was 20.5 days (median, 11; range, 6–71 days). Regarding early outcomes, the hospital and 30-day mortality rates were 2.5% (two patients). Six patients (7.5%) required reoperation for bleeding. Stroke occurred in one patient (1.2%), and spinal cord ischemic injury (paraplegia) occurred in one patient (1.2%). Renal failure requiring dialysis occurred in six patients (7.5%), and two of the six patients were receiving dialysis at the time of hospital discharge. Twelve patients (15%) required

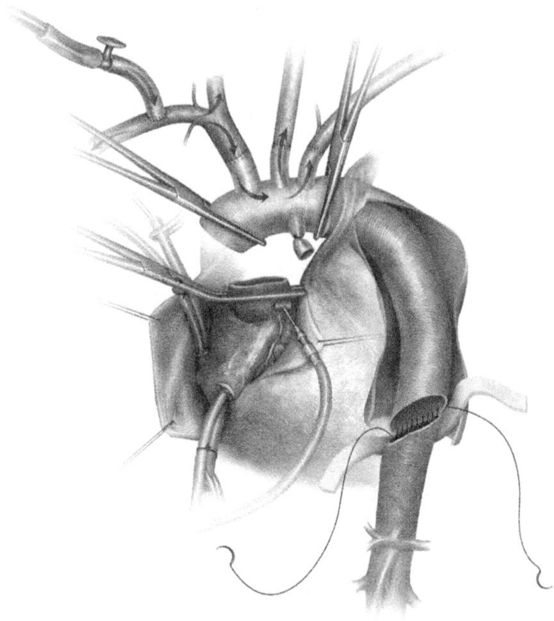

Fig. 8 After completion of the branch anastomoses, the aortic graft is clamped distal to the left subclavian artery. The clamps on the three branches are released, and after evacuation of air, the aortic graft is clamped just proximal to the innominate artery and antegrade flow is established through the three arteries (arrows). The fourth branch of the graft is ligated. Arterial flow from the femoral artery is discontinued, and the clamp on the distal thoracic aorta is removed. A segment of the septal tissue between the true and false lumens is excised to permit perfusion of both lumens, and the graft is cut to the appropriate length and sutured to the outer circumference of the aorta, incorporating a strip of polytetrafluoroethylene felt. Arterial flow from the femoral artery is discontinued, and antegrade flow is established from the axillary artery. (From Kouchoukos [33])

a tracheostomy, nine of whom had the tracheostomy in place at the time of discharge. One patient was treated conservatively for a deep chest wound infection.

At 1-year, the mortality rate was 12% (eight patients). During the follow-up interval, which extends to 18.2 years, there have been 42 late deaths. No patient whose cause of death was known died of aortic rupture. Actuarial survival at 5 and 10 years was 76.4% and 52.6%, respectively. Sixty-five of the 78 hospital survivors (83%) had serial imaging studies suitable for calculation of growth rates of the remaining dissected thoracic and abdominal aorta. The annual growth rate of the distal aorta for the entire cohort was 1.7 mm/year. The maximum aortic diameter increased in 40 patients (mean, 2.8 mm/year), remained unchanged in 16 patients, and decreased in 9 patients (mean, −0.6 mm/year). The growth rate was highest for the 12 patients whose initial aortic diameters were 4.5 cm or greater (2.5 mm/year). For the 8 patients in whom the dissection was confined to the thoracic aorta, the annual growth rate was −0.2 mm/year, whereas it was 1.9 mm/year for the 57 patients in whom the dissection extended into the abdominal aorta.

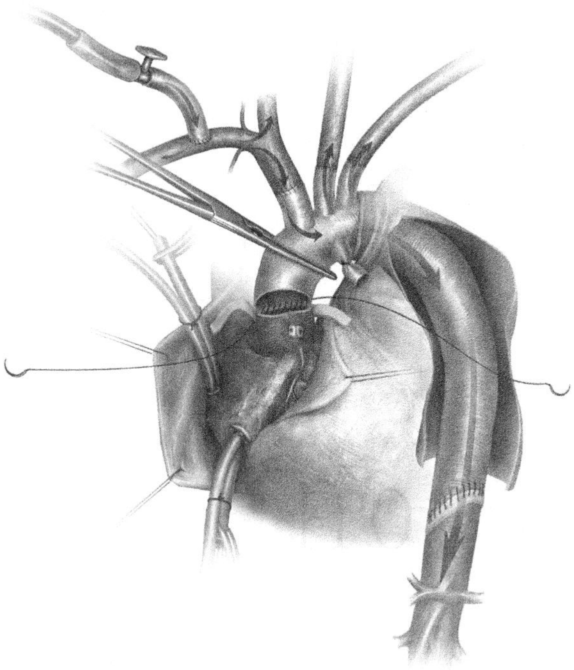

Fig. 9 The proximal end of the graft is cut to the appropriate length and sutured to the ascending aorta just above the aortic commissures, to an existing aortic graft, or to a composite graft. (From Kouchoukos [33])

Five patients required reoperation on the contiguous thoracic or abdominal aorta distal to the aortic graft for aneurysmal degeneration at 8, 27, 34, 51, and 174 months postoperatively. Four of the five patients had replacement of the remaining thoracic aorta and the abdominal aorta to a level just above the aortic bifurcation, while the fifth patient underwent a hybrid procedure with abdominal debranching followed by endovascular stent graft repair. No patient whose dissection was confined to the descending thoracic aorta has required reoperation. Actuarial freedom from reoperation for aneurysmal growth of the contiguous distal aorta at 5 and 10 years was 95.4% and 93% (Fig. 10). Seven additional patients required operations on the aorta or its major branches, on the aortic graft, or the aortic valve for indications unrelated to aneurysmal growth of the contiguous aorta. Actuarial freedom from any aortic reoperation was 89.2% at 5 years and 81.4% at 10 years (Fig. 11). Survival free of aortic reoperation at 5 and 10 years was 68.6% and 43.9%, respectively.

Discussion

We have used the 1-stage technique exclusively since 1995 for patients with chronic aortic dissection who require extensive resection of the thoracic aorta. The bilateral anterior thoracotomy incision provides excellent exposure of the heart, the

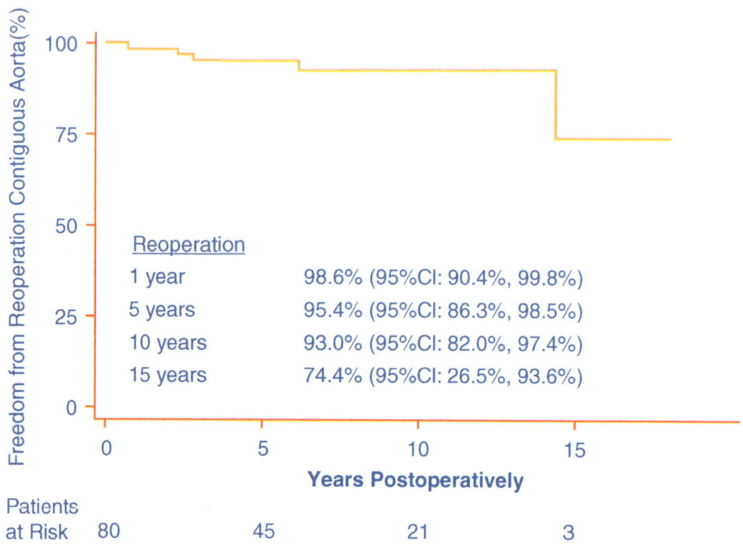

Fig. 10 Freedom from reoperation on the contiguous distal aorta for aneurysmal degeneration after the 1-stage surgical procedure. *CI* confidence interval. (From Kouchoukos et al. [27])

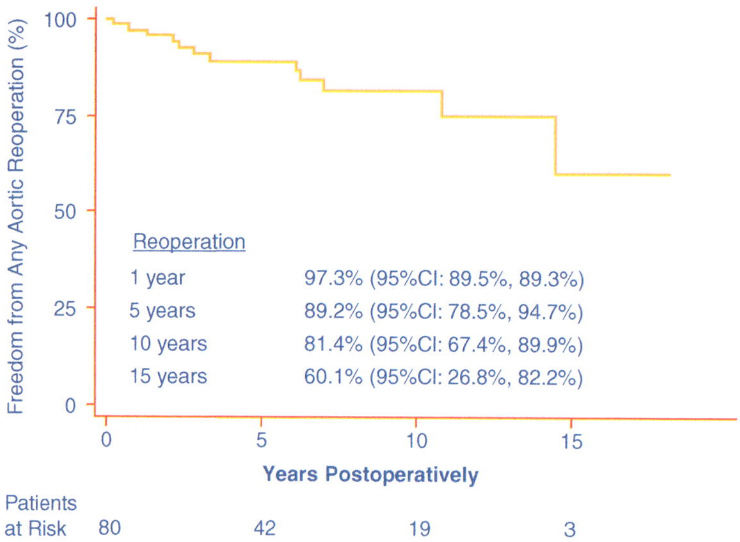

Fig. 11 Freedom from any aortic reoperation after the 1-stage surgical procedure. *CI* confidence interval. (From Kouchoukos et al. [27])

brachiocephalic arteries, both phrenic and the left vagus nerves, and the entire descending aorta. Injury to the dilated ascending aorta (that can occur with sternotomy during reoperation) is avoided because the transverse thoracotomy incision is generally made below this level. The wide exposure of the left pleural cavity helps avoid excessive manipulation of the left lung and the potential for intrapulmonary hemorrhage in a fully heparinized patient. In the usual scenario, mobilization of the heart from the pericardium is necessary only along the lateral surface of the right atrium and the interatrial groove. However, if concomitant CABG is required, exposure of the coronary arteries is easily accomplished. Tricuspid or mitral valve procedures can also be performed with exposure of the right atrium and the interatrial groove.

Use of the bilateral anterior thoracotomy technique permits resection of the entire thoracic aorta. This eliminates the need for two-stage procedures and the attendant mortality and morbidity that can occur in the interval between the stages or during the second thoracic aortic procedure [34–36]. While the traditional method for total arch replacement involves the distal aortic anastomosis first before the arch anastomosis [37–39], we apply an arch-first approach and implant a branched aortic graft. This differs from the older technique where a cuff of aorta surrounding the brachiocephalic arteries was sutured to the aortic graft. Since longer periods of circulatory arrest are associated with greater risk of perioperative stroke and death [39, 40], with the 1-stage technique described above, antegrade hypothermic cerebral perfusion is rapidly initiated to minimize the duration of brain ischemia, and the mean duration of circulatory arrest was 12.1 ± 6.7 min. Arterial brain perfusion is provided via the axillary artery, thus avoiding the need for direct cannulation of the brachiocephalic arteries (a potential cause of stroke) or a separate perfusion circuit for the brain.

Several alternative options exist for the management of chronic dissecting aneurysms confined to the thoracic aorta. These include a staged approach, commonly using the elephant trunk technique, or hybrid procedures using debranching and stent graft techniques [17–19, 36, 41, 42]. One of the major limitations of a staged approach relates to the cumulative risk of the two operations and the risk of aortic rupture in the interval between the stages. In four of the largest reported series of elephant trunk procedures, which contain a substantial number of patients with chronic aortic dissection (31–39% of the total), the cumulative mortality for the two procedures and the risk of death from aortic rupture in the interval between the two procedures exceeded 20% [18, 19, 34, 36]. Our mortality rate of 2.5% for the 1-stage operation compares favorably with the early mortality associated with the conventional elephant trunk procedure for the first stage of a two-stage procedure [18, 19, 34, 36, 43–46]. Applying newer techniques, the frozen elephant trunk operation has a reported mortality rate of 10.2–15.5% [21–23, 47, 48], and the early mortality associated with the hybrid debranching option has ranged from 3% to 17% in reported series [24–26].

Despite the sacrifice of both internal thoracic arteries using the bilateral anterior thoracotomy approach, we have noted excellent wound healing and only one deep wound infection in our series. With regards to other perioperative morbidity, the prevalence of stroke, renal failure, and left recurrent laryngeal nerve injury in our experience has not exceeded that reported for patients undergoing conventional first-stage elephant trunk procedures [17–19, 36, 46], and the intraoperative transfusion requirements have been substantially less [17, 19]. Our rates of stroke (1.2%) and renal failure requiring dialysis (7.5%) also compare favorably to those reported from series of patients undergoing the frozen elephant trunk procedure (2.2–9.8% and 12–22%, respectively) [20–23, 47, 48], or hybrid stent graft procedures (3–8% and 0–11%, respectively) [24–26]. Of note, in a recent meta-analysis summarizing the data from 1103 patients treated with the frozen elephant trunk procedure, the prevalence of spinal cord ischemic injury was 7.9% [49]. With the hybrid procedure, potentially fatal complications such retrograde aortic dissection can occur [24–26].

The relatively high prevalence of pulmonary dysfunction and need for tracheostomy rate have been considered by other groups to be significant limitations of the 1-stage procedure [20, 50, 51]. However, our rate of pulmonary complications does not exceed that reported for the first stage of a two-stage approach [39]. Among patients undergoing the conventional 2-stage elephant trunk procedure (sternotomy for the first stage), the prevalence of tracheostomy has been reported at 16.5% following the two procedures [46]. For patients undergoing the frozen elephant trunk procedure, the frequency of prolonged intubation for more than 72 h has been reported at 12–24% [21, 23]. In our experience with the 1-stage technique, tracheostomy was required in 15% of patients, and with increasing experience, this rate has decreased [27].

The fate of the distal aorta and the need for subsequent aortic interventions are important considerations for the management of patients after extensive thoracic aortic repair. For patients in whom the conventional elephant trunk procedure is used to treat patients with extensive chronic thoracic aortic dissection, a second open or endovascular procedure is almost always required, and there is a risk of death from aortic rupture during the interval between the operations. For patients treated with the frozen elephant trunk procedure, reintervention on the distal aorta during follow-up is not infrequent, ranging from 22% to 25% in two of the largest published series [21, 47]. In the largest series of patients with chronic aortic dissection treated with hybrid procedures, additional stent grafts were needed in 18% of patients for type I and type II endoleaks during a mean follow-up interval of only 2 years [26]. This may relate to the progressive thickening and stiffening of the septum between the true and false lumen, as well as the presence of multiple septal fenestrations, limiting the ability of stent grafts to fixate to the aortic wall and induce complete thrombosis of the false lumen [52, 53]. In the aggregate, a substantial number of aortic reinterventions are necessary following elephant trunk or hybrid techniques.

However, after the 1-stage procedure, we have noted a reoperation rate on the contiguous downstream aorta of only 7% at 10 years and a low overall rate of growth of the distal aorta. These findings indicate that after replacement of the more proximal aneurysmal aortic segments using this technique, distal aneurysm formation is infrequent. Possible explanations for the low rates of growth and aneurysm formation after the 1-stage procedure include stabilization of the aorta at the distal anastomosis that results from firm fixation to the aortic graft with felt buttressing, and maintenance of flow into both the true and false lumens. Despite the low rate of reoperation in our series, we continue to advocate annual surveillance with serial imaging studies after the 1-stage procedure, which is of particular importance in patients with Marfan syndrome and other genetically mediated conditions, especially since reoperations were required as late as 174 months postoperatively.

Conclusion

Our extended experience with the 1-stage open procedure confirms its safety and durability for the treatment of chronic aortic dissection with enlargement confined to the thoracic aorta. The procedure is associated with low operative risk and a low incidence of reoperation on the contiguous distal aorta. The prevalence of spinal cord ischemic injury is substantially less than that reported for the frozen elephant trunk and hybrid procedures. By limiting the duration of circulatory arrest and providing hypothermic cerebral perfusion with axillary cannulation, we have been able to achieve low rates of stroke and temporary neurologic dysfunction. It remains our treatment of choice for extensive chronic aortic dissection with aneurysmal dilatation confined to the thoracic aorta, and we believe it represents a suitable alternative to the 2-stage, frozen elephant trunk and hybrid procedures that are also used to treat this condition. Because growth of the distal aorta occurs at a variable rate, lifelong surveillance of patients with chronic aortic dissection is required.

References

1. Fattori R, Bacchi-Reggiani L, Bertaccini P, Napoli G, Fusco F, Longo M, et al. Evolution of aortic dissection after surgical repair. Am J Cardiol. 2000;86(8):868–72.
2. Immer FF, Krahenbuhl E, Hagen U, Stalder M, Berdat PA, Eckstein FS, et al. Large area of the false lumen favors secondary dilatation of the aorta after acute type A aortic dissection. Circulation. 2005;112(9 Suppl):I249–52.
3. Kirsch M, Soustelle C, Houel R, Hillion ML, Loisance D. Risk factor analysis for proximal and distal reoperations after surgery for acute type A aortic dissection. J Thorac Cardiovasc Surg. 2002;123(2):318–25.
4. Geirsson A, Bavaria JE, Swarr D, Keane MG, Woo YJ, Szeto WY, et al. Fate of the residual distal and proximal aorta after acute type a dissection repair using a contemporary surgical reconstruction algorithm. Ann Thorac Surg. 2007;84(6):1955–64; discussion 64.
5. Shiono M, Hata M, Sezai A, Niino T, Yagi S, Negishi N. Validity of a limited ascending and hemiarch replacement for acute type A aortic dissection. Ann Thorac Surg. 2006;82(5):1665–9.
6. Yeh CH, Chen MC, Wu YC, Wang YC, Chu JJ, Lin PJ. Risk factors for descending aortic aneurysm formation in medium-term follow-up of patients with type A aortic dissection. Chest. 2003;124(3):989–95.

7. Heinemann M, Laas J, Karck M, Borst HG. Thoracic aortic aneurysms after acute type A aortic dissection: necessity for follow-up. Ann Thorac Surg. 1990;49(4):580–4.
8. Kazui T, Yamashita K, Washiyama N, Terada H, Bashar AH, Suzuki T, et al. Impact of an aggressive surgical approach on surgical outcome in type A aortic dissection. Ann Thorac Surg. 2002;74(5):S1844–7; discussion S57-63.
9. Halstead JC, Meier M, Etz C, Spielvogel D, Bodian C, Wurm M, et al. The fate of the distal aorta after repair of acute type A aortic dissection. J Thorac Cardiovasc Surg. 2007;133(1):127–35.
10. Zierer A, Voeller RK, Hill KE, Kouchoukos NT, Damiano RJ Jr, Moon MR. Aortic enlargement and late reoperation after repair of acute type A aortic dissection. Ann Thorac Surg. 2007;84(2):479–86; discussion 86-7.
11. Gillinov AM, Lytle BW, Kaplon RJ, Casselman FP, Blackstone EH, Cosgrove DM. Dissection of the ascending aorta after previous cardiac surgery: differences in presentation and management. J Thorac Cardiovasc Surg. 1999;117(2):252–60.
12. von Kodolitsch Y, Simic O, Schwartz A, Dresler C, Loose R, Staudt M, et al. Predictors of proximal aortic dissection at the time of aortic valve replacement. Circulation. 1999;100(19 Suppl):II287–94.
13. Still RJ, Hilgenberg AD, Akins CW, Daggett WM, Buckley MJ. Intraoperative aortic dissection. Ann Thorac Surg. 1992;53(3):374–9; discussion 80.
14. Canaud L, Ozdemir BA, Patterson BO, Holt PJ, Loftus IM, Thompson MM. Retrograde aortic dissection after thoracic endovascular aortic repair. Ann Surg. 2014;260(2):389–95.
15. Preventza O, Garcia A, Moeller K, Cooley DA, Gonzalez L, Cheong BY, et al. Retrograde ascending aortic dissection after thoracic endovascular aortic repair for distal aortic dissection or with zone 0 landing: association, risk factors, and true incidence. Ann Thorac Surg. 2015;100(2):509–15.
16. Higashigawa T, Kato N, Chino S, Hashimoto T, Shimpo H, Tokui T, et al. Type A aortic dissection after thoracic endovascular aortic repair. Ann Thorac Surg. 2016;102(5):1536–42.
17. Safi HJ, Miller CC III, Estrera AL, Huynh TT, Porat EE, Allen BS, et al. Staged repair of extensive aortic aneurysms: long-term experience with the elephant trunk technique. Ann Surg. 2004;240(4):677–84; discussion 84-5.
18. Svensson LG, Kim KH, Blackstone EH, Alster JM, McCarthy PM, Greenberg RK, et al. Elephant trunk procedure: newer indications and uses. Ann Thorac Surg. 2004;78(1):109–16; discussion 16.
19. LeMaire SA, Carter SA, Coselli JS. The elephant trunk technique for staged repair of complex aneurysms of the entire thoracic aorta. Ann Thorac Surg. 2006;81(5):1561–9; discussion 9.
20. Sun LZ, Qi RD, Chang Q, Zhu JM, Liu YM, Yu CT, et al. Is total arch replacement combined with stented elephant trunk implantation justified for patients with chronic Stanford type A aortic dissection? J Thorac Cardiovasc Surg. 2009;138(4):892–6.
21. Di Eusanio M, Petridis FD, Pacini D, Di Bartolomeo R. Facilitated aortic arch repair with the frozen elephant trunk technique. Eur J Cardiothorac Surg. 2011;40(5):1261–2.
22. Leontyev S, Tsagakis K, Pacini D, Di Bartolomeo R, Mohr FW, Weiss G, et al. Impact of clinical factors and surgical techniques on early outcome of patients treated with frozen elephant trunk technique by using EVITA open stent-graft: results of a multicentre study. Eur J Cardiothorac Surg. 2016;49(2):660–6.
23. Weiss G, Tsagakis K, Jakob H, Di Bartolomeo R, Pacini D, Barberio G, et al. The frozen elephant trunk technique for the treatment of complicated type B aortic dissection with involvement of the aortic arch: multicentre early experience. Eur J Cardiothorac Surg. 2015;47(1):106–14; discussion 14.
24. Cochennec F, Tresson P, Cross J, Desgranges P, Allaire E, Becquemin JP. Hybrid repair of aortic arch dissections. J Vasc Surg. 2013;57(6):1560–7.
25. Bunger CM, Kische S, Liebold A, Leissner M, Glass A, Schareck W, et al. Hybrid aortic arch repair for complicated type B aortic dissection. J Vasc Surg. 2013;58(6):1490–6.
26. Faure EM, Canaud L, Marty-Ane C, Alric P. Hybrid aortic arch repair for dissecting aneurysm. J Thorac Cardiovasc Surg. 2016;152(1):162–8.

27. Kouchoukos NT, Kulik A, Castner CF. Clinical outcomes and rates of aortic growth and reoperation after 1-stage repair of extensive chronic thoracic aortic dissection. J Thorac Cardiovasc Surg. 2018;155(5):1926–35.
28. Minale C, Splittgerber FH, Wendt G, Messmer BJ. One-stage intrathoracic repair of extended aortic aneurysms. J Card Surg. 1994;9(5):604–13.
29. Doss M, Woehleke T, Wood JP, Martens S, Greinecker GW, Moritz A. The clamshell approach for the treatment of extensive thoracic aortic disease. J Thorac Cardiovasc Surg. 2003;126(3):814–7.
30. Kouchoukos NT, Masetti P, Mauney MC, Murphy MC, Castner CF. One-stage repair of extensive chronic aortic dissection using the arch-first technique and bilateral anterior thoracotomy. Ann Thorac Surg. 2008;86(5):1502–9.
31. Kouchoukos NT, Kulik A, Castner CF. Clinical outcomes and fate of the distal aorta following 1-stage repair of extensive chronic thoracic aortic dissection. J Thorac Cardiovasc Surg. 2013;146(5):1086–91.
32. Kulik A, Castner CF, Kouchoukos NT. Outcomes after total aortic arch replacement with right axillary artery cannulation and a presewn multibranched graft. Ann Thorac Surg. 2011;92(3):889–97.
33. Kouchoukos NT. One-stage repair of extensive thoracic aneurysm using the arch-first technique and bilateral anterior thoracotomy. Op Tech Thor Cardiovasc Surg. 2009;13:232–43.
34. Safi HJ, Miller CC 3rd, Estrera AL, Huynh TT, Rubenstein FS, Subramaniam MH, et al. Staged repair of extensive aortic aneurysms: morbidity and mortality in the elephant trunk technique. Circulation. 2001;104(24):2938–42.
35. Kieffer E, Koskas F, Godet G, Bertrand M, Bahnini A, Benhamou AC, et al. Treatment of aortic arch dissection using the elephant trunk technique. Ann Vasc Surg. 2000;14(6):612–9.
36. Schepens MA, Dossche KM, Morshuis WJ, van den Barselaar PJ, Heijmen RH, Vermeulen FE. The elephant trunk technique: operative results in 100 consecutive patients. Eur J Cardiothorac Surg. 2002;21(2):276–81.
37. Griepp RB, Stinson EB, Hollingsworth JF, Buehler D. Prosthetic replacement of the aortic arch. J Thorac Cardiovasc Surg. 1975;70(6):1051–63.
38. Crawford ES, Saleh SA. Transverse aortic arch aneurysm: improved results of treatment employing new modifications of aortic reconstruction and hypothermic cerebral circulatory arrest. Ann Surg. 1981;194(2):180–8.
39. Svensson LG, Crawford ES, Hess KR, Coselli JS, Raskin S, Shenaq SA, et al. Deep hypothermia with circulatory arrest. Determinants of stroke and early mortality in 656 patients. J Thorac Cardiovasc Surg. 1993;106(1):19–28; discussion 31.
40. Ergin MA, Galla JD, Lansman SL, Quintana C, Bodian C, Griepp RB. Hypothermic circulatory arrest in operations on the thoracic aorta. Determinants of operative mortality and neurologic outcome. J Thorac Cardiovasc Surg. 1994;107(3):788–97; discussion 97-9.
41. Chavan A, Karck M, Hagl C, Winterhalter M, Baus S, Galanski M, et al. Hybrid endograft for one-step treatment of multisegment disease of the thoracic aorta. J Vasc Interv Radiol. 2005;16(6):823–9.
42. Kato M, Kuratani T, Kaneko M, Kyo S, Ohnishi K. The results of total arch graft implantation with open stent-graft placement for type A aortic dissection. J Thorac Cardiovasc Surg. 2002;124(3):531–40.
43. Svensson LG, Rushing GD, Valenzuela ES, Rafael AE, Batizy LH, Blackstone EH, et al. Modifications, classification, and outcomes of elephant-trunk procedures. Ann Thorac Surg. 2013;96(2):548–58.
44. Shrestha M, Martens A, Kruger H, Maeding I, Ius F, Fleissner F, et al. Total aortic arch replacement with the elephant trunk technique: single-centre 30-year results. Eur J Cardiothorac Surg. 2014;45(2):289–95; discussion 95-6
45. Ius F, Hagl C, Haverich A, Pichlmaier M. Elephant trunk procedure 27 years after Borst: what remains and what is new? Eur J Cardiothorac Surg. 2011;40(1):1–11.
46. Etz CD, Plestis KA, Kari FA, Luehr M, Bodian CA, Spielvogel D, et al. Staged repair of thoracic and thoracoabdominal aortic aneurysms using the elephant trunk technique: a consecutive

series of 215 first stage and 120 complete repairs. Eur J Cardiothorac Surg. 2008;34(3):605–14; discussion 14-5

47. Pacini D, Tsagakis K, Jakob H, Mestres CA, Armaro A, Weiss G, et al. The frozen elephant trunk for the treatment of chronic dissection of the thoracic aorta: a multicenter experience. Ann Thorac Surg. 2011;92(5):1663–70; discussion 70
48. Jakob H, Tsagakis K, Pacini D, Di Bartolomeo R, Mestres C, Mohr F, et al. The International E-vita Open Registry: data sets of 274 patients. J Cardiovasc Surg (Torino). 2011;52(5):717–23.
49. Cao P, De Rango P, Czerny M, Evangelista A, Fattori R, Nienaber C, et al. Systematic review of clinical outcomes in hybrid procedures for aortic arch dissections and other arch diseases. J Thorac Cardiovasc Surg. 2012;144(6):1286–300, 300 e1-2.
50. Kazui T. Invited commentary. Ann Thorac Surg. 2008;86(5):1509.
51. Roselli EE, Sepulveda E, Pujara AC, Idrees J, Nowicki E. Distal landing zone open fenestration facilitates endovascular elephant trunk completion and false lumen thrombosis. Ann Thorac Surg. 2011;92(6):2078–84.
52. Swee W, Dake MD. Endovascular management of thoracic dissections. Circulation. 2008;117(11):1460–73.
53. Shimono T, Kato N, Yasuda F, Suzuki T, Yuasa U, Onoda K, et al. Transluminal stent-graft placements for the treatments of acute onset and chronic aortic dissections. Circulation. 2002;106(12 Suppl 1):I241–7.

Management of Complicated Type A Aortic Dissection: The Cornell-New York Presbyterian Approach

Erin Iannacone, Christopher Lau, Mario Gaudino, and Leonard N. Girardi

Introduction

Acute type A aortic dissection (ATAAD) is a potentially lethal disease, with a mortality estimated at 1% per hour for the first 48 h and a 30-day mortality of 90% without surgical intervention [1]. Despite improvements in diagnostic capabilities, surgical management, and critical care, the operative mortality for ATAAD remains significant even when performed at specialized centers reporting to large databases like the International Registry of Acute Aortic Dissections (IRAD), the German Registry for Acute Aortic Dissection Type A, or the Nordic Consortium for Acute Type A Aortic Dissection [1–3]. Malperfusion of aortic branch vessels complicates up to a third of ATAAD cases, and represents one of the most catastrophic sequela influencing outcomes [4]. The gold standard approach to ATAAD involves immediate repair of the ascending aorta [5, 6]. While there is some controversy surrounding the optimal approach for patients presenting with advanced malperfusion syndromes, the abysmal outcome for patients with medical management is not debatable.

Classification Systems, Definitions, and Epidemiology

The DeBakey classification system was the first nomenclature to define the extent of aortic dissection [7]. A type I dissection begins in the ascending aorta and extends into the descending aorta, while a DeBakey II dissection begins in the ascending aorta and often terminates in the aortic arch. Type III dissections begin distal to the left subclavian artery with a IIIa limited to the descending aorta and a IIIb extending

E. Iannacone (✉) · C. Lau · M. Gaudino · L. N. Girardi
Department of Cardiothoracic Surgery, Weill Cornell Medicine, New York, NY, USA
e-mail: eem9006@med.cornell.edu

J. S. Coselli et al. (eds.), *Aortic Dissection and Acute Aortic Syndromes*,
https://doi.org/10.1007/978-3-030-66668-2_25

into the abdominal aorta. The Stanford classification system is based more on the location of the primary tear and was first described in 1970 [8]. In 2009, Augoustides and colleagues introduced a clinical classification system for ATAAD that stratified patients according to their ischemic profile (Table 1) [9]. Penn Class "a" patients are characterized by the absence of branch vessel malperfusion or circulatory collapse. Penn Class "b" patients include those with localized branch vessel ischemia (visceral, central nervous system, renal, peripheral). Class "c" patients are those with circulatory collapse and generalized ischemia. Class "b and c" patients have both localized and generalized ischemia. This classification was predicated on an observational cohort of 221 patients, and later validated as a risk assessment tool for predicting operative mortality [10].

Some authors have since proposed modifications to include subcategories of end organ ischemia [11], while others have proposed a mortality risk score based on lactate levels, creatinine, and the presence of hepatic malperfusion [12]. Recent analysis of the large cohort of patients in the GERAADA led the authors to conclude that a simple preoperative stratification of "complicated" and "uncomplicated" groups based on the presence or absence of malperfusion best predicts risk and aids in the planning of therapeutic strategy [4]. Irrespective of the classification system used, the presence of end-organ malperfusion remains a preoperative risk factor highly associated with worse outcome for patients with ATAAD.

Malperfusion of a vascular bed is a direct result of the dissection process itself; either the dissection flap or resultant false-lumen thrombus compress or occlude the true lumen of the branch vessel resulting in coronary, cerebral, spinal, visceral, renal, or limb ischemia. Branch obstruction can be classified as dynamic, static, or both, and characterized by intermittent or persistent malperfusion [13–15]. Dynamic malperfusion is caused by a mobile intimal flap obstructing the orifice of a branch vessel and is responsive to hemodynamic forces and changes in blood pressure. Static malperfusion results from dissection of the branch vessel with obstruction of the true lumen, most often by the thrombosed false lumen (Fig. 1). Both dynamic and static malperfusion may resolve with immediate central repair. Patients with static lesions and a delay in diagnosis or treatment resulting in more advanced organ ischemia may be better managed by alternative strategies to the standard immediate ascending aortic repair. When assessing risk, it is important to distinguish between vascular compromise based on imaging alone, versus clinical end-organ ischemia, i.e., "malperfusion syndrome (MPS)." Imaging can be frightening to look at but it is the presence of end-organ dysfunction that portends a poor prognosis [16]. MPS can

Table 1 University of Pennsylvania acute type A dissection classification system [9]

Classification	Ischemic Profile
Class a	Absence of branch vessel malperfusion or circulatory collapse
Class b	Branch vessel malperfusion with ischemia
Class c	Circulatory collapse
Class b and c	Both branch vessel malperfusion and circulatory collapse

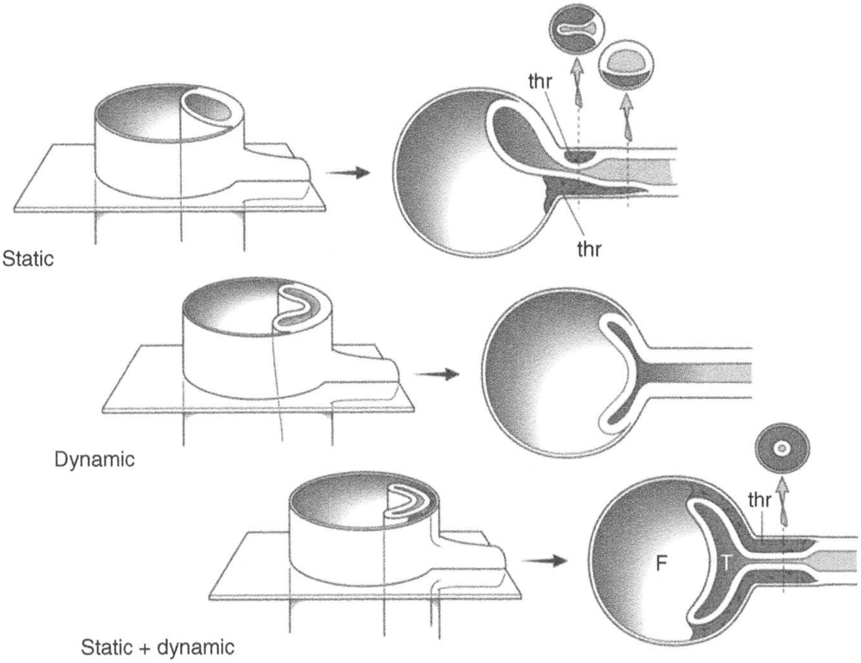

Fig. 1 Diagram depicting anatomical relationship of dissection flap with branch artery [15]. In static malperfusion, the dissection flap extends into the branch vessel and thrombus (thr) in the false lumen can compress and obstruct the true lumen. In dynamic malperfusion, the dissection flap prolapses over the vessel origin

manifest as changes in physical exam and/or abnormalities in laboratory data, but should also include radiographic evidence of vessel compromise.

The widespread use of computed tomographic (CT) scans performed on patients presenting to emergency departments with chest pain has contributed to an increase in the number of ATAAD cases identified with malperfusion. Even without detailed imaging, however, a simple vascular exam can be quite useful in risk assessment. Pulse deficits are a harbinger of malperfusion in other organs and are present in nearly a third of patients in the IRAD database [17]. They were demonstrated to be an independent predictor of mortality and in-hospital adverse events. Hospital mortality was directly correlated with the number of affected vessels: 24.7% with no deficits, 36.2% with one, 48.9% with two, and 55.9% with three. Similar to the results reported from IRAD, the GERAADA Registry also identified a linear correlation between operative mortality and the number of malperfused organs present at the time of diagnosis (Fig. 2) [4].

The incidence of the different forms of malperfusion are interestingly consistent across a wide spectrum of reports on ATAAD [4, 17–19]. Coronary perfusion and peripheral malperfusion are the most common forms occurring in 10–15% and 10–13% of patients, respectively. Cerebral malperfusion is the third most common form of this potentially lethal disease occurring in 6–14% of cases while spinal

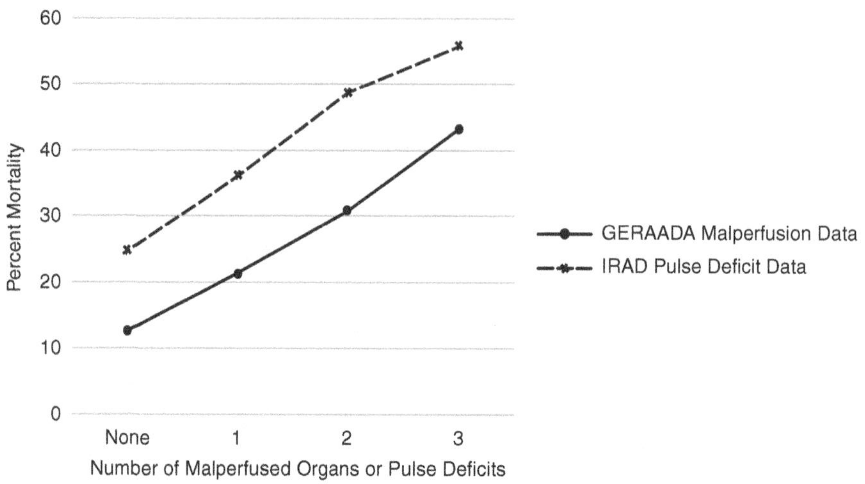

Fig. 2 Mortality per number of malperfused organs or pulse deficits at presentation [4, 17]

(2–5%), mesenteric (4–6%), and renal malperfusion (6–9%) occur in far fewer numbers. The prognostic implications of malperfusion very much depend on the involved vascular bed. The coronary, cerebral, and visceral circulations are the most sensitive to ischemia. MPS involving these vascular beds confers the greatest risk.

Coronary Malperfusion

Coronary artery malperfusion is thankfully a rare complication, occurring in 6.1–11.3% of ATAAD cases in single institution series and 10–15% in larger registries [4, 17, 20–23]. It may be easily confused with an acute coronary syndrome (ACS) leading to delays in diagnosis that are associated with a very high mortality. In the IRAD data, the presence of an abnormal ECG on presentation conferred a 77% increased risk of mortality, similar to the 88% increase seen in patients reported to GERAADA [4, 19]. As it is not uncommon for dissection patients to have concomitant coronary artery disease (CAD), differentiation between ischemia secondary to ATAAD and an ACS can be quite challenging. ECG changes, arrhythmias, wall motion abnormalities on echocardiogram, hemodynamic instability in the absence of pericardial tamponade, and acute valvular dysfunction are all common endpoints of myocardial ischemia regardless of etiology. The subsequent triage of a patient down an incorrect treatment pathway may result in catastrophic consequences.

In a recent series of 76 patients with coronary artery malperfusion due to ATAAD, 25% were originally diagnosed as having an acute myocardial infarction and were found to have a dissection only during diagnostic coronary angiography [21]. Further confusion may result from ischemic ECG changes that occur in the setting of global malperfusion often seen with ATAAD. Neri and colleagues found that, of the 18.9% of ATAAD patients presenting with ECG signs of myocardial ischemia, only 11.3% had dissection involving a coronary ostium. All patients found to have dissection-related coronary malperfusion, however, exhibited ST or T-wave abnormalities on ECG, with two thirds presenting with Q waves [20]. ECG changes identified in the setting of an established ATAAD should prompt a heightened awareness for the potential need to harvest conduit for coronary artery bypass grafting (CABG).

In general, patients presenting with ATAAD are not evaluated with coronary angiography prior to proceeding to the operating room even in the setting of ongoing myocardial ischemia. Patients who have undergone previous CABG and who are hemodynamically stable may be the exception. In a study of 103 patients with ATAAD after previous cardiac surgery, hemodynamically significant tamponade was rare, occurring in only 1% of patients presenting more than 30 days from their primary surgery. Nearly all patients in this series with prior CABG required operative management of CAD during their dissection repair. Preoperative coronary angiography and operative management of native and graft coronary disease had the strongest impact on survival, supporting its use in stable ATAAD patients with prior CABG [24]. A rapid evaluation for evidence of concomitant CAD should include a focused history with review of prior ECGs, when possible. Calcifications in the coronary arteries on CT scan should be noted, and an intraoperative evaluation comprised of direct visualization and manual palpation may identify areas with significant plaque. Wall motion abnormalities on intraoperative echocardiogram also alert one to the possible need for surgical revascularization.

Whenever the decision is made to cross-clamp and open the ascending aorta, direct visualization of the coronary ostia is mandatory to guide the operative strategy. Neri and colleagues identified the three main types of lesions that can cause coronary malperfusion [20]. Type A lesions are those where the dissection abuts the ostium and creates a bulging local flap, causing malperfusion by a trapdoor mechanism. Type B lesions are those in which the dissection extends along the length of the coronary artery, creating a false channel. Type C lesions are those in which the dissection results in detachment or complete avulsion of the coronary intima (Fig. 3). Once the presence of coronary malperfusion is identified, immediate considerations should be given to methods of myocardial protection, strategies for coronary revascularization, and available options for postoperative support of the heart after an ischemic insult.

In the setting of preoperative myocardial ischemia, the adequacy of myocardial perfusion during systemic cooling may be difficult to assess. Routine use of a myocardial temperature probe permits one to measure regional cooling of the myocardium even before cross-clamping. In those who do not routinely utilize retrograde cardioplegia, failure to achieve anticipated levels of myocardial hypothermia during the administration of antegrade cardioplegia may heighten one's awareness of the need for earlier surgical revascularization. While the use of an internal mammary artery graft provides optimal long-term survival, the need to deliver cardioplegia expeditiously may alter surgical planning and mandate the use of a rapidly harvested greater saphenous vein.

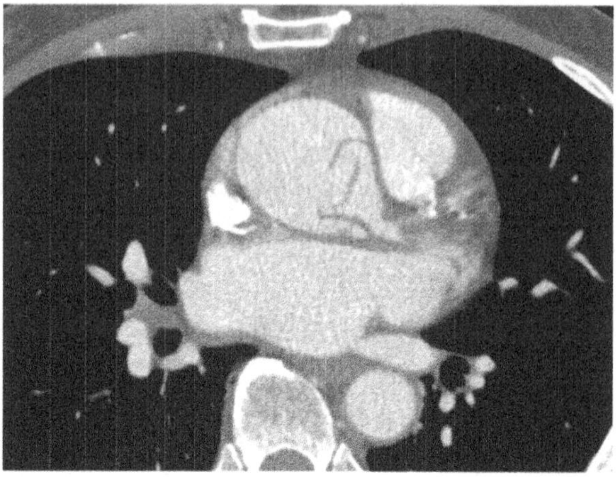

Fig. 3 Acute type A aortic dissection with a type B coronary lesion

Once the distal aorta anastomosis is completed, management turns to the proximal aorta and the coronary ostia. Patients with coronary malperfusion are more likely to need full root replacement rather than root preserving operations as the coronary ischemia is a marker of greater root destruction [25]. For those fortunate to have a single type A lesion, these potentially can be managed by resuspension of the commissures and reconstruction of the aorta at the sinotubular junction. However, one must be aware of the potential for persistent perfusion of the false lumen in the sinuses of Valsalva through needle holes in the aortic suture line, or through distal coronary re-entry tears on type B lesions. Should this occur, or for those with type C lesions, CABG with oversewing of the coronary ostia will be necessary.

There are a number of surgical options to consider when attempting to repair type A and B lesions in the setting of performing a full root replacement. Safe and hemostatic coronary button reimplantation mandates meticulous surgical technique and a proper evaluation of the integrity of the dissected tissue. After mobilizing buttons, one may decide to buttress the separated layers by a neo-media of Teflon felt before reattaching to the ascending aortic graft [26]. Alternatively, one may choose to reimplant the buttons directly with suture and to reinforce the suture lines with circumferential horizontal mattress, pledgetted sutures. In either case, the integrity and functionality of the reimplanted coronary arteries can be tested after reimplantation by pressurizing the aortic root graft with cardioplegia [27]. Failure to cool the myocardium under these circumstances should be concerning and may warrant CABG.

Algorithms for managing the affected coronaries vary in the literature. Some authors prefer bypass grafts to every coronary involved by dissection [23], while others attempt repair for all but the completely avulsed artery. Neri and colleagues report patch angioplasty and interposition grafts as options for managing type B and C lesions, while others question the time-consuming nature of these endeavors, in addition to the likelihood of early technical failures [21]. Our general practice involves repair of the coronary at the level of the ostium for most type A and focal type B lesions. For extended type B lesions and type C lesions there is a low threshold for proceeding with CABG. Similarly, should there be concerns about the integrity of an ostial repair, bypass grafting is performed. Regardless of the preferred mechanism of direct coronary repair or bypass, once the aorta is unclamped and an adequate period of reperfusion achieved, a heightened awareness for ongoing malperfusion is paramount. Refractory atrial or ventricular arrhythmias, unresolved wall motion abnormalities, and significant right or left ventricular dysfunction are indicative of ongoing ischemia and warrant the consideration of bypass grafts to the involved coronary distributions.

Mortality rates for patients with coronary malperfusion due to ATAAD are high, ranging from 20–33.3% [20–23]. All of the deaths in most series are due to uni- or biventricular failure. The preoperative factors heralding the worst prognoses include ejection fraction of less than 25% and elevated myocardial enzyme levels. Postoperative factors with significantly worse outcomes include the presence of ventricular arrhythmias, persistent mitral regurgitation, ejection fraction of less than 25%, and persistently elevated myocardial enzyme levels [20]. Many surviving patients require a prolonged period of myocardial recovery with inotropic support for low cardiac output syndrome. Most patients require a prolonged hospitalization. Few patients requiring mechanical support to leave the operating room survive [21]. Rapid treatment, aggressive myocardial protection, and stable revascularization are the cornerstones to rescuing patients from this often fatal complication of ATAAD.

Cerebral Malperfusion

There is considerable debate regarding the optimal management of patients with ATAAD presenting with cerebral malperfusion. Mechanisms for cerebral malperfusion include obstruction of the true lumen by the dissection flap, embolism from thrombus, and global ischemia from shock. In a recent IRAD review of 1873 patients diagnosed with ATAAD, Di Eusanio and colleagues found that 4.7% also presented with cerebrovascular accident (CVA) and 2.9% presented with coma. Definitions of cerebral malperfusion and its diagnostic criteria vary in the literature making interpretation of the data somewhat difficult. The altered consciousness with which many of the patients with cerebral malperfusion present may also lead to diagnostic challenges that delay treatment.

In the IRAD study, CVA was defined as persistent loss of neurologic function caused by an ischemic event. Coma was defined as completely unresponsive to stimulation. Scoring systems like the Glascow Coma Scale or National Institutes of Health Stroke Scale (NIHSS) can be helpful to classify patients preoperatively. In general, greater neurologic insults portend worse results, with mortality increasing two- to threefold for patients presenting with CVA or coma, respectively. Right-sided strokes appear to be the most common, suggesting that malperfusion often occurs from the dissecting flap or false lumen obstructing the ostia of the great vessels (Fig. 4) [28].

Some consider cerebral malperfusion itself to be a contraindication to immediate repair. The prominent concerns with immediate central repair, most often done with concurrent hypothermic circulatory arrest and with full anticoagulation, include the risk of hemorrhagic conversion and reperfusion injury worsening neurologic outcome. Patients with ATAAD and cerebral malperfusion are also more likely to present with other characteristics predictive of poor outcomes, including hypotension, shock, tamponade, renal failure, myocardial ischemia, and limb ischemia. The risk of delaying surgery for stabilization of the neurologic condition, however, includes rupture and death. According to recent IRAD data, surgery is significantly less likely to be performed in patients with coma (66.7%) or stroke (75.9%) than those without a brain injury (88.9%). However, patients with ATAAD and brain injury perform miserably when managed medically, with a 100% mortality if presenting with coma. Only 12.8% of those with CVA managed medically survive to discharge. Although CVA and coma predict at least a two- or threefold higher mortality, patients who receive surgical treatment have a 75% survival to discharge [29].

There are some reports of novel techniques for early cerebral reperfusion including direct carotid perfusion, endovascular stenting, or direct surgical fenestration, followed by central repair [30–32]. Our standard approach is immediate central repair of the dissection. Central cannulation of the true lumen is our preferred arterial cannulation strategy. We utilize a Seldinger technique and the guidance of both epiaortic ultrasound and transesophageal echocardiography to ensure true lumen perfusion [33]. Near-infrared spectroscopy (NIRS) confirms symmetric great vessel flow, thus eliminating the need to manipulate the great vessels. In the small number of patients in which we are unable to access the true lumen centrally, we utilize the femoral artery for arterial inflow and only use axillary artery cannulation as a last resort. In our experience, the depth of the axillary artery, fragility of the vessel, and the need to place a perfusion graft onto the artery a majority of the time leads to additional cerebral ischemic time that can be avoided.

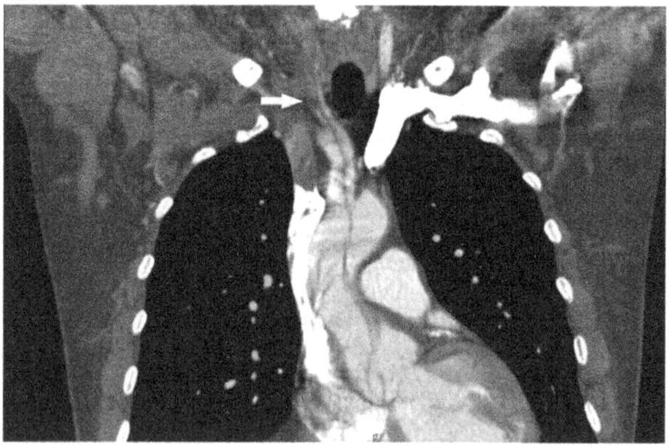

Fig. 4 Acute type A aortic dissection with innominate artery dissection and occlusion of right carotid artery (arrow)

Intraoperative cerebral monitoring can include any combination of electroencephalogram, NIRS, and transcranial Doppler ultrasound. We routinely use NIRS (Somanetics INVOS Cerebral/Somatic Oximeter, Covidien, IL, USA) to evaluate cerebral perfusion, particularly during the initiation of cardiopulmonary bypass or with aortic cross clamping. A sharp decrease in the cerebral oxygenation suggests the need for alternative arterial cannulation or removal of the cross clamp for the remainder of cooling. Although the optimal cerebral protection strategy during arch surgery is often debated, a recent network meta-analysis of 26,968 patients, in which dissections were included, compared deep hypothermic circulatory arrest with antegrade (ACP) and retrograde cerebral perfusion (RCP). The authors found no difference between ACP and RCP for stroke or operative mortality [34]. We prefer RCP and deep hypothermic circulatory arrest (DHCA) with a systemic temperature of 20 °C or less. In the setting of cerebral perfusion we prefer a conservative strategy of hemiarch reconstruction to limit cerebral ischemic time and quickly reestablish antegrade great vessel flow.

Patient selection has been crucial to improving surgical outcomes over the last two decades. Although quality of life data is not readily available for patients surviving immediate surgical management of ATAAD with cerebral malperfusion, several studies have reported favorable outcomes [28, 29, 32, 35]. Complete resolution of neurologic deficits have been reported in up to 84% of patients presenting with focal deficits. Patients with more devastating neurologic injury are significantly less likely to achieve neurologic improvement. Neither cerebral protection method nor extent of aortic arch repair appear to be predictive of neurologic improvement. Early intervention, however, particularly within 10 h of presentation of stroke, is integral to achieving neurologic recovery [28, 35]. This data should encourage surgeons to offer emergent surgery to selected patients, particularly those with focal deficits, despite their higher risk profile.

Spinal Malperfusion

Spinal malperfusion complicating ATAAD is rare, occurring in less than 5% of patients [4, 18]. It manifests as paraparesis or paraplegia, may present unilaterally, and may be accompanied by urinary or bowel incontinence. Immediate central aortic repair is the mainstay of treatment, with complete resolution of spinal cord injury occurring in 61% [18]. The presence of preoperative spinal malperfusion is associated with increased risk of postoperative complications, and significantly increased risk of mortality [4]. Resolution of spinal ischemia, however, is protective against the increased risk of early mortality seen by those who do not experience neurologic recovery [18]. The presence of preoperative spinal malperfusion should not deter surgeons from offering a potentially life-saving procedure. Although nearly 40% of patients do not experience complete resolution of their symptoms, there may be an opportunity for those with partial recovery to experience additional return of lower extremity function with extensive rehabilitation.

Mesenteric Malperfusion

Mesenteric malperfusion is fortunately a rare complication of ATAAD, occurring in 4–6% of patients [4, 36]. It can be insidious in presentation and frequently presents with malperfusion of other vascular territories. Patients with mesenteric MPS may present with abdominal pain, melena, metabolic acidosis, or elevated liver enzymes. The etiology may be dynamic obstruction, occlusive, or thromboembolic. The presence of mesenteric MPS is highly lethal, with nearly two-thirds of patients dying during hospitalization, a threefold increase over those without the complication [4, 36].

Management strategies for mesenteric malperfusion are perhaps the most strongly debated. The traditional approach of immediate aortic repair remains the most commonly utilized. Despite this, nearly one third of patients diagnosed with mesenteric ischemia are treated "medically" according to recent IRAD data. This likely reflects surgeons' acknowledgement that, even with repair, mesenteric malperfusion is one of the most threatening dissection-related complications. Without intervention, however, less than 5% survive [36].

Over recent decades, some groups have dedicated their efforts to a peripheral revascularization first strategy in order to resolve the MPS before moving on to primary aortic repair [37–41]. This approach relies heavily on early identification of patients who are at great risk of death from end-organ failure, and the availability of proceduralists and facilities skilled at performing complex interventional procedures. The theoretical benefit to this approach is that resolving the MPS will reduce systemic inflammation and metabolic derangements that otherwise would increase the risk of central repair [16]. It may also prevent a futile attempt at open aortic repair for the already unsalvageable patient who succumbs to organ failure despite reperfusion of the affected vascular bed. Avoiding preventable aortic rupture while awaiting resolution of MPS is the biggest challenge of the staged approach. Yang and colleagues were able to eliminate fatal aortic rupture with their modified algorithm (Fig. 5), noting that they enforced strict hemodynamic management during the endovascular phase and waited only for downtrending rather than normalization of ischemic markers before central repair. Despite this, total mortality for patients with mesenteric MPS remained high, 33.3–40.3% [38]. Those presenting with stroke (odds ratio [OR] 23), lactate >6 mmol/L (OR 13.5), or with bowel necrosis at laparotomy (OR 7) are the most difficult to salvage [37].

In many practices, including ours, the most expeditious means to restore end-organ function is rapid transfer to the operating room. We most often establish antegrade flow into the true lumen early by central cannulation, followed by rapid conservative aortic repair. The risk of rupture or fatal tamponade complicating delayed central repair is eliminated, and metabolic derangements can be corrected while on bypass. Persistently elevated lactates in the operating room after central aortic repair or high risk preoperative profile may warrant immediate laparotomy after central repair. Ongoing postoperative clinical or biochemical evidence of

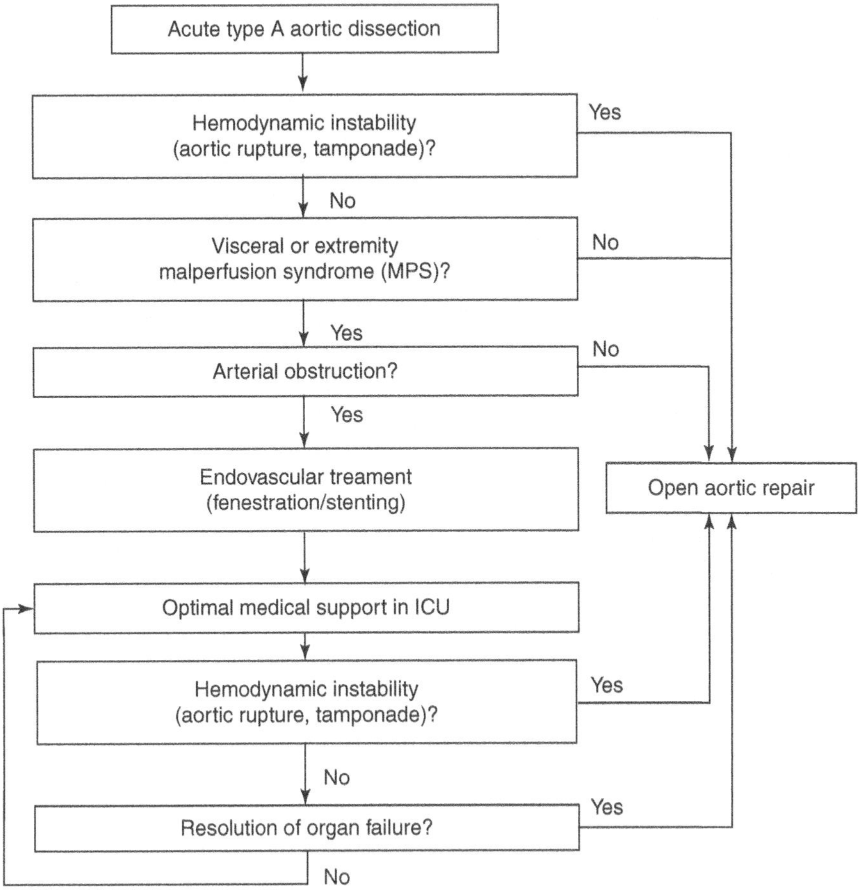

Fig. 5 Michigan algorithm for acute type A aortic dissection and mesenteric or extremity malperfusion syndrome (MPS). ICU indicates intensive care unit [38]

persistent bowel ischemia after central repair should prompt mesenteric angiography with interventional fenestration, angioplasty, or stenting, accompanied by abdominal exploration and resection of any ischemic bowel. Patients presenting with the particularly moribund risk factors of concomitant stroke or severely elevated lactate may be considered for a staged approach.

Mortality rates for patients with ATAAD complicated by mesenteric MPS are dismal with medical and endovascular therapies alone [36]. Disappointingly, however, when comparing the endovascular first to central repair first approaches, the overall mortality for patients with mesenteric MPS complicating ATAAD is still alarmingly high [42]. Ongoing efforts supporting more prompt detection and restoration of mesenteric blood flow is paramount to improving outcomes for this extremely high-risk cohort.

Peripheral Malperfusion

Peripheral malperfusion complicates ATTAD in 10–13% of patients in larger registries, and often accompanies malperfusion of other vascular beds [1, 3, 4, 17, 43]. Limb ischemia manifests early as a cool, pulseless extremity with mottled skin, later as sensory and motor deficits and, in its most advanced stage, as profound paralysis of the limb [44]. Significant preoperative elevations in creatine kinase may signal potentially irretrievable tissue damage [45]. Sequelae of limb reperfusion are not benign, and include shock, acidosis, rhabdomyolysis, and renal failure. For those with advanced limb ischemia, the need to amputate may remain despite reperfusion. Aggressive pursuit of fasciotomies after reperfusion are prudent to relieve or avoid development of compartment syndrome and to assess the viability of the muscle.

Hemodynamically stable ATAAD with isolated and advanced limb malperfusion as the presenting feature may benefit from prioritizing limb reperfusion with a brief period of recovery before central aortic repair [38]. For ATAAD patients with multiple vascular beds affected by malperfusion, and for those with isolated early peripheral MPS, our preference is for immediate central aortic repair. Several studies report favorable results with immediate proximal aortic repair alone relieving lower limb ischemia in 60–100% of patients [5, 46–48]. After central repair, intraoperative recognition of ongoing limb ischemia and expeditious revascularization produces excellent outcomes comparable to those of ATAAD patients without malperfusion syndromes [43].

Conclusions

The ideal approach to the patient with ATAAD and malperfusion includes rapid diagnosis and reperfusion of the ischemic vascular beds while minimizing the risk of aortic rupture. In cases where there is radiographic and clinical evidence of multiorgan malperfusion, or with ongoing hemodynamic instability, an aortic repair first strategy optimizes the timing of true lumen reperfusion throughout the aorta and eliminates the risk of rupture and influence of pericardial tamponade. However, when advanced single organ malperfusion syndromes are present (excluding coronary malperfusion), there may be opportunities to avoid the additional metabolic and inflammatory insult of open surgery by utilizing a percutaneous revascularization first approach. The operative mortality with all approaches remains disappointingly high but a gratifying rate of salvage can be anticipated when patients are triaged quickly to centers and surgeons with extensive experience caring for a wide variety of aortic pathology.

Conflicts No conflicts of interest to report.

Funding No outside funding received.

References

1. Berretta P, Patel HJ, Gleason TG, Sundt TM, Myrmel T, Desai ND, et al. IRAD experience on surgical type A acute dissection patients: results and predictors of mortality. Ann Cardiothorac Surg. 2016.
2. Conzelmann LO, Weigang E, Mehlhorn U, Abugameh A, Hoffmann I, Blettner M, et al. Mortality in patients with acute aortic dissection type A: analysis of pre- and intraoperative risk factors from the German Registry for Acute Aortic Dissection Type A (GERAADA). Eur J Cardiothorac Surg. 2016;49:e44–52.
3. Zindovic I, Gudbjartsson T, Ahlsson A, Fuglsang S, Gunn J, Hansson EC, et al. Malperfusion in acute type A aortic dissection: an update from the Nordic Consortium for Acute Type A Aortic Dissection. J Thorac Cardiovasc Surg. 2019;157:1324–1333.e6.
4. Czerny M, Schoenhoff F, Etz C, Englberger L, Khaladj N, Zierer A, et al. The impact of pre-operative malperfusion on outcome in acute type A aortic dissection: results from the GERAADA Registry. J Am Coll Cardiol. 2015;65:2628–35.
5. Girardi LN, Krieger KH, Lee LY, Mack CA, Tortolani AJ, Isom OW. Management strategies for type A dissection complicated by peripheral vascular malperfusion. Ann Thorac Surg. 2004;77:1309–14; discussion 1314.
6. Fann JI, Sarris GE, Mitchell RS, Shumway NE, Stinson EB, Oyer PE, et al. Treatment of patients with aortic dissection presenting with peripheral vascular complications. Ann Surg. 1990;212:705–13.
7. Debakey ME, Henly WS, Cooley DA, Morris GC, Crawford ES, Beall AC. Surgical management of dissecting aneurysms of the aorta. J Thorac Cardiovasc Surg. 1965;49:130–49.
8. Daily PO, Trueblood HW, Stinson EB, Wuerflein RD, Shumway NE. Management of acute aortic dissections. Ann Thorac Surg. 1970;10:237–47.
9. Augoustides JGT, Geirsson A, Szeto WY, Walsh EK, Cornelius B, Pochettino A, et al. Observational study of mortality risk stratification by ischemic presentation in patients with acute type A aortic dissection: the Penn classification. Nat Clin Pract Cardiovasc Med. 2009;6:140–6.
10. Olsson C, Hillebrant C-G, Liska J, Lockowandt U, Eriksson P, Franco-Cereceda A. Mortality in acute type A aortic dissection: validation of the Penn classification. Ann Thorac Surg. 2011;92:1376–82.
11. Chien T-M, Cheng Q-H, Chen C-W, Yu C-P, Chen H-M, Chen Y-F. Modification of Penn classification and its validation for acute type A aortic dissection. Am J Cardiol. 2014;114:497–9.
12. Ghoreishi M, Wise ES, Croal-Abrahams L, Tran D, Pasrija C, Drucker CB, et al. A novel risk score predicts operative mortality after acute type A aortic dissection repair. Ann Thorac Surg. 2018;106:1759–66.
13. Yang B, Patel HJ, Williams DM, Dasika NL, Deeb GM. Management of type A dissection with malperfusion. Ann Cardiothorac Surg. 2016;5:265–74.
14. Williams DM, Lee DY, Hamilton BH, Marx MV, Narasimham DL, Kazanjian SN, et al. The dissected aorta: percutaneous treatment of ischemic complications–principles and results. J Vasc Interv Radiol. 1997;8:605–25.
15. Kamman AV, Yang B, Kim KM, Williams DM, Michael Deeb G, Patel HJ. Visceral malperfusion in aortic dissection: the Michigan experience. Semin Thorac Cardiovasc Surg. 2017;29:173–8.
16. Goldberg JB, Lansman SL, Kai M, Tang GHL, Malekan R, Spielvogel D. Malperfusion in type A dissection: consider reperfusion first. Semin Thorac Cardiovasc Surg. 2017;29:181–5.
17. Berretta P, Trimarchi S, Patel HJ, Gleason TG, Eagle KA, Di Eusanio M. Malperfusion syndromes in type A aortic dissection: what we have learned from IRAD. J Vis Surg. 2018;4:65.
18. Sandhu HK, Charlton-Ouw KM, Jeffress K, Leake S, Perlick A, Miller CC, et al. Risk of mortality after resolution of spinal malperfusion in acute dissection. Ann Thorac Surg. 2018;106:473–81.

19. Mehta RH, Suzuki T, Hagan PG, Bossone E, Gilon D, Llovet A, et al. Predicting death in patients with acute type a aortic dissection. Circulation. 2002;105:200–6.
20. Neri E, Toscano T, Papalia U, Frati G, Massetti M, Capannini G, et al. Proximal aortic dissection with coronary malperfusion: presentation, management, and outcome. J Thorac Cardiovasc Surg. 2001;121:552–60.
21. Kreibich M, Bavaria JE, Branchetti E, Brown CR, Chen Z, Khurshan F, et al. Management of patients with coronary artery malperfusion secondary to type A aortic dissection. Ann Thorac Surg. 2019;107:1174–80.
22. Eren E, Toker ME, Tunçer A, Keles C, Erdogan HB, Anasiz H, et al. Surgical management of coronary malperfusion due to type A aortic dissection. J Card Surg. 2007;22:2–6.
23. Kawahito K, Adachi H, Murata S, Yamaguchi A, Ino T. Coronary malperfusion due to type A aortic dissection: mechanism and surgical management. Ann Thorac Surg. 2003;76:1471–6; discussion 1476.
24. Stanger O, Schachner T, Gahl B, Oberwalder P, Englberger L, Thalmann M, et al. Type A aortic dissection after nonaortic cardiac surgery. Circulation. 2013;128:1602–11.
25. Yang B, Norton EL, Hobbs R, Farhat L, Wu X, Hornsby WE, et al. Short- and long-term outcomes of aortic root repair and replacement in patients undergoing acute type A aortic dissection repair: twenty-year experience. J Thorac Cardiovasc Surg. 2019;157:2125–36.
26. Bavaria JE, Brinster DR, Gorman RC, Woo YJ, Gleason T, Pochettino A. Advances in the treatment of acute type A dissection: an integrated approach. Ann Thorac Surg. 2002;74:S1848–52; discussion S1857.
27. Lau C, Wingo M, Rahouma M, Ivascu N, Iannacone E, Kamel M, et al. Valve-sparing root replacement in patients with bicuspid aortopathy: an analysis of cusp repair strategy and valve durability. J Thorac Cardiovasc Surg. 2019.
28. Estrera AL, Garami Z, Miller CC, Porat EE, Achouh PE, Dhareshwar J, et al. Acute type A aortic dissection complicated by stroke: can immediate repair be performed safely? J Thorac Cardiovasc Surg. 2006;132:1404–8.
29. Di Eusanio M, Patel HJ, Nienaber CA, Montgomery DM, Korach A, Sundt TM, et al. Patients with type A acute aortic dissection presenting with major brain injury: should we operate on them? J Thorac Cardiovasc Surg. 2013;145:S213–21.e1.
30. Urbanski PP, Wagner M. Perfusion and repair technique in acute aortic dissection with cerebral malperfusion and damage of the innominate artery. J Thorac Cardiovasc Surg. 2012;144:982–4.
31. Heran MKS, Balaji N, Cook RC. Novel percutaneous treatment of cerebral malperfusion before surgery for acute type A dissection. Ann Thorac Surg. 2019;108:e15–7.
32. Sultan I, Bianco V, Patel HJ, Arnaoutakis GJ, Di Eusanio M, Chen EP, et al. Surgery for type A aortic dissection in patients with cerebral malperfusion: results from the International Registry of Acute Aortic Dissection. J Thorac Cardiovasc Surg. 2019.
33. Frederick JR, Yang E, Trubelja A, Desai ND, Szeto WY, Pochettino A, et al. Ascending aortic cannulation in acute type a dissection repair. Ann Thorac Surg. 2013;95:1808–11.
34. Hameed I, Rahouma M, Khan FM, Wingo M, Demetres M, Tam DY, et al. Cerebral protection strategies in aortic arch surgery: a network meta-analysis. J Thorac Cardiovasc Surg. 2019.
35. Morimoto N, Okada K, Okita Y. Lack of neurologic improvement after aortic repair for acute type A aortic dissection complicated by cerebral malperfusion: predictors and association with survival. J Thorac Cardiovasc Surg. 2011;142:1540–4.
36. Di Eusanio M, Trimarchi S, Patel HJ, Hutchison S, Suzuki T, Peterson MD, et al. Clinical presentation, management, and short-term outcome of patients with type A acute dissection complicated by mesenteric malperfusion: observations from the International Registry of Acute Aortic Dissection. J Thorac Cardiovasc Surg. 2013;145:385–390.e1.
37. Yang B, Norton EL, Rosati CM, Wu X, Kim KM, Khaja MS, et al. Managing patients with acute type A aortic dissection and mesenteric malperfusion syndrome: a 20-year experience. J Thorac Cardiovasc Surg. 2019;158:675–687.e4.
38. Yang B, Rosati CM, Norton EL, Kim KM, Khaja MS, Dasika N, et al. Endovascular fenestration/stenting first followed by delayed open aortic repair for acute type A aortic dissection with malperfusion syndrome. Circulation. 2018;138:2091–103.

39. Patel HJ, Williams DM, Dasika NL, Suzuki Y, Deeb GM. Operative delay for peripheral malperfusion syndrome in acute type A aortic dissection: a long-term analysis. J Thorac Cardiovasc Surg. 2008;135:1288–95; discussion 1295.
40. Yamashiro S, Arakaki R, Kise Y, Inafuku H, Kuniyoshi Y. Management of visceral malperfusion complicated with acute type A aortic dissection. Interact Cardiovasc Thorac Surg. 2015;21:346–51.
41. Tsagakis K, Konorza T, Dohle DS, Kottenberg E, Buck T, Thielmann M, et al. Hybrid operating room concept for combined diagnostics, intervention and surgery in acute type A dissection. Eur J Cardiothorac Surg. 2013;43:397–404.
42. Girardi LN. Commentary: Acute type A aortic dissection and mesenteric malperfusion syndrome: still a long way to go. J Thorac Cardiovasc Surg. 2019;158:688–9.
43. Preece R, Srivastava V, Akowuah E, Kendall S. Should limb revascularization take priority over dissection repair in type A aortic dissection presenting as isolated acute limb ischaemia. Interact Cardiovasc Thorac Surg. 2017;25:643–6.
44. Rutherford RB, Baker JD, Ernst C, Johnston KW, Porter JM, Ahn S, et al. Recommended standards for reports dealing with lower extremity ischemia: revised version. J Vasc Surg. 1997;26:517–38.
45. Currie IS, Wakelin SJ, Lee AJ, Chalmers RT. Plasma creatine kinase indicates major amputation or limb preservation in acute lower limb ischemia. J Vasc Surg. 2007;45:733–9.
46. Charlton-Ouw KM, Sritharan K, Leake SS, Sandhu HK, Miller CC, Azizzadeh A, et al. Management of limb ischemia in acute proximal aortic dissection. J Vasc Surg. 2013;57:1023–9.
47. Charlton-Ouw KM, Sandhu HK, Leake SS, Jeffress K, Miller CC, Durham CA, et al. Need for limb revascularization in patients with acute aortic dissection is associated with mesenteric ischemia. Ann Vasc Surg. 2016;36:112–20.
48. Girdauskas E, Kuntze T, Borger MA, Falk V, Mohr F-W. Surgical risk of preoperative malperfusion in acute type A aortic dissection. J Thorac Cardiovasc Surg. 2009;138:1363–9.

Management of Complicated Acute Type A Aortic Dissection: The Stanford Approach

Albert J. Pedroza and Michael P. Fischbein

Introduction

Acute aortic dissection is a rare, life-threatening condition with an incidence ranging from 5 to 10/100,000 person-years [1]. Cardiac surgeons have long recognized that this disease process is clinically challenging with a high mortality rate. Among the simplest and earliest classification systems, the Stanford paradigm proposed in 1970 by Dailey et al. established surgical repair as the standard of care for the 'Type A' variant involving the ascending aorta (Fig. 1) [2]. While the wealth of experience treating this entity over the subsequent five decades has reaffirmed the need for prompt surgical intervention, one central theme remains certain: not all aortic dissections are created equal. Within the cohort of patients referred for prompt surgical repair of acute type A aortic dissection (ATAAD), many potential complicating factors contribute to operative candidacy, optimal interventional strategy and morbidity/mortality risk. In particular, the presence of neurologic injury, mesenteric malperfusion, limb ischemia or shock mandate rapid decisive action. When present, these factors comprise a heterogeneous "complicated ATAAD" variant with heightened technical challenges and surgical risk. Whereas the debate around neurologic status reflects a question of 'if' an operation should be attempted, the presence of malperfusion or limb ischemia raises important considerations of 'how' it should be performed. Various institutional paradigms have been built around theories on optimal management, reflecting the lack of clear consensus across the specialty about how to optimally manage these difficult problems. The growing body of literature surrounding complicated aortic dissection management underscores the need for centralized cardiac surgery referral centers capable of interdisciplinary aortic interventions and the rapidly evolving practice of the modern aortic surgeon. This chapter presents pertinent lessons learned from institutional experience and multi-center

A. J. Pedroza · M. P. Fischbein (✉)
Cardiothoracic Surgery, Stanford University, Stanford, CA, USA
e-mail: alpedroz@stanford.edu; mfischbe@stanford.edu

J. S. Coselli et al. (eds.), *Aortic Dissection and Acute Aortic Syndromes*,
https://doi.org/10.1007/978-3-030-66668-2_26

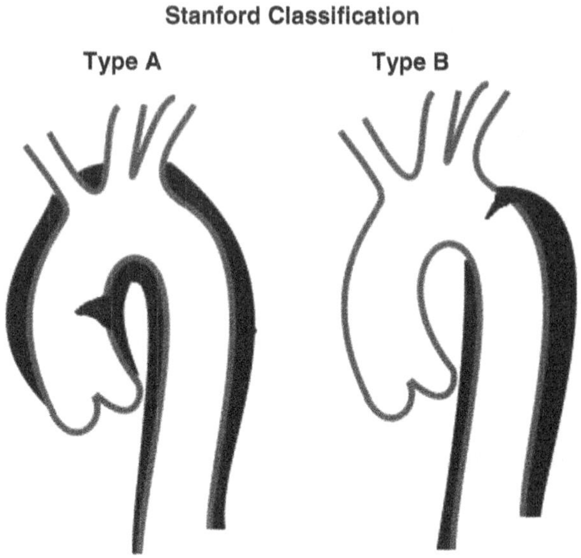

Fig. 1 Stanford classification for acute aortic dissection. In the "Type A" variant, the primary intimal tear occurs in the ascending aortic segment, while in "Type B", the tear occurs distal to the aortic arch, affecting the descending thoracic aorta

databases to highlight branch points in the treatment algorithm for complicated ATAAD.

Pre-Operative Evaluation

Operative Candidacy

Decisions on operative candidacy for ATAAD in general are made difficult by the very poor outcomes of medical management alone. While modern mortality estimates for medical management alone are implicitly limited by selection and reporting biases, data from the International Registry of Acute Aortic Dissection (IRAD) database showed 57% mortality for patients treated medically. Surgical outcomes have steadily improved since the inception of the IRAD database with reported multi-center surgical mortality rates falling from 25% to 18% between 1995 and 2013 [3]. Findings from the IRAD database also highlight age-dependent increases in mortality risk regardless of treatment modality but consistent superiority of surgical treatment up to 80 years of age [4]. The paucity of data for patients over 80 within this cohort precludes robust determination of optimal management for octogenarians. Given these dichotomous outcomes, every ATAAD patient should be considered for operative repair. With few exceptions, our default pathway is immediate transfer directly to a hybrid operating room and preparation for central aortic repair. The presence of distal malperfusion, which may affect one or multiple organ beds, represents a central branch point in treatment algorithm for patients presenting with ATAAD.

Malperfusion

Review of computed tomography imaging to confirm the diagnosis and determine the extent of dissection is critical to operative planning. In particular, the extent of dissection into the aortic arch vessels should be assessed to determine the feasibility of axillary artery perfusion strategies. Involvement of mesenteric, renal, and iliac artery branches should also be evaluated.

An important distinction related to the complicated ATAAD is the concept of "dynamic" versus "static" obstruction of the affected branch vessel [5]. Dynamic obstruction, which results from collapse of the true lumen by the pressurized false lumen, is rectified by central aortic repair and true lumen pressure/flow restoration. Conversely, static obstruction arises from tear entry or intussusception into the branch vessel and subsequent thrombosis (Fig. 2). In this scenario, central aortic repair does not resolve flow obstruction and delays reperfusion to the affected vascular bed until secondary branch vessel intervention is performed. Careful

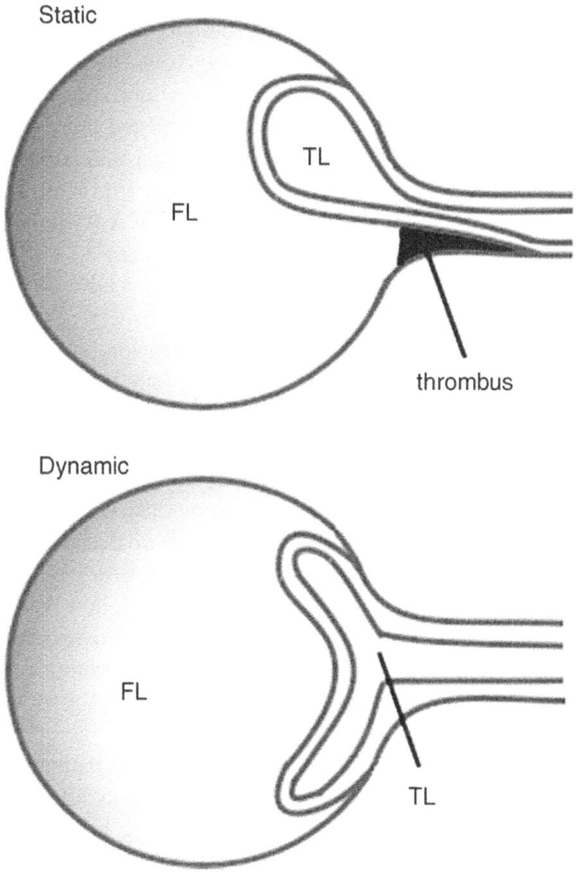

Fig. 2 Mechanisms of branch vessel malperfusion. In static cases, dissection into the branch leads to thrombosis. Ostial obstruction of branch vessels by the dissection flap may occur in dynamic malperfusion, which is resolved with true lumen pressurization. *TL* true lumen, *FL* false lumen

assessment of the celiac and superior mesenteric arteries on CTA imaging is imperative to determine whether static or dynamic malperfusion is present because delayed mesenteric reperfusion may be lethal following open aortic repair. This upfront distinction is less relevant to myocardial or cerebral malperfusion, both of which can be addressed via reconstruction or bypass of the affected branch vessels as part of the central repair strategy. Intervention for static renal malperfusion, typically via endovascular stenting or dissection flap fenestration can typically be delayed until after primary surgery in a staged approach. Iliac malperfusion can be managed intraoperatively with secondary arterial cannulation of the affected extremity during primary aortic repair and secondary bypass when necessary. Thus, we regard the combination of clinical mesenteric malperfusion syndrome with appearance of static SMA or celiac obstruction on CT imaging as the exception to the "central repair first" algorithm and treat these patients with upfront endovascular stenting.

While CTA imaging is helpful in identifying affected aortic branch vessels and vascular territories, malperfusion is a clinical diagnosis. The presence of peritonitis, hematochezia or ileus on pre-operative imaging should alert the surgeon to the possibility of ongoing mesenteric ischemia. Similarly, oliguria is suggestive of renal hypoperfusion. New neurologic deficits or pulseless extremities imply neurologic and limb malperfusion states, respectively. Unsurprisingly, both the extent and location of malperfusion syndromes affect mortality. In our own series, patients with visceral malperfusion had higher unadjusted mortality (28.6%) than renal or limb ischemia (16.1% and 14.5%, respectively), and patients with multiple affected vascular beds were at further increased risk [6]. Multi-center data from the German Registry for Acute Aortic Dissection Type A (GERAADA) demonstrated stepwise increases in operative mortality with increased number of malperfused vascular beds (12.6% with no malperfusion up to 43.4% with three affected systems) [7]. Lawton et al. demonstrated through retrospective review of their single institution series that the constellation of malperfusion and severe metabolic acidosis (base deficit or −10 or more) was uniformly fatal [8].

In light of these challenges, the group at University of Michigan has set forth an upfront reperfusion strategy utilizing endovascular fenestration or SMA stenting followed by an observation period prior to central aortic repair for ATAAD patients with visceral malperfusion syndromes [9]. Yang et al. reported outcomes for 82 patients treated with this approach over two decades at Michigan; for the 47 patients (57%) who survived to open repair they observed equivalent operative mortality compared to patients without malperfusion, however 31 patients (37%) died from aortic rupture or organ failure following endovascular treatment [10]. Our institutional philosophy remains centered around prompt central aortic repair as the primary strategy to restore true lumen flow and resolve malperfusion states except when clinical gut malperfusion and static celiac or SMA obstruction are encountered. We recently reported outcomes for 82 patients presenting with ATAAD and visceral, renal or peripheral malperfusion syndromes (26.9% of the all patients undergoing surgery for ATAAD extending beyond the ascending aorta) [6]. We observed no significant difference for in-hospital mortality in patients presenting with ATAAD with malperfusion (13.4%) compared to ATAAD alone (8.5%). Unsurprisingly, we observed increased need for aortic branch interventions for the malperfused group (12.3% versus 5.7% at 10 years, Fig. 3).

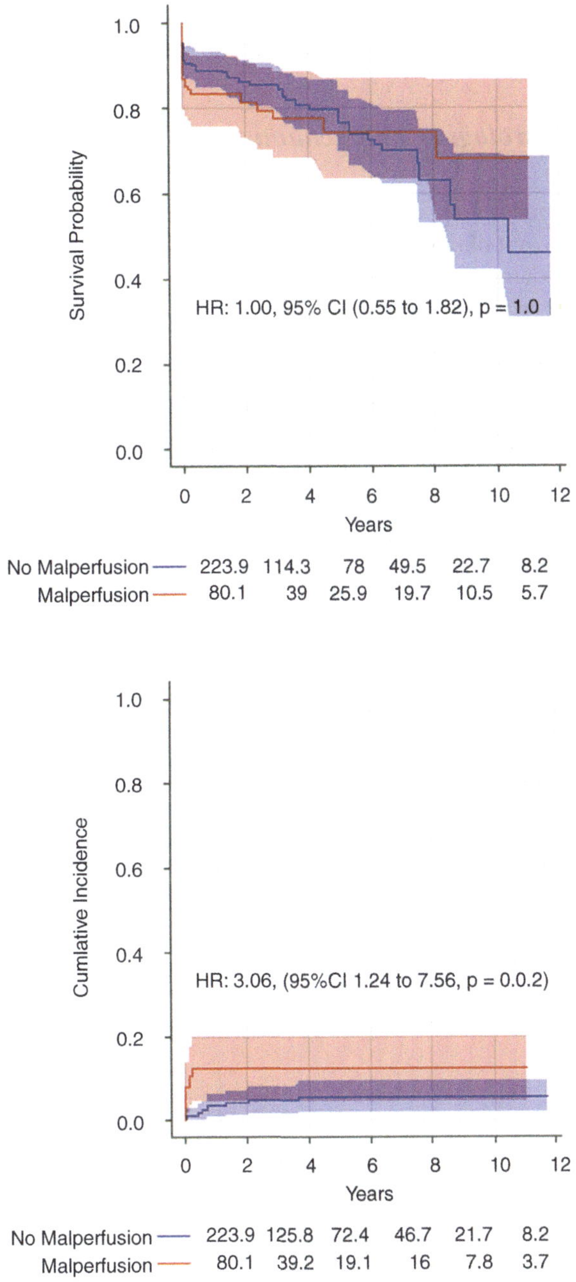

Fig. 3 Malperfusion did not confer increased mortality risk in ATAAD patients treated with central repair strategy (top) but did correlate with increased branch interventions (bottom). Reproduced with permission from [6]

Cumulatively, these studies highlight the difficulty in applying rigid treatment algorithms to this highly variable clinical entity and the importance of pre-operative evaluation for malperfusion states. Regardless of general philosophy about the best initial treatment approach for complicated ATAAD, these challenges underscore the importance of both open surgical and endovascular capabilities in major referral centers.

Neurologic Complications

Among complicating factors, neurologic injury (ranging from transient mild deficits to overt obtundation) is present in 10–15% of patients presenting with ATAAD in modern series and is associated with significantly higher mortality risk [11]. We do not withhold surgery for patients presenting with stroke or obtundation/coma. We recently reported our 10-year experience of 345 ATAAD repair cases, of which 50 (14.4%) presented with neurologic injury. While concerns exist about potential conversion of ischemic insults to hemorrhagic stroke following systemic heparinization, we observed intracranial hemorrhage in only 2 patients (4%) after aortic repair on cardiopulmonary bypass [12]. In our experience, time-to-operation did not predict neurologic or survival outcomes in ATAAD patients with stroke (Fig. 4). Conversely, Estrera et al. reported on 16 ATAAD patients treated surgically after presenting with stroke; post-operative neurologic improvement occurred only in patients who underwent repair within 10 h of symptoms [13]. Tsukube et al. analyzed outcomes in 27 ATAAD patients presenting with coma and found improved

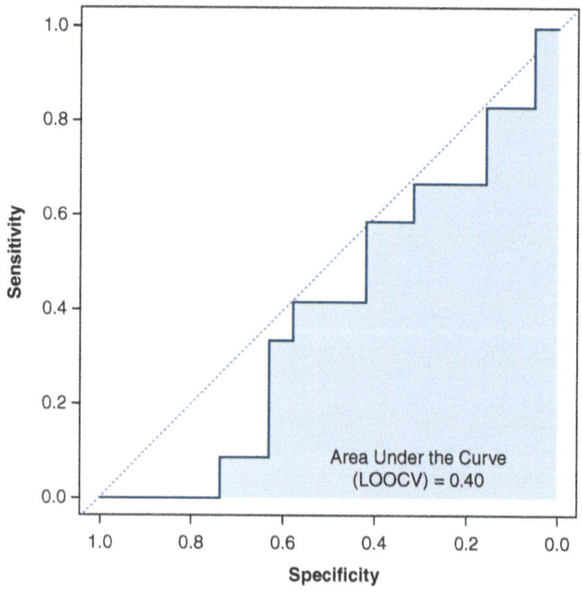

Fig. 4 Time-to-operation was a poor predictor for lack of neurologic recovery in ATAAD patients with neurologic insults. Reproduced with permission from [12]

mortality (14% vs. 67%) and neurologic recovery (86% vs. 17%) in patients who underwent surgery within 5 h of symptoms [14]. Furthermore, subset analysis of the International Registry of Acute Aortic Dissection (IRAD) database has revealed return of brain function in 84.3% of patients with stroke and 78.8% of those with coma after aortic repair [15]. Collectively, these data support an immediate operative approach to resolve dynamic obstruction of aortic branch vessels for ATAAD patients presenting with neurologic injury. We therefore do not advocate for operative delays for cerebrovascular imaging or clinical observation.

Physical Exam

The majority of ATAAD patients are transferred to central referral centers from peripheral hospitals, necessarily producing a delay of several hours between diagnosis and operation [16]. In complicated cases, this time period may present dynamic changes in hemodynamic status, acid/base balance, and neurologic exam. Upon arrival to the operating room, a rapid neurologic assessment, abdominal exam and determination of peripheral pulses should be performed. Hemodynamic assessment must occur in parallel with preparation for general anesthesia. Hypotension or overt shock, which may reflect impending tamponade physiology or aortic rupture, are independent predictors of mortality in ATAAD patients [17].

Operative Technique

Anesthetic Considerations

Induction of general anesthesia represents a period of vulnerability for patients with ATAAD. Nearly one-fifth of patients with ATAAD present with some degree of cardiac tamponade [18]. The surgical team should be present and ready to commence the operation at the time of induction. Blood products should be available and central intravenous access obtained. Transesophageal echocardiography after anesthesia induction is useful to confirm the diagnosis of dissection, determine the degree of pericardial effusion and assess aortic valve regurgitation. As a period of circulatory arrest is uniformly necessary during distal graft anastomosis with the unclamped aorta, EEG and monitoring of cerebral oxygen saturation with near-infrared spectroscopy (NIRS) is advisable.

Cerebral Protection Strategy

The goal of central aortic repair for complicated ATAAD is to re-establish true lumen flow, resect the primary intimal tear and reverse distal malperfusion. A variety of distal repair strategies may be employed depending on the extent of dissection and clinical scenario. Regardless of whether the operative approach calls for partial or total arch replacement, a period of hypothermic circulatory arrest is required to complete the repair. Systemic cooling is a mainstay of cerebral protection, though the extent of cooling varies among surgeons. Deep hypothermia (18–20 °C) can be safely employed for arch repairs with circulatory arrest times up to 50 min without adjunct cerebral perfusion with good long-term outcomes in elective cases, though short-term results in dissection patients are less favorable [19]. When combined with selective antegrade cerebral perfusion (SACP), Algarni et al. reported that moderate hypothermia (22–28 °C) was superior to deep cooling during ATAAD repair (circulatory arrest time 25.9 ± 14.3 versus 28.9 ± 19.9 min) [20]. Leshnower et al. similarly showed that moderate hypothermia with unilateral SACP was safe for patients undergoing total arch replacement in both elective cases and dissections [21].

Similarly, individual surgeons and institutions utilize multiple variations of cerebral perfusion strategies. While SACP comprises strategies to perfuse the cerebral vessels directly via ostial cannulation of the innominate and/or carotid artery or indirectly via the axillary artery, retrograde cerebral perfusion (RCP) utilizes reversed cardiopulmonary bypass flow through the superior vena cava. Some groups advocate for RCP, which is technically simpler and faster [22], but SACP is utilized more frequently worldwide and has been associated with better long-term outcomes in some studies [23, 24]. SACP may be performed using unilateral or bilateral approaches; advocates for bilateral cannulation argue that only a minority of patients have a functionally complete Circle of Willis (as few as 28% among aortic surgery patients as assessed by transcranial doppler) [25]. Nevertheless unilateral SACP was equivalent to bilateral cannulation in a German study of over 1000 patients undergoing aortic arch repair using mild hypothermia [26]. For ATAAD cases, we use moderate hypothermia and SACP via the right axillary artery with few exceptions (extensive dissection into axillary artery or hemodynamic instability). We employ cerebral oximetry intraoperatively to monitor left-sided perfusion and use bilateral cerebral perfusion only when concern for inadequate cerebral protection arises.

Arterial Cannulation Site

The choice of cannulation sites for cardiopulmonary bypass varies among surgeons and clinical scenarios. Our primary goal is to establish antegrade perfusion for CPB, which can be done via axillary, innominate, or carotid artery graft, direct aortic true lumen cannulation over a wire with TEE guidance [27], or transapical placement of an aortic cannula across the aortic valve [28]. Reestablishing true lumen pressure, which may reduce dynamic malperfusion while on cardiopulmonary bypass, is a central benefit of these antegrade strategies. Retrograde arterial perfusion via femoral cannulation is our last resort, given uncertainty about the relative pressurization of true and false lumens and increased stroke rate compared to central cannulation [29, 30]. Nevertheless, in an unstable patient, emergency percutaneous or open femoral cannulation may be required prior to sternotomy.

Our preferred arterial cannulation method is the creation of a right axillary artery chimney graft, which can be employed in most cases. This technique requires a separate infraclavicular incision ideally prior to sternotomy and is therefore best suited for hemodynamically stable patients. Direct cannulation of the axillary artery is not advisable. The vessel lumen should be inspected for evidence of dissection prior to end-to-side anastomosis using a Dacron graft.

An adjunct arterial graft may be added into the arterial circuit to address malperfusion states. This technique is particularly useful to perfuse an ischemic limb due to proximal iliac occlusion or provide unilateral cerebral perfusion distal to a proximally obstructed carotid takeoff [31]. Antegrade placement of a superficial femoral artery cannula may also be considered for distal perfusion of malperfused lower extremities [32].

Exposure and Dissection

Standard median sternotomy and pericardiotomy are performed, frequently releasing a bloody pericardial effusion which can improve hemodynamics in unstable patients. Following systemic heparinization, central venous cannulation is achieved via the right atrium and a retrograde cardioplegia catheter is directed into the coronary sinus. Dissection of the aorta can be performed prior to commencing cardiopulmonary bypass to minimize time on pump. The arch branches are dissected to achieve circumferential control. The axillary chimney graft is then connected to the bypass circuit with standard connectors and cardiopulmonary bypass commenced. Left ventricular vent placement via the right superior pulmonary vein is advisable given the likelihood of significant aortic regurgitation. Systemic cooling is then undertaken; we cool to a core temperature of 28 °C for limited arch operations and 24 °C if the need for total arch replacement is anticipated. Retrograde cardioplegia is administered via the coronary sinus and the distal ascending aorta is cross-clamped. Direct handheld cardioplegia administration should be used cautiously if the coronary ostia are involved with the proximal extent of dissection.

Limited Root Repair or Aortic Root Replacement

Following transection, the aorta is then resected down to one centimeter above the aortic valve commissures. Stay sutures above the commissures assist with exposure and evaluation of the aortic root and valve leaflets. Aortic valve resuspension and primary re-approximation of dissected aortic layers represents the standard proximal repair strategy in uncomplicated dissection. Frequently this can be completed while cooling prior to distal repair. Evaluation of the coronary ostia for involvement by the proximal extent of dissection requires close attention.

Decision-making about the extent of proximal repair must be predicated on maximizing each patient's chance of survival. While young patients with uncomplicated ATAAD may tolerate longer bypass runs for root replacement, a limited root operation to minimize bypass and operative times may be more appropriate in elderly patients or those with malperfusion syndromes. We performed retrospective review of 293 patients who underwent limited root repair or full root replacement for ATAAD [33]. While there was difference in mortality between groups (Fig. 5), patients who had limited root operations were more likely to require aortic root or aortic valve reoperation (11.8% vs 0%). A limited repair strategy may therefore be most appropriate for surgeons with limited experience performing aortic root replacements or in the setting of malperfusion syndromes with the understanding that reoperation may be required.

In some cases, performing a full aortic root replacement is appropriate or even necessary. Aortic rupture, valve degeneration, commissural destruction, root aneurysm, poor tissue integrity or known/suspected connective tissue disorder are indications for aortic root replacement during the index operation. We generally utilize a composite valve graft (CVG) prosthesis with a patient-appropriate selection of mechanical or biologic valve. Valve-sparing aortic root replacement using the reimplantation (David V) technique may be appropriate for young patients, particularly those with connective tissue disorders, but should be used only by surgeons with substantial experience in an elective setting [34]. When full aortic root replacement

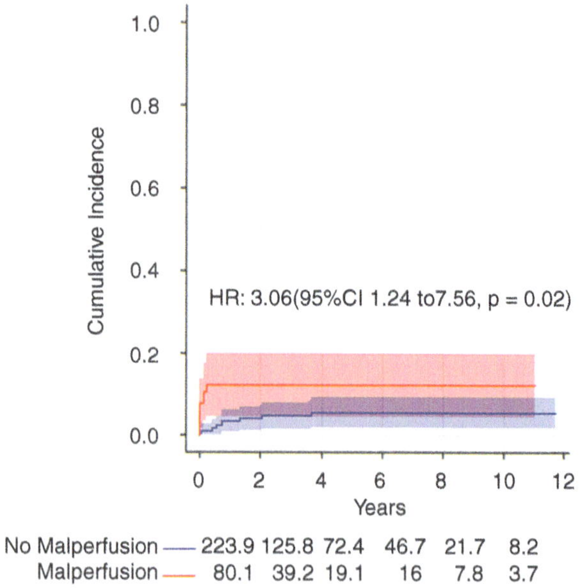

Fig. 5 Patients who underwent full aortic root replacement had equivalent mortality compared to those undergoing limited root repair. Reproduced with permission from [33]

(Bentall technique) is undertaken, buttons of coronary ostial tissue are fashioned for eventual reimplantation. The aortic valve leaflets are resected, annular mattress sutures are placed circumferentially, passed through the CVG prosthesis and tied down. The graft is then incised at the appropriate level for left coronary button reimplantation with end-to-side technique. We complete the graft-to-graft anastomosis prior to implanting the right coronary button to ensure appropriate height with the aortic graft in final position.

Aortic Arch Operations

Distal aortic repair commences once the desired systemic cooling threshold is reached. Adjunct cerebral protection measures such as cranial topical cooling with ice and administration of mannitol and furosemide may be used. Cardiopulmonary bypass flow is reduced to 10 mL/kg/min, the innominate and left common carotid arteries are clamped and the aortic cross-clamp is removed. Indicators of inadequate left-sided protection during SACP include discordant tympanic membrane temperatures or cerebral oxygen saturation reduction greater than 15%, which should prompt maneuvers to improve perfusion such as increasing SACP flow or transfusing to increase hematocrit. If necessary and deemed safe, a small retrograde cannula can be placed directly into the carotid artery orifice to provide bilateral cerebral perfusion.

Once adequate cerebral protection is ensured the primary intimal tear can be resected entirely. Frequently the tear can be entirely resected via excision the lesser curvature of the aortic arch and graft replacement using an extended "peninsula-style" repair (Fig. 6). The dissected layers of the distal aorta must be

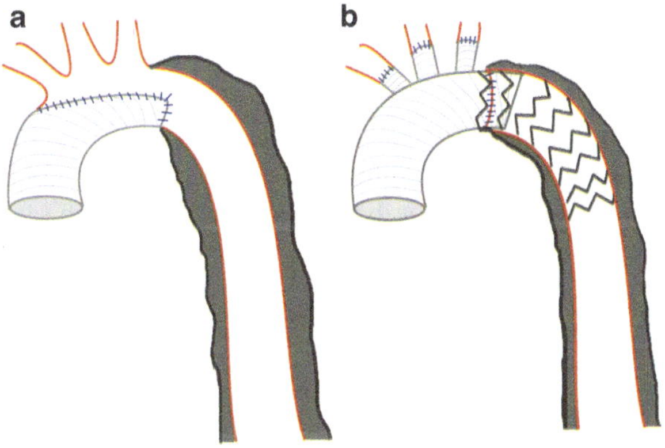

Fig. 6 Aortic arch reconstruction in ATAAD. (**a**) Extended 'peninsula' style hemi-arch repair includes resection of the lesser curvature to the level of the left subclavian. (**b**) Total arch with frozen elephant trunk (FET, left) comprises complete arch replacement with Dacron graft and antegrade stent-graft placement into the proximal descending aorta

reapproximated to obliterate flow into the false lumen. Total arch replacement is indicated if the primary intimal tear is located within the greater curvature, significant arch aneurysm is encountered, distal arch rupture, and for patients with connective tissue disorders. In some cases, the intimal tear may extend into or originate in the descending thoracic aorta (the "retrograde type A" variant). To completely treat the primary intimal tear in this scenario, especially in the setting of malperfusion, total arch replacement with frozen elephant trunk (FET) distal extension is indicated. An invaginated graft is placed into the descending thoracic aortic true lumen and end-to-end anastomosis is completed in running fashion. The proximal, branched graft portion is then withdrawn, leaving a 5 cm cuff of graft distally. A covered 10 cm thoracic endoprosthesis can then be deployed in an antegrade fashion distally to "freeze" the surgical graft in place. We deploy these devices antegrade over a wire introduced from the femoral artery using intravascular ultrasound (IVUS) to confirm true lumen landing distally. Newer generation off-the-shelf devices with combined multi-branch arch graft and endoprostheses may also be employed for this indication. Minimizing the distal length of the endoprosthesis is critical to prevent ischemic injury to the spinal cord during FET reconstruction. This technique has good aortic outcomes with acceptable neurologic complications in experienced hands and with spinal cord protective measures [35, 36].

After distal anastomosis, a variety of strategies for arch branch anastomosis may be employed. Typically, a multi-branch graft is used to anastomose each branch individually. While an "island" of arch tissue may be fashioned and reimplanted as a single anastomosis, we do not recommend this technique as it can be difficult to obtain hemostasis of bleeding from the posterior portion. After de-airing the graft, full cardiopulmonary bypass flow is resumed, ending hypothermic circulatory arrest. Systemic re-warming, proximal repair and graft-to-graft anastomosis are then completed.

Addressing Malperfusion

Coronary malperfusion due to involvement of the coronary ostia must be recognized early to prevent acute heart failure associated with high mortality. Coronary vessels may be affected by static or dynamic malperfusion or in severe cases completely avulsed or "sheared off". If the extent of dissection prohibits administration of handheld antegrade cardioplegia, we perform upfront coronary bypass prior to aortic repair to ensure adequate myocardial protection can be maintained.

Following central repair, attention is redirected to vascular beds with preoperative malperfusion. If abdominal distention is encountered, exploratory laparotomy should be considered to assess bowel viability. Similarly, peripheral pulses should be re-examined. Malperfused lower extremities should be closely monitored for swelling and compartment syndrome which may manifest following reperfusion.

Completion aortography may be considered to confirm mesenteric perfusion post-repair. Endovascular intervention (branch stenting, thoracic endograft distal extension, or flap fenestration) may then be performed as necessary. We do not routinely perform aortography following repair unless a specific concern persists.

Post-Operative Care

Aggressive resuscitation during and following central aortic repair is critical to reverse metabolic derangement resulting from malperfusion and cardiopulmonary bypass. Platelets and fresh frozen plasma are frequently required to address coagulopathy. Active warming may be required to maintain normothermia. Metabolic acidosis and elevated serum lactate are frequently present on arrival to the ICU and should be monitored for correction with ongoing volume resuscitation. Persistent metabolic acidosis should prompt re-evaluation for ongoing malperfusion or unrecognized bowel ischemia. A baseline neurologic status should be obtained within the first few hours in ICU; persistent obtundation or change in neurologic exam should prompt immediate head CT.

Renal malperfusion due to static obstruction may persist following central repair. Oliguria and rising serum creatinine from this entity is difficult to distinguish from more typical acute kidney injury after cardiopulmonary bypass and transient low-flow states. Devoted renal doppler ultrasound should be obtained in this setting. Delayed renal artery stenting can be undertaken following initial resuscitation in an attempt to salvage renal function.

Final Remarks

Complicated ATAAD represents a unique clinical challenge for aortic surgeons. The heterogeneous spectrum of presentation precludes the application of a "one size fits all" strategy. Despite specialized care at tertiary referral hospitals, surgical mortality remains frustratingly high. Effective management requires a broad range of skills, sound decision-making and institutional capability to perform both traditional open surgery and hybrid endovascular interventions. Care of the complicated ATAAD patient is frequently multidisciplinary, encompassing multiple consulting specialties to manage complications of malperfusion. Meticulous clinical decision-making is a central theme in the determination of operative candidacy, strategy, and extent of aortic repair in these patients, decisions which may mean the difference between life and death. Finally, ATAAD patients require lifelong surveillance with cross-sectional imaging for progressive aneurysmal dilation of the distal dissected aorta. We strongly advocate for institution-based aortic teams to manage surveillance and secondary interventions for the residual aorta. The "aortic team" consisting of cardiac and vascular surgeons and devoted cardiovascular Radiology specialists is a critical asset in the longitudinal management of this complex patient subset.

References

1. Mody PS, Wang Y, Geirsson A, Kim N, Desai MM, Gupta A, et al. Trends in aortic dissection hospitalizations, interventions, and outcomes among medicare beneficiaries in the United States, 2000–2011. Circ Cardiovasc Qual Outcomes. 2014 Nov;7(6):920–8.
2. Daily PO, Trueblood HW, Stinson EB, Wuerflein RD, Shumway NE. Management of acute aortic dissections. Ann Thorac Surg. 1970 Sep;10(3):237–47.
3. Pape LA, Awais M, Woznicki EM, Suzuki T, Trimarchi S, Evangelista A, et al. Presentation, diagnosis, and outcomes of acute aortic dissection: 17-year trends from the international registry of acute aortic dissection. J Am Coll Cardiol. 2015 Jul 28;66(4):350–8.
4. Trimarchi S, Eagle KA, Nienaber CA, Rampoldi V, Jonker FHW, Vincentiis CD, et al. Role of age in acute type A aortic dissection outcome: report from the International Registry of Acute Aortic Dissection (IRAD). J Thorac Cardiovasc Surg. 2010 Oct 1;140(4):784–9.
5. Williams DM, Lee DY, Hamilton BH, Marx MV, Narasimham DL, Kazanjian SN, et al. The dissected aorta: percutaneous treatment of ischemic complications – principles and results. J Vasc Interv Radiol. 1997 Aug;8(4):605–25.
6. Chiu P, Tsou S, Goldstone AB, Louie M, Woo YJ, Fischbein MP. Immediate operation for acute type A aortic dissection complicated by visceral or peripheral malperfusion. J Thorac Cardiovasc Surg. 2018;156(1):18–24.e3.
7. Czerny M, Schoenhoff F, Etz C, Englberger L, Khaladj N, Zierer A, et al. The impact of pre-operative malperfusion on outcome in acute type A aortic dissection: results from the GERAADA registry. J Am Coll Cardiol. 2015 Jun 23;65(24):2628–35.
8. Lawton JS, Moon MR, Liu J, Koerner DJ, Kulshrestha K, Damiano RJ, et al. The profound impact of combined severe acidosis and malperfusion on operative mortality in the surgical treatment of type A aortic dissection. J Thorac Cardiovasc Surg. 2018;155(3):897–904.
9. Patel HJ, Williams DM, Dasika NL, Suzuki Y, Deeb GM. Operative delay for peripheral malperfusion syndrome in acute type A aortic dissection: a long-term analysis. J Thorac Cardiovasc Surg 2008 Jun;135(6):1288–1295; discussion 1295–1296.
10. Yang B, Norton EL, Rosati CM, Wu X, Kim KM, Khaja MS, et al. Managing patients with acute type A aortic dissection and mesenteric malperfusion syndrome: a 20-year experience. J Thorac Cardiovasc Surg. 2019;158(3):675–687.e4.
11. Bossone E, Corteville DC, Harris KM, Suzuki T, Fattori R, Hutchison S, et al. Stroke and outcomes in patients with acute type A aortic dissection. Circulation. 2013 Sep 10;128(11_suppl_1):S175–9.
12. Chiu P, Rotto TJ, Goldstone AB, Whisenant JB, Woo YJ, Fischbein MP. Time-to-operation does not predict outcome in acute type A aortic dissection complicated by neurologic injury at presentation. J Thorac Cardiovasc Surg. 2019;158(3):665–72.
13. Estrera AL, Garami Z, Miller CC, Porat EE, Achouh PE, Dhareshwar J, et al. Acute type A aortic dissection complicated by stroke: Can immediate repair be performed safely? J Thorac Cardiovasc Surg. 2006 Dec 1;132(6):1404–8.
14. Tsukube T, Haraguchi T, Okada Y, Matsukawa R, Kozawa S, Ogawa K, et al. Long-term outcomes after immediate aortic repair for acute type A aortic dissection complicated by coma. J Thorac Cardiovasc Surg 2014 Sep;148(3):1013–1018; discussion 1018–1019.
15. Di Eusanio M, Patel HJ, Nienaber CA, Montgomery DM, Korach A, Sundt TM, et al. Patients with type A acute aortic dissection presenting with major brain injury: should we operate on them? J Thorac Cardiovasc Surg. 2013 Mar;145(3 Suppl):S213–221.e1.
16. Harris KM, Strauss CE, Eagle KA, Hirsch AT, Isselbacher EM, Tsai TT, et al. Correlates of delayed recognition and treatment of acute type A aortic dissection: the International Registry of Acute Aortic Dissection (IRAD). Circulation. 2011 Nov 1;124(18):1911–8.
17. Bossone E, Pyeritz RE, Braverman AC, Peterson MD, Ehrlich M, O'Gara P, et al. Shock complicating type A acute aortic dissection: Clinical correlates, management, and outcomes. Am Heart J. 2016;176:93–9.

18. Gilon D, Mehta RH, Oh JK, Januzzi JL, Bossone E, Cooper JV, et al. Characteristics and in-hospital outcomes of patients with cardiac tamponade complicating type A acute aortic dissection. Am J Cardiol. 2009 Apr 1;103(7):1029–31.
19. Damberg A, Carino D, Charilaou P, Peterss S, Tranquilli M, Ziganshin BA, et al. Favorable late survival after aortic surgery under straight deep hypothermic circulatory arrest. J Thorac Cardiovasc Surg. 2017;154(6):1831–1839.e1.
20. Algarni KD, Yanagawa B, Rao V, Yau TM. Profound hypothermia compared with moderate hypothermia in repair of acute type A aortic dissection. J Thorac Cardiovasc Surg. 2014 Dec;148(6):2888–94.
21. Leshnower BG, Kilgo PD, Chen EP. Total arch replacement using moderate hypothermic circulatory arrest and unilateral selective antegrade cerebral perfusion. J Thorac Cardiovasc Surg. 2014 May;147(5):1488–92.
22. Rylski B, Bavaria JE, Milewski RK, Vallabhajosyula P, Moser W, Kremens E, et al. Long-term results of neomedia sinus valsalva repair in 489 patients with type A aortic dissection. Ann Thorac Surg 2014 Aug;98(2):582–588; discussion 588–589.
23. Conzelmann LO, Weigang E, Mehlhorn U, Abugameh A, Hoffmann I, Blettner M, et al. Mortality in patients with acute aortic dissection type A: analysis of pre- and intraoperative risk factors from the German Registry for Acute Aortic Dissection Type A (GERAADA). Eur J Cardiothorac Surg. 2016 Feb;49(2):e44–52.
24. El-Hamamsy I, Ouzounian M, Demers P, McClure S, Hassan A, Dagenais F, et al. State-of-the-art surgical management of acute type A aortic dissection. Can J Cardiol. 2016 Jan;32(1):100–9.
25. Smith T, Jafrancesco G, Surace G, Morshuis WJ, Tromp SC, Heijmen RH. A functional assessment of the circle of Willis before aortic arch surgery using transcranial Doppler. J Thorac Cardiovasc Surg. 2019;158(5):1298–304.
26. Zierer A, El-Sayed Ahmad A, Papadopoulos N, Moritz A, Diegeler A, Urbanski PP. Selective antegrade cerebral perfusion and mild (28°C–30°C) systemic hypothermic circulatory arrest for aortic arch replacement: results from 1002 patients. J Thorac Cardiovasc Surg. 2012 Nov;144(5):1042–9.
27. Frederick JR, Yang E, Trubelja A, Desai ND, Szeto WY, Pochettino A, et al. Ascending aortic cannulation in acute type a dissection repair. Ann Thorac Surg. 2013 May;95(5):1808–11.
28. Wada S, Yamamoto S, Honda J, Hiramoto A, Wada H, Hosoda Y. Transapical aortic cannulation for cardiopulmonary bypass in type A aortic dissection operations. J Thorac Cardiovasc Surg. 2006 Aug;132(2):369–72.
29. Benedetto U, Raja SG, Amrani M, Pepper JR, Zeinah M, Tonelli E, et al. The impact of arterial cannulation strategy on operative outcomes in aortic surgery: evidence from a comprehensive meta-analysis of comparative studies on 4476 patients. J Thorac Cardiovasc Surg. 2014 Dec;148(6):2936–2943.e1–4.
30. Etz CD, von Aspern K, da Rocha E Silva J, Girrbach FF, Leontyev S, Luehr M, et al. Impact of perfusion strategy on outcome after repair for acute type a aortic dissection. Ann Thorac Surg. 2014 Jan;97(1):78–85.
31. Rylski B, Urbanski PP, Siepe M, Beyersdorf F, Bachet J, Gleason TG, et al. Operative techniques in patients with type A dissection complicated by cerebral malperfusion. Eur J Cardiothorac Surg. 2014 Aug;46(2):156–66.
32. Howe KL, Harlock J, Parry D. Management of lower extremity ischaemia during type A dissection repair. EJVES Short Rep. 2018;39:44–6.
33. Chiu P, Trojan J, Tsou S, Goldstone AB, Woo YJ, Fischbein M. Limited root repair in acute type A aortic dissection is safe but results in increased risk of reoperation. J Thorac Cardiovasc Surg. 2018 Jan;155(1):1–7.e1.
34. Rosenblum JM, Leshnower BG, Moon RC, Lasanajak Y, Binongo J, McPherson L, et al. Durability and safety of David V valve-sparing root replacement in acute type A aortic dissection. J Thorac Cardiovasc Surg. 2019;157(1):14–23.e1.

35. Poon SS, Tian DH, Yan T, Harrington D, Nawaytou O, Kuduvalli M, et al. Frozen elephant trunk does not increase incidence of paraplegia in patients with acute type A aortic dissection. J Thorac Cardiovasc Surg. 2020;159(4):1189–1196.e1.
36. Hohri Y, Yamasaki T, Matsuzaki Y, Hiramatsu T. Early and mid-term outcome of frozen elephant trunk using spinal cord protective perfusion strategy for acute type A aortic dissection. Gen Thorac Cardiovasc Surg. 2020 Mar 9;68(10):1119–27.

Management of Type B Aortic Dissection

Ali Khoynezhad, Tiffany Worthington, Raffat Jaber, Jeffrey Altshuler, and Rodney White

Introduction

Acute aortic dissection (AAD) is a devastating aortic catastrophe accounting for more than 20 cases per million per year. AAD begins with a tear in the intimal layer presumably due to existing wall weakness or an episode of high blood pressure. Blood under pulsatile pressure subsequently forces the intimomedial tear to open within the media of the aorta and dissects along into the media layers in the diseased aortic wall, forming a false lumen(s). Temporal classification of AAD includes hyperacute (within 24 hours of onset), acute (1–14 days after dissection), subacute (15–90 days) or chronic (greater than 90 days from onset. Additionally, AAD is classified by the location of the dissection. The Stanford classification system divides acute aortic syndromes into two location categories: type A, when the intimomedial tear is in the ascending aorta, and type B when the intimomedial tear is in the descending thoracic aorta [1]. This classification system is important for patient triage, as typically all type A dissections should be evaluated for surgical intervention; however, type B lesions can often be managed with medical therapy alone. Some experts disagree as to where the anatomic divide occurs for type A and type B classification. The consensus is the origin of the left subclavian establishes the divide, however other experts argue that arch dissection without a proximal extension should be managed conservatively [2].

In the absence of complicating factors such as rupture, malperfusion syndromes, rapid aortic expansion, and/or refractory pain (i.e., complicated acute type B aortic dissection), acute type B aortic dissection (TBAD) can often be treated with medical management alone. For those that exhibit these complications or high-risk features, immediate endovascular or open surgical intervention

A. Khoynezhad (✉) · T. Worthington · R. Jaber · J. Altshuler · R. White
Department of Cardiovascular Surgery, MemorialCare Heart and Vascular Institute, Long Beach, CA, USA
e-mail: akhoynezhad@memorialcare.org

J. S. Coselli et al. (eds.), *Aortic Dissection and Acute Aortic Syndromes*,
https://doi.org/10.1007/978-3-030-66668-2_27

is recommended. This chapter discusses the management of TBAD and when to consider additional interventions.

Presenting Signs and Symptoms

The typical patient with acute TBAD is a male patient, 60–70 years old, with a longstanding history of hypertension presenting to the emergency department with sudden onset, ripping/tearing back, or abdominal pain. Chest pain is more common for those with type A pathology; however up to 62% of those with TBAD may also present with this complaint [3]. Patients 40–50 years old with TBAD are less likely to have a history of hypertension; instead, they often have a history of the bicuspid aortic valve, Marfan syndrome, or another connective tissue disorder, or history of prior aortic surgery [4]. Of patients presenting to the emergency department, 90% reported this pain as severe or the worst pain of their lives [3]. One out of six patients with acute aortic dissection may also describe a migratory quality to the pain [3].

In addition to complaints of pain, patients with aortic dissection may also report more generalized complaints such as dyspnea, nausea, diaphoresis, nausea, and vomiting. In the event of malperfusion syndrome, patients also may present with symptoms specific to branch arteries that have been affected. Diminished perfusion to cerebral vessels may lead to stroke or coma. If intercostal or segmental arteries are affected, paraplegia or quadriplegia may be present. While patients with acute ischemia of the superior mesenteric artery typically have substantial abdominal pain and a poor prognosis, those with malperfusion to the lower extremities may take a while to exhibit symptoms [5].

Signs and symptoms consistent with malperfusion syndrome may be persistent or intermittent due to the dynamic nature of flow obstruction with the mobile intimal flap.

Physical exam findings are often nonspecific and are not sufficiently sensitive to rule out aortic dissection, but it can be useful for raising the index of suspicion for the presence of dissection and the need for emergent intervention [6]. ED physicians were able to correctly suspect aortic dissection in only 65% of cases according to one study [7]. Pulse deficits are present in up to 31% of patients with TBAD and significantly raise the likelihood ratio of aortic dissection (LR 5.7) [3, 6]. The majority of patients (70%) presenting with TBAD are hypertensive (SBP >150 mmHg) [2]. The presence of hypotension is an ominous sign in a patient with dissection.

Prognosis

Once a patient develops an aortic dissection, the usual survival curve is significantly compromised. Although type A dissection is associated with an early mortality rate of up to 50%, in patients with acute TBAD the mortality is 10–12% [8]. More recent studies show all-comer hospital mortality of 8.8% for all acute TBAD [9]. Most of these patients can be managed medically with antihypertensive medical therapy and close follow-up imaging. This cohort of completely uncomplicated type B aortic dissection do relatively well in early hospital stay with early mortality of 1.2–3% [9, 10]. This reduced mortality is mostly due to protocolization, dedicated aortic centers, and improved anti-impulsive management of these patients.

Patients with complicated acute TBAD have a substantially worse prognosis [11]. The early mortality is around 13% across North American medical centers and one-year survival of 81% [12]. Unfortunately, up to 80% of survivors develop aneurysmal dilatation of the false lumen in the follow-up period with intervention required in one-third of cases [13]. IRAD data suggest that about one in four patients with TBAD died at the three-year mark regardless of the mode of therapy [14]. Three-year survival for those treated medically, surgically, and with the endovascular intervention were 77.6%, 82.8%, and 76.2%, respectively [14]. Independent predictors of mortality include aortic diameter >4 cm, a patent false lumen, and partial thrombosis of the false lumen [15].

Diagnostic Imaging

The diagnosis of acute aortic dissection in the emergency department remains a clinical challenge. The classic presentation of dissection includes chest pain, which is the second most common complaint in the emergency department. Of the approximately 4.4 million patients who present annually to the ED for chest pain, only about 2000 have an aortic dissection [6, 16]. By this volume, an ED physician seeing 3000–4000 patients per year would encounter a patient with aortic dissection once every three to four years [16].

The selection of diagnostic imaging depends on several factors, including patient stability, availability of resources, and local expertise. The goals for imaging are to confirm (or rule out) dissection rapidly, to evaluate the extent of the aortic injury, locate intimal tears, confirm the presence of false lumen as well as any associated thrombus formation, assess arterial branch involvement, identify aortic regurgitation and locate any signs of local rupture including pericardial or pleural effusion.

Chest x-ray findings classically associated with aortic dissection include pleural effusion, displaced intimal calcification, abnormal aortic contour, and widened mediastinum. Unfortunately, sensitivity and specificity of chest X-ray for the diagnosis of aortic disease are limited (64% and 86% respectively); thus the presence or absence of these findings does not sufficiently rule out dissection [17]. In 12.4% of patients with aortic dissection, no chest X-ray abnormality was noted [3]. For this reason, a chest X-ray should be avoided in the patient with suspected aortic disease, as this may lead to further delay of definitive imaging.

Definitive imaging is crucial in the workup for aortic dissection. Imaging options available include computed tomography angiography (CTA), transesophageal echocardiography (TEE), aortography, and magnetic resonance angiography (MRA).

Aortography has lost popularity as a diagnostic imaging tool. Currently, angiography is used for diagnosis in <4% of cases [18]. It is associated with numerous disadvantages, including large contrast requirements (1 mg/kg), the time it takes to complete the procedure (up to 2 h), and the usual risks associated with an invasive procedure.

Sensitivity for CTA, TEE, and MRA are similar for the diagnosis of aortic dissection (98–100%). CTA is widely available and offers visualization of the entire aorta. It is the first choice for work up in aortic dissection and can often identify intimal flap location, the extent of branch vessel involvement, and is relatively rapid to perform. Disadvantages include the need for contrast administration and patient transportation to the imaging suite. Due to the static nature of imaging, functional assessment of the aortic valve cannot be performed with CTA.

MRA is not generally recommended as a first-line imaging choice for suspected acute dissection due to the extended duration of the study and the rarity of availability on an emergent basis.

TEE is an acceptable alternative for patients who are hemodynamically unstable and unable to leave the emergency department for alternate imaging [2]. Advantages include the ability to perform echocardiography at the patient bedside and acceptable sensitivity in identifying aortic pathology. TEE is more sensitive in detecting type A pathology than type B (93.5% v 88.1%, respectively) [19].

History of Surgical Versus Medical Management

Morgagni initially described aortic dissection in the 1700s. For two hundred years, although awareness persisted for the disease, treatment options for patients with dissection were limited. Hirst et al. published a case series in 1958 describing 505 patients noting the manifestations, pathologic correlations, and historical aspects to characterize further factors associated with aortic dissection [20]. Until the 1950s, the management of aortic dissection was limited. After the landmark aortic operation by Drs. DeBakey and Cooley in the 1950s, TBAD became a surgically managed condition [21]. During that time, most patients with acute TBAD were offered replacement of the descending thoracic aorta with an operative mortality of 30–40%. In the 1960s, Wheat et al. started research on the effects of anti-impulsive therapy [22]. To further evaluate medical treatments of aortic disease, researchers used a variety of animal models. Dog models were used to assess the effects of the force of contraction (dP/dT) and blood pressure control [23]. Male broad-breasted white turkeys, which are naturally quite prone to aortic dissection, were used to assess the effects of various medications on the elastin and collagen properties of aortic tissue. The turkeys were fed B-aminopropionitrile (BAPN), which would cause medial degeneration through the disruption of collagen cross-links and elastin fibers in the media of the turkey. The beneficial effects of propranolol and hydralazine on aortic elastin and collagen were identified through these models [24]. Through the 1970s, medical management of uncomplicated TBAD became the standard of care as availability of potent beta-blockers increased and comparative mortality to surgical intervention favored a more conservative approach.

Early experience with the thoracic endovascular aortic intervention was initially published in 1988 by Volodos et al. on the intervention of patients with a traumatic aortic aneurysm [25]. In 1991, Juan Parodi published his experience with endovascular intervention for the treatment of an abdominal aortic aneurysm [26]. The following year, Dake et al. published cases of endovascular intervention in the thoracic aorta [27]. Initial stent-grafts were designed using a 24F delivery system, were custom made for each case, and were used predominantly in patients with aortic aneurysm. White and co-workers used physicians-sponsored investigational device exemptions for early evaluation of TEVAR for acute and chronic dissection in the early 1990s [28]. This research laid the foundation for the studies that led to the first indication in the United States for thoracic endografts for patients with malperfusion by the FDA. This allowed Medtronic and Gore to obtain rapid approval for malperfusion indication and was later used to cover additional thoracic indications with the agreement to participate in post-market surveillance for other indications. This led to rapid approval for numerous indications, faster than what would be expected with individual studies. Cook is now doing a post-market study to get the same approvals.

Through the late 1990s, less than ten percent of patients with TBAD were treated with stent-grafts [29]. According to IRAD data in 2000, 20% of patients with type B dissection underwent surgical therapy, 4.3% underwent percutaneous fenestration or stenting [3]. In 2015, 8% underwent surgical intervention, 31% underwent endovascular intervention, and 63% were treated with medication alone [30]. This is in contrast to today's clinical practice, where the overwhelming majority of acute TBAD offered an intervention, undergo aortic stent grafting.

Initial Medical Management

Management options for patients with aortic dissection include medical, surgical, or endovascular interventions. Regardless of the treatment approach considered, initial intervention should be aimed at reducing the propagation of the dissection by decreasing aortic wall stress [31]. This is achieved by controlling blood pressure and left ventricular ejection force (dP/dT). Upon suspicion of aortic dissection in a patient in the ED, the patient should be emergently assessed by the ED provider with an abbreviated history and physical examination including the time of onset, risk factors for aortic dissection, and assessment for findings consistent with aortic dissection. Two large-bore IVs should be established, supplemental oxygen administered, and the patient placed on a cardiac monitor. EKG, portable chest x-ray, and lab work including type and cross are critical if massive transfusion is needed for hemodynamic collapse.

Patients with uncomplicated type B aortic dissection should be admitted to the cardiac intensive care unit with close monitoring including arterial line blood pressure monitoring, frequent neurologic status checks, urine output monitoring, telemetry, supplemental oxygen, and pain control.

Initial management of acute type B aortic dissection
In the emergency department
(1) Establish two large-bore IVs (>18 gauge)
(2) Administer supplemental oxygen
(3) Cardiac monitoring, EKG, chest X-ray
(4) Obtain CBC, chemistry panel, coagulation panel, UA, CK, troponin, d-dimer
(5) Type and cross 10 units packed red blood cells
(6) Early surgery consultation
Imaging
1. Computed tomography angiogram (CTA)
2. Echocardiogram
3. Magnetic resonance angiogram (MRA)
Blood pressure, heart rate, pain management Goals: heart rate < 60 beats/min, systolic blood pressure < 100 mmHg)
1. First line: beta-blockers
a. Esmolol (200–500 mcg/kg IV loading dose) + 25–50 mcg/kg/min infusion (up to 300 mcg/kg/min max dose)
b. Labetalol (20 mg IV bolus) + 0.5–2 mg/min IV infusion (up to 10 mg/min max dose)
2. If hypertension persists: vasodilators
a. Nicardipine (2.5–5 mg/h IV infusion titrated up to max dose 30 mg/r)
3. Pain relief: morphine
Hemodynamically unstable patients
1. Tracheal intubation, mechanical ventilation
2. Blood pressure support with IV fluids, PRBCs if rupture suspected

Studies suggest that 97% of patients with uncomplicated type B aortic dissection will require at least one parenteral antihypertensive during admission [9]. Most patients will require a regimen consisting of multiple antihypertensive medications that require frequent titration to achieve a systolic BP less than 120 mmHg [32]. All patients with type B aortic dissection should be discharged on antihypertensive medications.

First-line antihypertensive therapy includes beta-blockers such as labetalol, esmolol, and metoprolol to reduce left ventricular contraction force (dP/dT) [33].

Adequate hemodynamic stabilization will reduce the risk of progression of dissection and help to reduce the risk of rupture [34]. In patients with contraindication to beta-blockers such as asthma and heart failure, a trial of esmolol may be initiated, the short half-life is typically well tolerated in patients with a history of pulmonary disease. In the event esmolol is not well tolerated, non-dihydropyridine calcium channel blockers can be used as an acceptable alternative [35]. A labetalol is an attractive option for first-line therapy due to the alpha- and beta- characteristics which work to reduce both dP/dT as well as have vasodilatory properties. Caution should be used in using beta-blockers in the presence of significant acute aortic valve insufficiency due to the effects on compensatory mechanisms [2].

These medications also work to prevent reflex tachycardia which can occur with the use of vasodilator medications. In the event of contraindications to beta-blocker usages such as asthma and heart failure, calcium channel blockers can be used as an alternative. Heart rate should be kept below 60 bpm with systolic blood pressure below 120 mmHg [2].

Hydralazine and sodium nitroprusside were used historically for the management of blood pressure, however, are closely associated with reflex tachycardia and increasing left ventricular contractile force (dP/dT), thus should be avoided in patients with dissection. Nicardipine is a vasodilator of choice in patients with dissection. Patients often require multiple antihypertensive medications to achieve the guideline recommendation of <120 mmHg [35].

Pain control includes the use of morphine which also provides a reduction in stress-induced hypertension due to its sedative properties. Poorly controlled pain can lead to a hyperadrenergic state further potentiating the progression of dissection [36].

In the rare event of hypotension, it is crucial to confirm the absence of pseudohypotension as a result of measurement in an extremity with flow compromise. Blood pressure should be measured in both arms and both legs to determine the highest central blood pressure [2]. Fluid resuscitation should be performed with crystalloid, PRBCs, or other colloid solutions.

During hospitalization for the uncomplicated type B dissection patient, continued blood pressure control should be maintained with the goal of SBP between 100–120 mmHg and heart rate <60 bpm [2]. This is most commonly initially achieved through the use of parenteral medications, however during the hospital stay, the patient should be transitioned to oral antihypertensives as a bridge to discharge and long-term blood pressure control. Continued telemetry monitoring and arterial line monitoring are important measures during the patient's stay in the intensive care unit. As the patient stabilizes on oral medications, transfer to a telemetry unit, and subsequently to home is reasonable if there are no signs of end-organ ischemia or malperfusion, blood pressure has been stabilized to goal with oral medications, and repeat imaging is without significant progression of the disease.

Endovascular Repair

Optimal medical therapy remains the standard of care for uncomplicated dissection, however, this strategy fails to prevent long-term aortic-related morbidity and mortality. The paucity of supporting data has created controversy surrounding the optimal treatment strategy for acute type B dissection. Medical therapy has low early mortality in centers experienced in the management of acute aortic syndrome, however, 30% of the patients will require an operation due to enlargement of the chronic dissection within the first five years. Recent data and trends show a paradigm shift favoring early TEVAR in acute type B dissection. TEVAR improves the chance of reverse remodeling of the descending thoracic aorta and therefore reduced the rate of reoperations in the follow-up. TEVAR is a reasonable option for patients with aortic disease, however, some concern remains regarding reintervention rates and aneurysmal dilatation in the setting of dissection.

A meta-analysis was performed of 39 studies involving a total of 609 patients who underwent stent-graft placement for a type B dissection [37]. Procedural success was reported in 98% of patients. Major complications were reported in 11% with the most dreaded neurologic complications in 2.9% of patients. Periprocedural stroke was encountered more frequently than paraplegia (1.9% versus 0.8%). The major complication rate was significantly higher for acute compared with chronic dissection (21.7% versus 9.1%). Minor complications occurred in 2.5%. The rate of complications compared favorably with previous reported surgical series. The in-hospital mortality rate was 5.2%. Thirty-day mortality was 5.3% and was significantly higher for acute compared with chronic dissection (9.8% versus 3.2%) [37].

Outcomes were much better in centers that had performed more than 20 endovascular procedures compared with fewer. This included significantly lower rates of overall complications (7.7 versus 20.9 percent), neurologic complications (1.0 versus 5.7 percent), and 30-day mortality (3.2 versus 8.5 percent). One report evaluated 19 patients with an acute dissection (15 with type B) and an indication for surgery [37]. Complete thrombosis of the false lumen was achieved in 79 percent, and revascularization with a relief of ischemic symptoms occurred in 76 percent of obstructed aortic branch sites. The 30-day mortality rate was 16 percent, and morbidity was 21 percent morbidities included small bowel and renal infarction and lower extremity gangrene [37].

In an IRAD report of 384 type B dissections, 46 (12%) were managed with endovascular stent-grafting [38]. Stenting was only performed for patients who had at least eight weeks of medical management. Inpatient mortality was only in three patients (6.5%). Two-year follow up of 49 patients was performed for patients who underwent stent-graft placement for treatment of acute or chronic type B dissection. Serial computed tomography (CT) studies in the 32 patients with type B aortic dissection showed that, at two years, total occlusion of the false lumen was achieved with acute dissection in 76 percent of patients [39].

ADSORB is a randomized trial that compared outcomes between patients with acute uncomplicated TBAD who were treated with best medical therapy alone ($n = 31$) or medical treatment in addition to TEVAR ($n = 31$) [40]. The 30-day mortality and neurological complication rates were 0% for both groups, but a significantly higher rate of favorable remodeling (complete false lumen thrombosis) was reported at 1 year after stenting (57 vs. 3%, $p < .001$). The study was not powered for mortality or late aortic intervention.

INSTEAD is the larger trial that prospectively randomized patients with uncomplicated chronic TBAD to continuing optimal medical therapy ($n = 68$) or medical therapy in addition to stent-graft placement ($n = 72$) [41].

At 2 years, despite a higher rate of favorable remodeling in the stented group, all-cause and aorta-related mortality were similar between the two groups. There was also no significant difference in the rate of secondary interventions as cross-overs to endovascular repair in the medical therapy group were balanced by stent extensions and access-vessel repairs in the TEVAR group. Long-term analysis at 5 years did, however, demonstrate a significantly higher aorta-specific mortality in medically managed patients than those who underwent elective stenting (19.3 vs. 6.9%, $p = .045$) [41].

INSTEAD, XL was a follow-up study of the subjects enrolled in the INSTEAD trial and continued original analysis for 5 years following the original procedure [42]. Analysis for subjects managed with optimal medical therapy (OMT) and TEVAR ($n = 72$) versus OMT alone ($n = 68$) included all-cause mortality (0% versus 16.9%; $P = 0.0003$), aorta-specific mortality (0% versus 16.9%; $P = 0.0005$), and progression (4.1% versus 28.1%; $P = 0.004$). Stent graft induced false lumen thrombosis at 5 years after TEVAR was associated with both improved survival and less progression of disease in 90.6% of subjects ($P < 0.0001$) [42]. Despite this data, the treatment strategy for acute type B dissection remains controversial. Early treatment has been suggested to positively affect overall reverse aortic remodeling and visceral flow (Fig. 1). High-risk morphologic features including partial thrombosis in false lumen, total aortic diameter > 4 cm, false lumen diameter > 2.2 cm, and refractory pain should be considered

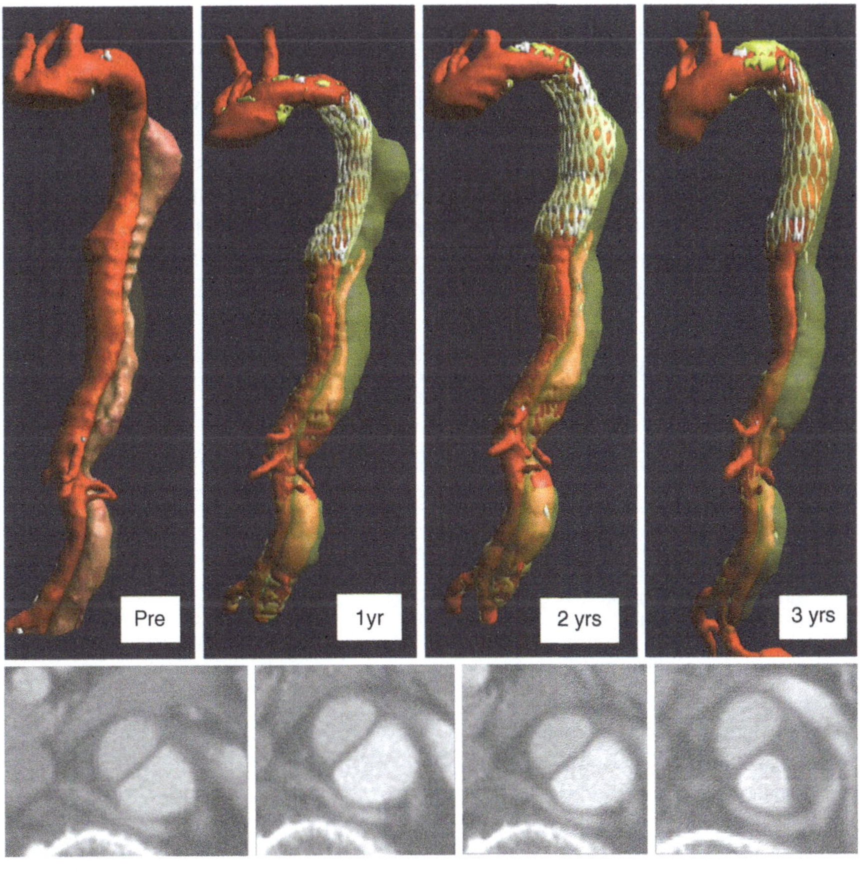

Fig. 1 Three year follow-up imaging on type B dissection following thoracic endovascular aortic repair (TEVAR). Positive aortic remodeling demonstrated in post-TEVAR images with progressive thrombosis of proximal false lumen over time

when evaluating a patient for early TEVAR versus OMT alone. Additionally, given that the benefit associated with early TEVAR is not achieved until years following the intervention as illustrated in the INSTEAD XL findings, patient age and comorbidities should be considered before deciding to proceed with TEVAR (Fig. 2).

Complicated Acute Type B Dissection

Up to 50% of patients with uncomplicated type B dissection will experience sequelae which can include further propagation of dissection either retrograde converting to a type A, or antegrade with risk for malperfusion syndromes. Additionally, aneurysm degeneration and possible rupture can occur during the long-term follow up of these patients [43]. Comorbidities that can be associated with the progression of an uncomplicated dissection to a complicated state include a bicuspid aortic valve, underlying connective tissue disorders (such as Marfan syndrome and Loeys Dietz), aortic coarctation, poorly controlled hypertension, and cocaine abuse [44].

There is an unpredictable variability to blood flow patterns in the dissected aorta, this can lead to spontaneous resolution of malperfusion syndromes in some cases. Dynamic obstruction from the prolapse of intimal flap blocking flow into branch vessels can lead to intermittent signs and symptoms. In the event of a direct extension of dissection into the branch vessel (static obstruction), a more sustained presentation may occur [2]. Additional contributors to the development of malperfusion post-dissection include arterial thrombosis, embolization, compression of branch vessels from false lumen expansion, rupture or leakage of the false lumen into surrounding structures, and distortion of the aortic valve leading to acute aortic valve insufficiency [2].

Aortic Dissection Acuity
Uncomplicated
1. No rupture 2. No malperfusion 3. No high-risk features
High-Risk Features
1. Refractory pain 2. Refractory hypertension 3. Bloody pleural effusion 4. Aortic diameter > 4 cm 5. Radiographic only malperfusion 6. Readmission 7. Entry tear: lesser curve location 8. False lumen diameter > 22 mm
Complicated
1. Rupture 2. Malperfusion

From: Lombardi JV, Hughes GC, Appoo JJ, Bavaria JE, Beck AW, Cambria RP, Charlton-Ouw K, Eslami MH, Kim KM, Leshnower BG, Maldonado T. Society for Vascular Surgery (SVS) and Society of Thoracic Surgeons (STS) reporting standards for type B aortic dissections. The Annals of Thoracic Surgery. 2020 Jan 27.

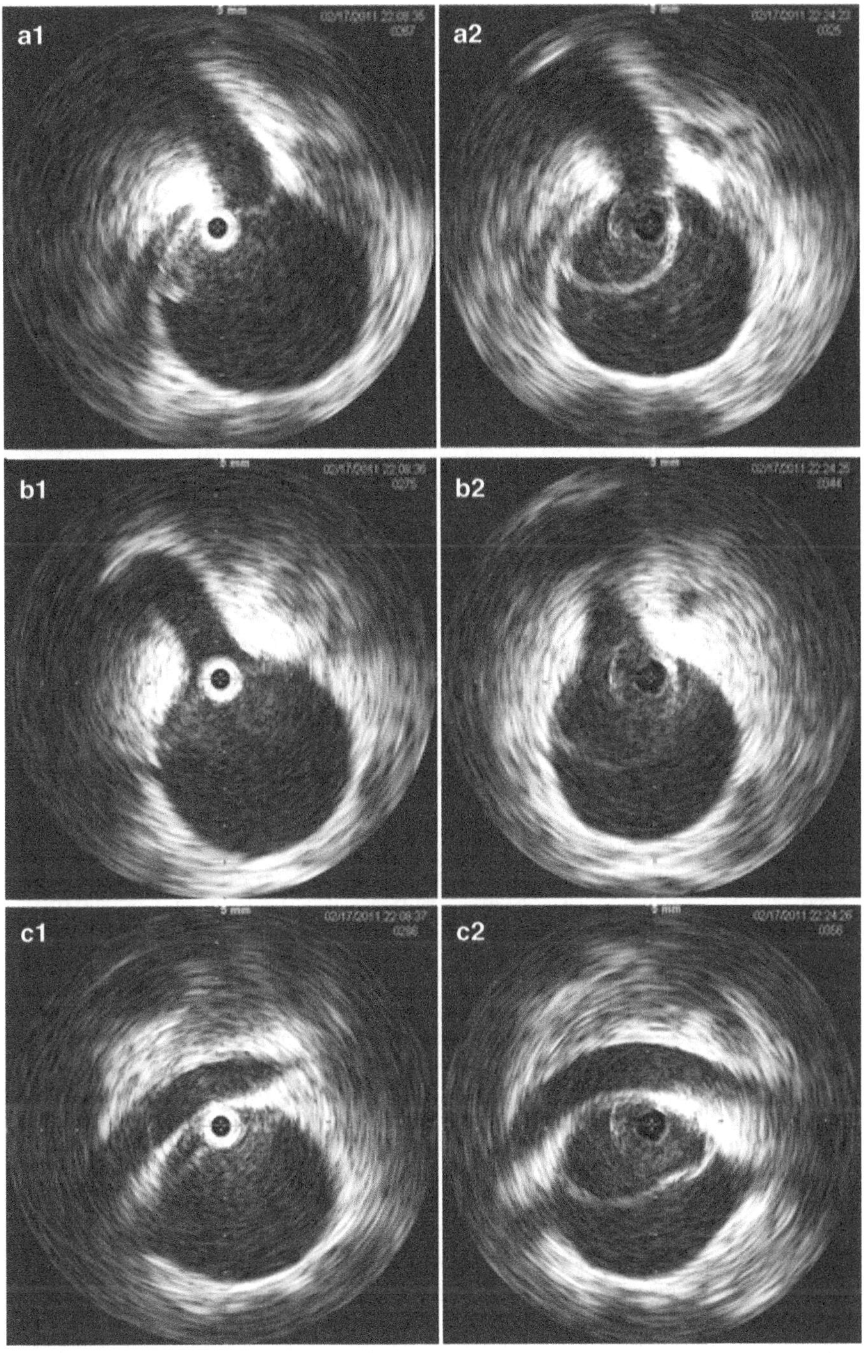

Fig. 2 Pre and post-treatment IVUS images of perivisceral true lumen of uncomplicated TBD dissection. True lumen in very small Celiac (**a1**) SMA (**b1**) and renal (**c1**) arteries, post-treatment the true lumen has dramatically expanded after covering the entry tear with a stent graft (**a2**, **b2**, **c2**)

The presence of malperfusion syndrome is a significant contributor to mortality in patients with type B aortic dissection. The most common cause of death in patients with type B aortic dissection is mesenteric ischemia [2]. Fortunately, mesenteric ischemia is uncommon, presenting in only 3.7% of cases [45].

Endovascular stent grafting has been used as a less invasive alternative to open surgery for the management of type B aortic dissection. The stent-graft is positioned to cover the intimal flap to seal the entry site of the dissection, resulting in thrombosis of the false lumen [46]. With successful coverage of the intimal tear, perfusion is restored in patients with dynamic aortic obstruction in approximately 95% of patients.

Initial repair of the dissection often resolves peripheral ischemia; however additional distal stenting of the aorta or rarely fenestration of the intimal flap may be required to achieve adequate perfusion in cases of persistent peripheral or visceral ischemia.

Despite the favorable aortic remodeling reported after TEVAR in patients with aortic dissection, a review of 1108 patients found that there is the continued growth of the thoracic aorta in 6.6–84% of patients [47]. In a review of 397 patients with TBAD, abdominal aorta growth was reported in 10–54% of cases [47].

Stabilization of the distal flap has been investigated using the PETTICOAT technique (provisional extension to induce complete attachment). In this approach, a proximal endograft is placed in the true lumen, with a bare-metal stent extension distally. With the deployment of the bare metal stent, the aim is to stabilize the distal intimal flap and allow blood flow to the visceral vessels [48]. In one review which investigated outcomes of acute (89 cases) and subacute (54) type B dissection, the PETTICOAT procedure had an overall 30-day mortality rate of 4.9% and a clinical success rate of 90.2% [49]. Early expansion of the true lumen of the thoracic and abdominal aorta was observed; however there was no evidence of improved short and mid-term survival when compared to standard stent-grafting [49].

The Study of Thoracic Aortic Type B Dissection Using Endoluminal Repair (STABLE I) trial is a nonrandomized multicenter prospective study that was performed to evaluate the safety and performance of the Zenith Dissection endovascular stent system. This system is specifically designed for the treatment of dissection and is comprised of a proximal stent-graft with distal bare-metal stent based on the PETTICOAT approach [50]. In this study, 86 patients were enrolled, inclusion criteria included acute phase and non-acute phase patients with TBAD presenting with branch vessel obstruction or compromise, impending rupture, resistant hypertension, persistent pain or symptoms, or rapid aortic growth [50]. During this feasibility study, 30-day mortality was 5.5% for acute patients and 3.2% for nonacute [50]. Kaplan-Meier estimate of freedom from dissection-related mortality at 5 years was 83.9% for acute patients and 90.1% for nonacute patients [50]. False lumen thrombosis was exhibited in 74.1% of acute patients and 58.8% of non-acute patients at 5 years, and a majority of patients experienced stable or reduced thoracic aortic size at 5 years (acute, 65.5%; nonacute, 81.3%) [50].

The STABLE II study pivotal study was a follow up prospective, nonrandomized multicenter study including 73 patients with acute type B aortic dissection again evaluating the Zenith Dissection Endovascular System based on the PETTICOAT procedure. Inclusion criteria were expanded in this trial to include rupture and malperfusion. The primary safety endpoint was freedom from adverse events at 30 days and the primary effectiveness endpoint was the rate of survival at 30 days. The Kaplan-Meier estimate of freedom from all-cause mortality was 80.3% (+/− 4.7%) at one year. One year follow up identified complete or partial thrombosis in 100% of patients at the stent site and 97.4% of the patient within the bare stent region. Thoracic aortic growth >5 mm after one year was observed in 14.9% of patients in the area of the stent-graft, 38.5% of patients within the bare stent site.

In a comparative analysis performed by Sobocinski et al., TEVAR alone was compared to the PETTICOAT technique for the treatment of acute complicated TBAD by use of secondary analyses to compare cohorts from high-volume aortic centers in Europe using TEVAR alone versus the STABLE cohorts [51]. Reintervention rates at one year were similar between the TEVAR and STABLE cohorts (11.1% TEVAR, 12.8% STABLE). Both cohorts exhibited positive thoracic aorta remodeling; however in the STABLE cohort, the investigators observed a statistically significant increase in true lumen volume at the abdominal aorta while the TEVAR group did not. Malperfusion related mortality was statistically lower in the STABLE group versus TEVAR (2.3% vs. 12.2%) [51].

Building on the foundation of the PETTICOAT technique and STABLE I and STABLE II, the concept of STABILISE was introduced. Stent assisted balloon induced disruption and relamination in aortic dissection repair (STABILISE) was first described by Hofferberth et al. in 2014 [52]. In this approach, a stent-graft is used to cover the proximal intimal tear with a bare-metal stent distally, with the added step of serial balloon dilatation to the point of intimal flap disruption to return the dissected intima to the aortic wall [52]. The 30-day mortality rate among the 41 patients treated was 2% with no aortic-related mortality at 12 months. All patients had complete aortic remodeling at the stent graft and bare stent level at follow up, 39% had complete aortic remodeling at the non-stented infrarenal aortoiliac level. Of those who experienced persistent false-lumen flow at the bare-stent level, the aortoiliac diameter remained stable in 92% at one year [53].

Fenestration

Intimal flap fenestration can be performed to equalize pressure between the true and false lumen as well as serving as an alternative to TEVAR in patients who are at high risk for spinal cord ischemia or when the false lumen is perfusing a large number of lumbar or intercostal branch vessels. Fenestration is rarely used in modern practice, and typically reserved for patients with significant peripheral or visceral malperfusion or cases where TEVAR may not be possible such as excessive aortic diameter or intimal tear near crucial branch vessels. Fenestration can be useful for the management of dynamic obstruction; however if a static obstruction is also present, stenting of the branch vessels should also be considered. It is technically demanding, time-consuming, and is associated with significant patient morbidity. The exact relationship of each major branch vessel to the intimal flap and false lumen should be reviewed before the beginning of the procedure. In one study, a 17% early mortality rate was reported after endovascular fenestration with 7% of these due to false lumen rupture and 10% to malperfusion complications [54]. Long term outcomes showed freedom from aortic rupture or repair at 1, 5, and 8 years of 80.2%, 67.7%, and 54.2% [54]. There are various techniques to achieve the fenestration of the dissection flap. Some authors report an approach by puncture through the flap with a wire or needle with the subsequent deployment of an angioplasty balloon to extend the fenestration. Other approaches described include a variety of techniques centered around wire access in the false and true lumen with subsequent downward traction to divide the flap longitudinally. These techniques are associated with significant potential risks, including intimal flap dehiscence as a result of "snag and drag" instead of the desired longitudinal fenestration effect [54].

Open Surgical Repair

Before the advent of TEVAR in the 1990s, open surgical repair provided the only treatment option that offered any meaningful survival. Surgical repair, similar to fenestration, is rarely used in modern practice. Since the advent of TEVAR, the treatment of acute TBAD has shifted to endovascular therapy [55].

The University of Michigan reviewed their outcomes with open or endovascular repair in patients with acute complicated TBAD. While there was statistically no difference between the two cohort's early and late survival, there was a higher rate of mortality, higher ventilation time, use of blood product, and longer hospital stays those patients treated with open repair. Also, the TEVAR were older with more comorbidities [55].

In a retrospective review of the University of Pennsylvania experience from 2002 to 2010, Zeehan et al. reported 77 complicated TBAD treated acutely comparing TEVAR to conventional treatment, including open surgical repair or optimal medical treatment [56]. 45 patients were treated with TEVAR (26 within 24 h of presentation), and 32 patients were in the open surgical repair and optimal medical treatment group. This group included 20 patients undergoing open surgery repair (10 of those within 24 h of presentation); the remainder were treated with medical therapy. In hospital, mortality was 4% in the TEVAR group vs 40% in the group treated with open and medical approaches [56]. Survival at 1, 3, and 5 years for those who underwent TEVAR versus those who underwent open surgical repair was 82%, 79%,79% versus 58%, 54%, 44% [56]. These findings were confounded by lumping open and medical treatment together.

In a series of complicated Type B dissections treated in the acute or subacute phase, Wilkinson showed no significant difference in hospital mortality, late mortality, or freedom from re-intervention [55]. The long term follow-up of the patients treated in the Zeehan series showed the best survival in those treated with TEVAR [56].

A combined retrospective and meta-analysis study showed no long-term survival or reintervention benefit to either open or endovascular repair of acute TBAD [57]. In the setting of chronic Type B dissections, van Bogerjen et al. showed no long-term survival benefit, although the lower re-intervention rate in open compared to endovascular repair [58]. They did note lower operative mortality in the chronic setting as compared to that reported for open repairs in the acute phase [58]. Using a slightly different treatment algorithm treating all complicated Type B with TEVAR and uncomplicated with optimal medical therapy followed by open or endovascular repair for OMT failures, Lou et al. found better long term survival in those patients receiving open repair compared to TEVAR in the chronic phase. Those receiving acute TEVAR fared better than those who underwent TEVAR for chronic dissection [59].

Despite the increased use of endovascular repair, there are still patients for whom open repair may be indicated or required. Those benefiting from open repair include younger patients with connective tissue disorder or patients with anatomic constraints for TEVAR, and as a bail-out for complications of TEVAR in the setting of acute TBAD.

Outpatient Follow Up

Regardless of the treatment approach, more than 60% of those with aortic dissection experience aneurysmal growth within 5 years [60]. In the outpatient setting, continued close surveillance is vital as aortic remodeling continues. Guidelines recommend repeat imaging at 1, 3, 6, and 12 months following the index event, and annually after that [2]. Those with stable findings after 5 years may be followed up in longer intervals. Lifestyle recommendations for the dissection patient should include the avoidance of strenuous lifting or other isometric exercises that increase intrathoracic pressures [2]. Additionally, avoidance of activities that put the patient at risk for sudden deceleration should be discussed. Blood pressure management is an essential factor in the continued stabilization of aortic dissection, patients should be counseled on the importance of following their prescribed regimen, as poorly controlled hypertension can have a disastrous consequence to the dissected aorta.

Future Perspective

Given the suboptimal results of purely medical or surgical therapy in uncomplicated type B AAD, there has been significant interest in the use of TEVAR in this patient cohort. The basis of endovascular therapy is the concept that obliteration and thrombosis of the false lumen may result in improved long-term outcomes and reduce the need for future reoperation. Furthermore, the newer generation of stent-grafts, including ones with a lower profile or with absorbable material are being evaluated.

Once the reverse remodeling after acute TBAD has completed, the stent-graft may become obsolete, and in these cases an absorb stent-graft would be very beneficial in reducing future complications including infection, migration, branch obstruction or retrograde dissection.

References

1. Khoynezhad A, Walot I, Kruse MJ, Rapae T, Donayre CE, White RA. Distribution of intimomedial tears in patients with type B aortic dissection. J Vasc Surg. 2010 Sep 1;52(3):562–8.
2. Hiratzka LF, Bakris GL, Beckman JA, Bersin RM, Carr VF, Casey DE, Eagle KA, Hermann LK, Isselbacher EM, Kazerooni EA, Kouchoukos NT. 2010 ACCF/AHA/AATS/ACR/ASA/SCA/SCAI/SIR/STS/SVM guidelines for the diagnosis and management of patients with thoracic aortic disease. J Am Coll Cardiol. 2010 Apr 6;55(14):e27–129.
3. Hagan PG, Nienaber CA, Isselbacher EM, Bruckman D, Karavite DJ, Russman PL, Evangelista A, Fattori R, Suzuki T, Oh JK, Moore AG. The International Registry of Acute Aortic Dissection (IRAD): new insights into an old disease. JAMA. 2000 Feb 16;283(7):897–903.
4. Januzzi JL, Isselbacher EM, Fattori R, Cooper JV, Smith DE, Fang J, Eagle KA, Mehta RH, Nienaber CA, Pape LA. Characterizing the young patient with aortic dissection: results from the International Registry of Aortic Dissection (IRAD). J Am Coll Cardiol. 2004 Feb 18;43(4):665–9.
5. Khoynezhad A, Rao R, Trento A, Gewertz B. Management of acute type B aortic dissections and acute limb ischemia. J Cardiovasc Surg. 2011 Aug;52(4):507–17.
6. Klompas M. Does this patient have an acute thoracic aortic dissection? JAMA. 2002 May 1;287(17):2262–72.
7. Rosman HS, Patel S, Borzak S, Paone G, Retter K. Quality of history taking in patients with aortic dissection. Chest. 1998 Sep 1;114(3):793–5.
8. Nienaber CA, Eagle KA. Aortic dissection: new frontiers in diagnosis and management: Part I: from etiology to diagnostic strategies. Circulation. 2003 Aug 5;108(5):628–35.
9. Estrera AL, Miller CC, Goodrick J, Porat EE, Achouh PE, Dhareshwar J, Meada R, Azizzadeh A, Safi HJ. Update on outcomes of acute type B aortic dissection. Ann Thorac Surg. 2007 Feb 1;83(2):S842–5.
10. Nienaber CA, Zannetti S, Barbieri B, Kische S, Schareck W, Rehders TC. INvestigation of STEnt grafts in patients with type B Aortic Dissection: design of the INSTEAD trial—a prospective, multicenter, European randomized trial. Am Heart J. 2005 Apr 1;149(4):592–9.
11. Khoynezhad A, Donayre CE, Omari BO, Kopchok GE, Walot I, White RA. Midterm results of endovascular treatment of complicated acute type B aortic dissection. J Thorac Cardiovasc Surg. 2009 Sep 1;138(3):625–31.
12. Khoynezhad A, Donayre CE, White RA. Techniques and results of endovascular management of acute complicated type B aortic dissection in North America. Rev Cardiovasc Med. 2012;13(4):e176–84.
13. Onitsuka S, Akashi H, Tayama K, Okazaki T, Ishihara K, Hiromatsu S, Aoyagi S. Long-term outcome and prognostic predictors of medically treated acute type B aortic dissections. Ann Thorac Surg. 2004 Oct 1;78(4):1268–73.
14. Tsai TT, Evangelista A, Nienaber CA, Trimarchi S, Sechtem U, Fattori R, Myrmel T, Pape L, Cooper JV, Smith DE, Fang J. Long-term survival in patients presenting with type A acute aortic dissection: insights from the International Registry of Acute Aortic Dissection (IRAD). Circulation. 2006 Jul 4;114(1_supplement):I–350.
15. Tsai TT, Evangelista A, Nienaber CA, Myrmel T, Meinhardt G, Cooper JV, Smith DE, Suzuki T, Fattori R, Llovet A, Froehlich J. Partial thrombosis of the false lumen in patients with acute type B aortic dissection. N Engl J Med. 2007 Jul 26;357(4):349–59.

16. Nawar EW, Niska RW, Xu J. National hospital ambulatory medical care survey: 2005 emergency department summary. Adv Data. 2007 Jun 29;386:1–32.
17. von Kodolitsch Y, Nienaber CA, Dieckmann C, Schwartz AG, Hofmann T, Brekenfeld C, Nicolas V, Berger J, Meinertz T. Chest radiography for the diagnosis of acute aortic syndrome. Am J Med. 2004 Jan 15;116(2):73–7.
18. Moore AG, Eagle KA, Bruckman D, Moon BS, Malouf JF, Fattori R, Evangelista A, Isselbacher EM, Suzuki T, Nienaber CA, Gilon D. Choice of computed tomography, transesophageal echocardiography, magnetic resonance imaging, and aortography in acute aortic dissection: International Registry of Acute Aortic Dissection (IRAD). Am J Cardiol. 2002 May 15;89(10):1235–8.
19. Mauban EC, Pyeritz R, Hutchison S, Ota T, Upchurch G, Nour K, Taylor B, Braverman A, Montgomery D, Nienaber C, Isselbacher E. Diagnostic imaging for acute aortic dissection: imaging sensitivity and preference revisited. J Am Coll Cardiol. 2018 Mar 10;71(11 Supplement):A2073.
20. HIRST AE, JOHNS VJ, KIME SW. Dissecting aneurysm of the aorta: a review of 505 cases. Medicine. 1958 Sep 1;37(3):217.
21. De Bakey ME, Beall AC Jr, Cooley DA, Crawford ES, Morris GC Jr, Garrett HE, Howell JF Jr. Dissecting aneurysms of the aorta. Surg Clin N Am. 1966 Aug 1;46(4):1045–55.
22. Wheat MW Jr, Palmer RF, Bartley TD, Seelman RC. Treatment of dissecting aneurysms of the aorta without surgery. J Thorac Cardiovasc Surg. 1965 Sep 1;50(3):364–73.
23. Prokop EK, Palmer RF, Wheat MW Jr. Hydrodynamic forces in dissecting aneurysms: in-vitro studies in a tygon model and in dog aortas. Circ Res. 1970 Jul;27(1):121–7.
24. Simpson CF, Boucek RJ. The B-aminopropionitrile-fed turkey: a model for detecting potential drug action on arterial tissue. Cardiovasc Res. 1983 Jan 1;17(1):26–32.
25. Volodos NL, Karpovich IP, Shekhanin VE, Trojan VI, Iakovenko LF. A case of distant transfemoral enodprosthesis of the thoracic artery using self-fixing synthetic prosthesis in traumatic aneurysm. Grudn Khir. 1988:84–6.
26. Parodi JC, Palmaz JC, Barone HD. Transfemoral intraluminal graft implantation for abdominal aortic aneurysms. Ann Vasc Surg. 1991 Nov 1;5(6):491–9.
27. Dake MD, Miller DC, Semba CP, Mitchell RS, Walker PJ, Liddell RP. Transluminal placement of endovascular stent-grafts for the treatment of descending thoracic aortic aneurysms. N Engl J Med. 1994 Dec 29;331(26):1729–34.
28. White RA, Miller DC, Criado FJ, Dake MD, Diethrich EB, Greenberg RK, Piccolo RS, Siami FS. Multidisciplinary Society for Vascular Surgery Outcomes Committee. Report on the results of thoracic endovascular aortic repair for acute, complicated, type B aortic dissection at 30 days and 1 year from a multidisciplinary subcommittee of the Society for Vascular Surgery Outcomes Committee. J Vasc Surg. 2011 Apr 1;53(4):1082–90.
29. Dake MD, Miller DC, Mitchell RS, Semba CP, Moore KA, Sakai T. The "first generation" of endovascular stent-grafts for patients with aneurysms of the descending thoracic aorta. J Thorac Cardiovasc Surg. 1998 Nov 1;116(5):689–704.
30. Pape LA, Awais M, Woznicki EM, Suzuki T, Trimarchi S, Evangelista A, Myrmel T, Larsen M, Harris KM, Greason K, Di Eusanio M. Presentation, diagnosis, and outcomes of acute aortic dissection: 17-year trends from the International Registry of Acute Aortic Dissection. J Am Coll Cardiol. 2015 Jul 28;66(4):350–8.
31. Tran TP, Khoynezhad A. Current management of type B aortic dissection. Vasc Health Risk Manag. 2009;5:53.
32. Khoynezhad A. Antihypertensive therapy in a patient with type B and de novo type A aortic dissection: case study. Crit Care Clin. 2007 Oct;23:29.
33. Khoynezhad A, Celis R, Hashemzadeh M, Movahed MR, Jalali Z. Current status of thoracic endografting and its adjunctive pharmacology. Expert Opin Pharmacother. 2009 Dec 1;10(17):2871–81.
34. Kodama K, Nishigami K, Sakamoto T, Sawamura T, Hirayama T, Misumi H, Nakao K. Tight heart rate control reduces secondary adverse events in patients with type B acute aortic dissection. Circulation. 2008 Sep 30;118(14_suppl_1):S167–70.

35. Eggebrecht H, Schmermund A, Von Birgelen C, Naber CK, Bartel T, Wenzel RR, Erbel R. Resistant hypertension in patients with chronic aortic dissection. J Hum Hypertens. 2005 Mar;19(3):227–31.
36. Feldman M, Shah M, Elefteriades JA. Medical management of acute type A aortic dissection. Ann Thorac Cardiovasc Surg. 2009 Oct 1;15(5):286–93.
37. Eggebrecht H, Nienaber CA, Neuhäuser M, Baumgart D, Kische S, Schmermund A, Herold U, Rehders TC, Jakob HG, Erbel R. Endovascular stent–graft placement in aortic dissection: a meta-analysis. Eur Heart J. 2006 Feb 1;27(4):489–98.
38. Suzuki T, Mehta RH, Ince H, Nagai R, Sakomura Y, Weber F, Sumiyoshi T, Bossone E, Trimarchi S, Cooper JV, Smith DE. Clinical profiles and outcomes of acute type B aortic dissection in the current era: lessons from the International Registry of Aortic Dissection (IRAD). Circulation. 2003 Sep 9;108(10_suppl_1):II–312.
39. Kusagawa H, Shimono T, Ishida M, Suzuki T, Yasuda F, Yuasa U, Onoda K, Yada I, Hirano T, Takeda K, Kato N. Changes in false lumen after transluminal stent-graft placement in aortic dissections: six years' experience. Circulation 2005 Jun 7;111(22):2951–2957.
40. Brunkwall J, Kasprzak P, Verhoeven E, Heijmen R, Taylor P, Trialists A, et al. Endovascular repair of acute uncomplicated aortic type B dissection promotes aortic remodelling: 1 year results of the ADSORB trial. Eur J Vasc Endovasc Surg. 2014;48(3):285e91.
41. Nienaber CA, Rousseau H, Eggebrecht H. Randomized comparison of strategies for type B aortic dissection: the INvestigation of STEent Grafts in Aortic Dissection (INSTEAD) trial. J Vasc Surg. 2010 May 1;51(5):1321–2.
42. Nienaber CA, Kische S, Rousseau H, Eggebrecht H, Rehders TC, Kundt G, Glass A, Scheinert D, Czerny M, Kleinfeldt T, Zipfel B. Endovascular repair of type B aortic dissection: long-term results of the randomized investigation of stent grafts in aortic dissection trial. Circ Cardiovasc Interv. 2013 Aug;6(4):407–16.
43. Gysi J, Schaffner T, Mohacsi P, Aeschbacher B, Althaus U, Carrel T. Early and late outcome of operated and non-operated acute dissection of the descending aorta. Eur J Cardiothorac Surg. 1997 Jun 1;11(6):1163–70.
44. Roberts WC. Aortic dissection: anatomy, consequences, and causes. Am Heart J. 1981 Feb 1;101(2):195–214.
45. Evangelista A, Isselbacher EM, Bossone E, Gleason TG, Eusanio MD, Sechtem U, Ehrlich MP, Trimarchi S, Braverman AC, Myrmel T, Harris KM. Insights from the International Registry of Acute Aortic Dissection: a 20-year experience of collaborative clinical research. Circulation. 2018 Apr 24;137(17):1846–60.
46. Tsai TT, Nienaber CA, Eagle KA. Acute aortic syndromes. Circulation. 2005 Dec 13;112(24):3802–13.
47. Famularo M, Meyermann K, Lombardi JV. Aneurysmal degeneration of type B aortic dissections after thoracic endovascular aortic repair: a systematic review. J Vasc Surg. 2017 Sep 1;66(3):924–30.
48. Rong D, Ge Y, Liu J, Liu X, Guo W. Combined proximal descending aortic endografting plus distal bare metal stenting (PETTICOAT technique) versus conventional proximal descending aortic stent graft repair for complicated type B aortic dissections. Cochrane Database Syst Rev. 2019;10
49. Bertoglio L, Rinaldi E, Melissano G, Chiesa R. The PETTICOAT concept for endovascular treatment of type B aortic dissection. J Cardiovasc Surg. 2019 Feb;60(1):91–9.
50. Lombardi JV, Cambria RP, Nienaber CA, Chiesa R, Teebken O, Lee A, Mossop P, Bharadwaj P. Prospective multicenter clinical trial (STABLE) on the endovascular treatment of complicated type B aortic dissection using a composite device design. J Vasc Surg. 2012 Mar 1;55(3):629–40.
51. Sobocinski J, Fabre D, Azzaoui, R, Haulon S. TEVAR alone versus the STABLE technique for acute complicated TBAD. Endovascular Today Supplement. 2019 Nov.

52. Hofferberth SC, Nixon IK, Boston RC, McLachlan CS, Mossop PJ. Stent-assisted balloon-induced intimal disruption and relamination in aortic dissection repair: the STABILISE concept. J Thorac Cardiovasc Surg. 2014 Apr 1;147(4):1240–5.
53. Faure EM, El Batti S, Rjeili MA, Julia P, Alsac JM. Mid-term outcomes of stent assisted balloon induced intimal disruption and relamination in aortic dissection repair (STABILISE) in acute type B aortic dissection. Eur J Vasc Endovasc Surg. 2018 Aug 1;56(2):209–15.
54. Patel HJ, Williams DM, Meekov M, Dasika NL, Upchurch GR Jr, Deeb GM. Long-term results of percutaneous management of malperfusion in acute type B aortic dissection: implications for thoracic aortic endovascular repair. J Thorac Cardiovasc Surg. 2009 Aug 1;138(2):300–8.
55. Wilkinson DA, Patel HJ, Williams DM, Dasika NL, Deeb GM. Early open and endovascular thoracic aortic repair for complicated type B aortic dissection. Ann Thorac Surg. 2013 Jul 1;96(1):23–30.
56. Zeeshan A, Woo EY, Bavaria JE, Fairman RM, Desai ND, Pochettino A, Szeto WY. Thoracic endovascular aortic repair for acute complicated type B aortic dissection: superiority relative to conventional open surgical and medical therapy. J Thorac Cardiovasc Surg. 2010;140(6 Suppl):S109–15.
57. Zhu Y, Wang B, Meng Q, Liu J, Zhai S, He J. Long-term efficacy of endovascular vs open surgical repair for complicated type-B aortic dissection: a single-center retrospective study and meta-analysis. Braz J Med Biol Res. 2016;49(6).
58. van Bogerijen GH, Patel HJ, Williams DM, Yang B, Dasika NL, Eliason JL, Deeb GM. Propensity adjusted analysis of open and endovascular thoracic aortic repair for chronic type B dissection: a twenty-year evaluation. Ann Thorac Surg. 2015 Apr 1;99(4):1260–6.
59. Lou X, Chen EP, Duwayri YM, Veeraswamy RK, Jordan WD Jr, Zehner CA, Leshnower BG. The impact of thoracic endovascular aortic repair on long-term survival in type B aortic dissection. Ann Thorac Surg. 2018 Jan 1;105(1):31–8.
60. Fattori R, Cao P, De Rango P, Czerny M, Evangelista A, Nienaber C, Rousseau H, Schepens M. Interdisciplinary expert consensus document on management of type B aortic dissection. J Am Coll Cardiol. 2013 Apr 23;61(16):1661–78.

Subacute and Chronic Type A Aortic Dissection

Lars G. Svensson

Current anatomic descriptions of aortic dissection categorize dissection based on where the original intimal tear is located (DeBakey classification) or whether the ascending aorta is involved (Stanford classification). Following a study of aortic dissection of 690 patients surgically treated by E Stanley Crawford et al. [1], subacute and chronic aortic dissections were defined as dissections operated on between two and six weeks and beyond six weeks after onset of symptoms, respectively [1–5]. Further, when dealing with subacute and chronic aortic dissection, it is worthwhile to recall classes of aortic dissection, particularly for intramural hematomas [6]. This chapter examines how course of treatment for aortic dissection is determined based on class, comorbidities, and time interval from dissection.

Our previous study [6] categorizing aortic dissection into subclasses was based on the appearance of the aortic dissection, apart from the well-known definitions of extent from DeBakey and Stanford (Fig. 1) [4, 5, 7]. Class I tears are associated with classic aortic dissection and two classical lumens for extent DeBakey I or II (recall Stanford A includes the ascending aorta, Stanford B does not). Class II tears are intramural hematomas. While some 15% are classified as such by computed tomography (CT) or magnetic resonance imaging (MRI), in actuality at postmortem evaluation, only 5% have no tear. We rarely see tears that do not involve an intimal tear; usually, if carefully looked for, even tears of 1–2 mm in diameter can be found or in the descending aorta with retrograde dissection or, more rarely, from the abdominal aorta. Of note, some institutions, particularly with older patients, treat intramural Class II aortic dissection conservatively and then perform surgery in the chronic phase, if needed. Class III tears involve limited areas of dissection with exposure of the tunica media or middle layer but without extensive dissection of the intimal flap that separates the false from the true lumen or undermining of the tunica intima, or

L. G. Svensson (✉)
Department of Thoracic and Cardiovascular Surgery, Heart, Vascular, and Thoracic Institute, Cleveland Clinic, Cleveland, OH, USA
e-mail: svenssl@ccf.org

J. S. Coselli et al. (eds.), *Aortic Dissection and Acute Aortic Syndromes*,
https://doi.org/10.1007/978-3-030-66668-2_28

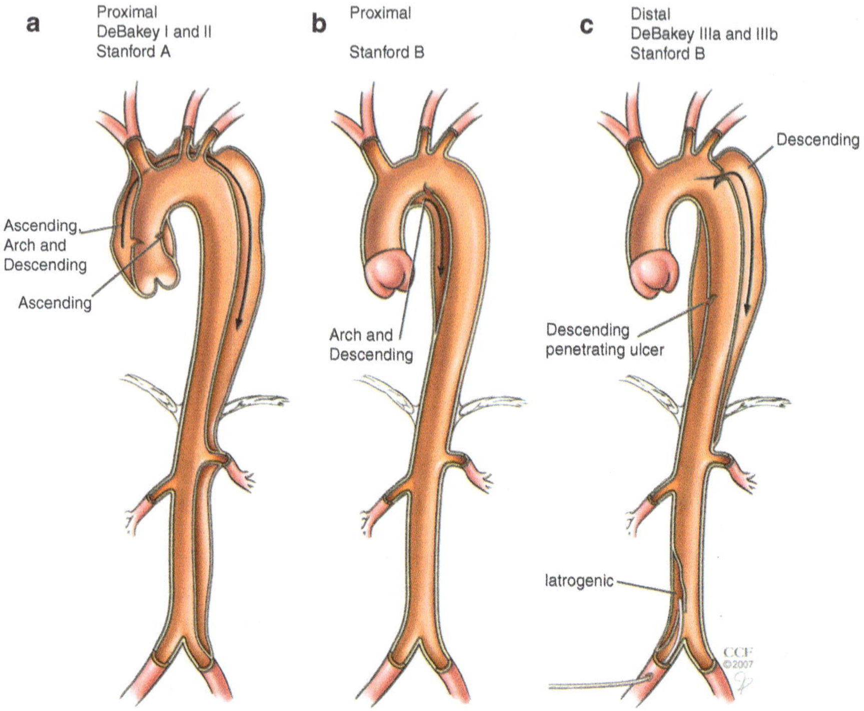

Fig. 1 (**a**) Proximal, DeBakey I and II, Stanford A. (**b**) Proximal, Stanford B. (**c**) Distal, DeBakey IIIa and IIIb, Stanford B. Reprinted from Svensson LG. Limited intimal aorta tears: Royalty torn asunder, and a nation was created, J Am Coll Cardiol. 2019;71:2786–2789. Copyright © 2019, with permission from Elsevier [7]

inner layer (Fig. 2) [7]. In earlier studies [6, 7], we described the difficulty in identifying limited Class III aortic dissection by imaging, noting that angiography of the ascending aorta and root from multiple angles shows the bulge. Subsequently, the Stanford group [7, 8] indicated that 4.8% of patients in their series had this Class III dissection. Aortic dissections in these patients are often missed and present in the subacute phase, for example, because of pericardial effusion or progression of dissection diagnosed in retrospect or at the time of frank aortic rupture. Class IV tears are penetrating ulcers that appear to have a different etiology, often associated with calcification of the aortic wall, frequently with infection. While they may be seen in the ascending aorta, more often, class IV tears are seen in the lesser curve of the aortic arch, proximal descending thoracic aorta, or opposite the visceral arteries. Of note, the natural history is often much more lethal than expected. Based on postmortem examinations done by the author many years ago, the plane of dissection is often between the tunica media and tunica adventitia, and hence, rupture occurs or patients present with large pleural effusions more often. Class V tears are iatrogenic dissections, typically seen after an attempted catheterization of the coronary ostia or after transcatheter aortic valve replacement.

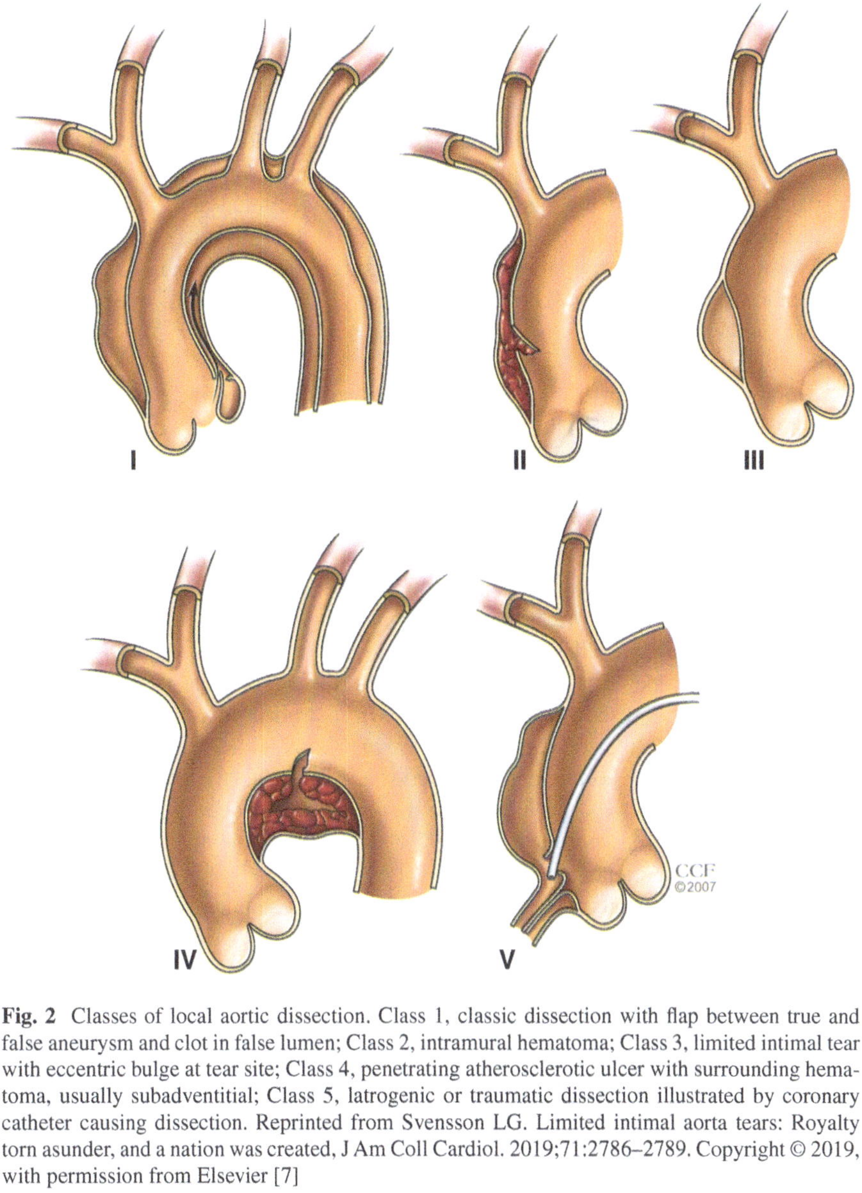

Fig. 2 Classes of local aortic dissection. Class 1, classic dissection with flap between true and false aneurysm and clot in false lumen; Class 2, intramural hematoma; Class 3, limited intimal tear with eccentric bulge at tear site; Class 4, penetrating atherosclerotic ulcer with surrounding hematoma, usually subadventitial; Class 5, Iatrogenic or traumatic dissection illustrated by coronary catheter causing dissection. Reprinted from Svensson LG. Limited intimal aorta tears: Royalty torn asunder, and a nation was created, J Am Coll Cardiol. 2019;71:2786–2789. Copyright © 2019, with permission from Elsevier [7]

Because not all patients with acute or chronic dissections are symptomatic, such as patients with Marfan syndrome, and the interval from dissection may be unknown, the question then becomes, do all subacute dissections or chronic dissections require surgical intervention? E Stanley Crawford, MD, believed that all Type A Class I aortic dissections, even if not dilated, should be treated surgically unless other serious comorbidities precluded surgery. We have followed that advice, particularly as it is not unusual to find healed tears with superimposed new acute dissections, particularly for Class III tears.

As more patients with Class II intramural hematomas are treated conservatively, including elderly patients or patients with diabetes, and many may resolve with the appearance of two lumens, when should these patients undergo surgery? Our general advice has been to operate if there are complications, like stroke perhaps related to platelet/thrombi or if the size exceeds the cross-sectional area to height ratio, exceeding a ratio of 10 [9, 10].

With modern imaging, it has become increasingly rare to see patients with Type A chronic Class I tears who have not had surgery. Nevertheless, in a series of 151 patients with Marfan syndrome, one patient was surgery-free for 27 years after a Type A dissection, a distinct outlier [11].

In emergency and urgent Type A aortic dissections, the priority is to save the patient's life and deal with a definitive procedure and the consequences of the aortic dissection later, if needed. Clearly, for emergency and urgent operations, acute dissection outcomes are not as positive. Our mortality rate of 595 patients with acute dissection was 8.1% and stroke risk was 7.6% following ascending/hemi-arch repairs; for total arch replacements, mortality and stroke were 9.7% and 8.4%, respectively, as reported at the 2018 American Association for Thoracic Surgery meeting on whether mortality could be reduced to less than 5% [12]. This was supported by a more detailed analysis [13] of our data, although the risks are higher in an analysis of STS data [14].

The definitive operations in these two time-related (subacute or chronic) subtypes should thus be used for dilated aortas without aortic dissection. Hence, for larger roots with trileaflet valves, an aortic valve reimplantation and replacement of the root and ascending aorta should be used if needed [15]. In our current series of over 1000 reimplantations, we have done this operation frequently for subacute or chronic dissection with no deaths and 97% overall freedom from reoperation at 10 years [15]. For patients with bicuspid valves, the procedure is chosen as appropriate for each individual case. For example, procedures can involve reimplantation, the inclusion technique type of remodeling, simple tricuspid valve repair, or ascending arch with separate tube graft replacement [16]. In some patients, the root can be left alone and only the ascending aorta and arch replaced [17]. How the arch and greater vessels are dealt with is a matter of getting the most durable repair, depending also if connective tissue disorder is present in the patient. An ascending aorta tube graft is all that is needed for many classic DeBakey Type 2 extent dissections. For most patients, a total arch with an elephant trunk procedure [18], even if prophylactic for a non dilated descending aorta [19], is the procedure of choice for more extensive dissections (DeBakey Type 1). If the patient has a connective tissue disorder, especially if young, the best option is an elephant trunk procedure distally. In this case, separate tube grafts for the innominate artery or separate right subclavian and right carotid artery with another tube graft to the left carotid artery, with or without grafting of the left subclavian artery are key depending on the distal elephant trunk anastomosis site.

For brain protection, key methods are cooling to a nasopharyngeal temperature below 20°C, CO_2 field flooding at 10 L/min, right subclavian artery perfusion, centrifugal pump with white cell filtration, steep Trendelenburg position, and meticulous de-airing of CO_2 from the arch by antegrade perfusion from the right subclavian artery. In our recent prospective, randomized trial of total arch replacements, there was no difference between antegrade and retrograde brain perfusion [20]; if circulatory arrest time is expected to be less than 30 minutes, neither is used based on our findings that risk of stroke increases after 40 minutes [21]. In the above-mentioned prospective, randomized trial of total arch replacements, 30-day mortality was 0.8% and stroke was also 0.8%, despite 39% being reoperations and 61% having elephant trunk procedures [20].

The management of patients with chronic Type A aortic dissections after previous repairs should be similar to those who have not had surgery for subacute or chronic dissection, with the exception of chest entry and perhaps valve reimplantation. Hence, the priority is definitive repair of the ascending aorta and arch. While some programs have chosen to treat a dilated descending thoracic aorta that is dissected by dealing with the enlarged descending segment first, our preference has been to do a total arch with elephant trunk procedure and then a second-stage descending aortic repair [18]. The root is treated as needed.

For chest re-entry, our preference is to place the patient on cardiopulmonary bypass using a side graft on the right subclavian artery and cannulating the right femoral vein with a venous cannula threaded into the right atrium with transesophageal echocardiography [22]. The patient is opened on pump and given lidocaine and atropine to delay fibrillation when cooling. For severe aortic valve regurgitation, a percutaneous retrograde cardioplegic cannula is placed by anesthesia to allow for arresting the heart until antegrade cardioplegia can be given.

In summary, because the management of subacute and chronic aortic dissection is typically completed by elective surgery, a definitive aortic operation should be performed as often as possible so that there is no need for another operation via median sternotomy [23].

Author Disclosures
The author declares no conflicts of interest.

Funding
The study was funded in part by the Delos M. Cosgrove, MD, Chair for Heart Disease Research.

References

1. Svensson LG, Crawford ES, Hess KR, Coselli JS, Safi HJ. Dissection of the aorta and dissecting aortic aneurysms: improving early and long-term surgical results. Circulation. 1990;82(suppl IV):IV-24–IV-48.
2. Crawford ES, Svensson LG, Coselli JS, Safi HJ, Hess KR. Aortic dissection and dissecting aortic aneurysms. Ann Surg. 1988;208:254–73.
3. Svensson LG, Crawford ES. Aortic dissection and aortic aneurysm surgery, II: clinical observations, experimental investigations, and statistical analyses. Curr Probl Surg. 1992;29:917–22.

4. Svensson LG, Adams DH, Bonow RO, Kouchoukos NT, Miller DC, O'Gara PT, Shahian DM, Schaff HV, Akins CW, Bavaria JE, Blackstone EH, David TE, Desai ND, Dewey TM, D'Agostino RS, Gleason TG, Harrington KB, Kodali S, Kapadia S, Leon MB, Lima B, Lytle BW, Mack MJ, Reardon M, Reece TB, Reiss GR, Roselli EE, Smith CR, Thourani VH, Tuzcu EM, Webb J, Williams MR. Aortic valve and ascending aorta guidelines for management and quality measures. Ann Thorac Surg. 2013;95(6 Suppl):S1–66.
5. Hiratzka LF, Bakris GL, Beckman JA, Bersin RM, Carr VF, Casey DE Jr, Eagle KA, Hermann LK, Isselbacher EM, Kazerooni EA, Kouchoukos NT, Lytle BW, Milewicz DM, Reich DL, Sen S, Shinn JA, Svensson LG, Williams DM, American College of Cardiology Foundation; American Heart Association Task Force on Practice Guidelines; American Association for Thoracic Surgery; American College of Radiology; American Stroke Association; Society of Cardiovascular Anesthesiologists; Society for Cardiovascular Angiography and Interventions; Society of Interventional Radiology; Society of Thoracic Surgeons; Society for Vascular Medicine. 2010 ACCF/AHA/AATS/ACR/ASA/SCA/SCAI/SIR/STS/SVM guidelines for the diagnosis and management of patients with thoracic aortic disease: executive summary. A report of the American College of Cardiology Foundation/American Heart Association Task Force on Practice Guidelines, American Association for Thoracic Surgery, American College of Radiology, American Stroke Association, Society of Cardiovascular Anesthesiologists, Society for Cardiovascular Angiography and Interventions, Society of Interventional Radiology, Society of Thoracic Surgeons, and Society for Vascular Medicine. Catheter Cardiovasc Interv. 2010;76:E43–86.
6. Svensson LG, Labib SB, Eisenhauer AC, Butterly JR. Intimal tear without hematoma: an important variant of aortic dissection that can elude current imaging techniques. Circulation. 1999;99:1331–6.
7. Svensson LG. Limited intimal aorta tears: Royalty torn asunder, and a nation was created. J Am Coll Cardiol. 2019;71:2786–9.
8. Chin AS, Willemink MJ, Kino A, Hinostroza V, Sailer AM, Fischbein MP, Mitchell RS, Berry GJ, Miller DC, Fleischmann D. Acute limited intimal tears of the thoracic aorta. J Am Coll Cardiol. 2018;71:2773–85.
9. Svensson LG, Kim K-H, Lytle BW, Cosgrove DM. Relationship of aortic cross-sectional area to height ratio and the risk of aortic dissection in patients with bicuspid aortic valves. J Thorac Cardiovasc Surg. 2003;126:892–3.
10. Masri A, Kalahasti V, Svensson LG, Roselli EE, Johnston D, Hammer D, Schoenhagen P, Griffin BP, Desai MY. Aortic cross-sectional area/height ratio and outcomes in patients with a trileaflet aortic valve and a dilated aorta. Circulation. 2016;134:1724–37.
11. Svensson LG, Crawford ES, Coselli JS, Safi HJ, Hess KR. Impact of cardiovascular operation on survival in the Marfan patient. Circulation. 1989;80(suppl I):I-233–I-242.
12. Svensson LG. How to repair an uncomplicated Type A dissection with <5% mortality. Presented at the American Association for Thoracic Surgery 98th Annual Meeting. April 29–May 1, 2018; San Diego, CA.
13. Rosinski BF, Idrees JJ, Roselli EE, Germano E, Pasadyn SR, Lowry AM, Blackstone EH, Johnston DR, Soltesz EG, Navia JL, Desai MY, Mick SL, Bakaeen FG, Svensson LG. Cannulation strategies in acute type A dissection repair: A systematic axillary artery approach. J Thorac Cardiovasc Surg. 2019;158:647–659.e5.
14. Ghoreishi M, Sundt TM, Cameron DE, Holmes SD, Roselli EE, Pasrija C, Gammie JS, Patel HJ, Bavaria JE, Svensson LG, Taylor BS. Factors associated with acute stroke after type A aortic dissection repair: an analysis of the Society of Thoracic Surgeons National Adult Cardiac Surgery Database. J Thorac Cardiovasc Surg. 2020 Jun;159(6):2143–2154.e3.
15. Svensson LG. Root reimplantation with leaflet repair. Semin Thorac Cardiovasc Surg. 2019;31:153–4.
16. Zeeshan A, Idrees JJ, Johnston DR, Rajeswaran J, Roselli EE, Soltesz EG, Gillinov AM, Griffin B, Grimm R, Hammer DF, Pettersson GB, Blackstone EH, Sabik JF 3rd, Svensson

LG. Durability of aortic valve cusp repair with and without annular support. Ann Thorac Surg. 2018;105:739–48.
17. Svensson LG, Al Kindi AH, Vivacqua A, Pettersson GB, Gillinov AM, Mihaljevic T, Roselli EE, Sabik JF 3rd, Griffin B, Hammer DF, Rodriguez L, Williams SJ, Blackstone EH, Lytle BW. Long-term durability of bicuspid aortic valve repair. Ann Thorac Surg 2014;97:1539–1547; discussion 1548.
18. Svensson LG, Rushing GD, Valenzuela ES, Rafael AE, Batizy LH, Blackstone EH, Roselli EE, Gillinov AM, Sabik JF 3rd, Lytle BW. Modifications, classification, and outcomes of elephant-trunk procedures. Ann Thorac Surg. 2013;96:548–58.
19. Idrees JJ, Roselli EE, Wojnarski CM, Feng K, Aftab M, Johnston DR, Soltesz EG, Sabik JF 3rd, Svensson LG. Prophylactic stage 1 elephant trunk for moderately dilated descending aorta in patients with predominantly proximal disease. J Thorac Cardiovasc Surg. 2015;150:1150–5.
20. Svensson LG, Blackstone EH, Apperson-Hansen C, Ruggieri PM, Ainkaran P, Naugle RI, Lima B, Roselli EE, Cooper M, Somogyi D, Tuzcu EM, Kapadia S, Clair DG, Sabik JF 3rd, Lytle BW. Implications from neurologic assessment of brain protection for total arch replacement from a randomized trial. J Thorac Cardiovasc Surg. 2015;150:1140–7.e11.
21. Svensson LG, Crawford ES, Hess KR, Coselli JS, Raskin S, Shenaq SA, Safi HJ. Deep hypothermia with circulatory arrest. Determinants of stroke and early mortality in 656 patients. J Thorac Cardiovasc Surg 1993;106:19–28; discussion 28–31.
22. Svensson LG, Blackstone EH, Rajeswaran J, Sabik JF 3rd, Lytle BW, Gonzalez-Stawinski G, Varvitsiotis P, Banbury MK, McCarthy PM, Pettersson GB, Cosgrove DM. Does the arterial cannulation site for circulatory arrest influence stroke risk? Ann Thorac Surg. 2004;78:1274–84. discussion 1274-1284
23. Svensson LG. Are we there yet? Emerging milestones in aortic dissection care. J Am Heart Assoc. 2019;8:e012402.

Management of Chronic Descending Thoracic and Thoracoabdominal Dissection and Aneurysm - Stent Grafting, Debranching

Roland Assi and Wilson Y. Szeto

Introduction

In the late 1990's, sentinel reports demonstrated the safety and feasibility of endovascular stent-grafting for the management of acute type B aortic dissection (ATBAD) [1, 2]. Over the following decade, endovascular repair replaced open surgery as the treatment of choice of complicated acute type B aortic dissection due to the superior perioperative survival [3–7]. Medical management remains the treatment of choice for uncomplicated ATBAD. However, in certain uncomplicated ATBAD cases, endovascular repair in addition to optimal medical therapy (OMT) might have a role to improve long-term survival and favor late aortic reverse remodeling by achieving early false lumen thrombosis [8, 9].

In chronic type B aortic dissection (CTBAD), OMT is the mainstay of therapy for non-aneurysmal and asymptomatic cases. Open surgical repair is indicated for aneurysms that reach operative threshold or in the presence of symptoms or complications. OMT includes blood pressure control and anti-impulse therapy with beta blocking agents, the use of statins to stabilize the endothelial layer, and smoking cessation among other cardiovascular risk profile interventions. The endovascular treatment of chronic type B aortic dissection (CTBAD) continues, however, to present challenges to the surgeon. Conceptually, the treatment strategy is centered around the principle of coverage of entry tears and all degenerative aortic segments. Technically, this concept translates into difficulty finding distal landing zones, complexity of reperfusing visceral branches originating from the false lumen, and the

R. Assi
Division of Cardiac Surgery, Department of Surgery, Yale University, New Haven, CT, USA
e-mail: roland.assi@yale.edu

W. Y. Szeto (✉)
Division of Cardiovascular Surgery, Department of Surgery, University of Pennsylvania, Philadelphia, PA, USA
e-mail: wilson.szeto@pennmedicine.upenn.edu

J. S. Coselli et al. (eds.), *Aortic Dissection and Acute Aortic Syndromes*,
https://doi.org/10.1007/978-3-030-66668-2_29

stiffness of the intimal flap that precludes re-expansion of the true lumen. In the remainder of this chapter we explore the technical success, challenges and outcomes of endovascular repair of CTBAD.

Goals of Therapy and Defining CTBAD Disease Spectrum

Based on data from the International Registry of Acute Aortic Dissection (IRAD), 1 out of 4 patients with ATBAD surviving to hospital discharge were deceased at 3 years (data from 1996 to 2003) [10]. Risk factors for adverse outcomes were non-treatment specific and included female gender, a history of prior aortic aneurysm, a history of atherosclerosis, in-hospital renal failure, pleural effusion on chest radiograph, and in-hospital hypotension/shock. The primary therapeutic goal is to alter the natural history of CTBAD and improve long term survival. In ATBAD, TEVAR is a safe and technically successful in the vast majority of cases; it is now considered the standard of care. But what about TEVAR in the chronic phase?

The role of TEVAR in CTBAD remains somewhat controversial.

"Chronic" is not well defined. It appears that most studies consider any dissection older than 2 weeks as chronic. This would include a wide variety of dissected aortas in various stages of remodeling. The intimal flap in a dissected aorta of 2 weeks is much more flexible than a thickened calcified septum of many years. A relatively recent dissection in an aneurysmal aorta behaves very differently from an old dissected aorta that degenerated into a large complex aneurysm.

For the late chronic dissecting aneurysms of the aorta, the technical challenges are related to the characteristics of the degenerated aorta. The stiffness of the intimal flap may preclude true lumen expansion and create a very narrow space for wire and catheter navigation. The presence of multiple distal re-entry tears makes it difficult to achieve complete coverage and creates channels for retrograde filling of the false lumen. In addition, the deployment of a stent-graft in a small true lumen against a rigid dissecting flap may create new tears, known as stent-induced new entry tears (SINE), which could be devastating. Another challenge is encountered when one or more visceral branches are originating from the false lumen. Rapid or progressive occlusion of the false lumen by the stent-graft would result in new end-organ malperfusion. Pre-operative planning for TEVAR in a chronically dissected aorta requires careful consideration of the above-mentioned technical barriers.

TEVAR Feasibility

With the understanding that CTBAD includes a wide spectrum of progressive aortic pathology, we now have growing body of data on the feasibility of TEVAR in CTBAD from clinical trials and real-world experience.

In a meta-analysis of 17 reports of 567 patients (mostly retrospective cohorts) who underwent TEVAR for CTBAD between 1994 and 2009, technical success rate was 89.9% (range 77.6–100%) with a re-intervention rate ranging between 0 and 60%. The data was very variable in between studies and most likely represented early experience with TEVAR for CTBAD. The type and brand of stent-grafts used were also variable. It is remarkable, however, that perioperative stroke and spinal cord injury were only 0.82% (range 0–6.7%) and 0.43% (range 0–2.8%), respectively [11].

In a prospective comparative study of TEVAR (208 patients) vs OMT (95 patients) from 4 centers in China between 2007 and 2010, technical success rate was 100% and there was no index hospitalization mortality in either groups. The rate of type I endoleak was 12%, paraplegia 0.9% and retrograde type A dissection 0.9% [12].

In a report from the Vascular Quality Initiative Registry, 125 patients underwent TEVAR for CTBAD between 2010 and 2015. Technical success rate was 98.4%, in-hospital mortality was 2.4%, stroke 0.8% and spinal cord ischemia 2.4% [13].

In the widely cited European INSTEAD trial randomizing 140 CTBAD patients to elective TEVAR with OMT vs OMT only between 2003 and 2005, technical success was 95.7% and there was no operative mortality. Stroke was 1.5% and spinal cord injury 2.9% [14].

Other studies from smaller series reported technical success between 96% and 100%, operative mortality between 0% and 5%, stroke rate between 0% and 1.3%, and no spinal cord injury [15, 16].

Based on the data above, it is reasonable to conclude that in selected patients with CTBAD, TEVAR is feasible and can be accomplished with high success rate and acceptable operative morbidity and mortality.

Effect on Late Aortic Reverse Remodeling and Survival Benefit

The effect on aortic reverse remodeling and late survival is difficult to assess due in part to the lack of large databases with long term follow-up and the variable definition of aortic reverse remodeling. In general, the desired TEVAR effect is the sustainable reduction of the total aortic size with preferential true lumen perfusion, eliminating the risk of rupture or malperfusion. This is usually accomplished by completely eliminating blood flow through the false lumen whether it is origination from intimal primary and re-entry tears or from false lumen branches (type II endoleak). To achieve this goal, the initial approach is usually a descending thoracic aorta (DTA) stent-graft to cover all primary tears, with the hope of inducing reverse remodeling in the stented aorta and the downstream visceral aorta. Multiple re-interventions and distal stent-graft extensions may be required and lifelong surveillance is mandatory. Conceptually, the assumption is that aortic reverse remodeling would translate into late survival benefit.

In the INSTEAD trial, there was no survival benefit at 2 years with TEVAR despite significant rate of complete false lumen thrombosis (91.3%) and larger true lumen compared to the OMT group [14]. The survival advantage was however demonstrated in the follow-up INSTEAD-XL trial. At 5 years, all end-points were superior in the TEVAR group compared with the OMT group. All-cause mortality was 11.1% vs 19.3%, aorta-specific mortality was 6.9% vs 19.3%, and progression was 27% vs 46.1%. An important finding was that survival and reverse remodeling were associated with stent graft induced false lumen thrombosis in 90.6% of cases [9].

In the Chinese multicenter comparative study, survival at 2 and 4 years did not differ between the TEVAR and OMT groups; however, freedom from aorta-related death at 2 and 4 years was higher in the TEVAR vs OMT groups (91.6% and 88.1% vs 82.8% and 73.8%). Reverse remodeling of the thoracic aorta occurred in 88.7% in the TEVAR group compared to only 11.8% in the OMT group. This effect was not seen in the untreated abdominal aorta; the aorta continued to increase in diameter similarly in both groups (1 mm/year), likely caused by distal re-entry sites [12].

In a study from the University of Pennsylvania that included 48 patients who underwent TEVAR for CTBAD between 2005 and 2015, 60.4% of patients failed to show regression of aortic size of the DTA at 1 year. Predictors of poor late aortic reverse remodeling included increasing number of visceral vessels off the false lumen, maximum preoperative aortic size, and location of the primary tear on the greater curve [17].

Other studies reported variable degrees of aortic reverse remodeling in the short and mid-terms. In general, the true lumen tends to expand in most cases while the false lumen regresses depending on the presence of distal re-entry tears [18–20]. Distal re-entry tears are probably underdiagnosed because they are not easily detectable on traditional early arterial phase CT angiograms; delayed-phase imaging is required to confirm that no entry tear is left behind [21, 22].

In summary, TEVAR is successful in inducing reverse aortic remodeling at a much higher rate than OMT, particularly when false lumen flow is completely interrupted. Late survival data is not available for large numbers of patients, but conceptually it appears that at least aorta-related deaths could be prevented when reverse aortic remodeling is sustained.

Perioperative Management

a. Preoperative evaluation

   Evaluation of patients with CTBAD includes a complete cardiovascular and neurologic examination and routine blood tests to check organ function, particularly renal. Echocardiography is generally helpful and any myocardial functional abnormalities should be evaluated with a stress test and coronary catheterization when indicated. Significant rapid hemodynamic changes may occur during the procedure and may induce myocardial demand ischemia. Another important element is a focused family history to rule out hereditary aortopathies. The most important diagnostic test is a CT angiogram with early and delayed arterial phases to determine aortic anatomy and suitability for TEVAR.

b. Spinal cord injury (SCI) prevention

   The role of spinal cord drainage and avoidance of perioperative hypotension has been demonstrated repeatedly in large studies of open thoracoabdominal aortic repair [23, 24]. Practices vary widely between centers, but in general the same considerations apply to TEVAR. Spinal cord drainage perioperatively is recommended whenever large segments of the aorta are covered, particularly when a collateral circuit is compromised (left subclavian artery, intercostal arteries, lumbar arteries and internal iliac arteries). Open or endovascular reconstruction of the left subclavian artery or the internal iliac arteries is desirable whenever coverage is anticipated [25–31].

c. Stroke prevention

   In most cases, access to the aortic arch and ascending aorta with stiff wires is required to provide a stable endovascular platform for stent-grafting of the thoracoabdominal aorta. Very meticulous wire and catheter manipulation and avoiding repetitive wire exchanges in the aortic arch are critical, particularly in the presence of arch calcifications. For complex TEVAR, stroke rate may be as high as 20%. Other important considerations for stroke prevention include: the use of heparin for ACT >250 seconds, cardiac output reduction during stent-graft deployment, ICU surveillance postoperatively and the use of general anesthesia for proximal aortic interventions [32].

Treatment Strategies

Different approaches to the endovascular treatment of CTBAD have been described.

a. TEVAR for DTAA, with or without coverage of the left subclavian artery.

   Coverage of the thoracic aorta from the left subclavian artery to the celiac artery is the most common surgical modality of treatment for type B aortic dissection. Since most common primary tears originate from the proximal DTA, coverage would restore true lumen perfusion and induce false lumen thrombosis. This is accomplished relatively easily in the acute and subacute settings. In CTBAD, distal re-entry tears originating in the abdominal aorta are common, precluding false lumen thrombosis. In this sense, DTA TEVAR is best suited for the treatment of CTBAD limited to the thoracic aorta (DeBakey type IIIA) (Fig. 1). Even then, treatment failure may still occur despite full coverage of the dissected aorta. Failure of distal reverse aortic remodeling has been linked to a large size aorta at the level of the distal landing zone and failure to extend the repair to the level of the celiac trunk [17, 33].

   A key technical aspect of TEVAR for CTBAD is sizing of the stent-graft. In ATBAD stent-grafts are generally oversized 10% to the total aortic size at the proximal landing zone. The optimal sizing for CTBAD is not well known. Stent-

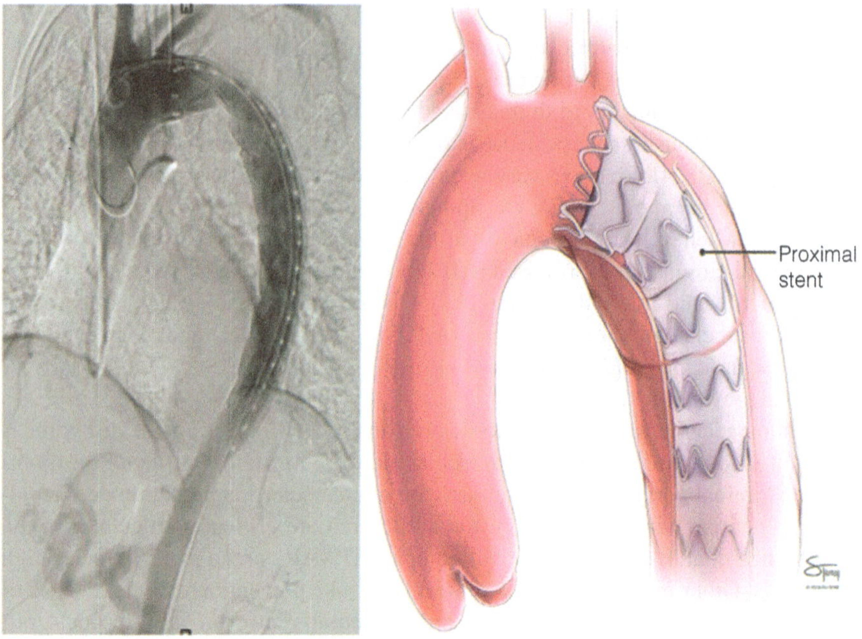

Fig. 1 TEVAR extending from the left subclavian artery to the celiac artery with coverage of a large proximal intimal tear

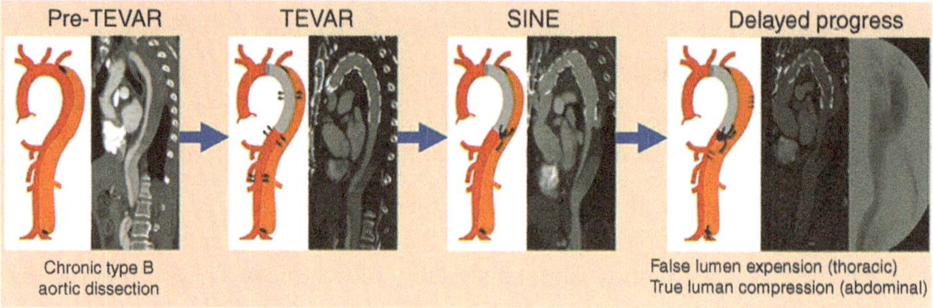

Fig. 2 Stent-graft induced new entry tear (SINE). Note the improvement in the true to false lumen size ratio immediately after TEVAR (left 2 panels). Note the late occurrence of SINE followed by true lumen compression and false lumen expansion (right 2 panels)

induced new entry tears (SINE) is a TEVAR-related complication that is associated with increased morbidity, re-interventions, conversion to open surgery and lack of reverse remodeling (Fig. 2). It could be lethal in cases of retrograde type A dissection and may require urgent open intervention. The occurrence of stent-induced new entry tears (SINE) in CTBAD has been linked to oversizing, however, the pathological mechanism is far more complex and is most likely related to the biomechanical properties of the stent-graft used versus the pathologic aorta. Hereditary aorthopathies are also a risk factor. Other factors such as ballooning and the use non-tapered stent-grafts may play a role. In fact, SINE can still occur even in the absence of oversizing [34–36]. In general, 10% oversizing based on the total aortic diameter—not the compressed true lumen—is considered safe.

b. Fenestrated or branched TEVAR/EVAR (F/BEVAR) for dissecting thoracoabdominal aortic aneurysms (TAAA)

Early experience with F/BEVAR showed that the approach is technically successful in selected cases. These techniques offer elegant total endovascular solutions for complex TAAA dissecting aneurysms. In general, for visceral branches taking off at a right angle and when the stent-graft is against the aortic wall, fenestration is preferred. For larger aortic diameters, especially when the visceral branch take-off is at a steep angle, a branched graft is preferred (Fig. 3).

In an early series of 6 patients, technical success was achieved in all patients, with no operative mortality or paraplegia. Most patients, however, required re-interventions for endoleaks or stent occlusion [37].

A more recent study from physician-sponsored investigational device exemption databases showed similar technical success and early outcomes of F/BEVAR for post-dissection TAAA compared to degenerative TAAA [38]. Endoleaks, however were frequent and more prevalent in the post-dissection TAAA F/BEVAR (76% vs 43%).

Verhoeven et al. reported the long-term outcomes of the largest European series of endovascular TAAA repair using fenestrated and branched stent grafts (166 patients between 2004–2013). The series included 9% emergent operation for contained rupture or symptoms and 65% were refused open surgery earlier. 11% were aneurysms secondary to chronic type B dissection. 47% had prior open or endovascular aortic procedures. Technical success was 95% and operative mortality was 9%. SCI was 9% (permanent paraplegia in 1.2%). Survival at 1, 2 and 5 years was 83%, 78%, and 66.6%, respectively. Reintervention rate was 24% mostly by endovascular means. Freedom from reintervention at 1 and 3 years was 88.3% and 78.4% [39].

In patients with marginal proximal landing zones, experience with branched aortic arch TEVAR in conjunction with TAAA repair is growing and contemporary series have shown promising results. These techniques offer elegant endovascular solutions, particularly to patients with high risk for open proximal thoracic aortic repair [40, 41] (Fig. 4).

In general, F/BEVAR is feasible and safe in selected cases of CTBAD. Extensive aortic coverage should be staged whenever possible. Most patients may require multiple re-interventions for endoleaks or target vessel occlusion.

c. Hybrid procedures

A visceral hybrid approach for the treatment of complex post-dissection TAAA may simplify the TEVAR approach and decrease the opportunity for endoleaks by decreasing the stent-branch and stent-stent interface. Many approaches may be utilized. In general, any large aortic branch may be chosen as inflow to bypass the visceral/renal vessels, which are then ligated at their origin. The entire length of the aorta is then covered with a multiple overlapping TEVAR

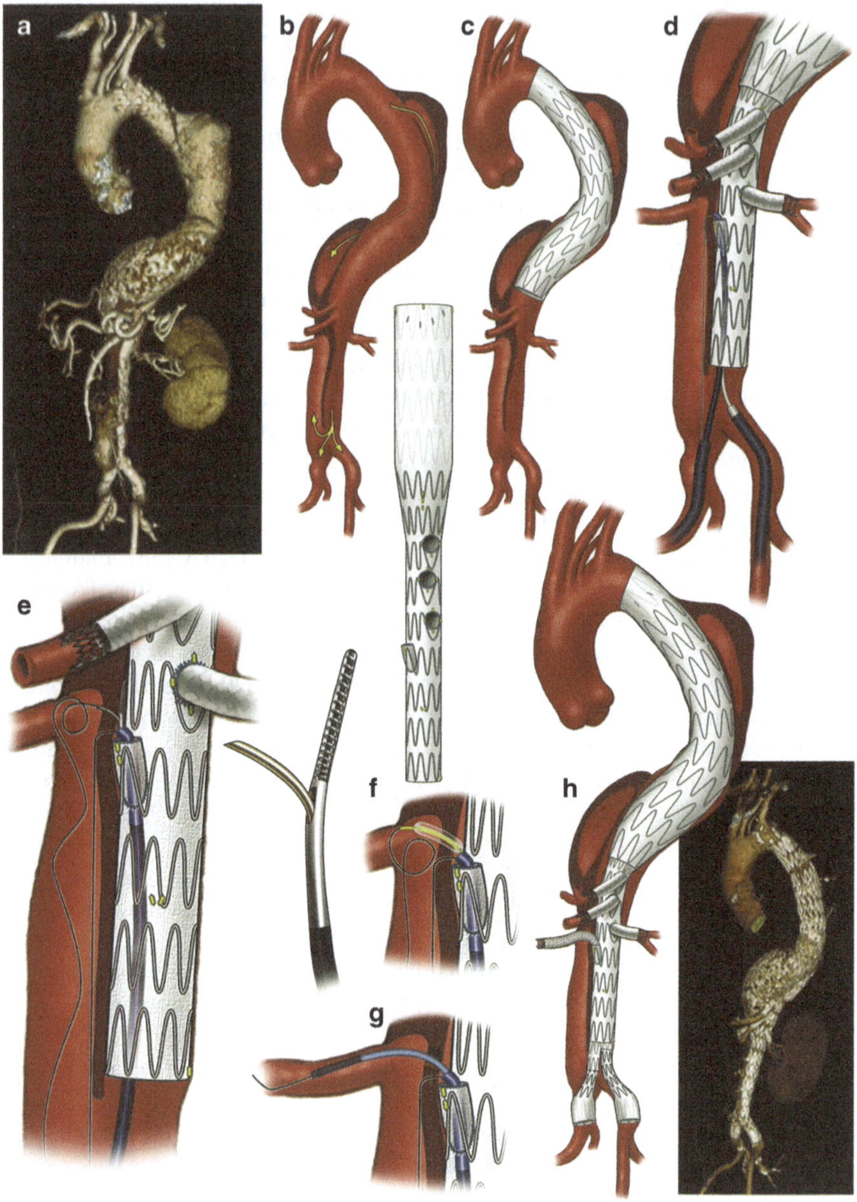

Fig. 3 Endovascular treatment of complex dissecting TAAA with multiple re-entry tears (**a**, **b**). A straight tubular graft was used for the treatment of DTA as a first stage (**c**). Then a fenestrated stent-graft in the peri-visceral segment (**d**, **e**, **f**, **g**) and a branched stent-graft in the aorto-iliac segment (**h**) were used to complete the repair

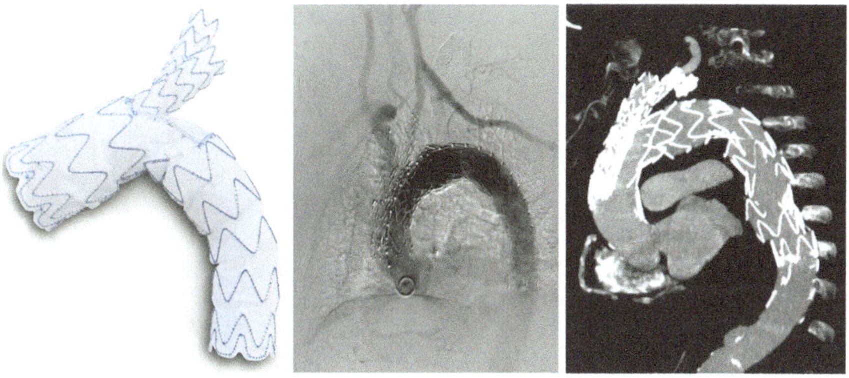

Fig. 4 Aortic arch stent-grafting using a dual branch device. A Terumo Aortic dual branch platform was used (Left panel). The branches were deployed in the innominate artery and the left carotid artery. Note the revascularization of the left subclavian artery using a carotid-subclavian bypass graft (Middle panel). Postoperative CT angiogram (Right panel)

stent-grafts [42]. The iliac arteries are most commonly used, but if pathologic, the ascending aorta may be used as inflow and the graft tunneled to the abdominal cavity through the anterior mediastinum.

Hybrid aortic arch approaches are particularly useful in young patients with suboptimal proximal landing zones due to residual arch dissecting aneurysms and who are fit to undergo open proximal aortic repair. Aortic arch replacement with a Dacron graft provides an excellent and stable proximal landing zone for TEVAR and eliminates the risk of retrograde dissection (Fig. 5). Multiple open procedures have been described with or without cardiopulmonary bypass to either replace the proximal aorta or debranch the aortic arch [43].

In general, when total or near-total thoraco-abdominal aortic coverage is anticipated, data from experimental animal studies suggest reduced SCI when the procedure is staged over time [44].

d. False lumen interventions

Interventions on the false lumen have been described during the index TEVAR operation or later for persistent false lumen perfusion. The goal is to induce false lumen thrombosis and improve the chances of reverse aortic remodeling. Multiple techniques have been described including coil embolization, the candy-plug technique, cork in the bottleneck technique, deployment of detachable balloon, and injection of thrombogenic solutions. Another solution for immediate false lumen obliteration is the use of an oversized thoracic tubular endograft in conjunction with controlled balloon fracture of the dissecting septum (the knickerbrocker technique). This allows for the oversized TEVAR to reach the outer aortic wall and occlude the false lumen. In general, false lumen obliteration is achieved successfully in most cases but the long-term effects are unknown [45–52] (Fig. 6).

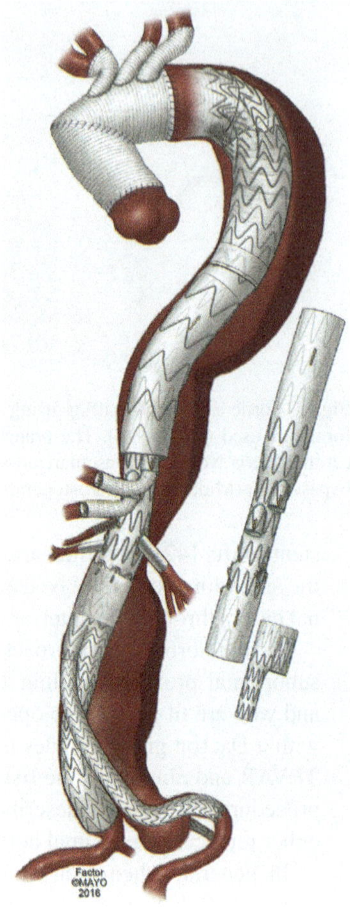

Fig. 5 Staged hybrid repair of complex dissecting TAAA. Note the proximal landing zone of the stent-graft in a prosthetic arch graft

Summary

Careful patient selection based on aortic anatomy is the most important factor for TEVAR success in the treatment of CTBAD. The long-term durability is not well known and lifelong imaging surveillance is necessary. Endovascular re-interventions are common, particularly after complex repairs.

The best therapeutic effect of TEVAR is seen in the stented portion of the aorta, in general the DTA. The downstream dissected aorta is not well treated by DTA TEVAR, most likely due to distal filling channels. In general, the distal landing zone is key to predicting downstream aortic remodeling. If the distal landing zone at the celiac artery is not a healthy normal size aorta, poor distal aortic reverse remodeling should be expected.

With these limitations in mind, we recommend that older patients with CTBAD who have suitable anatomy be considered for TEVAR as a first-line therapy. For younger patients with unfavorable anatomy, open surgery offers the most durable solution. For younger patients with suitable anatomy, TEVAR is reasonable, usually

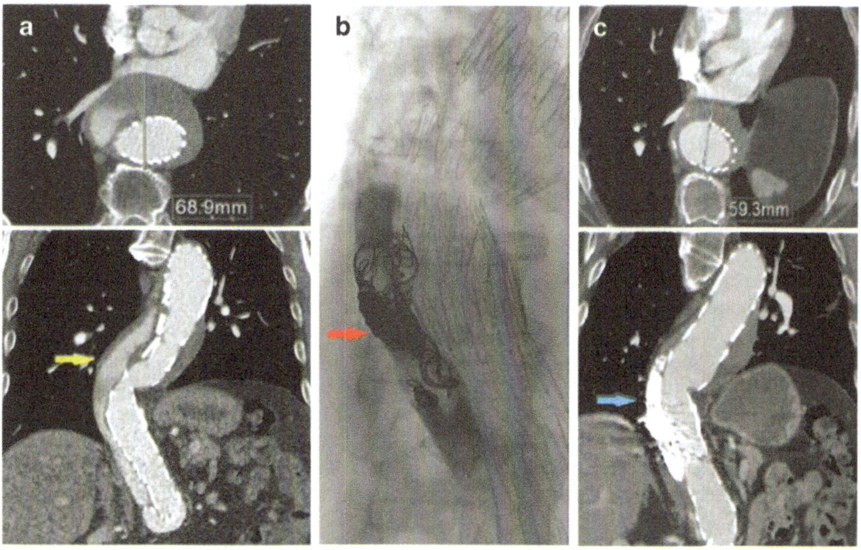

Fig. 6 Coil embolization and glue injection of a patent false lumen. Large patent false lumen following TEVAR (**a**). Deployment of coils and injection of glue in the false lumen (**b**, red arrow). Postoperative CTA showing thrombosed false lumen and decreased total aortic diameter (**c**)

in combination with open surgery. In our opinion, for most patients, TEVAR and open surgery are complimentary, not competitive, in the treatment of CTBAD.

The future of TEVAR for CTBAD probably lies in the proper use of fenestrated and/or branched stent-grafts proximally and distally and at the peri-visceral level. This would eliminate suboptimal landing zones. Proximal thoracic aortic operations may hold the key to the technical success of TEVAR by creating the ideal proximal landing zone. This could be accomplished with open arch debranching operations or with the use of branched arch stent-grafts. When total aortic coverage is planned, staging the procedure may decrease the risk of spinal cord injury.

Disclosures
Terumo Aortic: investigator, advisory board, speaker.

WL Gore: investigator.

Medtronic: investigator, advisory board, speaker.

References

1. Dake MD, Kato N, Mitchell RS, Semba CP, Razavi MK, Shimono T, et al. Endovascular stent-graft placement for the treatment of acute aortic dissection. N Engl J Med. 1999;340(20):1546–52.
2. Nienaber CA, Fattori R, Lund G, Dieckmann C, Wolf W, Von Kodolitsch Y, et al. Nonsurgical reconstruction of thoracic aortic dissection by stent-graft placement. N Engl J Med. 1999;340(20):1539–45.

3. Szeto WY, Mcgarvey M, Pochettino A, Moser GW, Hoboken A, Cornelius K, et al. Results of a new surgical paradigm: endovascular repair for acute complicated type b aortic dissection. Ann Thorac Surg. 2008;86(1):87–93; Discussion-4.
4. Conrad MF, Ergul EA, Patel VI, Paruchuri V, Kwolek CJ, Cambria RP. Management of diseases of the descending thoracic aorta in the endovascular era: a medicare population study. Ann Surg. 2010;252(4):603–10.
5. Bavaria JE, Appoo JJ, Makaroun MS, Verter J, Yu ZF, Mitchell RS, et al. Endovascular stent grafting versus open surgical repair of descending thoracic aortic aneurysms in low-risk patients: a multicenter comparative trial. J Thorac Cardiovasc Surg. 2007;133(2): 369–77.
6. Eggebrecht H, Nienaber CA, Neuhauser M, Baumgart D, Kische S, Schmermund A, et al. Endovascular stent-graft placement in aortic dissection: a meta-analysis. Eur Heart J. 2006;27(4):489–98.
7. Zeeshan A, Woo EY, Bavaria JE, Fairman RM, Desai ND, Pochettino A, et al. Thoracic endovascular aortic repair for acute complicated type b aortic dissection: superiority relative to conventional open surgical and medical therapy. J Thorac Cardiovasc Surg. 2010;140(6 Suppl):S109–15; Discussion S42–S46.
8. Brunkwall J, Lammer J, Verhoeven E, Taylor P. Adsorb: a study on the efficacy of endovascular grafting in uncomplicated acute dissection of the descending aorta. Eur J Vasc Endovasc Surg. 2012;44(1):31–6.
9. Nienaber CA, Kische S, Rousseau H, Eggebrecht H, Rehders TC, Kundt G, et al. Endovascular repair of type B aortic dissection: long-term results of the randomized investigation of stent grafts in aortic dissection trial. Circ Cardiovasc Interv. 2013;6(4):407–16.
10. Tsai T, Fattori R, Trimarchi S, Isselbacher E, Myrmel T, Evangelista A, et al. Long-term survival in patients presenting with type B acute aortic dissection: insights from the international registry of acute aortic dissection. Circulation. 2006;114(21):2226–31.
11. Thrumurthy SG, Karthikesalingam A, Patterson BO, Holt PJ, Hinchliffe RJ, Loftus IM, et al. A systematic review of mid-term outcomes of thoracic endovascular repair (Tevar) of chronic type B aortic dissection. Eur J Vasc Endovasc Surg. 2011;42(5):632–47.
12. Jia X, Guo W, Li TX, Guan S, Yang RM, Liu XP, et al. The results of stent graft versus medication therapy for chronic type B dissection. J Vasc Surg. 2013;57(2):406–14.
13. Conway AM, Qato K, Mondry LR, Stoffels GJ, Giangola G, Carroccio A. Outcomes of thoracic endovascular aortic repair for chronic aortic dissections. J Vasc Surg. 2018;67(5):1345–52.
14. Nienaber CA, Rousseau H, Eggebrecht H, Kische S, Fattori R, Rehders TC, et al. Randomized comparison of strategies for type B aortic dissection: the investigation of stent grafts in aortic dissection (instead) trial. Circulation. 2009;120(25):2519–28.
15. Kang WC, Greenberg RK, Mastracci TM, Eagleton MJ, Hernandez AV, Pujara AC, et al. Endovascular repair of complicated chronic distal aortic dissections: intermediate outcomes and complications. J Thorac Cardiovasc Surg. 2011;142(5):1074–83.
16. Parsa CJ, Williams JB, Bhattacharya SD, Wolfe WG, Daneshmand MA, Mccann RL, et al. Midterm results with thoracic endovascular aortic repair for chronic type B aortic dissection with associated aneurysm. J Thorac Cardiovasc Surg. 2011;141(2):322–7.
17. Sultan I, Siki MA, Bavaria JE, Dibble TR, Savino DC, Kilic A, et al. Predicting distal aortic remodeling after endovascular repair for chronic debakey iii aortic dissection. Ann Thorac Surg. 2018;105(6):1691–6.
18. Andacheh ID, Donayre C, Othman F, Walot I, Kopchok G, White R. Patient outcomes and thoracic aortic volume and morphologic changes following thoracic endovascular aortic repair in patients with complicated chronic type B aortic dissection. J Vasc Surg 2012;56(3):644–650; Discussion 50.
19. Leshnower BG, Szeto WY, Pochettino A, Desai ND, Moeller PJ, Nathan DP, et al. Thoracic endografting reduces morbidity and remodels the thoracic aorta in Debakey III aneurysms. Ann Thorac Surg. 2013;95(3):914–21.

20. Yang CP, Hsu CP, Chen WY, Chen IM, Weng CF, Chen CK, et al. Aortic remodeling after endovascular repair with stainless steel-based stent graft in acute and chronic type B aortic dissection. J Vasc Surg. 2012;55(6):1600–10.
21. Flors L, Leiva-Salinas C, Norton PT, Patrie JT, Hagspiel KD. Imaging follow-up of endovascular repair of type B aortic dissection with dual-source, dual-energy CT and late delayed-phase scans. J Vasc Interv Radiol. 2014;25(3):435–42.
22. Pellenc Q, Girault A, Roussel A, Castier Y. Regarding "outcomes of thoracic endovascular aortic repair for chronic aortic dissections". J Vasc Surg. 2018;67(6):1942–3.
23. Coselli JS, Lemaire SA, Koksoy C, Schmittling ZC, Curling PE. Cerebrospinal fluid drainage reduces paraplegia after thoracoabdominal aortic aneurysm repair: results of a randomized clinical trial. J Vasc Surg. 2002;35(4):631–9.
24. Estrera AL, Rubenstein FS, Miller CC, 3rd, Huynh TT, Letsou GV, Safi HJ. Descending thoracic aortic aneurysm: surgical approach and treatment using the adjuncts cerebrospinal fluid drainage and distal aortic perfusion. Ann Thorac Surg 2001;72(2):481–486.
25. Griepp RB, Griepp EB. Spinal Cord perfusion and protection during descending thoracic and thoracoabdominal aortic surgery: the collateral network concept. Ann Thorac Surg. 2007;83(2):S865–9; Discussion S90–2.
26. Cina CS, Abouzahr L, Arena GO, Lagana A, Devereaux PJ, Farrokhyar F. Cerebrospinal fluid drainage to prevent paraplegia during thoracic and thoracoabdominal aortic aneurysm surgery: a systematic review and meta-analysis. J Vasc Surg. 2004;40(1):36–44.
27. Yang GK, Misskey J, Arsenault K, Gagnon J, Janusz M, Faulds J. Outcomes of a spinal drain and intraoperative neurophysiologic monitoring protocol in thoracic endovascular aortic repair. Ann Vasc Surg. 2019;61:124–33.
28. Suarez-Pierre A, Zhou X, Gonzalez JE, Rizwan M, Fraser CD 3rd, Lui C, et al. Association of preoperative spinal drain placement with spinal cord ischemia among patients undergoing thoracic and thoracoabdominal endovascular aortic repair. J Vasc Surg. 2019;70(2):393–403.
29. Malloy PC, Raghavan A, Elder T, Wright J, Wright CH, Burant C, et al. Cerebrospinal fluid drainage during endovascular aortic aneurysm repair: a systematic review of the literature and treatment recommendations. Vasc Endovasc Surg. 2020;54(3):205–13.
30. Kato M, Motoki M, Isaji T, Suzuki T, Kawai Y, Ohkubo N. Spinal cord injury after endovascular treatment for thoracoabdominal aneurysm or dissection. Eur J Cardiothorac Surg. 2015;48(4):571–7.
31. Etz CD, Weigang E, Hartert M, Lonn L, Mestres CA, Di Bartolomeo R, et al. Contemporary spinal cord protection during thoracic and thoracoabdominal aortic surgery and endovascular aortic repair: a position paper of the vascular domain of the european association for cardiothoracic surgerydagger. Eur J Cardiothorac Surg. 2015;47(6):943–57.
32. Rohlffs F, Haulon S, Kolbel T, Greenhalgh R, Collaborators S. Stroke from thoracic endovascular procedures (step) collaboration. Eur J Vasc Endovasc Surg. 2020.
33. Andersen ND, Keenan JE, Ganapathi AM, Gaca JG, Mccann RL, Hughes GC. Current management and outcome of chronic type B aortic dissection: results with open and endovascular repair since the advent of thoracic endografting. Ann Cardiothorac Surg. 2014;3(3):264–74.
34. Dong Z, Fu W, Wang Y, Wang C, Yan Z, Guo D, et al. Stent graft-induced new entry after endovascular repair for stanford type B aortic dissection. J Vasc Surg. 2010;52(6):1450–7.
35. Huang CY, Hsu HL, Chen PL, Chen IM, Hsu CP, Shih CC. The impact of distal stent graft-induced new entry on aortic remodeling of chronic type B dissection. Ann Thorac Surg. 2018;105(3):785–93.
36. Neuhauser B, Greiner A, Jaschke W, Chemelli A, Fraedrich G. Serious complications following endovascular thoracic aortic stent-graft repair for type B dissection. Eur J Cardiothorac Surg. 2008;33(1):58–63.
37. Verhoeven EL, Paraskevas KI, Oikonomou K, Yazar O, Ritter W, Pfister K, et al. Fenestrated and branched stent-grafts to treat post-dissection chronic aortic aneurysms after initial treatment in the acute setting. J Endovasc Ther. 2012;19(3):343–9.

38. Tenorio ER, Oderich GS, Farber MA, Schneider DB, Timaran CH, Schanzer A, et al. Outcomes of endovascular repair of chronic postdissection compared with degenerative thoracoabdominal aortic aneurysms using fenestrated-branched stent grafts. J Vasc Surg. 2019.
39. Verhoeven EL, Katsargyris A, Bekkema F, Oikonomou K, Zeebregts CJ, Ritter W, et al. Editor's choice – ten-year experience with endovascular repair of thoracoabdominal aortic aneurysms: results from 166 consecutive patients. Eur J Vasc Endovasc Surg. 2015;49(5):524–31.
40. Spear R, Hertault A, Van Calster K, Settembre N, Delloye M, Azzaoui R, et al. Complex endovascular repair of postdissection arch and thoracoabdominal aneurysms. J Vasc Surg. 2018;67(3):685–93.
41. Czerny M, Rylski B, Morlock J, Schrofel H, Beyersdorf F, Saint Lebes B, et al. Orthotopic branched endovascular aortic arch repair in patients who cannot undergo classical surgery. Eur J Cardiothorac Surg. 2018;53(5):1007–12.
42. Patel HJ, Upchurch GR Jr, Jl E, Criado E, Rectenwald J, Williams DM, et al. Hybrid debranching with endovascular repair for thoracoabdominal aneurysms: a comparison with open repair. Ann Thorac Surg. 2010;89(5):1475–81.
43. Bavaria J, Milewski RK, Baker J, Moeller P, Szeto W, Pochettino A. Classic hybrid evolving approach to distal arch aneurysms: toward the zone zero solution. J Thorac Cardiovasc Surg. 2010;140(6 Suppl):S77–80; Discussion S6–91.
44. Bischoff MS, Scheumann J, Brenner RM, Ladage D, Bodian CA, Kleinman G, et al. Staged approach prevents spinal cord injury in hybrid surgical-endovascular thoracoabdominal aortic aneurysm repair: an experimental model. Ann Thorac Surg. 2011;92(1):138–146; Discussion 46.
45. Ogawa Y, Nishimaki H, Chiba K, Murakami K, Sakurai Y, Fujiwara K, et al. Candy-Plug technique using an excluder aortic extender for distal occlusion of a large false lumen aneurysm in chronic aortic dissection. J Endovasc Ther. 2016;23(3):483–6.
46. Zhang H, Ge YY, Lu K, Cao L, Liu P, Liu XP, et al. Coil embolization for persistent thoracic false lumen of type B aortic dissection after thoracic endovascular aortic repair. Ann Vasc Surg. 2019;57:60–8.
47. Riga C, Bicknell C, Jenkins M, Hamady M. Coil embolization of an aneurysmal type B dissection persistent false lumen after visceral hybrid repair. J Vasc Interv Radiol. 2009;20(1):130–2.
48. Nakayama T, Hattori K, Hashizume T, Asano M. Staged coil embolization after thoracic endovascular stent grafting for aneurysmal chronic type b aortic dissection: a case report. Sage Open Med Case Rep. 2019;7:2050313x19828903.
49. Rakestraw S, Feghali A, Nguyen K, Salvatore D, Dimuzio P, Abai B. False lumen embolization as a rescue technique in the setting of acute and chronic dissecting aneurysms as adjunct to thoracic endovascular aortic repair. J Vasc Surg Cases Innov Tech. 2020;6(1):110–7.
50. Kolbel T, Lohrenz C, Kieback A, Diener H, Debus ES, Larena-Avellaneda A. Distal false lumen occlusion in aortic dissection with a homemade extra-large vascular plug: the candy-plug technique. J Endovasc Ther. 2013;20(4):484–9.
51. Loubert MC, Van Der Hulst VP, De Vries C, Bloemendaal K, Vahl AA. How to exclude the dilated false lumen in patients after a type B aortic dissection? The cork in the bottleneck. J Endovasc Ther. 2003;10(2):244–8.
52. Kolbel T, Carpenter SW, Lohrenz C, Tsilimparis N, Larena-Avellaneda A, Debus ES. Addressing persistent false lumen flow in chronic aortic dissection: the knickerbocker technique. J Endovasc Ther. 2014;21(1):117–22.

Management of Chronic Dissection of the Descending Thoracic and Thoracoabdominal Aorta: Open Approach

Cuneyt Köksoy, Alice Le Huu, and Joseph S. Coselli

Introduction

Although the chronic phase of aortic dissection is generally considered to begin 2 weeks after the onset of dissection-related symptoms, open repair of chronic distal aortic dissection is typically performed a few years after the acute precipitating event. The dissection process itself substantially weakens the outer aortic wall, leading to aortic dilatation; thus, over a highly variable period, a dissected aorta that is originally of normal diameter often dilates and becomes aneurysmal. Chronic dissection in the distal aorta occurs in survivors of acute DeBakey type I and III dissection events (Fig. 1). Regardless of type, chronic aortic dissection is a progressive disease that necessitates lifelong management to avoid late rupture and ischemic events.

C. Köksoy
Division of Cardiothoracic Surgery, Michael E. DeBakey Department of Surgery, Baylor College of Medicine, Houston, TX, USA

A. Le Huu
Division of Cardiothoracic Surgery, Michael E. DeBakey Department of Surgery, Baylor College of Medicine, Houston, TX, USA

Department of Cardiovascular Surgery, Texas Heart Institute, Houston, TX, USA

J. S. Coselli (✉)
Division of Cardiothoracic Surgery, Michael E. DeBakey Department of Surgery, Baylor College of Medicine, Houston, TX, USA

Department of Cardiovascular Surgery, Texas Heart Institute, Houston, TX, USA

Department of Cardiovascular Surgery, CHI St. Luke's Health—Baylor St. Luke's Medical Center, Houston, TX, USA
e-mail: jcoselli@bcm.edu

J. S. Coselli et al. (eds.), *Aortic Dissection and Acute Aortic Syndromes*,
https://doi.org/10.1007/978-3-030-66668-2_30

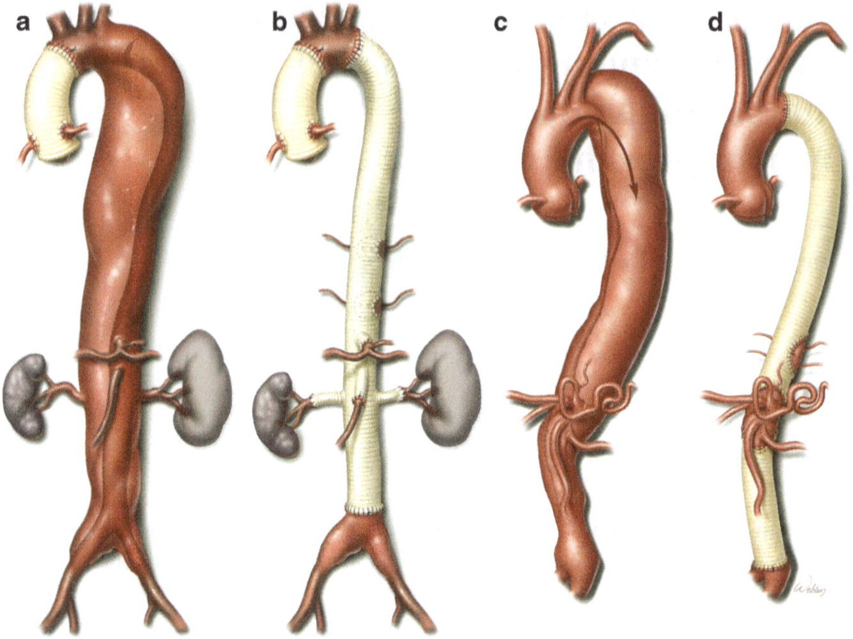

Fig. 1 Drawings showing the repair of chronic aortic dissection. (**a**) Gross dilatation of the distal aorta, 6 years after proximal aortic repair in a survivor of DeBakey type I aortic dissection. (**b**) The completed extent II thoracoabdominal aortic repair; a 4-branched graft was used to replace widely displaced visceral arteries. (**c**) A narrow true lumen (double arrows) within a dilatated distal aorta in a survivor of DeBakey type III aortic dissection, 5 years after onset. (**d**) The completed extent II thoracoabdominal aortic repair; a single patch incorporates the 4 visceral arteries. Used with permission of Baylor College of Medicine

Chronic distal aortic dissection affects roughly 15–40% of patients who undergo open repair of the descending thoracic (DTA) and thoracoabdominal aorta (TAAA) [1–5]. Our review of 4275 DTA and TAAA repairs performed between 1986 and 2019 identified 1362 (31.9%) chronic aortic dissections of DeBakey types I (n = 578, 13.5%), IIIa (n = 150, 3.5%), and IIIb (n = 634, 14.8%). Compared with the majority of patients who undergo open repair for degenerative aneurysm, patients with chronic dissection tend to be a decade younger (i.e., 50s vs 60s) and have far fewer comorbidities related to the atherosclerotic process. Additionally, approximately 1 in 4 patients with chronic distal aortic dissection has Marfan syndrome (MFS) or a related heritable thoracic aortic disease, as compared to 1 in 10 patients with degenerative aneurysm without dissection [1, 6, 7].

Factors suggested to significantly affect chronic aneurysm development after aortic dissection include poorly controlled hypertension and anatomic factors such as a maximal aortic diameter ≥4 cm in the acute phase, continued patency of the false lumen, partial thrombosis of the distal false lumen, and a proximal entry tear ≥10 mm [8–11].

Natural History

The chronically dissected aorta tends to dilate at a faster rate than a non-dissected one. Although it is generally assumed that both DeBakey types of chronically dissected aorta dilate at similar rates, evidence suggests otherwise [12, 13]. In survivors of DeBakey type I dissection, the persistence of a pressurized false lumen has been associated with subsequent distal aneurysm formation, need for intervention, and greater mortality [10, 14]. In an attempt to thrombose the false channel and thereby decrease the risk of late aneurysm formation, endovascular strategies have been developed to exclude segments of the false lumen in both acute (≤2 weeks since onset) [15] and chronic [16] aortic dissection. The effectiveness of such approaches is dependent on a variety of factors, including the extent of aortic dissection, because downstream portions of the false lumen—those without endovascular obliteration—continue to be pressurized and may perfuse upstream portions in a retrograde fashion.

Indications for Repair

Even if the entire distal aorta is dissected, dissection alone is not a sufficient indication for open graft replacement. Managing chronic dissection typically requires regularly repeated imaging studies and enhanced awareness of emerging symptoms through patient-education and optimization efforts (including, at a minimum, smoking cessation and strict blood pressure control).

Current US practice guidelines [17] recommend elective open aortic repair in asymptomatic patients with chronic dissection of the distal aorta when its diameter exceeds 5.5 cm (Class I recommendation; level of evidence B). Although the guidelines do not expressly state it, a lower diameter-based threshold is generally recommended if the patient has a heritable thoracic aortic disease (e.g., MFS) or if the rate of dilatation exceeds 0.5 cm/year.

Patients who develop symptoms and can withstand open repair should undergo it regardless of distal aortic diameter. Common indications for emergency repair of chronic distal aortic dissection include rupture or acute dissection superimposed on an existing chronic dissection (because such "double" dissection tends to progress rapidly to aortic rupture). Specific symptoms, when present, are usually related to aortic expansion and consequent compression of surrounding structures, or to malperfusion related to aortic dissection. Rarely, fistulas develop in patients with chronic distal aortic dissection, especially those who have been previously treated with endovascular aortic repair. The onset of symptoms is usually considered an indication of impending rupture or significant malperfusion and should prompt urgent evaluation. Pain is the most common symptom and may arise in the chest, back, abdomen, or left flank; it may be described as sharp or stabbing acute pain or as refractory pain. Additional symptoms may be related to embolization, frank rupture, or either acute-onset dissection or expanding chronic dissection. Plaque and thrombus may embolize distally, causing occlusion and thrombosis of the visceral, renal, or lower-extremity branches and subsequent malperfusion. Cold, blue, or painful extremities, spontaneous paraplegia, abdominal pain, nausea, vomiting, incontinence, and abnormal urination can all signify malperfusion caused by aortic dissection.

Indications for Reoperation

Because chronic aortic dissection is progressive, treating it commonly requires more than one aortic procedure. Elective repairs are generally limited to aneurysmal portions of the dissected aorta. In contrast, emergency repairs are generally limited to symptomatic portions of the aorta, even if other segments are aneurysmal; this strategy is undertaken in hopes of reducing operative risk.

For many years, the treatment paradigm for patients with acute DeBakey type III dissection dictated medical management. Today, however, such patients are often treated with thoracic endovascular aortic repair (TEVAR). Likewise, patients with chronic distal aortic dissection are now candidates for TEVAR. Recent reports suggest that in nearly 70% of patients who undergo TEVAR for chronic distal aortic dissection, the aortic diameter does not regress afterward [18, 19]. Evidence also suggests that reintervention after TEVAR is more common in patients with chronic dissection than in patients with aneurysm; 17–18% of patients who undergo TEVAR to treat chronic aortic dissection need additional open or endovascular repair, as compared to 10–15% of aneurysm patients [20, 21]. The most serious failures, such as continued aortic expansion, type I endoleak, and infection (with or without fistula), are typically treated with open repair [22]. Reportedly, open repair rates after TEVAR for acute and chronic dissection are 10% and 15%, respectively [23]. Therefore, open aortic repair as a secondary procedure after previous endovascular aortic therapy constitutes an important treatment option, even in the endovascular era.

Surgical Management

Preoperative Evaluation

Comorbidities that are typically considered to contribute to operative risk should be carefully evaluated and modified whenever possible to mitigate risk; likewise, preoperatively evaluating patients' physiologic reserve is critical to obtaining a beneficial outcome. A history and physical exam constitute the initial assessment. All patients, except those who require emergency repair, should undergo a thorough preoperative evaluation emphasizing cardiac, pulmonary, and renal function, as well as a careful review of imaging studies. We routinely obtain a transthoracic echocardiogram, a coronary angiogram, pulmonary function tests, and a carotid duplex scan, as well as laboratory panels to assess coagulation, liver, and kidney function. The most common complication after thoracic and thoracoabdominal aortic repairs is pulmonary dysfunction, including that necessitating prolonged ventilator dependence [1, 24]. Therefore, pulmonary function testing, including arterial blood gases and spirometry, is routinely performed before surgery. Also, because patients with severely impaired renal function are at elevated risk of death, kidney function should be evaluated [25].

Preoperative imaging with computed tomography is a cornerstone of surgical decision making. The diameter of the aorta is measured throughout the diseased and non-aneurysmal portions. Potential sites for aortic clamping and cannulation are reviewed for calcification, dissection, and mural thrombus. Branching vessels, such as the visceral and renal arteries, are carefully assessed for stenotic origins and their spatial orientation relative to each other; close attention is paid to anatomic variants. In chronic aortic dissection, it is especially important to determine whether blood entering branching arteries is supplied by the true lumen, the false lumen, or both. The extent of the aneurysmal portions of the chronically dissected aorta is identified proximally and distally; the degree of calcification and atheroma dictates the sites for clamping the aorta and cannulation for left heart bypass (LHB). The lumen of each artery is examined for areas of stenosis that may require endarterectomy or stenting.

Surgical Treatment and Adjuncts

Open distal aortic repair necessitates clamping the descending thoracic aorta, which creates downstream ischemic conditions that affect the spinal cord and abdominal viscera. To alleviate these complications, we routinely use a multimodal approach to organ protection during these operations that is largely based on the extent of repair (Fig. 2) [26]. However, because patients with chronic aortic dissection tend to have higher rates of distal aortic reoperation (which is thought to increase the likelihood of postoperative spinal cord deficit from further interruption of feeding arteries), protective adjuncts are more liberally used to benefit select patients (Table 1) [27]. To protect the spinal cord, we use mild passive hypothermia, cerebrospinal fluid drainage (CSFD), LHB, sequential cross-clamping, and selective reimplantation of intercostal or lumbar arteries [28–30]. We use CSFD for extent I and II repairs, for extent IV repair in patients who have had a previous DTA or extent I TAAA repair, and for extent III repair when we anticipate replacing the iliac vessels. We intermittently deliver cold renal solution to the kidneys to protect them from ischemic damage and prevent acute renal failure [31]. We also deliver isothermic blood from the LHB circuit to the celiac axis and the superior mesenteric artery (SMA) to minimize ischemic times for the abdominal organs.

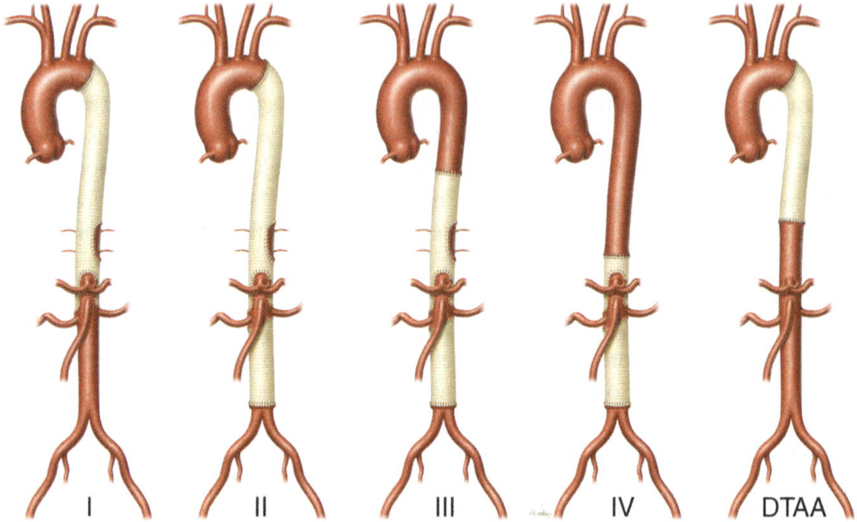

Fig. 2 Illustration of repairs. The Crawford classification system describing the 4 extents of thoracoabdominal aortic aneurysm (TAAA) repair is shown, along with a more limited descending thoracic aortic aneurysm (DTAA) repair (here, repair does not extend beyond the diaphragmatic hiatus or involve the visceral arteries). Crawford extent II TAAA repair carries the greatest operative risk. Used with permission of Baylor College of Medicine

Table 1 The use of adjuncts for organ protection during open repair of chronic distal aortic dissection

Extent of repair	CSFD	LHB	Isothermic blood to SMA/celiac artery	Cold renal perfusion	Reimplantation of segmental arteries
DTA	+/−	+/−	−	−	+/−
TAAA I	+	+	+/−	+/−	+/−
TAAA II	+	+	+	+	+
TAAA III	+/−	+/−	+/−	+	+/−
TAAA IV	+/−	−	−	+	+/−

CSFD cerebrospinal fluid drainage, *DTA* descending thoracic aneurysm, *LHB* left heart bypass, *SMA* superior mesenteric artery, *TAAA* thoracoabdominal aortic aneurysm
+: Generally use; −: Generally do not use; +/−: May use depending on patient characteristics and intraoperative findings
Adapted from Ouzounian et al. [27]

Preoperative Preparations

The perfusion team sets up a cell saver, as well as the LHB circuit. Standard intravenous access includes a large-bore peripheral intravenous line and a central venous catheter. Hemodynamic monitoring requires a Swan-Ganz catheter and a right radial or brachial arterial line. A temperature probe in the nasopharynx is used to guide permissive hypothermia. A Foley catheter facilitates monitoring kidney function and controlling fluid balance. Patients are intubated with a double-lumen endobronchial tube for single-lung ventilation during the procedure. A CSFD catheter is inserted by the anesthesia team at the L3–4, L4–5, or L5–S1 level. The patient is administered prophylactic antibiotics—vancomycin and cefepime—1 hour before the initial incision. In patients with prior elephant trunk repair, ultrasonography is used to locate the graft that is hanging within the proximal portion of the descending thoracic aorta.

Positioning

The patient is commonly arranged in a right lateral decubitus position, with the upper body at a 60° angle in relation to the operating table. The hips are then angled 30° to the horizontal (Fig. 3). The lower limbs are positioned to allow rapid access to the femoral arteries if cannulation becomes necessary. A beanbag is inflated to maintain this position.

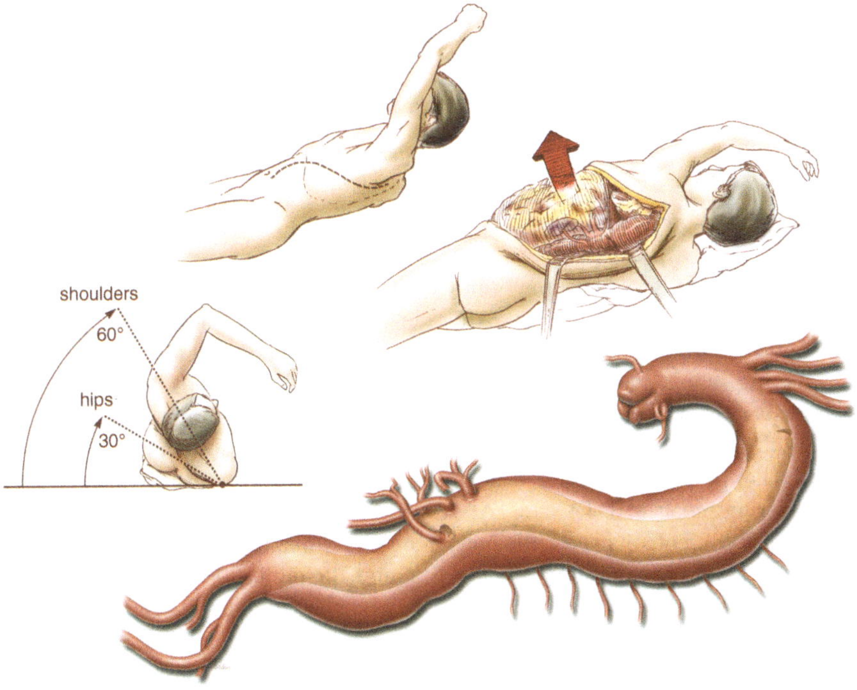

Fig. 3 Positioning of the patient, incision, and exposure of thoracoabdominal aorta to prepare for repair of chronic aortic dissection. Used with permission of Baylor College of Medicine

Exposure

Our surgical approach to open repair of DTA and TAAA has been described previously [32]. Briefly, for isolated DTA repair, the segment to be replaced is approached through a posterolateral thoracotomy through the fifth or sixth intercostal space, depending on the extent of repair. For Crawford extent I and II TAAAs, a sigmoid-shaped skin incision is made from behind the left scapula, along the seventh rib, across the costal margin, and toward the left periumbilical region. The chest is entered through the sixth intercostal space. For extent III TAAA repairs, the seventh or eighth intercostal space is entered; for extent IV TAAA repairs, a straight oblique incision is made through the ninth or tenth intercostal space. Left medial visceral rotation and circumferential division of the diaphragm enable exposure of the entire thoracoabdominal aorta. Using table-mounted self-retaining retractors maintains stable exposure throughout the procedure. The entire thoracoabdominal aorta is exposed by medial visceral rotation and circumferential division of the diaphragm. Possible clamp sites are dissected. In patients with chronic DeBakey type I aortic dissection, prior adhesions related to previous proximal aortic surgery necessitate more dissection, which makes preparing the proximal clamp site more challenging; however, if the patient underwent prior aortic arch replacement with an elephant trunk extension, the trunk is used as the proximal clamp site, which lessens preparation. In cases with no appropriate proximal site (e.g., contained rupture, an extremely large aneurysm, extension into the distal transverse arch), hypothermic circulatory arrest is used.

Left Heart Bypass

Left heart bypass is used routinely in Crawford extent I and II repairs and selectively in other distal aortic repairs. After heparin (1 mg/kg) is administered, a cannula is placed in the left atrium via left inferior pulmonary venotomy, held with a purse-string suture, and connected to the drainage line of the LHB circuit. Another cannula is placed in the distal descending thoracic aorta and connected to the circuit's inflow line. After LHB flow is initiated, the proximal aortic clamp is placed just distal or proximal to the left subclavian artery. Performing the proximal anastomosis during repair of DTA and TAAA is technically challenging; establishing a proximal aortic cuff that is sufficiently long and suitable for suturing is critical. Most commonly, this anastomosis is made immediately beyond the clamp placed distal to the left subclavian artery. However, in cases involving substantial dilatation of the distal arch (which is not uncommon in patients with DeBakey type I aortic dissection), the clamp is placed across the transverse aortic arch proximal to the left subclavian artery, and a bulldog clamp is used to occlude the left subclavian artery (Fig. 4). Once proximal control is established, a second aortic clamp is placed across the mid-descending thoracic aorta, and LHB flows are increased.

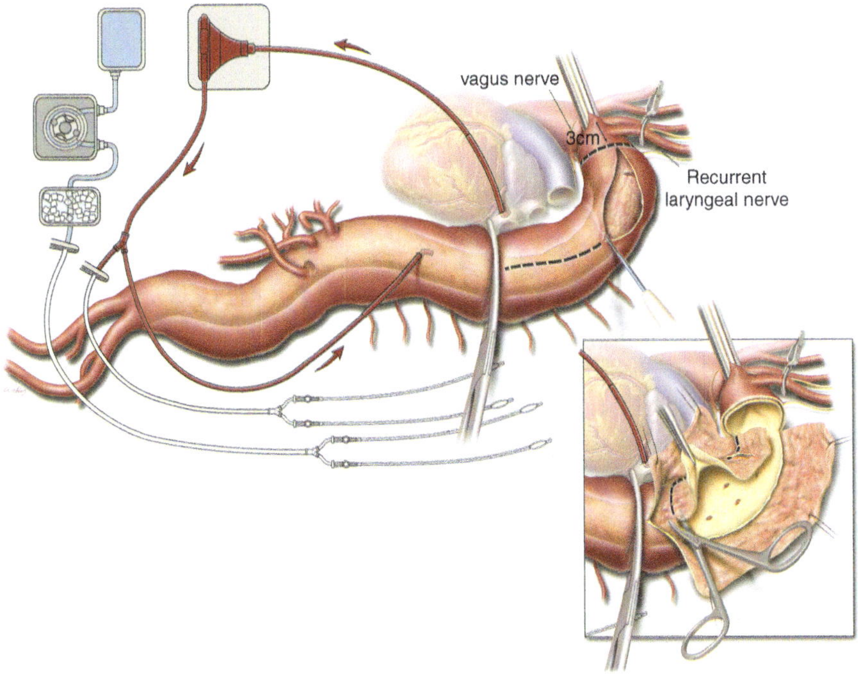

Fig. 4 Initiation of left heart bypass, placement of aortic clamps, and opening of the proximal descending thoracic aorta. (Inset) In repairs involving chronic dissection, the dividing septum is removed. Used with permission of Baylor College of Medicine

Proximal Anastomosis

The isolated segment of the proximal descending thoracic aorta is longitudinally opened, and the aorta is completely divided at the level of the proximal anastomosis. All shed blood is collected and returned to the patient through a cell saver system. Then, the thick dissecting membrane between the true and false lumens is excised (Fig. 4). Meanwhile, patent intercostal arteries at this level are oversewn with 2–0 silk sutures. For the proximal anastomosis, the aorta is transected, which allows full-thickness suturing through the aortic wall without risk of injuring the esophagus, pulmonary artery, or recurrent laryngeal nerve and allows absolute confirmation of all channels in the dissected aorta (Fig. 5).

To perform the proximal anastomosis, we typically use continuous 3–0 polypropylene suture; however, in patients with heritable disorders like MFS, we prefer finer suture material, either 4–0 or 5–0. The graft material of choice for aortic surgery is Dacron impregnated with either collagen or gelatin; the graft is soaked tableside in rifampin. For distal aortic repair, usually, a 24-, 26-, or 28-mm graft is used. The first stitch is placed at the posterolateral corner of the aorta and tied. Because it is difficult to rotate

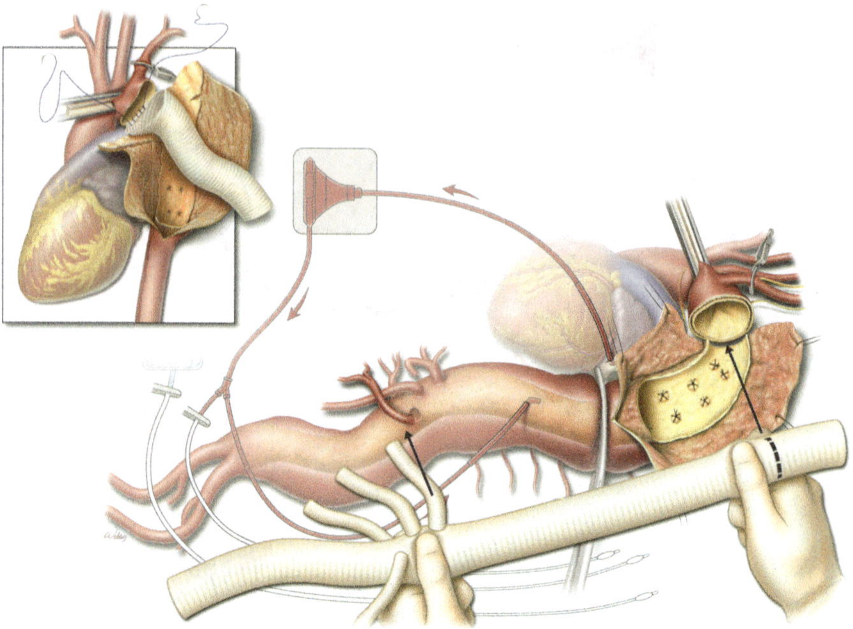

Fig. 5 An aortic replacement graft is sized to length to prepare for the proximal anastomosis. In this segment, the spinal arteries are ligated. (Inset) For repairs limited to the descending thoracic aorta (DTA), left heart bypass is typically not used. Beginning with the difficult-to-rotate posterior portion, the proximal anastomosis is first sutured transluminally; DTA repair is typically performed without using a distal aortic clamp (i.e., using an open distal anastomosis approach)

the aorta, we perform the posterior half of the suturing transluminally (Fig. 5). The suture is passed through all layers, with particular care taken to include the intima. The posterior part of the anastomosis is accomplished by running the suture medially (away from the surgeon) (Fig. 6). After the primary suture line is completed and the suture ends are tied, the graft is gently lifted up and the posterior portion of the anastomosis is carefully examined. Pledgeted mattress sutures are applied to areas with widely separated sutures, overlapping sutures, or tears in the aorta. In patients with notable dilation or residual dissection of the aortic arch, a reversed elephant trunk approach may be undertaken to facilitate subsequent proximal aortic repair; an extended (approximately 8-cm) portion of the replacement graft is invaginated to create the reversed elephant trunk, and the folded edge is used to create the proximal anastomosis.

Sequential Graft Clamping

Once the proximal anastomosis is complete, LHB is tapered and then discontinued. The aortic cross-clamp is removed and placed further distal on the graft (Fig. 7). Moving the clamp is especially crucial if it was originally placed proximal to the left

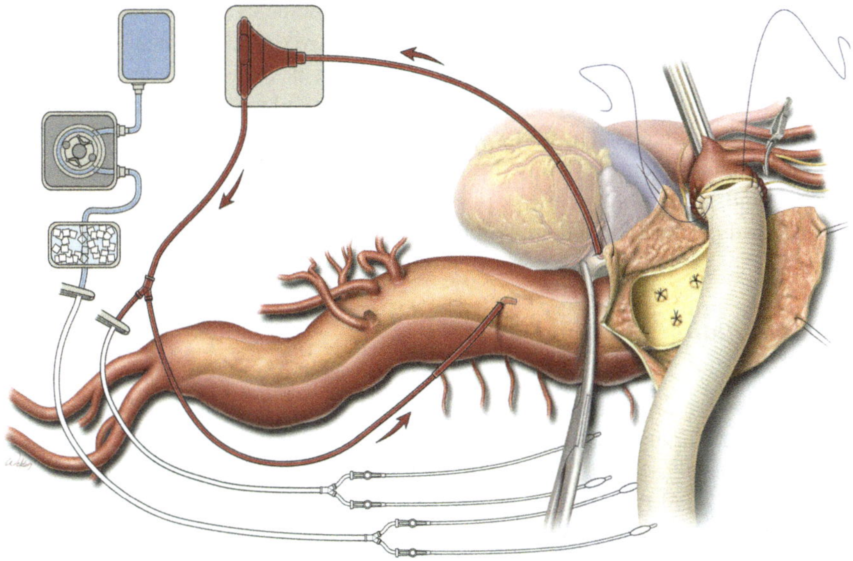

Fig. 6 Construction of the proximal anastomosis. Used with permission of Baylor College of Medicine

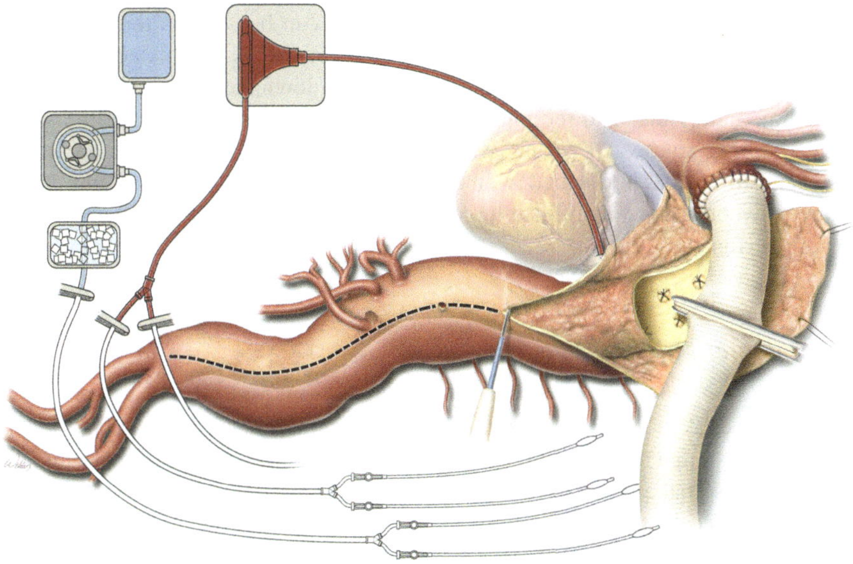

Fig. 7 Extension of the aortic incision after the aortic cross-clamp is moved down onto the graft. Used with permission of Baylor College of Medicine

subclavian artery, because moving it distally re-establishes flow to the subclavian and vertebral arteries. The distal cannula can be removed, and the distal cross-clamp released. With scissors or electrocautery, the aorta is opened longitudinally; the length of the incision depends on the extent of repair and may extend to the bifurcation of the iliac arteries. The aortic wall is prepared by excising the dissecting septum and manually removing any thrombus; this allows exposure of all intercostal, visceral, and lumbar branches. As possible throughout repair, the clamp is repositioned to aid perfusion and thereby reduce ischemic conditions.

Reimplantation of Spinal Arteries

Any rapidly bleeding spinal arteries are ligated. If there is good backflow, the inferior mesenteric artery is ligated with 2–0 silk suture. Of the remaining spinal arteries, a pair is selected for reimplantation into the aortic graft. These arteries should be between T7 and L2, close to each another, and large in caliber, and they should have no back-bleeding. Two techniques can be used to reattach the spinal arteries: an island patch or a small-diameter (8-mm) interposition graft. If the patient's anatomy is favorable, we prefer to implant the arteries as a patch, while incorporating a minimal amount of native aortic tissue. To reattach the arteries, a hole is cut into the Dacron graft, and the graft and island patch are anastomosed side-to-side with 3–0 polypropylene suture (Fig. 8). In areas where the native aortic tissue is fragile, a 3–0 or 4–0 pledgeted mattress suture can be used as reinforcement. After the patch reimplantation of the intercostal arteries is completed, whenever possible, the proximal aortic cross-clamp is moved down the aortic graft to a position immediately distal to the intercostal patch to allow reperfusion of the reimplanted spinal arteries. If repair is limited to the descending thoracic aorta, the distal anastomosis is performed as an open procedure (Fig. 5); the dissecting membrane between the true and false lumen is fenestrated to ensure that both lumens remain perfused.

Management of Visceral Arteries

Care must be taken to identify the renal and visceral arteries. In particular, the left renal artery is often displaced in patients with chronic dissection. During reimplantation of the spinal arteries, if any of the renal artery ostia are accessible, 9-Fr balloon perfusion catheters are placed in the renal arteries to infuse with cold perfusate via a standalone circuit (Fig. 8). If LHB was used, the celiac trunk and SMA are perfused with isothermic blood at 400–500 mL/min from a modified circuit. Endarterectomy of branching arteries is performed as needed. When dissection extends into the origins of the visceral vessels, the septum is excised or fenestrated, or the false lumen is sutured closed or obliterated by placing a balloon-expandable

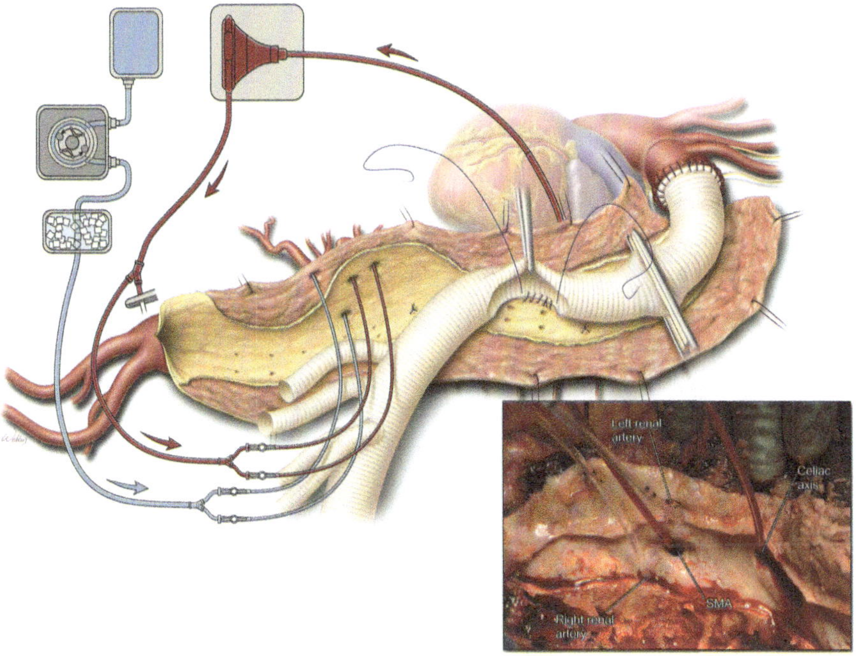

Fig. 8 Initiation of visceral perfusion and the intercostal patch anastomosis. (Inset) Isothermic blood is used to perfuse the celiac axis and the superior mesenteric artery (SMA); cold solution is used to perfuse the renal arteries. Used with permission of Baylor College of Medicine

stent (7 × 15 mm) inside the true lumen. These stents are positioned and expanded within the affected branch under direct vision and without guidewires, as detailed elsewhere [33].

If distal aortic repair ends at the level of the renal and visceral vessels (i.e., an extent I TAAA repair), the distal end of the graft can be tailored in a beveled fashion and sutured end-to-end with 3–0 polypropylene suture; distal fenestration is performed to ensure that both lumens remain perfused. Otherwise, repair necessitates reimplanting visceral arteries by using an island patch, bypass grafts, or both. Although a single patch can be used to reimplant all 4 visceral arteries, more commonly, the celiac, superior mesenteric and right renal arteries are reimplanted together as a 3-vessel patch to an opening made in the side of the graft. The remaining left renal artery is subsequently addressed and continues to undergo cold renal perfusion. Once the celiac, superior mesenteric, and right renal arteries are reimplanted, the cross-clamp is moved distally to a position below the visceral patch, thereby restoring perfusion to these arteries.

Single or multiple bypass grafts (including a prefabricated 4-branched graft) are used more frequently in repairs of chronic dissection than in repairs of aneurysm because of a tendency toward displacement of visceral artery origins and in efforts to minimize the residual aortic tissue associated with MFS. The 4-branched graft

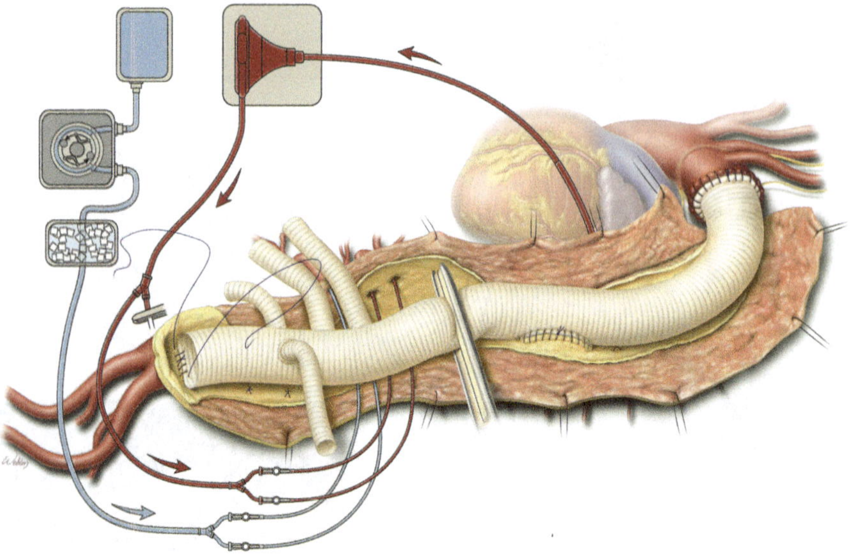

Fig. 9 The distal anastomosis is performed, which, when a branched graft is used, is typically performed before the visceral arteries are reattached. Visceral perfusion is continued. Used with permission of Baylor College of Medicine

technique affords a durable repair in patients with heritable thoracic aortic disease by eliminating residual native aorta in the visceral segment, thereby preventing the future development of patch aneurysm; additionally, anastomotic tension is reduced in this approach, which decreases the likelihood of late pseudoaneurysm formation. Because of the extended lower-extremity ischemic time necessitated by completing 4 separate anastomoses, the distal aortic anastomosis is performed before the visceral arteries are attached to the graft, enabling distal perfusion (Fig. 9). Meanwhile, visceral arteries are separately perfused. The order of visceral artery anastomosis usually is the right renal artery, the SMA, the celiac trunk, and the left renal artery as detailed elsewhere [34] (Fig. 10). Additional adjustments for repair in patients with MFS include using a finer suture (e.g., 4–0 instead of 3–0 polypropylene suture) and directly incorporating sutures into the visceral artery rather than merely approaching the ostia [34].

Distal Anastomosis

The distal aortic anastomosis usually is constructed at the level of the aortic bifurcation (or, occasionally, to each iliac or femoral artery separately). If the chronic dissection continues distally, the septum is fenestrated by resecting wedges of the dissecting membrane proximally and distally from within the aortic cuffs,

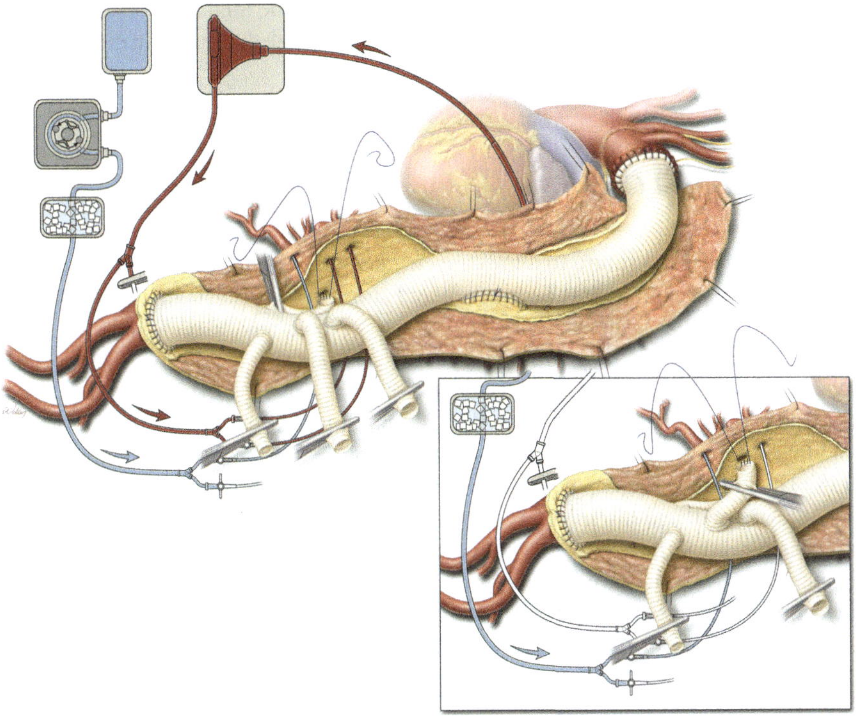

Fig. 10 Right renal artery anastomosis with a branched aortic graft, created after the distal aortic anastomosis was completed. (Inset) Superior mesenteric artery anastomosis to the branched aortic graft. Used with permission of Baylor College of Medicine

allowing blood to flow through both true and false channels after the reconstruction is completed. As needed, a bifurcated graft is anastomosed to the junction of the internal and external iliac arteries or more distally. The distal end of the aortic graft is trimmed to the appropriate length, and the distal anastomosis is performed end-to-end with continuous 3–0 or 4–0 polypropylene suture (depending on the quality of the tissue). The circumference of the distal anastomosis is selectively reinforced with pledgeted 3–0 polypropylene sutures in an interrupted mattress fashion. Then the patient is placed in Trendelenburg position, a 27-gauge needle is used to puncture multiple de-airing holes in the graft, and the aortic cross-clamp is slowly removed to re-establish blood flow to the pelvis and both lower extremities.

If the left renal artery is still receiving perfusate, it is now mobilized. A side-biting clamp is placed on the aortic graft, and flame cautery is used to make a 1-cm hole in the Dacron. The balloon perfusion catheter is removed, and an end-to-side anastomosis is completed with a 5–0 polypropylene suture and reinforced as need with pledgeted mattress suture. If the artery is of inadequate length, a small-diameter (8-mm) graft is used to bridge the distance. Before the suture is tied down, the side-biting clamp is released to deair the aorta through the final anastomosis. At this time, the inferior pulmonary vein is decannulated, and the purse-string suture is tied down.

Hemostasis and Closure

All anastomoses and suture ligatures are checked for bleeding and are reinforced as needed. After protamine has been given and surgical hemostasis has been secured, blood products are transfused as necessary to reverse any coagulopathy. The cut edges of the opened native aorta are cauterized. The completed repair is inspected to make sure that the main graft and its branches lie properly without kinking (Fig. 11). Both femoral arteries, both left renal arteries, the proper hepatic artery, and intestinal arterial branches are palpated for pulses and to ensure adequate blood flow. The kidneys are palpated for turgor, the bowel is visualized to confirm that it is well perfused, and the spleen is inspected for injury. A closed-suction abdominal drain is placed in the upper left retroperitoneal space. The left hemidiaphragm is reapproximated up to the costal margin with a continuous 1–0 polypropylene suture. Two straight 36-Fr chest tubes are placed in an anteroapical and posterobasal position within the left chest cavity. The abdominal fascia and chest are closed.

Postoperative Care

Distal aortic dissection repair is a tremendous undertaking, requiring supportive care in the postoperative period. The patients are kept intubated overnight to control parameters and achieve optimal outcomes. Standard intensive care monitoring and volume resuscitation are essential; in addition, the patients' neurological status is verified every hour. The CSF pressure should be 15–20 mmHg. To achieve this goal, the CSF can be drained up to 10 mL/h, with a maximum quantity of 25 mL/4 h. Exceeding this amount can lead to intracranial hemorrhage or herniation. In the event of emerging spinal cord deficit, the target CSF pressure is lowered to 10 mmHg, the goal mean arterial pressure (MAP) is increased to 90–110 mmHg, and the target hemoglobin level is raised to >10 g/dL. The patient is administered intravenous mannitol (12.5 g/L) and dexamethasone (10 mg/L) every 12 h for 24–48 h. If the CSF drain was removed before the onset of paraparesis or paraplegia, it should be quickly reinserted. In the absence of spinal cord complications, the CSF drain can be removed between 24–48 h postoperatively. Before removal, the drain can be clamped for 12–24 h to ensure the absence of neurological sequalae.

Patients can be extubated the morning after surgery when they are alert, oriented, and capable of protecting their airway. Typically, on postoperative day 4, the patient

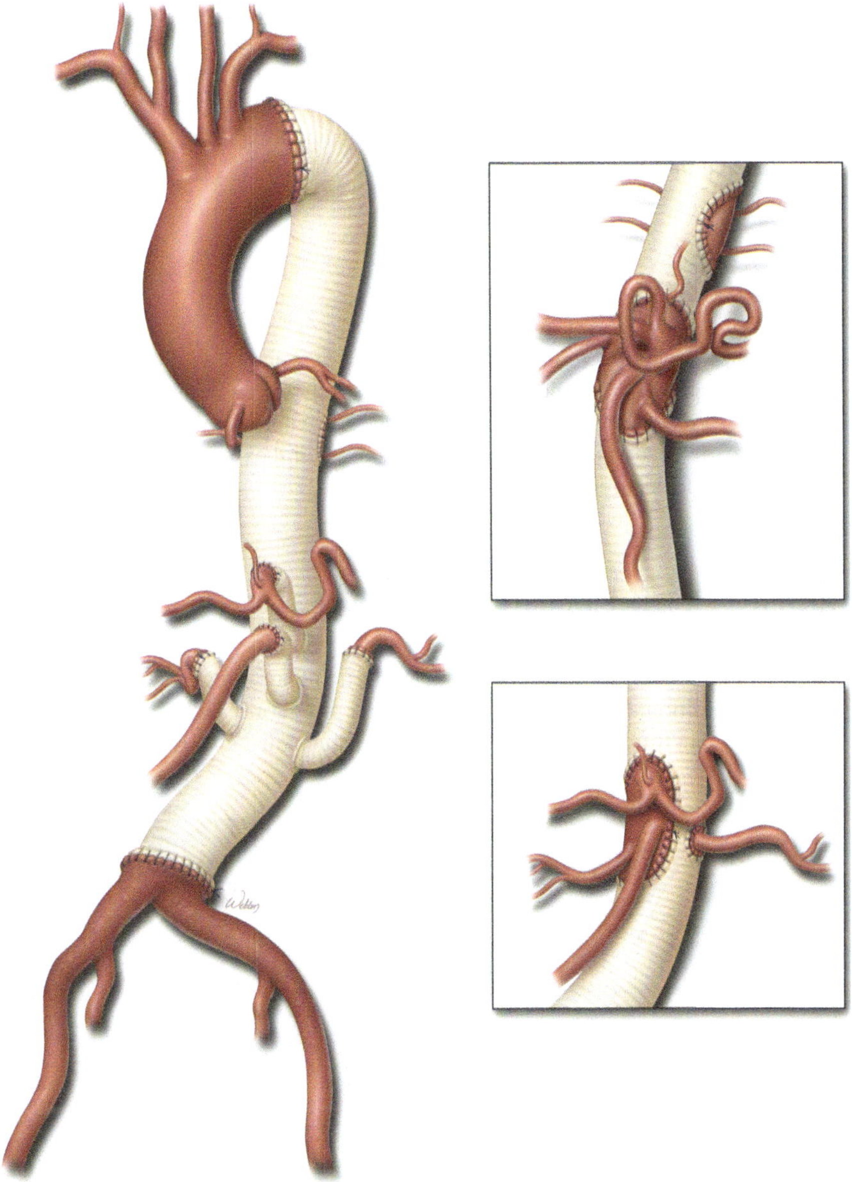

Fig. 11 Completed repair of DeBakey type III dissection in which a branched graft was used to reattach the visceral arteries. (Upper inset) A single visceral patch incorporates the celiac axis, superior mesenteric artery, and both renal arteries. (Lower inset) A three-vessel patch incorporates the celiac axis, superior mesenteric artery, and right renal arteries; the left renal artery is reattached as a button. Used with permission of Baylor College of Medicine

is slowly started on a solid diet, in conjunction with stool softeners and laxatives. Patients can be discharged from the hospital 7–10 days after surgery in ideal circumstances. If the patient has normal renal function, then a computed tomography scan with intravenous contrast of the chest, abdomen, and pelvis is requested for baseline measurements. Higher MAP goals are maintained for 4–6 weeks after surgery to prevent late neurological complications.

Follow-up

After repair, the patients remain at risk for further aortic pathology. A repeat computed tomography scan should be performed annually for 2–3 years after surgery. In the absence of disease, the frequency of scans can be decreased to every 2–3 years. For young patients, magnetic resonance imaging to limit exposure to ionizing radiation should be considered.

Open Repair After Endovascular Repair

Serious complications of prior endovascular aortic repair often necessitate an open procedure. Additionally, patients who underwent prior aortic arch replacement with a frozen elephant trunk extension may need subsequent distal aortic repair (Fig. 12).

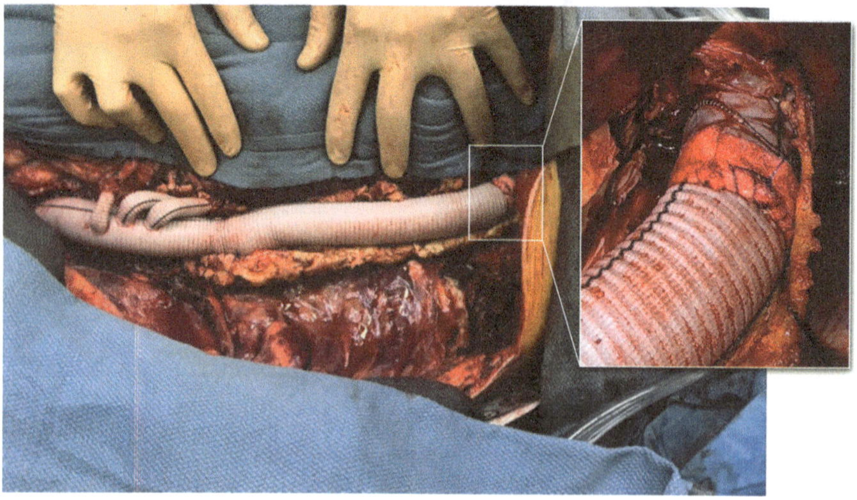

Fig. 12 Intraoperative photo of an extent II thoracoabdominal aortic aneurysm repair performed after a frozen elephant trunk repair of the transverse aortic arch. (Inset) The stent-graft–to-graft anastomosis is secured with a strip of felt. Used with permission of Baylor College of Medicine

To account for the presence of a stent-graft, we modify our standard incision to maximize exposure (i.e., enter through the fifth intercostal space rather than the sixth, or use a thoracoabdominal approach either to revise a prior endovascular abdominal aortic repair or, often, to remove the endovascular stent-graft all together). Many times, the proximal landing zone of the stent-graft impinges on the brachiocephalic vessels branching off the aortic arch; in such cases, it is often difficult to safely clamp the aorta, so it may be necessary to use hypothermic circulatory arrest, which at our center is atypical for this procedure.

Stent-grafts can be fully or partly extirpated [22, 35, 36]. Partial extirpation of the stent-graft may be a useful strategy in patients without infection (Fig. 13). Partial extirpation should be considered when the stent-graft is found to be well-incorporated, when the patient's hemodynamics are unstable in the operating room, or when inflammation or scar tissue is found in the area, making it unsafe to separate the endograft from the aortic wall. For example, if a portion of an endograft cannot be removed from the aortic arch without causing undue tissue trauma, it is preferable to leave it in place and trim off the rest of the stent-graft. It is not thought that partial extirpation leads to migration of the remaining portion of the endograft, device failure, component separation, or rupture during follow-up.

Outcomes

When performed in specialized centers, surgical repair of distal aortic dissection achieves good survival with acceptable morbidity [37]. In contemporary studies of chronic distal dissection repair, the rate of early mortality is 6–8%; stroke, 1–4%; paraplegia, 1–3%; and renal failure necessitating dialysis, 4–5% [5, 7, 38–43]. Our own outcomes have been generally good, with greater risk for patients undergoing Crawford extent II repair (Table 2). Early outcomes are comparable after open repair for chronic DeBakey type I and type III aortic dissections. Recently, our series of 466 patients with either chronic type I or type III aortic dissection, we determined that mortality was 6% for both types (n = 14 for each group) [41]. In patients with chronic DeBakey type I dissection undergoing open distal aortic aneurysm repair, factors reportedly associated with early death are greater age, chronic obstructive pulmonary disease, and clamping proximal to the left subclavian artery [6]. Acceptable results have been also observed in patients with MFS dissection [12, 44].

Regarding late survival, Conway and colleagues [5] reported 77% survival at 7 years, and Estrera and coauthors [39] reported 60% survival at 10 years. Preventza et al. [41] associated DeBakey types I and II with similar rates of survival (74% at 6 years). Open repair appears durable; Zoli et al. [45] reported 83% freedom from distal aortic reoperation at 10 years, and Estrera et al. [39] reported 94% freedom from reoperation at 20 years. However, the risk of disease progression requiring subsequent repair in an adjacent aortic segment is not insignificant; we reported

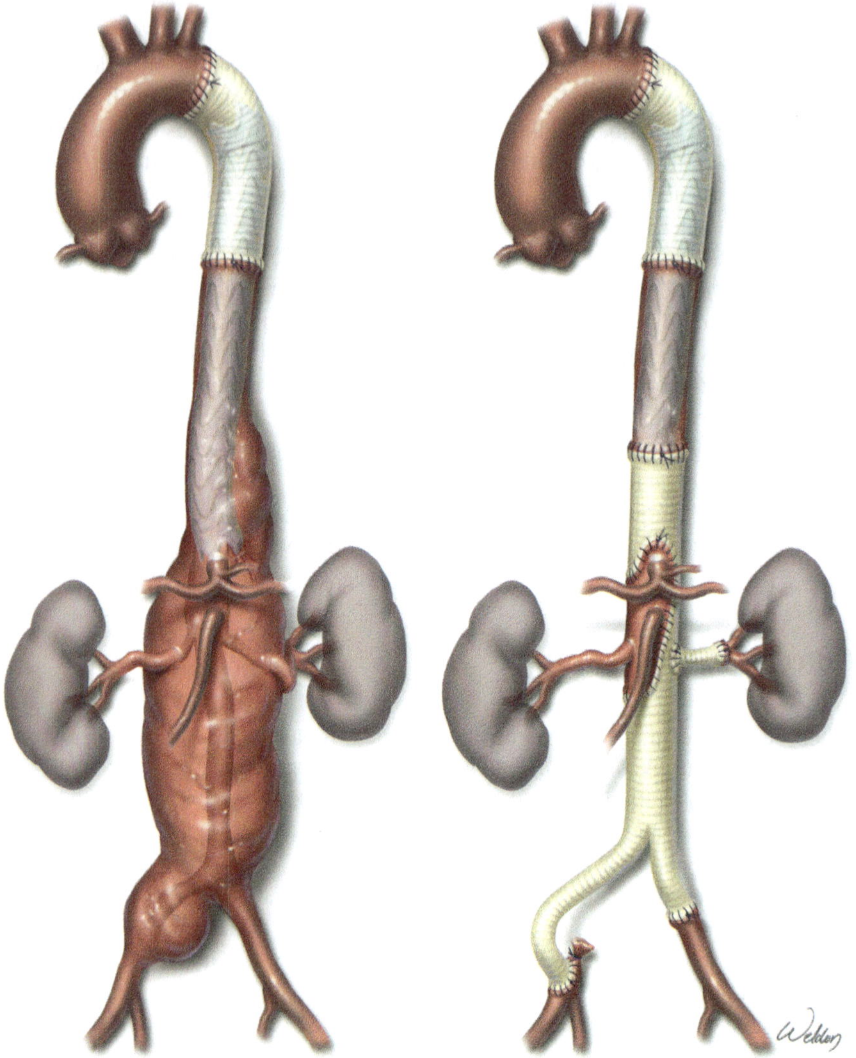

Fig. 13 Illustrations depicting partial endograft explantation in a patient with chronic DeBakey type III aortic dissection after previous open replacement of the proximal portion of the descending thoracic aorta (left). Afterward, the distal aorta dilated progressively; therefore, the patient underwent endovascular repair 3 years later. However, progressive expansion continued, necessitating further repair. (Right) Extent III thoracoabdominal aortic aneurysm (TAAA) repair was performed. Because the proximal portion of the stent-graft was well-adhered to the aortic wall, it was incorporated into the repair, and only the distal portion was removed. Used with permission of Baylor College of Medicine

Table 2 Results of 1362 open descending thoracic or thoracoabdominal aortic aneurysm repairs (1986–2019)

Extent of repair	No. patients	Operative deaths	Paraplegia[a]	Stroke[a]	Renal failure[a]
DTA	211	9 (6.5%)	2 (0.9%)	4 (1.9%)	4 (1.9%)
TAAA I	391	23 (5.9%)	4 (1.0%)	11 (2.8%)	12 (3.1%)
TAAA II	539	39 (7.2%)	13 (2.4%)	14 (2.6%)	34 (6.3%)
TAAA III	139	11 (7.9%)	4 (2.9%)	1 (0.7%)	10 (7.2%)
TAAA IV	85	4 (4.7%)	0	0	2 (2.4%)
Total	1362	86 (6.3%)	23 (1.7%)	30 (2.2%)	62 (4.6%)

DTA descending thoracic aneurysm, *TAAA* thoracoabdominal aortic aneurysm
[a]Persisting at the time of hospital discharge or operative death. Operative deaths include 30-day deaths and any deaths during the initial hospitalization period, including after transfer to another hospital

85% freedom from progressive aortic repair at 7 years, and Estrera et al. [39] reported 82% freedom at 20 years.

In conclusion, open repair of chronic descending thoracic or thoracoabdominal aortic dissection generally has good patient outcomes and tends to be durable. However, the progressive nature of residual chronic dissection often necessitates subsequent repair of nearby aortic segments.

Acknowledgments The authors express gratitude to Stephen N. Palmer, PhD, ELS (of the Texas Heart Institute), and Susan Y. Green, MPH, for editorial assistance, and to Scott A. Weldon, MA, CMI, for creating the illustrations and assisting with image selection.

References

1. Coselli JS, LeMaire SA, Preventza O, de la Cruz KI, Cooley DA, Price MD, et al. Outcomes of 3309 thoracoabdominal aortic aneurysm repairs. J Thorac Cardiovasc Surg. 2016;151:1323–37. https://doi.org/10.1016/j.jtcvs.2015.12.050.
2. Estrera AL, Sandhu HK, Charlton-Ouw KM, Afifi RO, Azizzadeh A, Miller CC 3rd, et al. A quarter century of organ protection in open thoracoabdominal repair. Ann Surg. 2015;262:660–8. https://doi.org/10.1097/SLA.0000000000001432.
3. Kouchoukos NT, Kulik A, Castner CF. Outcomes after thoracoabdominal aortic aneurysm repair using hypothermic circulatory arrest. J Thorac Cardiovasc Surg. 2013;145:S139–41. https://doi.org/10.1016/j.jtcvs.2012.11.077.
4. Conrad MF, Chung TK, Cambria MR, Paruchuri V, Brady TJ, Cambria RP. Effect of chronic dissection on early and late outcomes after descending thoracic and thoracoabdominal aneurysm repair. J Vasc Surg 2011;53:600–607; discussion 7. https://doi.org/10.1016/j.jvs.2010.09.053.
5. Conway AM, Sadek M, Lugo J, Pillai JB, Pellet Y, Panagopoulos G, et al. Outcomes of open surgical repair for chronic type B aortic dissections. J Vasc Surg. 2014;59:1217–23. https://doi.org/10.1016/j.jvs.2013.11.002.

6. Coselli JS, Green SY, Zarda S, Nalty CC, Price MD, Hughes MS, et al. Outcomes of open distal aortic aneurysm repair in patients with chronic DeBakey type I dissection. J Thorac Cardiovasc Surg. 2014;148:2986–93 e1–2. https://doi.org/10.1016/j.jtcvs.2014.07.048.
7. Kouchoukos NT, Kulik A, Castner CF. Open thoracoabdominal aortic repair for chronic type B dissection. J Thorac Cardiovasc Surg. 2015;149:S125–9. https://doi.org/10.1016/j.jtcvs.2014.07.064.
8. Bernard Y, Zimmerman H, Chocron S, Litzler J, Kastler B, Etievent J, et al. False lumen patency as a predictor of late outcome in aortic dissection. Am J Cardiol. 2001;87:1378–82. https://doi.org/10.1016/S0002-9149(01)01556-9.
9. Durham CA, Aranson NJ, Ergul EA, Wang LJ, Patel VI, Cambria RP, et al. Aneurysmal degeneration of the thoracoabdominal aorta after medical management of type B aortic dissections. J Vasc Surg. 2015;62:900–6. https://doi.org/10.1016/j.jvs.2015.04.423.
10. Fattouch K, Sampognaro R, Navarra E, Caruso M, Pisano C, Coppola G, et al. Long-term results after repair of type A acute aortic dissection according to false lumen patency. Ann Thorac Surg. 2009;88:1244–50. https://doi.org/10.1016/j.athoracsur.2009.06.055.
11. Schwartz SI, Durham C, Clouse WD, Patel VI, Lancaster RT, Cambria RP, et al. Predictors of late aortic intervention in patients with medically treated type B aortic dissection. J Vasc Surg. 2018;67:78–84. https://doi.org/10.1016/j.jvs.2017.05.128.
12. Coselli JS, Green SY, Price MD, Hash JA, Ouyang Y, Volguina IV, et al. Results of open surgical repair in patients with Marfan syndrome and distal aortic dissection. Ann Thorac Surg. 2016;101:2193–201. https://doi.org/10.1016/j.athoracsur.2015.11.008.
13. Schoenhoff FS, Jungi S, Czerny M, Roost E, Reineke D, Matyas G, et al. Acute aortic dissection determines the fate of initially untreated aortic segments in Marfan syndrome. Circulation. 2013;127:1569–75. https://doi.org/10.1161/circulationaha.113.001457.
14. Kirsch M, Legras A, Bruzzi M, Louis N. Fate of the distal aorta after surgical repair of acute DeBakey type I aortic dissection: a review. Arch Cardiovasc Dis. 2011;104:125–30. https://doi.org/10.1016/j.acvd.2010.11.009.
15. Moulakakis KG, Mylonas SN, Dalainas I, Kakisis J, Kotsis T, Liapis CD. Management of complicated and uncomplicated acute type B dissection. A systematic review and meta-analysis. Ann Cardiothorac Surg. 2014;3:234–46. https://doi.org/10.3978/j.issn.2225-319X.2014.05.08.
16. Nienaber CA, Kische S, Rousseau H, Eggebrecht H, Rehders TC, Kundt G, et al. Endovascular repair of type B aortic dissection: long-term results of the randomized investigation of stent grafts in aortic dissection trial. Circ Cardiovasc Interv. 2013;6:407–16. https://doi.org/10.1161/circinterventions.113.000463.
17. Hiratzka LF, Bakris GL, Beckman JA, Bersin RM, Carr VF, Casey DE, Jr, et al. 2010 ACCF/AHA/AATS/ACR/ASA/SCA/SCAI/SIR/STS/SVM guidelines for the diagnosis and management of patients with thoracic aortic disease: a report of the American College of Cardiology Foundation/American Heart Association Task Force on Practice Guidelines, American Association for Thoracic Surgery, American College of Radiology, American Stroke Association, Society of Cardiovascular Anesthesiologists, Society for Cardiovascular Angiography and Interventions, Society of Interventional Radiology, Society of Thoracic Surgeons, and Society for Vascular Medicine. Circulation. 2010;121:e266–369. https://doi.org/10.1161/CIR.0b013e3181d4739e.
18. Conway AM, Qato K, Mondry LR, Stoffels GJ, Giangola G, Carroccio A. Outcomes of thoracic endovascular aortic repair for chronic aortic dissections. J Vasc Surg. 2018;67:1345–52. https://doi.org/10.1016/j.jvs.2017.08.098.
19. Sultan I, Siki MA, Bavaria JE, Dibble TR, Savino DC, Kilic A, et al. Predicting distal aortic remodeling after endovascular repair for chronic DeBakey III aortic dissection. Ann Thorac Surg. 2018;105:1691–6. https://doi.org/10.1016/j.athoracsur.2018.01.006.
20. Nozdrzykowski M, Luehr M, Garbade J, Schmidt A, Leontyev S, Misfeld M, et al. Outcomes of secondary procedures after primary thoracic endovascular aortic repair. Eur J Cardiothorac Surg. 2016;49:770–7. https://doi.org/10.1093/ejcts/ezv279.

21. Patterson B, Holt P, Nienaber C, Cambria R, Fairman R, Thompson M. Aortic pathology determines midterm outcome after endovascular repair of the thoracic aorta: report from the Medtronic Thoracic Endovascular Registry (MOTHER) database. Circulation. 2013;127:24–32. https://doi.org/10.1161/circulationaha.112.110056.
22. Spiliotopoulos K, Preventza O, Green SY, Price MD, Amarasekara HS, Davis BM, et al. Open descending thoracic or thoracoabdominal aortic approaches for complications of endovascular aortic procedures: 19-year experience. J Thorac Cardiovasc Surg. 2018;155:10–8. https://doi.org/10.1016/j.jtcvs.2017.08.023.
23. Giles KA, Beck AW, Lala S, Patterson S, Back M, Fatima J, et al. Implications of secondary aortic intervention after thoracic endovascular aortic repair for acute and chronic type B dissection. J Vasc Surg. 2019;69:1367–78. https://doi.org/10.1016/j.jvs.2018.07.080.
24. Girardi LN, Lau C, Munjal M, Elsayed M, Gambardella I, Ohmes LB, et al. Impact of preoperative pulmonary function on outcomes after open repair of descending and thoracoabdominal aortic aneurysms. J Thorac Cardiovasc Surg. 2017;153:S22–S9. e2. https://doi.org/10.1016/j.jtcvs.2016.10.055.
25. Coselli JS, Amarasekara HS, Zhang Q, Preventza O, de la Cruz KI, Chatterjee S, et al. The impact of preoperative chronic kidney disease on outcomes after Crawford extent II thoracoabdominal aortic aneurysm repairs. J Thorac Cardiovasc Surg. 2018;156:2053–64.e1. https://doi.org/10.1016/j.jtcvs.2018.05.101.
26. MacArthur RG, Carter SA, Coselli JS, LeMaire SA. Organ protection during thoracoabdominal aortic surgery: rationale for a multimodality approach. Semin Cardiothorac Vasc Anesth. 2005;9:143–9. https://doi.org/10.1177/108925320500900207.
27. Ouzounian M, LeMaire SA, Weldon SA, Coselli JS. Current open treatment of thoracoabdominal aortic aneurysms. In: Stanger OH, Pepper JR, Svensson LG, editors. Surgical management of aortic pathology: current fundamentals for the clinical management of aortic disease. 1st ed. New York, NY: Springer; 2019. p. 1075–89.
28. Coselli JS, Green SY, Price MD, Zhang Q, Preventza O, de la Cruz KI, et al. Spinal cord deficit after 1114 extent II open thoracoabdominal aortic aneurysm repairs. J Thorac Cardiovasc Surg. 2019;159:1–13. https://doi.org/10.1016/j.jtcvs.2019.01.120.
29. Coselli JS, LeMaire SA. Left heart bypass reduces paraplegia rates after thoracoabdominal aortic aneurysm repair. Ann Thorac Surg 1999;67:1931–1934; discussion 53–8. https://doi.org/10.1016/s0003-4975(99)00390-2.
30. Coselli JS, LeMaire SA, Koksoy C, Schmittling ZC, Curling PE. Cerebrospinal fluid drainage reduces paraplegia after thoracoabdominal aortic aneurysm repair: results of a randomized clinical trial. J Vasc Surg. 2002;35:631–9. https://doi.org/10.1067/mva.2002.122024.
31. Koksoy C, LeMaire SA, Curling PE, Raskin SA, Schmittling ZC, Conklin LD, et al. Renal perfusion during thoracoabdominal aortic operations: cold crystalloid is superior to normothermic blood. Ann Thorac Surg. 2002;73:730–8. https://doi.org/10.1016/s0003-4975(01)03575-5.
32. Coselli JS, de la Cruz KI, Preventza O, LeMaire SA, Weldon SA. Extent II thoracoabdominal aortic aneurysm repair: How I do it. Semin Thorac Cardiovasc Surg. 2016;28:221–37. https://doi.org/10.1053/j.semtcvs.2016.07.005.
33. LeMaire SA, Jamison AL, Carter SA, Wen S, Alankar S, Coselli JS. Deployment of balloon expandable stents during open repair of thoracoabdominal aortic aneurysms: a new strategy for managing renal and mesenteric artery lesions. Eur J Cardiothorac Surg. 2004;26:599–607. https://doi.org/10.1016/j.ejcts.2004.04.035.
34. de la Cruz KI, LeMaire SA, Weldon SA, Coselli JS. Thoracoabdominal aortic aneurysm repair with a branched graft. Ann Cardiothorac Surg. 2012;1:381–93. https://doi.org/10.3978/j.issn.2225-319X.2012.08.05.
35. Coselli JS, Spiliotopoulos K, Preventza O, de la Cruz KI, Amarasekara H, Green SY. Open aortic surgery after thoracic endovascular aortic repair. Gen Thorac Cardiovasc Surg. 2016;64:441–9. https://doi.org/10.1007/s11748-016-0658-8.

36. LeMaire SA, Green SY, Kim JH, Sameri A, Parenti JL, Lin PH, et al. Thoracic or thoracoabdominal approaches to endovascular device removal and open aortic repair. Ann Thorac Surg 2012;93:726–732; discussion 33. https://doi.org/10.1016/j.athoracsur.2011.10.080.
37. Constantinou J, Kelay A, Mastracci TM. Open surgery for chronic dissection. J Vasc Surg. 2016;63:1377–83. https://doi.org/10.1016/j.jvs.2016.01.025.
38. Alfonsi J, Murana G, Smeenk HG, Kelder H, Schepens M, Sonker U, et al. Open surgical repair of post-dissection thoraco-abdominal aortic aneurysms: early and late outcomes of a single-centre study involving over 200 patients. Eur J Cardiothorac Surg. 2018;54:382–8. https://doi.org/10.1093/ejcts/ezy050.
39. Estrera AL, Jan A, Sandhu H, Shalhub S, Medina-Castro M, Nguyen TC, et al. Outcomes of open repair for chronic descending thoracic aortic dissection. Ann Thorac Surg 2015;99:786–793; discussion 94. https://doi.org/10.1016/j.athoracsur.2014.08.077.
40. Fujikawa T, Yamamoto S, Sekine Y, Oshima S, Kasai R, Mochida Y, et al. Operative results and clinical features of chronic stanford type B aortic dissection: Examination of 234 patients over 6 years. Eur J Vasc Endovasc Surg. 2015;50:738–43. https://doi.org/10.1016/j.ejvs.2015.07.012.
41. Preventza O, Price MD, Amarasekara HS, Tullos A, Chen P, Reidy MR, et al. Chronic Type I and Type III aortic dissections: a propensity analysis of outcomes after open distal repair. Eur J Cardiothorac Surg. 2018;54:510–6. https://doi.org/10.1093/ejcts/ezy039.
42. Pujara AC, Roselli EE, Hernandez AV, Vargas Abello LM, Burke JM, Svensson LG, et al. Open repair of chronic distal aortic dissection in the endovascular era: Implications for disease management. J Thorac Cardiovasc Surg. 2012;144:866–73. https://doi.org/10.1016/j.jtcvs.2012.01.021.
43. Tanaka A, Sandhu HK, Afifi RO, Miller CC 3rd, Ray A, Hassan M, et al. Outcomes of open repairs of chronic distal aortic dissection anatomically amenable to endovascular repairs. J Thorac Cardiovasc Surg. 2019; https://doi.org/10.1016/j.jtcvs.2019.09.083.
44. Ghanta RK, Green SY, Price MD, Arredondo CC, Wainwright D, Preventza O, et al. Midterm survival and quality of life after extent II thoracoabdominal aortic repair in Marfan syndrome. Ann Thorac Surg 2016;101:1402–1409; discussion 9. https://doi.org/10.1016/j.athoracsur.2015.10.018.
45. Zoli S, Etz CD, Roder F, Mueller CS, Brenner RM, Bodian CA, et al. Long-term survival after open repair of chronic distal aortic dissection. Ann Thorac Surg. 2010;89:1458–66. https://doi.org/10.1016/j.athoracsur.2010.02.014.

Diagnosis and Management of Ruptured Thoracic Aortic Aneurysms

Christopher Lau, Mario Gaudino, Erin Iannacone, and Leonard N. Girardi

Introduction

A ruptured thoracic aortic aneurysm (rTAA) is a lethal entity associated with a high rate of mortality. A majority of patients with rTAA die before reaching a hospital and those who survive the initial event often have ruptured aortas contained by the mediastinal tissues. Population level studies have found the incidence of rTAA to be 5 per 100,000 and only 41% of patients were alive upon arrival to a hospital. Fifty-four percent of patients die within 6 h of symptom onset and 76% die within 24 h. The most common location of rupture is the ascending aorta (54%) followed by the descending aorta (30%), and aortic arch (15%) [1].

Thoracic aneurysm ruptures in the various segments of the aorta require different operative approaches and skillsets for a successful repair. Similarly, the outcomes and operative risks of repair in different segments varies considerably. In the ascending aorta, most ruptures are associated with an aortic dissection and there is little controversy that the preferred surgical approach is with open repair via median sternotomy [2]. In the descending thoracic aorta, controversy exists regarding the optimal approach, whether that is an endovascular or traditional open repair. Both solutions have their limitations and unfortunately, there does not seem to be an ideal solution to date [3].

C. Lau (✉) · M. Gaudino · E. Iannacone · L. N. Girardi
Department of Cardiothoracic Surgery, Weill Cornell Medicine, New York, NY, USA
e-mail: chl9077@med.cornell.edu

J. S. Coselli et al. (eds.), *Aortic Dissection and Acute Aortic Syndromes*,
https://doi.org/10.1007/978-3-030-66668-2_31

Clinical Presentation

Thoracic aneurysms have a protracted, indolent clinical course and aneurysms remain asymptomatic until there is a catastrophic aortic event, such as rupture or dissection. For this reason, the clinical presentation of thoracic aneurysms occurs in two extremes: an asymptomatic incidentally discovered aneurysm or an acutely symptomatic aortic rupture or dissection. Those who present with pain are considered to have symptomatic aneurysms and surgical repair is indicated. Ruptured TAA fall into this latter category and the most common symptom upon presentation is severe chest pain, often radiating to or in association with back pain. Other clinical signs including a tearing sensation, dyspnea, tachycardia, and hemodynamic compromise.

While a majority of patients with rTAA likely expire in the field due to hemodynamic collapse, those who survive to reach the hospital have a broad spectrum of clinical presentation. In the best case scenario, there is a contained rupture and the presenting symptom is pain. These patients may even be severely hypertensive, which is sometimes itself the inciting cause of the rupture. These patients require immediate anti-impulse therapy with heart rate and blood pressure management in order to prevent further progression of the rupture while diagnostic and operative planning ensues. On the other end of the spectrum, patients may present with instability and impending hemodynamic collapse due to cardiac tamponade or free rupture. This group requires immediate volume resuscitation, support with vasoactive medications, and operative repair.

For asymptomatic TAA, current practice guidelines recommend surgical repair of aortic aneurysms with diameter >5.5 cm in the general population, with exceptions made for populations with increased risk of aortic events at smaller diameters. Patients at higher risk of aortic events, such as those with connective tissue disorder, family history of aortic dissection/rupture, or bicuspid aortopathy, are recommended for surgery at smaller diameters of 5 cm or less. On the other hand, patients with complex TAA disease, such as thoracoabdominal aortic aneurysms (TAAA), who are expected to have higher operative risk are given a higher threshold of 6 cm [4]. These recommendations are based on accumulating evidence that there exists an inflection point at 6 cm where the risk of rupture or dissection dramatically increases [5] (Fig. 1). Thus a recommendation for prophylactic surgery at 5.5 cm would decrease the rate of aortic events significantly but does not eliminate this risk.

In fact, a significant number of patients who present with aortic events have aneurysms of smaller sizes, which would not normally indicate a need for surgery. At the smaller diameters of less than 5 cm, aortic events mostly consist of dissection rather than rupture. At 5.0–5.9 cm, rupture risk begins to increase in prominence and the rate of rupture/dissection is 3% while rupture alone is 1.7%. With increasing diameter to over 6.0 cm, the rate of rupture alone increases significantly to 3.6% per year and rupture/dissection/death exceeds 10% [5]. Thus, continued monitoring for aortic growth and prophylactic surgery once aneurysms reach size thresholds is necessary to decrease the rate of fatal aortic events.

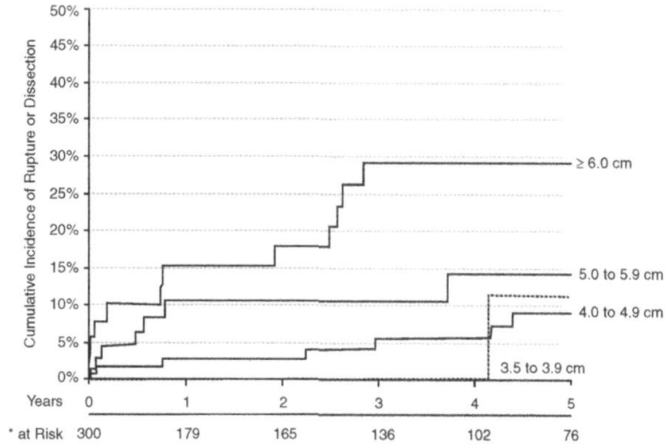

Fig. 1 Kaplan-Meier cumulative hazard function of rupture or dissection. Five-year hazard estimates are illustrated for patients as a function of initial aneurysm size (p = 0.006)

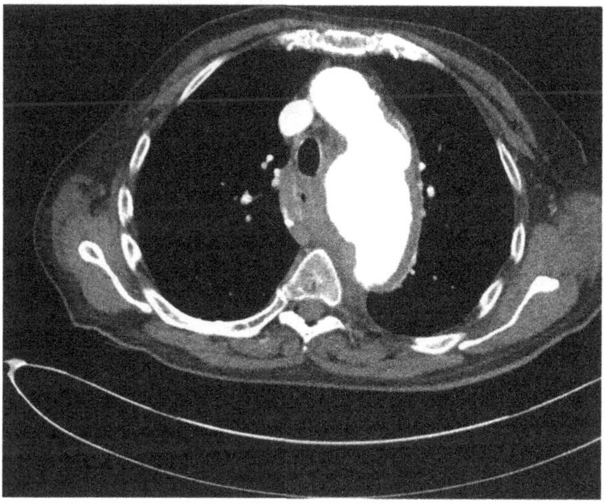

Fig. 2 Ruptured descending thoracic aneurysm

Diagnosis

Rupture of TAA may be suggested by clinical presentation but the diagnosis must be confirmed by cross-sectional imaging. The modality of choice is computed tomographic (CT) angiography due to the rapidity of image acquisition and highly detailed imaging resolution. While it may be difficult to get an unstable patient to the scanner, the imaging is absolutely necessary for identifying the cause and location of rupture, and for operative planning.

The etiology of rTAA is most often from aortic aneurysmal disease or aortic dissection (Figs. 2 and 3). A smaller proportion of ruptured aortas are due to blunt force trauma and rapid deceleration injuries causing tearing and pseudoaneurysm formation at the aortic isthmus. CT can clearly identify whether aortic dissection is present and it can give a sense of the chronicity of the dissection if present. It

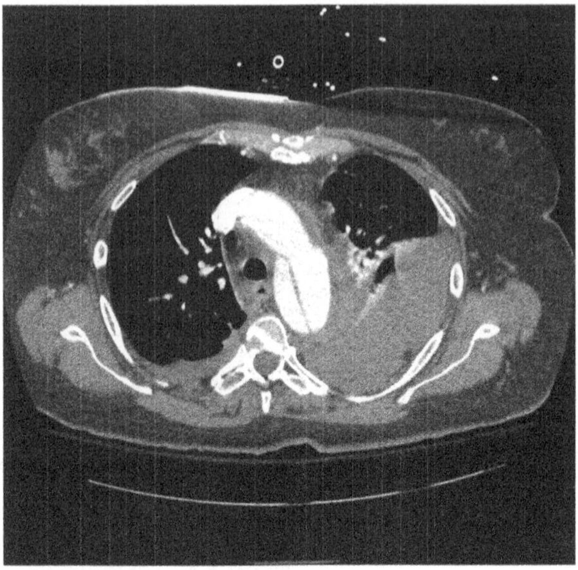

Fig. 3 Ruptured type B aortic dissection

characterizes the location and nature of the ruptured area, which is important information for planning the operation. Knowledge of the location of rupture is clearly of utmost importance to determine whether sternotomy, thoracotomy or endovascular approach is appropriate. The extent of aorta that is involved or aneurysmal will also dictate the amount of aorta that is replaced and specific technique that is used.

Aside from cross-sectional imaging of the aorta, a baseline echocardiogram documenting the ventricular function and any valvular pathology is helpful for risk stratification. Valvular pathology may require additional valve repair or replacement while regional wall motion abnormalities may imply a potential need for concomitant coronary artery bypass grafting. Usually the luxury of a cardiac catheterization to identify coronary disease and anatomy is not available due to the urgency of the need for surgical intervention.

Surgical Management

Ruptured TAA located in the ascending aorta are usually associated with an acute type A aortic dissection while ruptured aneurysms of the descending or thoracoabdominal aorta are comprised of a mix of pure aneurysmal disease, acute dissection, and chronic dissection. While rTAA of the ascending aorta are almost exclusively approached with open surgical repair via a sternotomy, ruptured descending thoracic aneurysm (DTA) may be repaired with either endovascular or open surgical techniques, depending on the situation.

Ruptured Ascending/Arch Aneurysm

The available data on ruptured ascending aortas is limited. A majority of patients with ruptured ascending aortas likely die in the field due to cardiac tamponade. The data that is available is difficult to compare due to differing definitions of "rupture." Rupture may be defined as bloody pericardial effusion, presence of cardiac tamponade physiology, or evidence of frank blood or clot in the pericardium. In our experience, rupture may also occur on the aortic wall adjacent to another structure such as the pulmonary artery, thus containing the blood in the epicardial tissues. Those with ruptured ascending aortas who survive to surgery have usually sealed or contained the rupture. The sternotomy and pericardiotomy often actually improve hemodynamics by relieving some degree of tamponade physiology.

In these cases, the priority is to get the patient on cardiopulmonary bypass in order to decrease the impulse pressure, which reduces the risk of worsening rupture. Secondly, if the rupture is located in the ascending aorta or aortic root, crossclamping and cardioplegic arrest will resolve the rupture issues. Aortic arch ruptures require repair with hypothermic circulatory arrest, which we routinely perform with adjunctive retrograde cerebral perfusion [6], although selective antegrade cerebral perfusion may be substituted depending on surgeon and institutional preferences.

Rupture defined as bloody pericardial effusion has not been found to be a risk factor for in-hospital mortality but may have some detrimental effect on long-term survival [7]. However, in an analysis of the International Registry of Acute Aortic Dissection database, 18% of patients with type A dissection had cardiac tamponade and the mortality in this group was significantly higher than in those without cardiac tamponade (44% versus 20%, $p < 0.001$). Additionally, periaortic hematoma is found in 45% of patients with cardiac tamponade and this itself is an independent predictor of mortality in patients with aortic dissection [2]. The presence of cardiac tamponade warrants emergent surgical intervention in order to prevent the later sequelae of prolonged low cardiac output, such as vasoplegia, renal failure, and hepatic failure.

Ruptured Descending/Thoracoabdominal Aorta

The management of ruptured DTA depends heavily on a number of factors including the etiology of the rupture, the experience and expertise of the operating surgeon and institution, the appropriateness of the aortic anatomy for thoracic endovascular aortic repair (TEVAR), and the availability of the appropriate implants. The need to proceed rapidly with repair limits these options. While some centers are equipped for expedient open aortic surgery, others may only have endovascular repair options available. Aneurysmal involvement of the visceral segment of the thoracoabdominal aorta further limits endovascular options. Endovascular repair in the visceral segment currently requires custom-made branched or fenestrated grafts that are not available on an emergent basis. Off-the-shelf options are not widely available at this time. Most centers do not have the resources and experience required to offer reasonable outcomes with both open repair and endovascular repair. There is a clear volume-outcome relationship at both the center and the surgeon level [8, 9]. Therefore, surgeons should use the approach that they are most familiar, whether that is endovascular or open repair. If the aortic anatomy precludes that approach then they should send the patient to a center experienced in the matter. At our center, we perform open aortic repair on all patients presenting with ruptured DTA with inadequate TEVAR landing zones or TAAA with involvement of the visceral branch vessels [10]. We employ TEVAR for ruptured aneurysms isolated to the DTA with adequate proximal and distal landing zones. In the setting of ruptured aneurysm with aortic dissection, we often perform open aortic repair rather than TEVAR due to the difficulty of permanently sealing off false lumen flow due to the inevitable presence of downstream fenestrations that perpetuate false lumen flow.

Aneurysm Versus Dissection

Consideration must be given to the primary aortic pathology causing the ruptured aorta, whether it is due to degenerative aneurysm, acute dissection, or chronic dissection. Degenerative aneurysms may be approached with either open surgical repair or TEVAR depending on the anatomy of the aneurysm and landing zones. Acute dissections with rupture may benefit from a TEVAR approach due to the fragile nature of acutely dissected aorta and the difficulty of open surgery in this setting. However, TEVAR may be more applicable in aortas that are not severely aneurysmal. With a rupture, one must be sure that the primary tear is covered and that there is complete obliteration of the false lumen in the area of the rupture to ensure that there is no perfusion to the ruptured area. With chronic aortic dissection and rupture, we would not recommend an endovascular approach. The indications for TEVAR have been expanding and some groups have had early success with TEVAR for chronic type B aortic dissections when anatomic criteria are appropriate (suitable proximal and distal landing zones, visceral vessels originating from the true lumen, absence of extremely small true lumen, presence of large proximal entry tear, and absence of connective tissue disorder) [11]. In follow up studies, reverse aortic remodeling and false lumen thrombosis have been seen in 86–91% of patients [12]. However, in the setting of aortic rupture, acute obliteration of false lumen flow cannot be guaranteed due to the stiff nature of the intimal septum and continued blood loss through the area of rupture may be possible. In this setting we prefer open surgical repair.

Open Repair

Open surgical repair is a versatile method of treating rTAA that can be used for all types of aortic anatomy, including aneurysms extending into the aortic arch and/or involving the visceral segment and abdominal aorta. However, it remains a formidable surgical challenge with morbidity and mortality that remain significantly higher than in elective situations [10]. Historical data from the Nationwide Inpatient Sample from 1988–1998 showed that open repair of rTAAA carried a 53% mortality but this sample included low-volume centers and both surgical technique and critical care have improved significantly since that time [13]. In contemporary single-center series, operative mortality ranges from 12% to 26% [10, 14–18]. However, centers with less experience who decide to attempt repair given the near certain risk of death without surgery likely contribute to the overall poor nationwide results.

Our algorithm for treating rTAAA is based on that we have described for intact TAAA [19] and modified according to the hemodynamic stability of the patient and the anatomy of the aneurysm. In unstable patients we skip the preoperative lumbar spinal drain and proceed straight to surgery. We perform a 5th–6th interspace thoracotomy and obtain proximal control immediately. Care is taken not to mobilize the lung off of the aneurysm aggressively because the rupture is often contained by the mediastinal tissues or lung itself. If proximal control is not attainable then cooling for circulatory arrest is initiated, usually via femoral cannulation. If proximal control is obtained, we almost exclusively use a clamp-and-sew technique for unstable patients in order to proceed as rapidly as possible. A lumbar spinal drain is then placed postoperatively in the operating room for spinal cord protection.

In stable patients, attempt is made to place a preoperative lumbar spinal drain given the strong evidence showing a reduction in spinal cord injury and minimal adverse effects of drainage [20, 21]. Hypothermic circulatory arrest is utilized when proximal control is lacking. When proximal control is attainable either between the left common carotid artery and left subclavian artery or distal to the left subclavian artery, then repair is completed with mild hypothermia with or without left heart bypass support. Simpler repairs such degenerative aneurysms limited to the thoracic aorta are repaired with a clamp-and-sew technique. Complex repairs, such as extent II TAAA or aortic dissections are repaired with the support of left heart bypass due to the increased time necessary to perform the repair and the increased risk of spinal cord injury. In these cases there is often an abundance of patent intercostal arteries that require time-consuming ligation. Left heart bypass is initiated from the left inferior pulmonary vein to the distal aorta or femoral artery. The proximal anastomosis is performed on partial bypass and then bypass is discontinued to perform an open distal anastomosis often with reimplantation of one to two sets of intercostal arteries in the lower thoracic region.

Using these techniques, our group recently reported on the repair of 100 consecutive rTAAA with an operative mortality of 14% [10], which represents an improvement from 18.5% in our prior series [22]. Improvement in surgeon experience, surgical technique, and perioperative care likely contributed to the improvements in outcomes. However, the results in the rupture group still remained over threefold worse than in the intact aneurysm group, which had a mortality of only 4.2% ($p = 0.01$) (Fig. 4). Additionally, the incidence of major postoperative adverse events was significantly higher in the rupture group. Myocardial infarction (7.0% vs 0.8%, $P < 0.004$), respiratory failure (19% vs 5.7%, $P < 0.001$), and the need for postoperative dialysis (11% vs 4.2%, $P = 0.01$) were all more prevalent in those presenting with rupture. Fortunately, spinal cord injury was not more common (5%

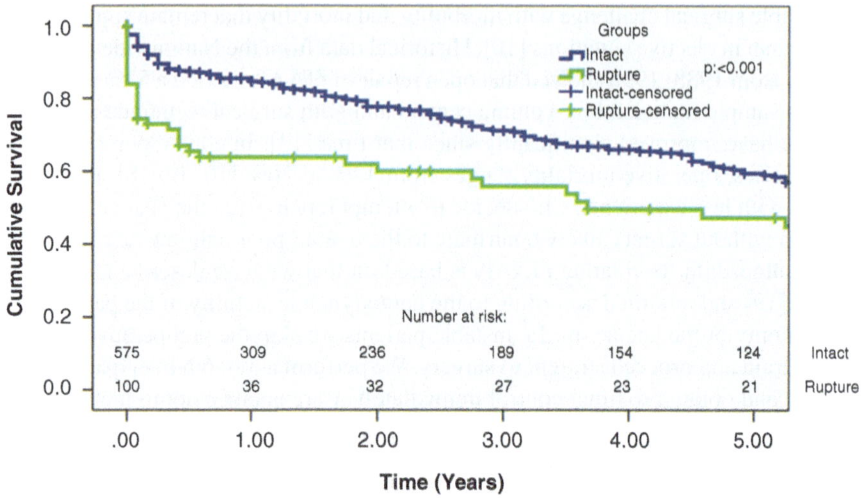

Survival	30 days (95% CI)	3- Year (95% CI)	5- Year (95% CI)
Intact	94.0% (92.0%-96.0%)	71.2% (66.5%-75.9%)	59.5% (53.8%-65.2%)
Rupture	73.5% (64.3%-82.7%)	56.0% (44.2%-67.8%)	47.5% (35.0%-60.0%)

Fig. 4 Kaplan-Meier survival curves, rupture versus intact, in the unmatched series. CI, Confidence interval

vs 2.4%, P = 0.16). Similar to findings from other groups, the 5-year survival was lower (47.5% vs 59.5%, P < 0.001) than for our nonruptured group [10].

Endovascular Repair

TEVAR has become a viable alternative to open surgical repair and it is being used with increasing frequency for rTAA. A majority of patients with rTAA present to hospitals that do not perform open DTA/TAAA repair in high volume and lack the infrastructure to achieve optimal results with open surgery. However, a growing number of surgeons have learned and developed endovascular skills, making successful treatment with TEVAR a possibility for a larger number of patients, even in a smaller hospital center. Potential advantages of TEVAR are the minimally invasive nature of the procedure, avoidance of thoracotomy incisions, more rapid recovery, and lower incidence of respiratory complications. While one might expect a minimally invasive endovascular procedure to have significantly better outcomes compared to open aortic repair, in reality, the incidence of major postoperative adverse events is quite similar, with the exception of reduced pulmonary complications. However, the trade-off is a high incidence of endoleaks, increased need for re-intervention, and poorer long-term survival [3, 23–31] (Fig. 5).

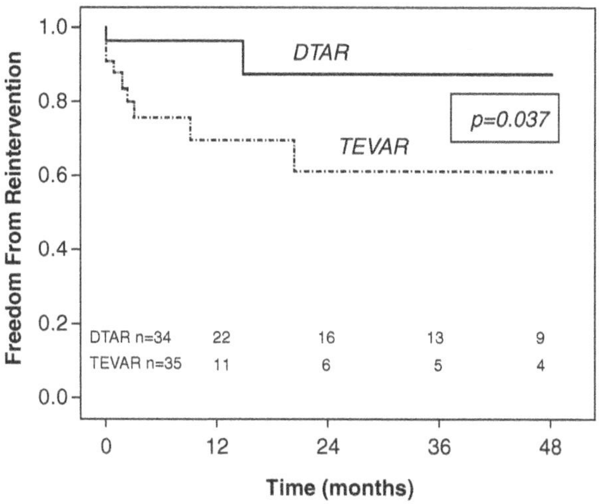

Fig. 5 A Kaplan-Meier analysis describing the need for reintervention in any aortic segment. This analysis suggests that the need for aortic reintervention at any aortic segment (treated, adjacent, or remote) is significantly higher in the TEVAR group. Freedom from reintervention at 4 years was 87.4% for DTAR vs 61.2% for TEVAR (P = 0.037). In this analysis, if patients were deemed to be nonoperative, or refused further intervention, the date at which point the need for reintervention was identified was used as the time of treatment failure

In our practice, we employ TEVAR for rTAA when the anatomy is ideal. These are patients with aneurysm and rupture isolated to the DTA, who have adequate proximal and distal landing zones and reasonable iliofemoral arterial access. If debranching of the arch will be necessary to obtain an adequate proximal landing zone, our preference is open repair. We also exclude chronic dissections from TEVAR while acute complicated type B dissections are approached with endovascular repair when anatomically feasible.

Operative mortality associated with TEVAR for rTAA has varied widely from 3% to 48% [3, 23–31] highlighting the importance of operator and institutional experience as well as the high-risk nature of these patients regardless of the repair methods chosen. The incidences of stroke and spinal cord injury were similar to most open surgical series, ranging from 0–11% and 4–26%, respectively [23–31]. The rate of endoleaks with TEVAR is quite prominent, occurring in approximately 16–18% of patients in a majority of series resulting in need for re-intervention in up to 24% of cases [23, 25, 26, 28, 29, 31]. The need for re-interventions in those surviving the initial procedure remains disappointing and negates the early mortality benefit of TEVAR in rTAAs in large data sets where late survival is actually worse with TEVAR then open repair [3].

Although pulmonary complications are less common with TEVAR than open surgery, in the setting of rTAA, it is still a common complication occurring in at least 18% of patients partly due to the presence of retained hemothorax [23, 32]. Undrained blood in the thorax may contribute to respiratory complications. At a minimum, the presence of hemothorax should indicate a thoracostomy tube and nearly a quarter of patients may require a thoracic drainage procedure [23]. If chest tube drainage fails to evacuate clotted blood, this could lead to fibrothorax.

Traumatic Aortic Rupture

One entity particularly well-suited for TEVAR rather than open repair is traumatic aortic rupture (Fig. 6). A majority of these patients have suffered from blunt force trauma causing injury at the isthmus of the aorta and have significant other associated traumatic injuries. Obtaining proximal aortic control can be hazardous during open repair due to the location of injury near the crossclamp site. Additionally, the higher amount of heparin necessary could worsen other injuries. TEVAR is well-suited since a majority of these patients have normal-sized aortas and landing zones are usually not an issue, although some patients will require coverage of the left subclavian artery. Direct comparisons between open repair and TEVAR for traumatic aortic rupture favor TEVAR in this situation [33, 34].

Comparison of Open Versus Endovascular Repair of Ruptured DTA

Comparisons between open repair and TEVAR for rTAA are skewed by confounding factors that affect patient selection. Thus, comparisons of the two groups are often not between evenly matched patient cohorts with similar risk factors and

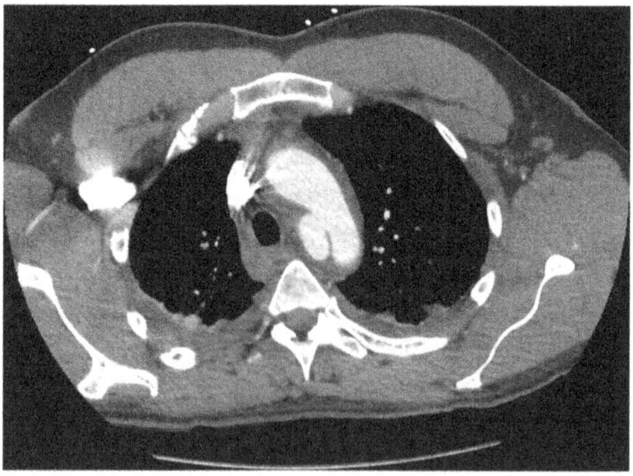

Fig. 6 Traumatic aortic rupture with pseudoanuerysm at the aortic isthmus after blunt trauma

anatomy. For example, patients with favorable anatomy and thus lesser risk, such as a mid-descending aneurysm with normal proximal and distal landing zones, are more likely to be repaired by TEVAR. Older patients, who may be higher risk would also be considered for TEVAR in order to avoid a risky open procedure, even if landing zones are suboptimal. Some difficult anatomies, such as distal arch aneurysm or perivisceral aneurysms, are not candidates for routine TEVAR and these higher risk patients can only be repaired by open surgery. These anatomic risk factors are often not captured even when patients are matched for baseline characteristics in studies. Despite this, a risk adjusted study from the US nationwide Inpatient Sample found that that the odds of mortality, complications, and failure to rescue were similar for TEVAR and open repair. Additionally, results of TEVAR were similar in smaller compared to larger hospitals but the results of open repair were poorer in smaller hospitals, where open repair expertise may have been lacking [35] (Table 1).

Single-center studies comparing open repair to TEVAR have often found TEVAR to be associated with a lower operative mortality and more favorable discharge disposition [16, 36]. However, other series from centers experienced in open repair have reported operative mortality as low as 14%, which is favorable compared to most TEVAR series [10]. A recent meta-analysis reported lower operative mortality with TEVAR (19% versus 33%, $p = 0.016$) but TEVAR was associated with a significant number of aneurysm-related deaths in follow-up, largely due to stent-graft related complications such as endoleak [17]. A study of the Medicare database showed similar findings. There was lower operative mortality with TEVAR compared to open repair (28.4% vs 45%, $P < 0.001$). However, this survival advantage disappeared by 1.5 years after the procedure, due to aortic events and need for re-intervention [3] (Fig. 7).

Table 1 Backward stepwise regression: final iterations of subgroup analysis

Predictor	Outcome	Group	OR	95% CI Lower	95% CI Upper	*P* value
Smaller (vs larger) hospital	Mortality	OAR	2.39	1.13	5.09	0.023
	Complications	OAR	3.96	1.78	8.79	0.001
	FTR	OAR	51.11	9.73	268.35	<0.001
Smaller (vs larger) hospital	Mortality	TEVAR	1.00	0.30	3.30	0.997*
	Complications	TEVAR	0.58	0.21	1.56	0.283*
	FTR	TEVAR	1.05	0.21	5.16	0.951*
Renal comorbidity	Mortality	TEVAR	10.81	3.54	32.99	<0.001
	FTR	TEVAR	309.54	47.97	1997.15	<0.001

CI Confidence interval; *OAR* open aortic repair; *FTR* failure to rescue; *TEVAR* thoracic endovascular aortic repair

*Represents *P* value when covariate was excluded, not final iteration

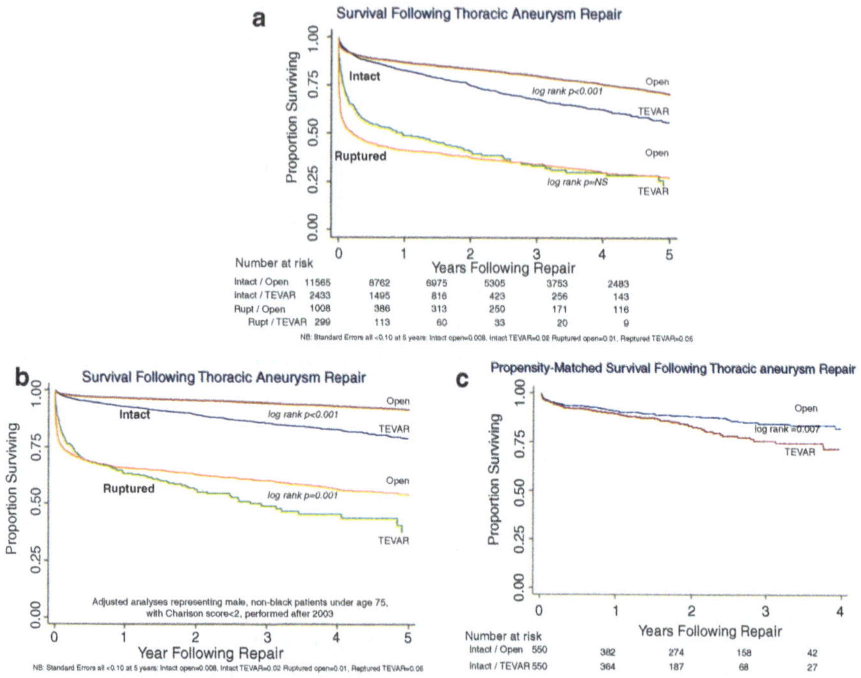

Fig. 7 (**a**) Unadjusted 5-year survival in thoracic aneurysms by procedure type and diagnosis. (**b**) Adjusted 5-year survival in thoracic aneurysms by procedure type and diagnosis. Results represent male, nonblack patients <75 years of age with a Charlson score < 2 performed after 2003. (**c**) Propensity-matched 5-year survival in thoracic aneurysms by procedure type. These patients represent a randomly selected, propensity-matched sample of low-risk patients who are at equal likelihood of undergoing either open repair or thoracic endovascular repair (TEVAR)

Conclusions

The answer to the question of whether open aortic repair or TEVAR is the preferred method for repairing rTAA is not straightforward. Fortunately, the results of both techniques are improving with experience. Surgeons experienced in either open aortic repair or TEVAR can achieve excellent results using their respective techniques. Thus the ideal repair technique in any single situation is the one with which the surgeon and institution has the best chance of success. With open aortic repair, experienced centers achieve results comparable to TEVAR but with excellent long-term durability. With TEVAR, even smaller, less experienced centers can achieve good results but long-term durability may be compromised due to endograft-related complications.

Conflicts of Interest No conflicts of interest to report.

Funding No outside funding received.

References

1. Johansson G, Markström U, Swedenborg J. Ruptured thoracic aortic aneurysms: a study of incidence and mortality rates. J Vasc Surg. 1995;21:985–8.
2. Evangelista A, Isselbacher EM, Bossone E, Gleason TG, Eusanio MD, Sechtem U, et al. Insights from the international registry of acute aortic dissection: a 20-year experience of collaborative clinical research. Circulation. 2018;137:1846–60.
3. Goodney PP, Travis L, Lucas FL, Fillinger MF, Goodman DC, Cronenwett JL, et al. Survival after open versus endovascular thoracic aortic aneurysm repair in an observational study of the medicare population. Circulation. 2011;124:2661–9.
4. Hiratzka LF, Bakris GL, Beckman JA, Bersin RM, Carr VF, Casey DE, et al. 2010 ACCF/AHA/AATS/ACR/ASA/SCA/SCAI/SIR/STS/SVM guidelines for the diagnosis and management of patients with Thoracic Aortic Disease: a report of the American College of Cardiology Foundation/American Heart Association Task Force on Practice Guidelines, American Association for Thoracic Surgery, American College of Radiology, American Stroke Association, Society of Cardiovascular Anesthesiologists, Society for Cardiovascular Angiography and Interventions, Society of Interventional Radiology, Society of Thoracic Surgeons, and Society for Vascular Medicine. Circulation. 2010;121:e266–369.
5. Davies RR, Goldstein LJ, Coady MA, Tittle SL, Rizzo JA, Kopf GS, et al. Yearly rupture or dissection rates for thoracic aortic aneurysms: simple prediction based on size. Ann Thorac Surg. 2002;73:17–27.
6. Lau C, Gaudino M, Iannacone EM, Gambardella I, Munjal M, Ohmes LB, et al. Retrograde cerebral perfusion is effective for prolonged circulatory arrest in arch aneurysm repair. Ann Thorac Surg. 2018;105:491–7.
7. Ehrlich MP, Grabenwöger M, Kilo J, Kocher AA, Grubhofer G, Lassnig AM, et al. Surgical treatment of acute type A dissection: is rupture a risk factor? Ann Thorac Surg. 2002;73:1843–8.
8. Cowan JA, Dimick JB, Henke PK, Huber TS, Stanley JC, Upchurch GR. Surgical treatment of intact thoracoabdominal aortic aneurysms in the United States: hospital and surgeon volume-related outcomes. J Vasc Surg. 2003;37:1169–74.
9. Patel VI, Mukhopadhyay S, Ergul E, Aranson N, Conrad MF, Lamuraglia GM, et al. Impact of hospital volume and type on outcomes of open and endovascular repair of descending thoracic aneurysms in the United States Medicare population. J Vasc Surg. 2013;58:346–54.
10. Gaudino M, Lau C, Munjal M, Girardi LN. Open repair of ruptured descending thoracic and thoracoabdominal aortic aneurysms. J Thorac Cardiovasc Surg. 2015;150:814–21.
11. Burke CR, Bavaria JE. The role of thoracic endovascular repair in chronic type B aortic dissection. Semin Thorac Cardiovasc Surg. 2019;32(1):21–4.
12. Khoynezhad A, Toluie S, Al-Atassi T. Treatment of the chronic type B aortic dissection: the pro-endovascular argument. Semin Thorac Cardiovasc Surg. 2017;29:131–6.
13. Cowan JA, Dimick JB, Wainess RM, Henke PK, Stanley JC, Upchurch GR. Ruptured thoracoabdominal aortic aneurysm treatment in the United States: 1988 to 1998. J Vasc Surg. 2003;38:319–22.
14. Lewis ME, Ranasinghe AM, Revell MP, Bonser RS. Surgical repair of ruptured thoracic and thoracoabdominal aortic aneurysms. Br J Surg. 2002;89:442–5.
15. Barbato JE, Kim JY, Zenati M, Abu-Hamad G, Rhee RY, Makaroun MS, et al. Contemporary results of open repair of ruptured descending thoracic and thoracoabdominal aortic aneurysms. J Vasc Surg. 2007;45:667–76.
16. Jonker FHW, Verhagen HJM, Lin PH, Heijmen RH, Trimarchi S, Lee WA, et al. Open surgery versus endovascular repair of ruptured thoracic aortic aneurysms. J Vasc Surg. 2011;53:1210–6.
17. Jonker FHW, Trimarchi S, Verhagen HJM, Moll FL, Sumpio BE, Muhs BE. Meta-analysis of open versus endovascular repair for ruptured descending thoracic aortic aneurysm. J Vasc Surg. 2010;51:1026–32.
18. Zanetti PP, Krasoń M, Walas R, Cebotaru T, Popa C, Vintila B, et al. "Open" repair of ruptured thoracoabdominal aortic aneurysm (experience of 51 cases). Kardiochir Torakochirurgia Pol. 2015;12:119–25.

19. Lau C, Gaudino M, Gambardella I, Mills E, Munjal M, Elsayed M, et al. Reoperative repair of descending thoracic and thoracoabdominal aneurysms. Eur J Cardiothorac Surg. 2017;52:501–7.
20. Coselli JS, LeMaire SA, Köksoy C, Schmittling ZC, Curling PE. Cerebrospinal fluid drainage reduces paraplegia after thoracoabdominal aortic aneurysm repair: results of a randomized clinical trial. J Vasc Surg. 2002;35:631–9.
21. Riley SP, Donnelly MJ, Khatib D, Warren C, Schroeder KM. Post-dural puncture headaches following spinal drain placement during thoracoabdominal aortic aneurysm repair: incidence, associated risk factors, and treatment. J Anesth. 2015;29:544–50.
22. Girardi LN, Krieger KH, Altorki NK, Mack CA, Lee LY, Isom OW. Ruptured descending and thoracoabdominal aortic aneurysms. Ann Thorac Surg. 2002;74:1066–70.
23. Jonker FHW, Verhagen HJM, Lin PH, Heijmen RH, Trimarchi S, Lee WA, et al. Outcomes of endovascular repair of ruptured descending thoracic aortic aneurysms. Circulation. 2010;121:2718–23.
24. Mitchell ME, Rushton FW, Boland AB, Byrd TC, Baldwin ZK. Emergency procedures on the descending thoracic aorta in the endovascular era. J Vasc Surg. 2011;54:1298–302.
25. Alsac J-M, Pierard T, El Batti S, Achouh P, Julia P, Fabiani J-N. Applicability and mid-term results of endovascular treatment for descending thoracic acute aortic syndromes. Ann Vasc Surg. 2013;27:1029–35.
26. Minami T, Imoto K, Uchida K, Karube N, Yasuda S, Choh T, et al. Thoracic endovascular aortic repair for ruptured descending thoracic aortic aneurysm. J Card Surg. 2015;30:163–9.
27. Doss M, Wood JP, Balzer J, Martens S, Deschka H, Moritz A. Emergency endovascular interventions for acute thoracic aortic rupture: four-year follow-up. J Thorac Cardiovasc Surg. 2005;129:645–51.
28. Geisbüsch P, Kotelis D, Weber TF, Hyhlik-Dürr A, Böckler D. Endovascular repair of ruptured thoracic aortic aneurysms is associated with high perioperative mortality and morbidity. J Vasc Surg. 2010;51:299–304.
29. Etienne H, Majewski M, Cochennec F, Segaux L, Becquemin J-P. Emergency endovascular interventions for ruptured descending thoracic aortic aneurysm. Ann Vasc Surg. 2017;39:160–6.
30. Hellgren T, Wanhainen A, Steuer J, Mani K. Outcome of endovascular repair for intact and ruptured thoracic aortic aneurysms. J Vasc Surg. 2017;66:21–8.
31. Hammo S, Larzon T, Hultgren R, Wanhainen A, Mani K, Resch T, et al. Outcome after endovascular repair of ruptured descending thoracic aortic aneurysm: a national multicentre study. Eur J Vasc Endovasc Surg. 2019;57:788–94.
32. Ju MH, Nooromid MJ, Rodriguez HE, Eskandari MK. Management of hemothorax after thoracic endovascular aortic repair for ruptured aneurysms. Vascular. 2018;26:39–46.
33. Buz S, Zipfel B, Mulahasanovic S, Pasic M, Weng Y, Hetzer R. Conventional surgical repair and endovascular treatment of acute traumatic aortic rupture. Eur J Cardiothorac Surg. 2008;33:143–9.
34. Amabile P, Collart F, Gariboldi V, Rollet G, Bartoli J-M, Piquet P. Surgical versus endovascular treatment of traumatic thoracic aortic rupture. J Vasc Surg. 2004;40:873–9.
35. Gopaldas RR, Dao TK, LeMaire SA, Huh J, Coselli JS. Endovascular versus open repair of ruptured descending thoracic aortic aneurysms: a nationwide risk-adjusted study of 923 patients. J Thorac Cardiovasc Surg. 2011;142:1010–8.
36. Patel HJ, Williams DM, Upchurch GR, Dasika NL, Deeb GM. A comparative analysis of open and endovascular repair for the ruptured descending thoracic aorta. J Vasc Surg. 2009;50:1265–70.

Monitoring and Medical Treatment of Chronic Thoracic, Abdominal, and Thoracoabdominal Aortic Aneurysms

Melinda S. Schaller, Winona W. Wu, and Marc L. Schermerhorn

Introduction

Aortic disease can be attributed as the cause of death in nearly 10,000 individuals a year in the United States [1]. Thoracic aortic aneurysms (TAA) are those of the aortic root, ascending aortic, aortic arch and descending aorta above the diaphragm (Fig. 1). In some individuals, multiple segments may be involved. When both the thoracic segment and the abdominal segment of the aorta are aneurysmal, this is referred to as a thoracoabdominal aneurysm (TAAA) (Fig. 2). Normal diameters of the different thoracic aortic segments vary based on age and gender, but generally, any localized dilation greater than 50% of predicted is considered aneurysmal [2]. Of TAA, 60% involve the root/ascending aorta, 10% involve the arch, 40% involve the descending portion, and 10% are TAAA [3]. The overall incidence of thoracic aneurysms is approximately 10 per 100,000 person years, though incidence rates increase substantially with age [4]. The average age at diagnosis is 69 years, but women are often older than their male counterparts, with women on average being diagnosed at the age of 76 years and men at the age of 63 years [4]. There are several conditions that predispose individuals to the development of a TAA, including genetic syndromes such as Marfan syndrome, Loeys-Dietz syndrome, Ehlers-Danlos syndrome, and Turner syndrome; inflammatory diseases such as Takayasu and Behcet disease; and anatomic variants such as a bicuspid aortic valve, right-sided aortic arch, or aberrant right subclavian artery [2].

Abdominal aortic aneurysms (AAA) involve the segment of the aortic below the diaphragm. Abdominal aortic aneurysms are defined by an increase in the aortic diameter by 50% compared with normal, adjacent aorta; in most individuals, this would be a size greater than 3 cm [5]. The majority of AAA, approximately 90%, involve the infrarenal segment, but any abdominal segment can be involved

M. S. Schaller · W. W. Wu · M. L. Schermerhorn (✉)
Division of Vascular Surgery, Beth Israel Deaconess Medical Center, Boston, MA, USA
e-mail: mscherm@bidmc.harvard.edu

J. S. Coselli et al. (eds.), *Aortic Dissection and Acute Aortic Syndromes*,
https://doi.org/10.1007/978-3-030-66668-2_32

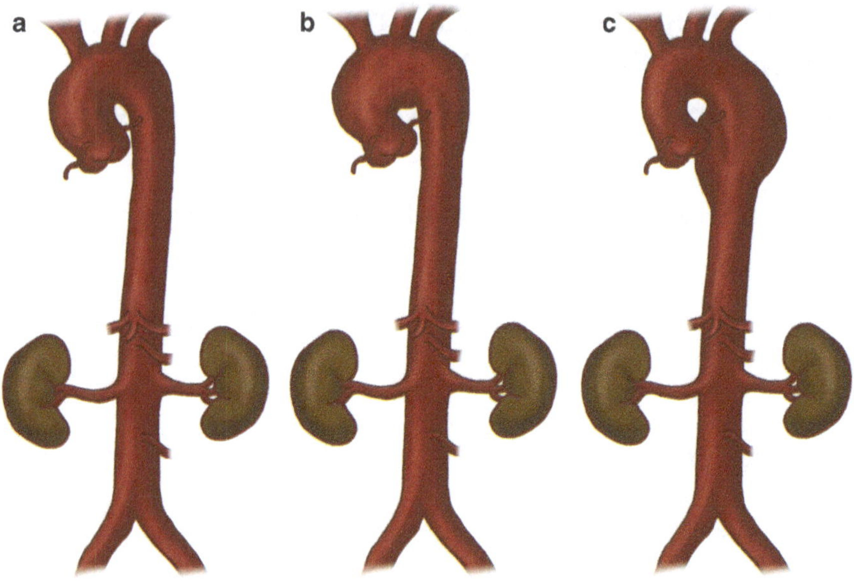

Fig. 1 Thoracic aortic aneurysms. These include (a) the aortic root and ascending aorta, (b) the aortic arch, and (c) the descending aorta

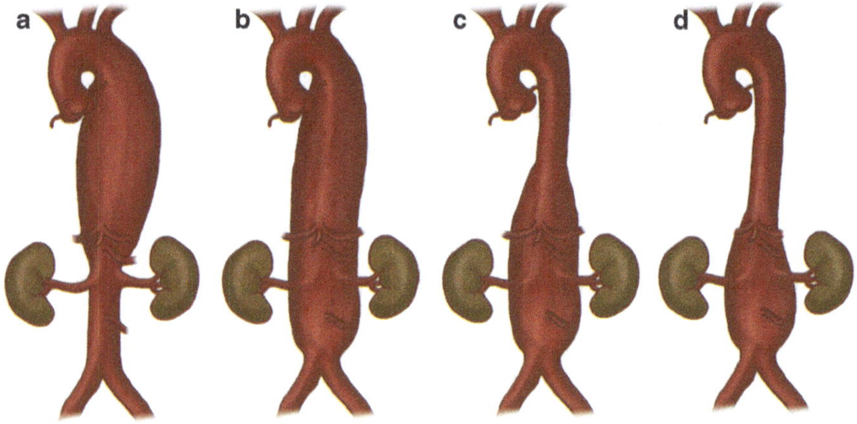

Fig. 2 The Crawford classification of thoracoabdominal aortic aneurysms (TAAA). (a) Type I TAAA, extends from the left subclavian (LSA) to the suprarenal aorta; (b) Type II TAAA, extends from the LSA to the aortic bifurcation; (c) Type III TAAA, extends from the distal descending thoracic aorta to the aortic bifurcation; (d) Type IV TAAA, extends from the supraceliac aorta to the aortic bifurcation

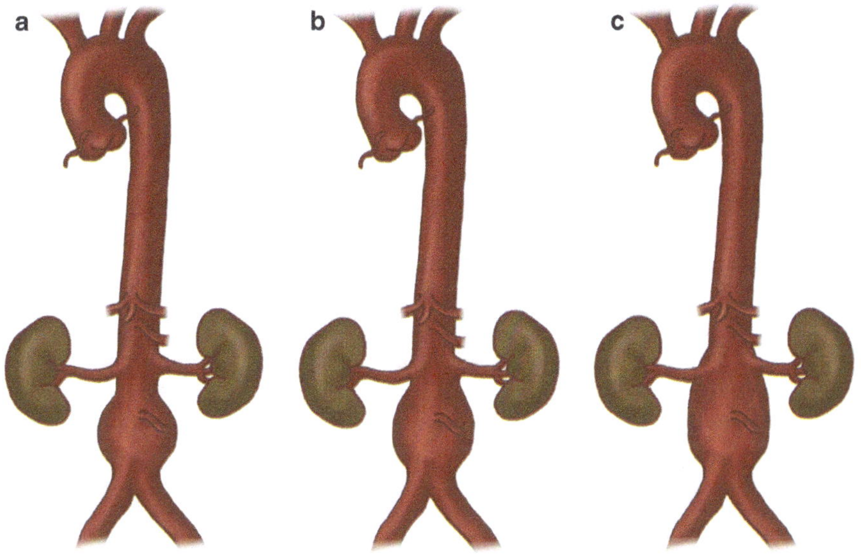

Fig. 3 Abdominal aortic aneurysms. These include (**a**) infrarenal, (**b**) juxtarenal, and (**c**) suprarenal

(Fig. 3) [6]. The prevalence of AAA is likely between 3% and 10% of those older than 50 years, but this will vary in populations depending on the prevalence of associated risk factors [7]. The most relevant modifiable risk factor for AAA is smoking [8]. Risk of developing an AAA increases with age and is substantially greater in men [9].

Clinical Manifestations, Screening, and Diagnosis

The majority of patients with either chronic TAA or AAA are asymptomatic and these aneurysms are diagnosed incidentally when imaging studies are obtained for other reasons. TAA can occasionally be recognized on chest x-rays as a widened mediastinum, increased girth of the aortic knob, or as a cause of tracheal deviation. Aneurysms of the root can lead to aortic regurgitation, which can occasionally be identified on physical exam. When TAA become large, they can sometimes lead to local compressive symptoms, such as that of the trachea or bronchus, which can lead to cough, shortness of breath, or wheezing. If the esophagus is compressed, this can lead to dysphagia [3]. If a TAA is suspected, the diagnostic studies of choice are either a CT or MR angiogram (CTA or MRA). Additionally, transthoracic or transesophageal echocardiography is useful for imaging and surveillance of the aortic root and can diagnose the degree of regurgitation, if present.

Aneurysms of the abdominal aorta are occasionally diagnosed on x-rays of the spine or abdominal cavity. They may also be appreciated on physical exam, although this is not a reliable way to exclude an aneurysm. An important aspect of the evaluation of a patient with an AAA is to palpate the aorta to elicit the presence of tenderness, necessitating expeditious repair. Like their thoracic counterparts, AAA are best imaged with a CT or MR angiogram, as this will give the clinician the most information about anatomic features that would impact the timing and technical aspects regarding repair. Abdominal ultrasound is also an important imaging modality for AAA, as it can be used for both screening and following growth of the aneurysm over time. Abdominal ultrasound is a useful modality for surveillance as it is reproducible, readily attainable, and non-invasive. Several studies have demonstrated that a single, ultrasound-based screening exam for AAA can effectively reduce mortality related to aneurysms as well as rupture risk [10–13]. These studies found that screening decreased aneurysm-related mortality by 40% and reduced aneurysm rupture by 50% [12, 13].

Natural History

The natural history of TAA is to increase in size with an average growth rate of about 0.1–0.42 cm/year [14, 15]. Smaller TAA (4 cm) typically grow around 0.08 cm/year whereas large aneurysms grow at a faster rate [16]. The rate of growth is also affected by the location of the TAA, with those of the ascending aorta growing more slowly than those of the descending thoracic aorta [16, 17]. Abdominal aortic aneurysms between 3 and 4 cm grow slowly with a < 10% increase in size per year [18, 19]. Those AAA 4 cm and larger tend to grow approximately 10% per year, although there is substantial variability among individuals [18, 20].

As aneurysms increase in size, the overall risk of rupture also increases. For TAA the yearly risk of rupture of aneurysms smaller than 5 cm is less than 5% compared to a yearly risk of approximately 16% for those greater than 6 cm [16]. A similar trend holds true for AAA. In the Aneurysm Detection and Management (ADAM) trial which reported the rupture risk for those with AAA who declined or were unfit for repair, the annual risk of rupture for aneurysms between 4 and 5 cm was 0.5–5%, for those between 5.5 and 5.9 cm was 9%, for those between 6 and 6.9 cm was 10%, and for those greater than 7 cm was 33% [21, 22].

Medical Management Strategies

The most important risk factor modification that can be made during aneurysm surveillance is smoking cessation [23, 24]. While risk factor modification in cardiovascular disease is well-established and often includes lipid-lowering agents such as statins and hemodynamic control with agents such as beta blockers and ACE inhibitors, data to support their use to decrease aneurysm expansion or rupture risk are lacking [25–28]. Although, perioperative statin therapy has been found to improve long-term survival in patients undergoing AAA repair, so their use is recommended in this patient population unless contraindications exist [29]. Investigations into the use of medications such as doxycycline, which can inhibit matrix metalloproteinases, have demonstrated no benefit to reduce aneurysm growth [30, 31]. During an aneurysm surveillance period, patients should be encouraged to stop smoking and their general health optimized when possible, including treatment of hypertension, dyslipidemia, and participation in a regular exercise regimen [32–34].

Surveillance Strategies

For both thoracic and abdominal aortic aneurysms, the timing and modality of surveillance imaging will depend on the initial size of the aortic aneurysm, its location, and its rate of expansion during the surveillance period. For ascending aortic aneurysms that are degenerative in nature, those smaller than 4 cm can be followed yearly with echocardiography, to reduce cumulative radiation exposure, or cross-sectional imaging. Once the ascending aorta reaches 4.5 cm, or the rate of growth is greater than 0.5 cm/year, one should obtain surveillance imaging every 6 months [2]. Operative repair should be considered once the ascending aorta reaches 5.5 cm in size [17, 35], though some have proposed using an aortic sizing index that takes into consideration variation in aortic size by gender and body size [36]. In individuals with connective tissue disorders, such as Marfan syndrome, the diameter for consideration of operative repair is smaller, at 4–5 cm [2, 17]. Size criteria and timing for surveillance of aneurysms of the aortic arch are similar to those of the ascending aorta, with operative repair being recommended in appropriate candidates at a size of 5.5 cm [15]. For the descending thoracic aorta and for TAAA, elective repair for asymptomatic degenerative aneurysms is recommended at a diameter of 5.5–6 cm, depending on patient health factors and anatomic and technical considerations; if an endovascular option exists, one may consider repair at a diameter of 5.5 cm versus waiting to 6 cm for those who will require an open repair due to the increased morbidity and mortality associated with open repairs [37]. Once an aneurysm is approaching a size where operative repair would be recommended, those who have been screened with ultrasound or MRA should have a CTA performed. This is the ideal study for identifying anatomic features that can impact repair strategies and is the best study for delineating the distribution of aortic calcification.

Once an aneurysm of the abdominal aorta is identified, these individuals should enter into a regular surveillance program. Regular surveillance has been found to be safe until the aneurysm reaches a size of 5.5 cm in men and between 5 and 5.4 cm in women [9, 38, 39]. Surveillance intervals of 3 years have been recommended for abdominal aneurysms measuring 3–3.9 cm, 1 year for aneurysms measuring 4–4.9, with intervals of 6 months being recommended for those larger than 5 cm [9, 40]. The majority of the recommendations for surveillance and repair of aortic aneurysms have been based on datasets in which women are underrepresented. Other strategies for aneurysms in women have been developed which may be more accurate for determining overall risk, and associated timelines for repair, including the aortic size index (aneurysm diameter (cm)/body surface area (m^2)) [41]. There are certain circumstances when one may recommend operative repair prior to the aneurysm size threshold criteria being met, including rapid aneurysm expansion, combined iliac aneurysms, and aneurysm-related embolic events.

References

1. Benjamin EJ, Virani SS, Callaway CW, Chamberlain AM, Chang AR, Cheng S, et al. Heart disease and stroke statistics-2018 update: a report from the American Heart Association. Circulation. 2018 Mar 20;137(12):e67–e492.
2. Hiratzka LF, Bakris GL, Beckman JA, Bersin RM, Carr VF, Casey DE Jr, et al. 2010 ACCF/AHA/AATS/ACR/ASA/SCA/SCAI/SIR/STS/SVM guidelines for the diagnosis and management of patients with thoracic aortic disease: a report of the American College of Cardiology Foundation/American Heart Association Task Force on Practice Guidelines, American Association for Thoracic Surgery, American College of Radiology, American Stroke Association, Society of Cardiovascular Anesthesiologists, Society for Cardiovascular Angiography and Interventions, Society of Interventional Radiology, Society of Thoracic Surgeons, and Society for Vascular Medicine. Circulation. 2010 Apr 6;121(13):e266–369.
3. Isselbacher EM. Thoracic and abdominal aortic aneurysms. Circulation. 2005 Feb 15;111(6):816–28.
4. Clouse WD, Hallett JW Jr, Schaff HV, Gayari MM, Ilstrup DM, Melton LJ 3rd. Improved prognosis of thoracic aortic aneurysms: a population-based study. JAMA. 1998 Dec 9;280(22):1926–9.
5. Wanhainen A. How to define an abdominal aortic aneurysm—influence on epidemiology and clinical practice. Scand J Surg. 2008;97(2):105–9. discussion 9
6. Moritz JD, Rotermund S, Keating DP, Oestmann JW. Infrarenal abdominal aortic aneurysms: implications of CT evaluation of size and configuration for placement of endovascular aortic grafts. Radiology. 1996 Feb;198(2):463–6.
7. Forsdahl SH, Singh K, Solberg S, Jacobsen BK. Risk factors for abdominal aortic aneurysms: a 7-year prospective study: the Tromsø Study, 1994-2001. Circulation. 2009 Apr 28;119(16):2202–8.
8. Wilmink TB, Quick CR, Day NE. The association between cigarette smoking and abdominal aortic aneurysms. J Vasc Surg. 1999 Dec;30(6):1099–105.
9. Chaikof EL, Dalman RL, Eskandari MK, Jackson BM, Lee WA, Mansour MA, et al. The society for vascular surgery practice guidelines on the care of patients with an abdominal aortic aneurysm. J Vasc Surg. 2018 Jan;67(1):2–77.
10. Collin J. Influence of screening on the incidence of ruptured abdominal aortic aneurysm: 5-year results of a randomized controlled study. Br J Surg. 1996 Jan;83(1):135.
11. Ashton HA, Buxton MJ, Day NE, Kim LG, Marteau TM, Scott RA, et al. The Multicentre Aneurysm Screening Study (MASS) into the effect of abdominal aortic aneurysm screening on mortality in men: a randomised controlled trial. Lancet (London, England). 2002 Nov 16;360(9345):1531–9.
12. Thompson SG, Ashton HA, Gao L, Buxton MJ, Scott RA. Final follow-up of the Multicentre Aneurysm Screening Study (MASS) randomized trial of abdominal aortic aneurysm screening. Br J Surg. 2012 Dec;99(12):1649–56.

13. Cosford PA, Leng GC. Screening for abdominal aortic aneurysm. Cochrane Database Syst Rev. 2007 Apr;18(2):CD002945.
14. Cambria RA, Gloviczki P, Stanson AW, Cherry KJ Jr, Bower TC, Hallett JW Jr, et al. Outcome and expansion rate of 57 thoracoabdominal aortic aneurysms managed nonoperatively. Am J Surg. 1995 Aug;170(2):213–7.
15. Coady MA, Rizzo JA, Hammond GL, Mandapati D, Darr U, Kopf GS, et al. What is the appropriate size criterion for resection of thoracic aortic aneurysms? J Thorac Cardiovasc Surg. 1997 Mar;113(3):476–91.
16. Davies RR, Goldstein LJ, Coady MA, Tittle SL, Rizzo JA, Kopf GS, et al. Yearly rupture or dissection rates for thoracic aortic aneurysms: simple prediction based on size. Ann Thoracic Surg. 2002 Jan;73(1):17–27.
17. Elefteriades JA. Natural history of thoracic aortic aneurysms: indications for surgery, and surgical versus nonsurgical risks. Ann Thoracic Surg. 2002 Nov;74(5):S1877–80.
18. Vardulaki KA, Prevost TC, Walker NM, Day NE, Wilmink AB, Quick CR, et al. Growth rates and risk of rupture of abdominal aortic aneurysms. Br J Surg. 1998 Dec;85(12):1674–80.
19. Santilli SM, Littooy FN, Cambria RA, Rapp JH, Tretinyak AS, d'Audiffret AC, et al. Expansion rates and outcomes for the 3.0-cm to the 3.9-cm infrarenal abdominal aortic aneurysm. J Vasc Surg. 2002 Apr;35(4):666–71.
20. Limet R, Sakalihassan N, Albert A. Determination of the expansion rate and incidence of rupture of abdominal aortic aneurysms. J Vasc Surg. 1991 Oct;14(4):540–8.
21. Lederle FA, Johnson GR, Wilson SE, Ballard DJ, Jordan WD Jr, Blebea J, et al. Rupture rate of large abdominal aortic aneurysms in patients refusing or unfit for elective repair. JAMA. 2002 June 12;287(22):2968–72.
22. Lederle FA, Johnson GR, Wilson SE, Chute EP, Littooy FN, Bandyk D, et al. Prevalence and associations of abdominal aortic aneurysm detected through screening. Aneurysm Detection and Management (ADAM) Veterans Affairs Cooperative Study Group. Ann Intern Med. 1997 Mar 15;126(6):441–9.
23. Sweeting MJ, Thompson SG, Brown LC, Powell JT. Meta-analysis of individual patient data to examine factors affecting growth and rupture of small abdominal aortic aneurysms. Br J Surg. 2012 May;99(5):655–65.
24. Brady AR, Thompson SG, Fowkes FG, Greenhalgh RM, Powell JT. Abdominal aortic aneurysm expansion: risk factors and time intervals for surveillance. Circulation. 2004 Jul 6;110(1):16–21.
25. Takagi H, Yamamoto H, Iwata K, Goto S, Umemoto T. Effects of statin therapy on abdominal aortic aneurysm growth: a meta-analysis and meta-regression of observational comparative studies. Eur J Vasc Endovasc Surg. 2012 Sep;44(3):287–92.
26. Wemmelund H, Høgh A, Hundborg HH, Thomsen RW, Johnsen SP, Lindholt JS. Statin use and rupture of abdominal aortic aneurysm. Br J Surg. 2014 Jul;101(8):966–75.
27. Propanolol Aneurysm Trial Investigators. Propranolol for small abdominal aortic aneurysms: results of a randomized trial. J Vasc Surg. 2002 Jan;35(1):72–9.
28. Sweeting MJ, Thompson SG, Brown LC, Greenhalgh RM, Powell JT. Use of angiotensin converting enzyme inhibitors is associated with increased growth rate of abdominal aortic aneurysms. J Vasc Surg. 2010 Jul;52(1):1–4.
29. O'Donnell TFX, Deery SE, Shean KE, Mittleman MA, Darling JD, Eslami MH, et al. Statin therapy is associated with higher long-term but not perioperative survival after abdominal aortic aneurysm repair. J Vasc Surg. 2018 Aug;68(2):392–9.
30. Baxter BT, Matsumura J, Curci JA, McBride R, Larson L, Blackwelder W, et al. Effect of doxycycline on aneurysm growth among patients with small infrarenal abdominal aortic aneurysms: a randomized clinical trial. Jama. 2020 May 26;323(20):2029–38. PubMed PMID: 32453369. Pubmed Central PMCID: PMC7251450 National Institute on Aging, National Institutes of Health (NIA-NIH). Dr Matsumura reported receiving grants from the NIH, Abbott, Cook, Medtronic, Gore, and Endologix. Dr Curci reported receiving grants from the NIH. Dr McBride reported receiving grants from the University of Maryland. Dr Larson reported receiving grants from the National Institute of Allergy and Infection Diseases. Dr Blackwelder reported receiving grants from the NIH. Dr Lam reported that she is employed

by Genentech, although the majority of the work was completed before employment began, and that she owns stock in Genentech and Merck. Dr Terrin reported receiving grants from NIH. No other disclosures were reported.
31. Meijer CA, Stijnen T, Wasser MN, Hamming JF, van Bockel JH, Lindeman JH. Doxycycline for stabilization of abdominal aortic aneurysms: a randomized trial. Ann Intern Med. 2013 Dec 17;159(12):815–23.
32. Leurs LJ, Visser P, Laheij RJ, Buth J, Harris PL, Blankensteijn JD. Statin use is associated with reduced all-cause mortality after endovascular abdominal aortic aneurysm repair. Vascular. 2006 Jan–Feb;14(1):1–8.
33. Ogden LG, He J, Lydick E, Whelton PK. Long-term absolute benefit of lowering blood pressure in hypertensive patients according to the JNC VI risk stratification. Hypertension (Dallas, TX: 1979). 2000 Feb;35(2):539–43.
34. Myers J, McElrath M, Jaffe A, Smith K, Fonda H, Vu A, et al. A randomized trial of exercise training in abdominal aortic aneurysm disease. Med Sci Sports Exerc. 2014 Jan;46(1):2–9.
35. Booher AM, Eagle KA. Diagnosis and management issues in thoracic aortic aneurysm. Am Heart J. 2011 Jul;162(1):38–46.
36. Davies RR, Gallo A, Coady MA, Tellides G, Botta DM, Burke B, et al. Novel measurement of relative aortic size predicts rupture of thoracic aortic aneurysms. Ann Thorac Surg. 2006 Jan;81(1):169–77.
37. Svensson LG, Kouchoukos NT, Miller DC, Bavaria JE, Coselli JS, Curi MA, et al. Expert consensus document on the treatment of descending thoracic aortic disease using endovascular stent-grafts. Ann Thorac Surg. 2008 Jan;85(1 Suppl):S1–41.
38. Cao P, De Rango P, Verzini F, Parlani G, Romano L, Cieri E. Comparison of surveillance versus aortic endografting for small aneurysm repair (CAESAR): results from a randomised trial. Eur J Vasc Endovasc Surg. 2011 Jan;41(1):13–25.
39. Powell JT, Brady AR, Brown LC, Fowkes FG, Greenhalgh RM, Ruckley CV, et al. Long-term outcomes of immediate repair compared with surveillance of small abdominal aortic aneurysms. N Engl J Med. 2002 May 9;346(19):1445–52.
40. Wanhainen A, Verzini F, Van Herzeele I, Allaire E, Bown M, Cohnert T, et al. Editor's choice - European Society for Vascular Surgery (ESVS) 2019 clinical practice guidelines on the management of abdominal aorto-iliac artery aneurysms. Eur J Vasc Endovasc Surg. 2019 Jan;57(1):8–93.
41. Lo RC, Lu B, Fokkema MT, Conrad M, Patel VI, Fillinger M, et al. Relative importance of aneurysm diameter and body size for predicting abdominal aortic aneurysm rupture in men and women. J Vasc Surg. 2014 May;59(5):1209–16.

External Aortic Support and Other Alternative Strategies in the Management of Aortic Pathology of Patients with Connective Tissue Disorders

John Pepper

Introduction

Due to an increasing awareness of thoracic aortopathy and an exponential growth in genetic diagnostic services, patients with Marfan syndrome and other connective tissue disorders are presenting earlier in their natural history seeking advice on how to prevent aortic dissection, aortic aneurysm, rupture and death. As the disease is usually inherited, the patients are generally well informed and want to understand the risks and benefits of all options available.

There is a long history of the use of drugs to delay aortic root dilatation. The effectiveness of beta-blockers has not been tested in large clinical trials and the justification for their use is expert opinion based on small studies and the reassurance that at least they will not cause harm. The initial enthusiasm for angiotensin receptor blockers (ARBs), specifically Losartan, has met with scepticism following four large international randomised controlled trials [1]. Except for the first trial report from the Netherlands, the subsequent three trials all showed no effect on the rate of aortic dilatation, although Losartan appears to be a reasonable alternative to a beta-blocker for those patients unable to tolerate the drug. Using a more potent ARB, Irbesartan, the latest results from the AIMS trial, reported at the ESC 2018, showed a modest treatment effect on the rate of dilatation of the Sinus of Valsalva, which was from placebo 0.74 mm/year to Irbesartan 0.52 mm/year.

A manuscript submitted for a chapter in **Aortic Dissection and Acute Aortic Syndromes** edited by Frank Sellke, Thoralf Sundt, Joseph Coselli, Joseph Bavaria and Neel Sodha to be published by Springer.

J. Pepper (✉)
Department of Surgery, Royal Brompton Hospital, London, UK
e-mail: j.pepper@rbht.nhs.uk

J. S. Coselli et al. (eds.), *Aortic Dissection and Acute Aortic Syndromes*,
https://doi.org/10.1007/978-3-030-66668-2_33

The current strategy for the prevention of ascending aortic dissection depends on aortic root replacement surgery. The Bentall total root replacement is well-established, has a low mortality and excellent long-term results. But the need for valve replacement imposes a risk of either long-term anticoagulation for a mechanical prosthesis or structural valve degeneration in the case of a tissue valve. The valve-sparing root replacement (VSRR) has been developed to deal with these issues and in the hands of very experienced surgeons excellent results have been obtained [2]. But it is difficult to judge the generalisability of these outcomes. The report from a multi-centre registry by Coselli and co-workers [3] showed a substantial risk of significant aortic regurgitation at a rate of 7% at one-year follow-up in Marfan patients. The meta-analysis of Benedetto [4] who compared Bentall and VSRR operations showed a re-intervention rate of 1.3% per year after VSRR in Marfan patients.

Personalised External Aortic Root Support (PEARS) may provide an alternative to aortic root replacement in selected patients and thus complement the existing armamentarium. The implantation of a personalised external aortic root support, computer designed and manufactured to match the aortic root morphology of the individual patient, was introduced in 2004 as a conservative approach for Marfan patients [5]. The device manufacture and operative method were the result of research and development between 2000 and 2004 when the first operation was performed. The computer aided design (CAD), the rapid prototyping (RP) manufacturing method and the surgical technique have all remained consistent without the iterative development which has characterised the evolution of both TRR and VSRR. After proof of principle [6] and prospective evaluation in the first 20 patients [7], the technique has undergone Health Technology Appraisal by the British National Institute for Health and Care Excellence (NICE).

Methods

The implant required for the PEARS operation is an ExoVasc mesh support made from the same polymer (polyethylene terephthalate) as standard vascular prostheses. (See Fig. 1 and its legend) The fabric of the ExoVasc has an open mesh structure with 0.7 mm pores compared with the familiar low porosity corrugated vascular grafts. Technical efficacy was reported in the first 10 patients [6], a comparative analysis of bypass, operative times and blood product usage in the first 20 [7], and clinical results up to 9 years in the first 30 patients [5]. Technical details of the methods of manufacture have remained consistent throughout the series [8]. The primary indication remains prophylactic treatment of root aneurysms to prevent further expansion with the intention of averting the risk of dissection and rupture.

Experimental implantation in sheep [9–11], and autopsy examination of one patient who died with an intact sleeved aorta [12], have shown that the mesh is consistently incorporated to form a neo-aorta with conservation of the endothelium/blood interface. In one of the sheep studies [11] a histological comparison was made

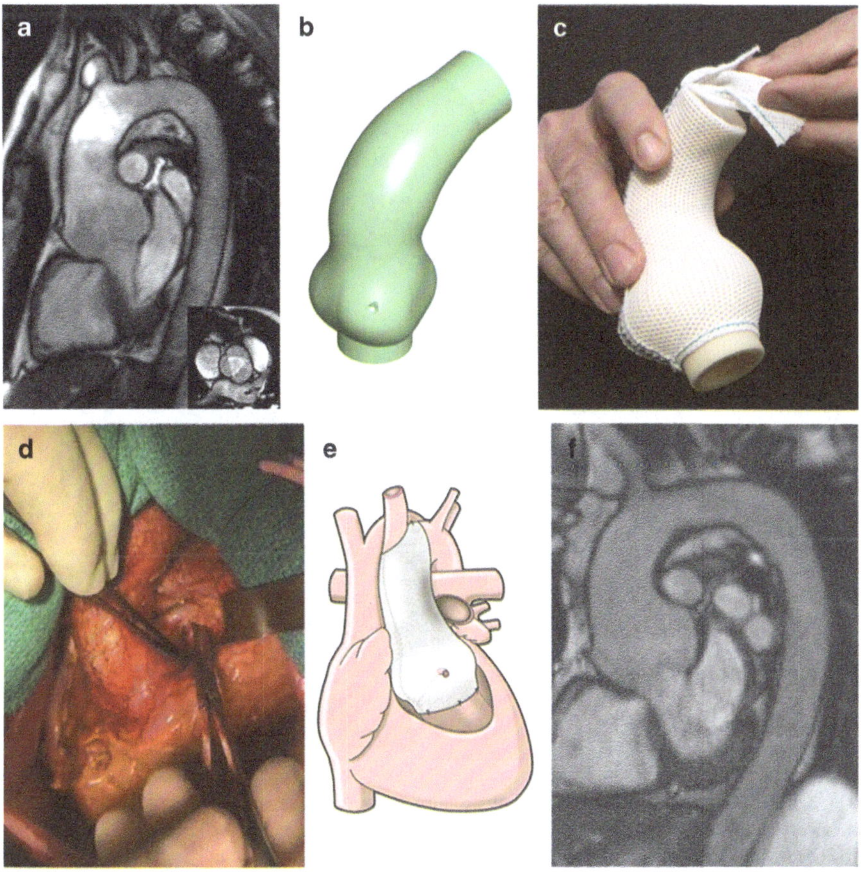

Fig. 1 From left to right the figure illustrates the design, manufacture and implantation of the ExoVasc personalised mesh support. Digital image (**a**) is used to make a 3D replica (**b**) of the patient's ascending aorta and aortic root. Small holes mark the position of the coronary ostia. On this a customised sleeve of an open mesh fabric is manufactured (**c**). Each stage requires expertise and time measured in hours. The aorta is dissected down to the aorto-ventricular junction (**d**). Here the surgeon is demonstrating that the dissection extends below (that is proximal to) the left main coronary artery. The mesh longitudinal seam is opened and incisions are made to the point where the main coronary arteries must pass through, making asterisk shaped incisions to conserve the mesh support. It extends from the aorto-ventricular junction proximally to the brachiocephalic artery distally (**e**). The final image (**f**) is that of the first recipient 14 years after implantation

between the microporous mesh of PEARS and the standard low-porosity Dacron graft (Fig. 2). In the first 24 patients, all operated in the lead hospital and with high quality imaging available, the three commissure-to-cusp diameters were measured after an average of 50 months [7]. Based on 72 (24 × 3) measurements, there was a small but significant reduction of the mean of the diameters from 4.4 to 4.3 cm ($P = 0.01$). The cross-sectional area was also reduced (NS) from 16.3 ± 1.9 cm^2 to 15.7 ± 2.7 cm^2. In none of the patients was there an increase in the severity of aortic

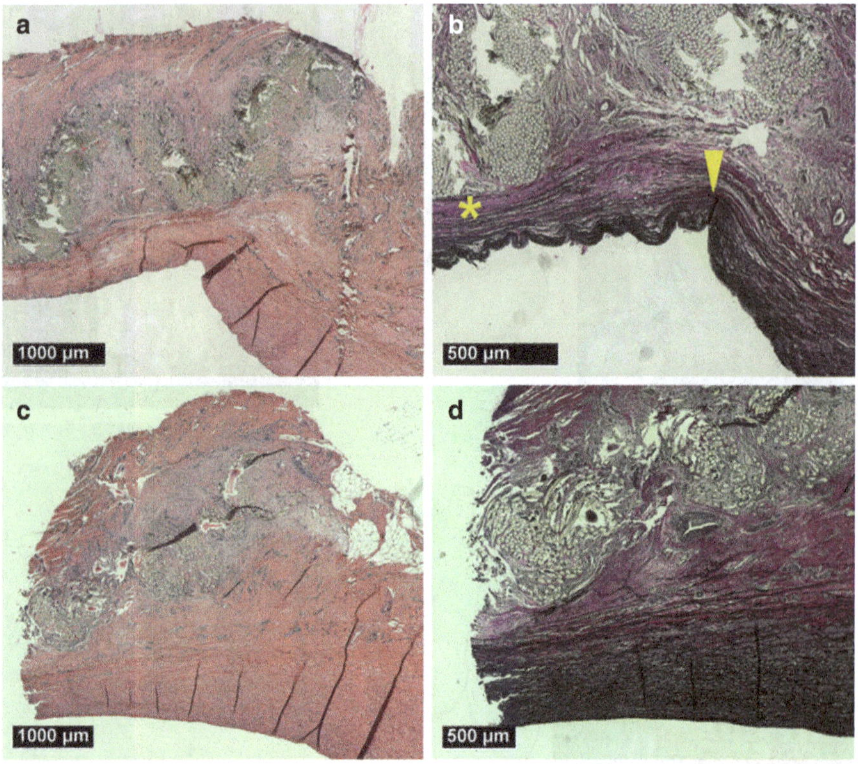

Fig. 2 Sheep study: transition zone, reconstruction of images taken at 10× magnification, longitudinal slices. (**a**) low-porosity graft (LPG) overview, Haematoxylin and Eosin. Buckling of the wall. (**b**) LPG detail with Verhoeff's elastic stain. Buckling of highly atrophic tunica media (arrowhead) and compression of adventitia underneath ridges with severed structural fibres (*). (**c**) macroporous mesh (MPM) overviews Haematoxylin and Eosin. Gradual transition of architectural changes. (**d**) MPM detail with Verhoeff's elastic stain. Gradual compression with well-preserved architecture

regurgitation or more than mild aortic regurgitation at follow-up. In the 24 patients studied, finite enlargement was seen in the descending aortic dimensions during a median period of under 2 years, while the aortic root was held at smaller size than that prior to surgery.

In 2003 an application was made to the Local Research & Ethics Committee and subsequently approved by the Clinical Practice Committee of our hospital Trust. Twenty operations were to be performed on patients with Marfan syndrome and the results reported to the Committee. The inclusion criteria agreed at that time were an Aortic Root/Sinus of Valsalva and Ascending Aorta with asymptomatic dilation of between 40 and 50 mm in diameter in patients aged 18+ years old. In 2010 after 23 patients had this operation, approval was given to continue the observational study and to recruit surgeons at other centres. The development group allowed widening of the criteria, accepting some younger patients. Patients eligible for inclusion in this report all had surgery for the primary indication: prophylactic treatment of life-threatening aortic root aneurysm, usually with a recognised and diagnosed syndrome. Patients considered for the technique have been assessed by clinical members of the study team. Surgeons wishing to join the programme underwent proctoring from one of the experienced PEARS surgeons, who went to their unit to assist in surgery, usually on at least two patients.

In 2018 we undertook an audit of all 117 operations who had their PEARS operation before the end of December 2017. We had access to the full manufacturing records and CAD models which were available from the secure file server at Exstent Ltd. The surgery case report forms (CRFs) were available from the operating surgeons and kept securely by Exstent. The Exstent records, the Royal Brompton Hospital database, and correspondence from the operating teams, were used to compile a full data set of demography, aetiology, aortic dimensions, the operation performed, operating time, cardiopulmonary bypass time (if used), and hospital stay (Table 1). Intraoperative adverse events, and any adjunctive surgery were recorded and any later cardiac, aortic, neurological or infective events were tabulated. The follow-up interval was from the date of operation to the date on which the patient was last clinically assessed and/or had cardiac investigations. The Kaplan Meier method was used to obtain estimates of patient survival and reoperation.

Results

180 PEARS procedures have been successfully carried out at 19 units internationally. As of January 1st 2019, 183 patients have received a PEARS implant representing 584 postoperative patient years. 41 patients have been followed for more than 5 years and 14 for more than 10 years. Of the 183 who had the operation 134 were

Table 1 Table of distributions

		Minimum	25%	Median	75%	Maximum
Age (years)						
All patients	N = 117	15	23	34	46	75
Females	N = 30	15	27	38	46	65
Males	N = 87	15	22	32	46	75
Aortic root (mm)						
All patients	N = 117	31	43	47	48	60
Females	N = 30	31	42	44	47	49
Males	N = 87	35	45	47	52	60
Operation time minutes	N = 116[a]	60	130	165	236	840
Bypass time minutes	N = 32[b]	22	46	70	90	245
Length of stay days	N = 116[a]	5	5	6	7	25
Follow-up months	N = 116[c]	2	7	20	89	166

[a]Cardiopulmonary bypass not used in 85/117 (73%)
[b]Not available in one case
[c]One death in hospital (no PEARS implanted) excluded

carried out for Marfan syndrome, 8 for Loeys-Dietz syndrome, 12 for bicuspid aortic valve, 2 for an enlarged aortic root identified more than 20 years following the arterial switch operation for TGA, 1 Tetralogy of Fallot, 11 Ross operations and 15 for non-syndromic enlargement of the ascending aorta and aortic root. The accrual of patient numbers and of units joining the programme are shown in Figs. 2 and 3. The operating time in 75% of the procedures was less than 4 h. The majority of the operations (73%) were undertaken without the use of cardiopulmonary bypass. The length of hospital stay was no longer than 7 days in 75% of patients. Further details with ranges and frequency distributions are provided in Table 1.

The breakdown by aetiology of the aortic disease in the 180 operated patients is shown in the flow chart (Fig. 3). Some patients have undergone adjunctive operations such as mitral valve repair in 12 and coronary artery bypass grafting in 3. The gender and age distribution of the operated patients is given in Table 2 with the aortic diameter at the level where the leaflets meet each other. Surgeons changed the operative plan from PEARS intraoperatively in 4 patients as indicated in the flow chart (Fig. 3).

There has been one early postoperative death. The patient suffered damage to his left main coronary artery at operation. This was repaired and coronary artery grafts were performed. Myocardial function was severely compromised and he required ECMO. He died from complications of this on post-operative day 5.

There have been two late deaths. One was unrelated to the PEARS operation at 4.5 years after operation [12]. In 2008, a 26-year old man had personalized external aortic root support (PEARS) with a macro-porous mesh. He was the 16th of 46 patients to have this operation. He had a typical Marfan habitus. His mother died of this disease as did his brother, with an aortic dissection. The patient himself died suddenly 4.5 years after his PEARS operation. At autopsy, there was no blood in the pericardium. The coronary orifices and proximal arteries were normal. His bicuspid aortic valve was minimally regurgitant as it was prior to operation and remained throughout follow-up. Macroscopically the implanted mesh was embedded in the adventitia and not separable from the aortic wall. Microscopically it was fully incorporated with collagen fibres as has been seen in our animal studies. The unsupported aortic arch showed some focal fragmentation of elastic fibres and a mild increase in mucopolysaccharides consistent with Marfan syndrome (Fig. 4). These appearances were not present in the supported aortic root, which had the histological appearance of a normal aorta. He was the first patient to die with an implant. The histological appearances suggest the possibility that the incorporated support of the aortic root allowed recovery of the microstructure of the media.

A further patient died 8 months after a PEARS procedure due to heart failure from cardiomyopathy.

Seven patients had significant perioperative events from which they made a full recovery as listed in the flow chart. There were no major bleeding events and only one superficial wound infection. Two patients had intraoperative ischaemic events resulting in 19 and 25-day hospital stays, but both made a full recovery. The survival

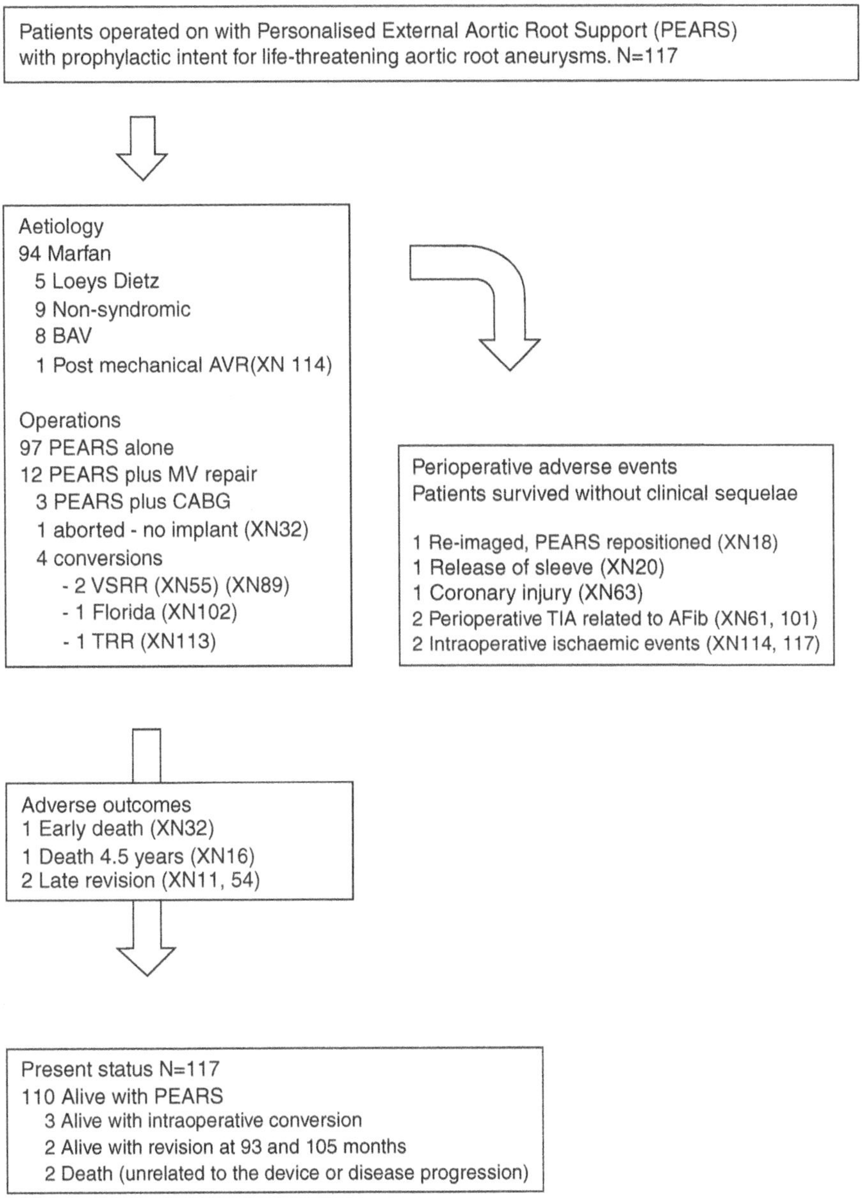

Fig. 3 This flow chart includes all 117 consecutive patients for whom there was an intention to treat and who had surgery before the end of December 2017. All perioperative adverse events [10], conversions [4] and adverse outcomes [4] are described in the Appendix of Clinical Events. There is 100% follow up and all patients are traceable

Table 2 Table comparing PEARS with VSRR in AVOOMPS

				AVOOMPS
		PEARS		VSRR
		N = 117		N = 239
Age (years)		34(23–46)		33 ± 13
Sex, % male		87 (74%)		148 (62%)
Sinus diameter		47 (43–48)		49 (46–52)
Aortic regurgitation				
	None	84 (72%)	None/trivial	106 (46%)
	Trivial/mild	28 (24%)	Grade 1	86 (37%)
	Moderate	5 (4%)	Grade 2	27 (12%)
			Grade 3	4 (2%)
			Grade 4	8 (4%)
Operation time (min)		165 (130–236)		340 (275–441)
Bypass time (32/117)	None for 73%	70 (46–90)		194 (148–270)
Hospital stay (days)		6 (5–7)		6 (5–9)
Conversions		4 (3.4%)		6 (2.5%)
30 day mortality		1 (0.9)		1 (0.4)

and re-operation-free survival for all 117 operated patients are shown in the Kaplan-Meier analysis (Fig. 5) which includes two deaths and two re-operations, one at 9 years and one at 6 years.

Other Applications of the PEARS Operation

We have used the mesh material to surround the pulmonary autograft in a Ross operation. In each instance, the autograft has been implanted in the aortic root as a free-standing graft with the coronary arteries anastomosed to the autograft root. The mesh was placed around the root prior to construction of the coronary anastomoses. We modelled the mesh on the pulmonary root using the same method of CTscan, CAD and RP. To allow for the effect of systemic pressure on the autograft, formers were made at 110% before the mesh was heat shrunk against it. In a limited number of operations, 8, we have found this approach to be satisfactory. We anticipate that the benefit of encasing the autograft root in the mesh will be to prevent late dilatation of the neo-sino-tubular junction and consequent aortic regurgitation. We do not yet have sufficient length of follow-up to see whether this is a fact.

A limited number of complex cardiac operations in infancy or early childhood can lead to a late complication of ascending aortic enlargement with a competent aortic valve. One such procedure was reported in 2016 [13] which involved a 28 years old man who was born with transposition of the great vessels and underwent a Mustard operation at the age of 3 years, when a delayed arterial switch operation was performed. Cardiological surveillance 24 years later revealed an enlarging aortic root with compression of the left anterior descending artery. A reduction plasty of the dilated anterior sinus of Valsalva was performed which

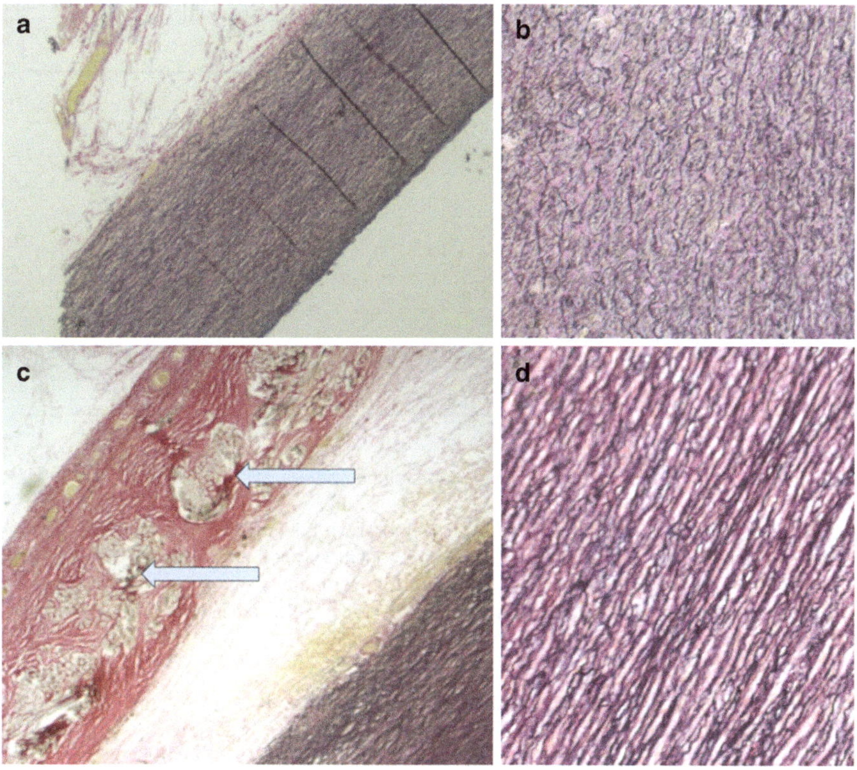

Fig. 4 (**a**) Sections from the unsupported aortic arch shows focal fragmentation of elastic fibres and a mild increase in mucopolysaccharides (mag. ×2.5). There is no root in contrast to (**c**) and the adventitia is not clearly defined as it is in the ascending aorta. (**b**) A high-power view of the media of the unsupported aortic arch (mag. ×10). The appearances are of medial degeneration consistent with Marfan syndrome. (**c**) Section of the aortic root of a total thickness of 4.5 mm. Collagen fibres (red staining) pass through the interstices between the filaments of the root (blue arrows) embedding it in the adventitia. Foreign body-type giant cells and a few scattered chronic inflammatory cells are present (mag. ×2.5). (**d**) High-power view of the protected aortic root wall (mag. ×10). The underlying media shows well preserved elastic lamellae with no fragmentation, loss or pooling of mucopolysaccharides

released a stretched left anterior descending coronary artery to allow normal flow and a PEARS implant was fitted around the aortic root and ascending aorta. The patient and the surgical repair remain intact 3 years later.

Discussion

The objective of all three operations performed electively on the aortic root is to prevent aortic dissection. According to natural history data reported in 1972 for 257 people with Marfan syndrome, median survival was 40–41 years for men and 48–49 years for women [14]. Among 72 patients who were dead at the time of

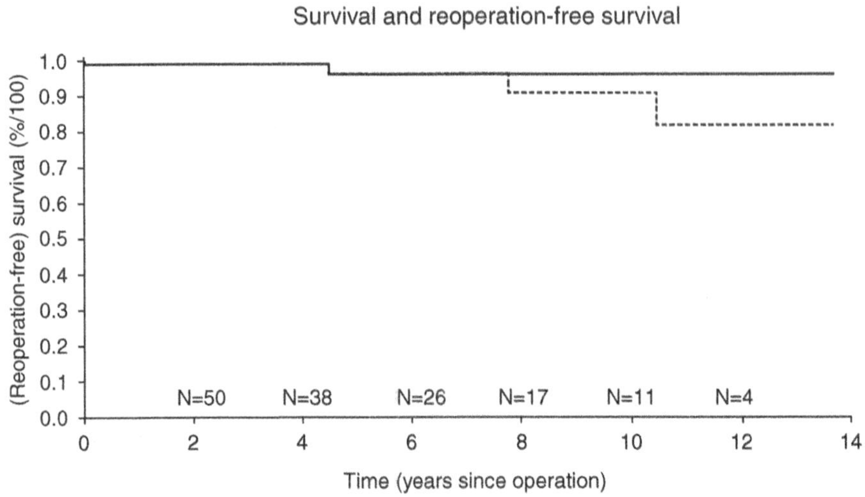

Fig. 5 Kaplan Meier analysis prepared by Professor JJM Takkenberg. Time to event analysis shows two deaths at 5 days and 4.5 years and two re-operations at 6 and 9 years. The small numbers of patients 'at risk' with more than 2 years of follow up affects the appearance of the chart. The single event at 9 years has a large impact on the overall analysis of survival because of the few patients operated on that long ago

life-table analysis, the average age at death was 32 years. As monitoring has become easier, operative risks have reduced, and awareness of the risk of dissection is heightened, root replacement has been advocated at a smaller size. The criterion has come down from 60 mm through 55 and 50 to the present recommendation of 45 mm for Marfan patients in the 2014 ESC Guidelines [15]. Earlier intervention introduces a new problem for patients and those advising them. It has always been possible that some patients having elective root replacement were never destined to have root dissection, and so, as the size criterion was lowered there is likely to be an increasing number of patients who undergo operation without gaining any years of life because their survival is determined by other factors. To illustrate the problem, we can consider carotid endarterectomy for which there are randomised controlled trials to evaluate the reduction in the risk of stroke. Using the "number needed to treat" (NNtT) calculation, the number of patients who have an operation in order to prevent one stroke is 6. These are patients with neurological symptoms and a carotid stenosis of greater than 70%, for whom the evidence for benefit is most compelling, yet 5 out of 6 patients having the operation gain no benefit from it. For clinical recommendations and comparative health economic evaluation, the number needed to treat to prevent a dissection in Marfan syndrome would be a useful statistic, but is not presently available. An attempt at decision analysis relied on best guesses from a handful of clinicians and thus failed for want of objective data [16, 17].

When we began to develop and evaluate PEARS we ensured that the innovation was evaluated by NICE [18]. We also thoroughly explored the possibility of a randomised controlled trial (RCT). The project development team worked with experienced clinical research scientists, established research agencies and grant giving bodies including the British National Institute for Health Research (NIHR), the research wing if the NHS, the British Heart Foundation, and the Medical Research Council to devise a controlled study to compare this novel approach with the established operations. The NIHR Research Design Service helped us identify two decision-making nodes which might be amenable to testing. One was the timing: put bluntly to 'go for it' or to procrastinate, or to put it more gently, the 'early/defer' dilemma. The other was whether to have the more predictable mechanical solution and accept life-long anticoagulation or accept the less durable but more attractive valve sparing operation. We published these considerations in an attempt to organise a trial [19, 20]. There was no prospect of professional equipoise as has been illustrated by arguments made in opposition to this conservative approach [21–23]. It should be noted that neither total root replacement nor valve sparing root replacement have been evaluated with animal experiments or controlled trials.

We then focussed on establishing an informed patients' perspective. The decision nodes were explored, along with other factors, using the Ottawa decision support framework. We found that people have cogently weighted and strongly expressed preferences on both the 'early/defer' question and the 'conserve/replace' choice [24]. Evidence concerning thromboembolism and bleeding with mechanical valves is plentiful and includes randomised trials [25, 26] and there has been a meta-analysis of the two approaches for root replacement [3, 4]. The decision is amenable to evidence based balancing of the pros and cons and is thus realistically not a matter for random assignment. The absence of randomly derived control data is therefore a limitation we have to live with for now. What we can do is to ensure that patients who are to have a prophylactic operation face perioperative risks as low as are achievable. They should be given evidence-based estimates of the durability of the operations available and reliable estimates of future failure and complications from the best available observational data.

A further limitation of our current knowledge of the PEARS operation is that because of the skewed accrual of patients with a recent upsurge there are relatively few patients with long-term follow-up. The best available data is on VSRR, especially the 1-year report of the Aortic Valve Operative Outcomes in the Marfan Patients Study [AVOOMPS] [3]. A strength shared by PEARS and AVOOMPS is that both kept a record on 'intention to treat'. All patients scheduled for PEARS (N = 117) and VSRR (N = 239) have been reported (Table 2). The age, gender and aneurysm diameters for PEARS are similar to those for VSRR. There was one early death in each group. The differences in operation time and the use of cardiopulmonary bypass are evident.

While the median and inter-quartile range (IQR) of aortic dimensions are comparable between PEARS and VSRR in AVOOMPS, the IQR excludes 25% of patients which is a large number to be regarded as statistical 'outliers' for a potentially lethal disease. There were 7 patients in the PEARS series with aortic root dimensions <40 cm and were below the 6th centile. These were from 66th to 122nd in the series and as can be seen from Fig. 3, they were the more recent patients operated on in the last 2 years. Further comparisons can be made but are difficult because of the variations in the nature and severity of aortic disease, comorbidity, use of cardiopulmonary bypass, myocardial ischaemia and circulatory arrest. Patients included in the AVOOMPS study would not all have been eligible for PEARS. Because

CAD modelling and rapid prototyping, loosely referred to as 3D printing, are prerequisites for the procedure, PEARS is an elective operation. Interestingly, a quarter of PEARS patients had some aortic regurgitation before operation and this was deliberately corrected in some by using an undersized (95%) ExoVasc mesh. This possibility is being explored further and there are reasons to believe that this is feasible in a wider group of patients [27].

In two patients we have seen progression of aortic regurgitation following PEARS. The point of note is that parts of the right and non-coronary sinuses were not covered by the mesh for clinical reasons. Over years these areas expanded resulting in regurgitation due to single leaflet prolapse thus providing an accidental experiment comparing supported and unsupported sinuses in the same patient. This is in line with earlier evidence where only the more accessible part of the aortic root was covered with prosthetic material. This part was stabilised while the uncovered part continued to dilate [28]. Stabilising the aortic root dimension and architecture has preserved aortic leaflet function well. There has been freedom from valve and aortic related events in longer term follow-up. There have been no bleeding or embolic events or endocarditis.

Early in the experience we used conservative criteria. A relatively early departure was in patients in whom mitral valve regurgitation was determining the need for surgery. PEARS was used rather than leave the aortic root unprotected and presenting trouble at a later date [29]. Other possible indications for the PEARS procedures include Loeys-Dietz Syndrome (LDS), complex congenital cardiac corrections presenting later in life, and an enlarging ascending aorta in patients with a bicuspid aortic valve but normal haemodynamics. The nature of LDS is such that it may be a prime indication for the PEARS operation because the event of rupture or dissection is rarely preceded by slow dilatation.

We have recently monitored 24 consecutive patients who underwent the PEARS procedure in the lead hospital from 2004 to 2012 [30]. Mean follow-up was 6.3 ± 2.6 years with 19 of the 24 patients (80%) completing at least 5 years review. The PEARS implant keeps the aortic root size stable and prevents dilatation in Marfan patients. At the same time, it was observed that the unsupported segments, the aortic arch and the descending aorta, remain prone to dilatation over time and so close follow-up is mandatory as is the case in Bentall and VSRR operations.

Conflict of Interest J. Pepper has no financial interest whatever in the company which manufacture the PEARS implant, Exostent Ltd.

References

1. Groenink M, Mulder BJM. How to treat Marfan syndrome: an update. Eur Heart J. 2016;37:986–7.
2. David TE. Aortic valve repair and aortic valve sparing operations. J Thorac Cardiovasc Surg. 2015;149:9–11.
3. Coselli JS, Volguina IV, Lemaire SA, Sundt TM, Connolly HM, Stephens EH, et al. Early and 1-year outcomes of aortic root surgery in patients with Marfan syndrome: a prospective, multicenter, comparative study. J Thorac Cardiovasc Surg. 2014 Jun;147(6):1758–67.

4. Benedetto U, Melina G, Takkenberg JJ, Roscitano A, Angeloni E, Sinatra R. Surgical management of aortic root disease in Marfan syndrome: a systematic review and meta-analysis. Heart. 2011 Jun;97(12):955–8.
5. Golesworthy T, Lamperth M, Mohiaddin R, Pepper J, Thornton W, Treasure T. A jacket for the Marfan's aorta. Lancet. 2004 Oct 30;364(9445):1582.
6. Pepper J, Golesworthy T, Utley M, Chan J, Ganeshalingam S, Lamperth M, Mohiaddin R, Treasure T. Manufacturing and placing a bespoke support for the Marfan aortic root: description of the method and technical results and status at one year for the first ten patients. Interact Cardiovasc Thorac Surg. 2010 Mar 5;10(3):360–5.
7. Treasure T, Crowe S, Chan KM, Ranasinghe A, Attia R, Lees B, Utley M, Golesworthy T, Pepper J. A method for early evaluation of a recently introduced technology by deriving a comparative group from existing clinical data: a case study in external support of the Marfan aortic root. BMJ Open. 2012;2(2):e000725. https://doi.org/10.1136/bmjopen-2011-000725.
8. Treasure T, Takkenberg JJ, Golesworthy T, Rega F, Petrou M, Rosendahl U, et al. Personalised external aortic root support (PEARS) in Marfan syndrome: analysis of 1-9 year outcomes by intention-to-treat in a cohort of the first 30 consecutive patients to receive a novel tissue and valve-conserving procedure, compared with the published results of aortic root replacement. Heart. 2014 June;100(12):969–75.
9. Verbrugghe P, Verbeken E, Pepper J, Treasure T, Meyns B, Meuris B, Herijgers P, Rega F. External aortic root support: a histological and mechanical study in sheep. Interact Cardiovasc Thorac Surg. 2013 Aug;17(2):334–9.
10. Van Hoof L, Verbrugghe P, Verbeken E, Treasure T, Famaey N, Meuris B, Herijgers P, Rega F. Support of the aortic wall: a histological study in sheep comparing a macroporous mesh with low-porosity vascular graft of the same polyethylene terephthalate material. Interact Cardiovasc Thorac Surg. 2017 July 1;25(1):89–95.
11. Vastmans J, Fehervary H, Verbrugghe P, Verbelen T, Vanderveken E, Vander SJ, et al. Biomechanical evaluation of a personalized external aortic root support applied in the Ross procedure. J Mech Behav Biomed Mater. 2018;78:164–74.
12. Pepper J, Goddard M, Mohiaddin R, Treasure T. Histology of a Marfan aorta 4.5 years after personalized external aortic root support. Eur J Cardiothorac Surg. 2015 Sep;48(3): 502–5.
13. Austin C, Mathur SK, Pepper J. Personalised external aortic root support (PEARS): utilisation in dilatational aortopathies after the arterial switch operation. Int J Cardiol. 2016;220: 772–4.
14. Murdoch JL, Walker BA, Halpern BL, Kuzma JW, McKusick VA. Life expectancy and causes of death in the Marfan syndrome. N Engl J Med. 1972 Apr 13;286(15):804–8.
15. Erbel R, et al. 2014 ESC guidelines on the diagnosis and treatment of aortic diseases. The task force for the diagnosis and treatment of aortic diseases of the European Society of Cardiology (ESC). Eur Heart J. 2014;35:2873–926.
16. Treasure T, Golesworthy T, Pepper J. Prophylactic surgery of the aortic root in Marfan syndrome: reconsideration of the decision making process in the era of a customised external aortic root support. J Vasc Endovasc Surg. 2011;18:215–23.
17. Kim SY, Martin N, Hsia EC. Management of aortic disease in Marfan syndrome: a decision analysis. Arch Intern Med. 2005;165:749–55.
18. Treasure T, Pepper J, Golesworthy T, Mohiaddin R, Anderson RH. External aortic root support: NICE guidance. Heart. 2012 Oct 14;98(1):65–8.
19. Treasure T. Options for pre-emptive aortic root surgery for people with Marfan syndrome. Eur Heart J. 2013;34(26):1947–9.
20. Treasure T, Pepper J. A call for expressions of interest in a comparative study of the options for pre-emptive aortic root surgery for people with Marfan syndrome. Eur J Cardiothorac Surg. 2013;44(3):588.
21. Cameron D. External support of the dilated aorta: back to the future? Heart. 2014;100:908.
22. Jahangiri M, Leigh B, Cameron D. External aortic support: a viable alternative treatment option? Consent and duty of candour. Eur J Cardiothorac Surg. 2017;51(5):1020.
23. Treasure T, Pepper J. Reply to Jahangiri et al. Eur J Cardiothorac Surg. 2017 May 1;51(5):1021.

24. Treasure T, King A, Hidalgo LL, Golesworthy T, Pepper J, Takkenberg JJ. Developing a shared decision support framework for aortic root surgery in Marfan syndrome. Heart. 2018;104:480–6.
25. Oxenham H, Bloomfield P, Wheatley DJ, Lee RJ, Cunningham J, Prescott RJ. Twenty year comparison of a Bjork-Shiley mechanical heart valve with porcine bioprostheses. Heart. 2003;89(7):715–21.
26. Murday AJ, Hochstitzky A, Mansfield J, Miles J, Taylor B, Whitley E, Treasure T. A prospective controlled trial of St. Jude versus Starr-Edwards aortic and mitral valve prostheses. Ann Thorac Surg. 2003;76:66–73.
27. Plonek T, Dumanski A, Obremska M, Kustrzycki W. First beating-heart valve-sparing aortic root repair: a "corset" technique. Ann Thorac Surg. 2015 Apr;99(4):1464–6.
28. Cohen O, Odim J, De la Zerda DJ, Ukatu C, Vyas R, Vyas N, Palatnik K, Laks H. Long-term experience of girdling the ascending aorta with Dacron mesh as definitive treatment for aneurysmal dilatation. Ann Thorac Surg. 2007;88(3):S780–4.
29. Benedetto U, Jin XY, Hill E, Treasure T, Petrou M. An option for concomitant management of moderate Marfan root aneurysm at the time of mitral valve repair: a role for personalized external aortic root support. Ann Thorac Surg. 2016 Dec;102(6):e499–501.
30. Izgi C, Newsome S, Alpendurada F, Nyktari E, Boutsikou M, Pepper J, Treasure T, Mohiaddin R. External aortic root support to prevent aortic dilatation in patients with Marfan syndrome. J Am Coll Cardiol. 2018;72(10):1095–105.

Management of Operative Complications After Type A Aortic Dissection Repair

Michael P. Robich and Jennifer S. Lawton

Introduction

Acute aortic syndromes often require urgent operation and these can be among the most technically challenging operations that cardiac surgeons perform. Specifically, patients with type A aortic dissection (TAD) are often taken to the operating room without the complete evaluation afforded to elective cardiac surgery patients, and often in a less than ideal physiologic state (Fig. 1). The decision to move forward with surgical intervention must be made with the essence of time in mind. Acute co-morbidities such as shock, cardiac tamponade, aortic regurgitation, myocardial ischemia, cerebral ischemia, paraplegia, renal/mesenteric ischemia, and limb ischemia may make the decision to operate more challenging. Careful recognition and prompt management of these complications can also make TAD operations some of the most rewarding operations that cardiac surgeons perform (Table 1).

While much of the patient's post-operative course will be determined in the operating room, the acute and chronic co-morbidities of the patient will also impact the types and severity of complications encountered after surgery. The in-hospital mortality rate has been reported to be 10–35% [1–3]. The morbidity rate after surgery is higher. Common complications after operative management of type A aortic dissections (TAD) include: bleeding, malperfusion, myocardial ischemia, aortic complications, neurologic complications, and multisystem organ failure.

M. P. Robich
Department of Cardiac Surgery, Heart and Vascular Institute, Tufts University Medical Center, Boston, MA, USA

J. S. Lawton (✉)
Division of Cardiac Surgery, Department of Surgery, Johns Hopkins Medical University, Baltimore, MD, USA
e-mail: Jlawton4@jhmi.edu

J. S. Coselli et al. (eds.), *Aortic Dissection and Acute Aortic Syndromes*,
https://doi.org/10.1007/978-3-030-66668-2_34

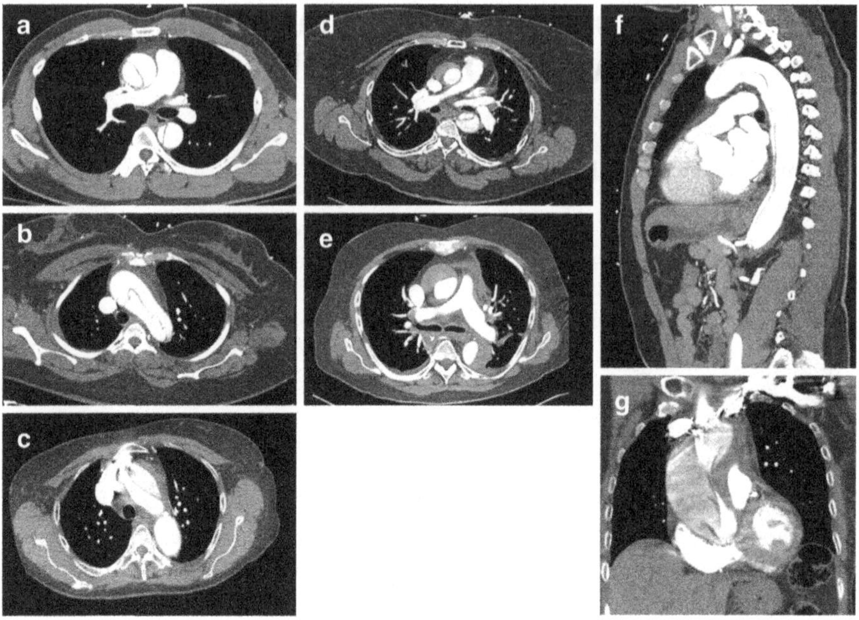

Fig. 1 Representative computed tomography images demonstrating acute type A aortic dissection. First panel top (**a**) Axial view with type A aortic dissection visible in ascending and descending aorta. First panel middle (**b**) Axial view with type A aortic dissection visible in the aortic arch (Previously published in Lawton JS. Acute type A aortic dissection 101. J Thorac Cardiovasc Surg 2015;150:769–770). First panel bottom (**c**) Axial view with type A aortic dissection visible in the proximal aortic arch. Second panel top (**d**) Axial view with type A aortic dissection with classic flap visible in the descending aorta and intramural hematoma in the ascending aorta. Second panel bottom (**e**) Axial view with type A aortic dissection with intramural hematoma visible in the ascending and descending aorta. Third panel top (**f**) Sagittal view with type A aortic dissection visible in the descending aorta. Third panel bottom (**g**) Coronal view with type A aortic dissection visible in the ascending aorta and proximal arch

Bleeding/Coagulopathy

Bleeding and coagulopathy after repair of a type A aortic dissection are common. Aortic surgery has been associated with more blood utilization than any other cardiac operation [4]. In a 2001 single center study, the average patient undergoing elective aortic surgery under DHCA received 4 units of red blood cells in the operating room, 2.6 units post-operatively and 58% of patients required five of more units of blood [5]. A number of factors contribute to bleeding including: raw surface area of the exposed false lumen, disseminated intravascular coagulopathy (DIC), hypothermia, thrombocytopenia, extent of aortic replacement (long length of suture line), and duration of the operation. Reported rates of takeback for bleeding after urgent aortic surgery are 20–25%. In one study, 56% of patients required return to the operating room for re-exploration after type A aortic dissection repair [6]. In this paper, independent predictors of massive post-operative bleeding after multivariable

Table 1 Complications of Type A aortic dissection repair

Complications of Type A aortic dissection repair
Bleeding—hypothermia, platelet destruction, DIC, acidosis
Malperfusion—coronary, limb, abdominal, brain
Neurologic complications—stroke, spinal cord ischemia, neuropathy, delirium
Myocardial ischemia—malperfusion, dissection, embolism, obstruction
Aortic complications—root, descending thoracic

Complications discussed in this chapter are listed (No abbreviations)

logistic regression included: hypertension (increased the odds of bleeding threefold), coronary artery disease (increased bleeding by 6 times), organ malperfusion (increased bleeding twofold) and preoperative dual antiplatelet therapy (sixfold increased risk). Increased time on cardiopulmonary bypass also led to a higher risk of massive bleeding. Another study of TAD patients showed a re-exploration rate of 24% and reported risk factors for bleeding included: aortic arch replacement (relative risk (RR) 1.4), cardiac tamponade (RR 4), age less than 70 years (RR 2), preexisting cardiac disease (RR 2) and need for CPR (RR 5). The Mayo clinic has described a stable 8% re-operation rate for bleeding after TAD surgery over a 20-year period [7].

Preoperatively, the patient with type A aortic dissection is likely to be in DIC as the exposed non-endothelial surface of the false lumen can drive a consumptive coagulopathy [8, 9]. This has been demonstrated in aortic dissection by a decrease in factors II, V, VII, X and XII with a significant elevation in fibrin/fibrinogen split products [10]. Cardiopulmonary bypass (CPB) causes similar disruptions in the coagulation cascade potentially compounding the consumptive coagulopathy [11], and platelets are destroyed in several ways leading to low quantity and poor function. Additionally, exposure to collagen in the false lumen results in further platelet consumption and decreased aggregation [12, 13].

Hypothermic circulatory arrest is a strategy often employed in the repair of TAD. Traditionally, deep hypothermic circulatory arrest (DHCA) with cooling core body temperature to 18 °C was standard. The major goal of this technique was to protect the brain and avoid neurologic injury during circulatory standstill [14, 15]. The coagulopathy associated with cooling is initially due to platelet dysfunction when temperatures are mildly reduced (35 °C). At temperatures below 33 °C however, there are more significant platelet effects and alterations in the kinetics of proteins in the coagulation cascade [16]. The presence of acidosis significantly worsens the coagulopathy associated with hypothermia, as suggested in the "lethal triad" in trauma—shock, acidosis and hypothermia [17]. While DDAVP and fibrinogen can be used to treat the coagulopathy of hypothermia, acidosis will negate the effects [18].

The use of moderate hypothermic arrest (MHCA) (core body temperature > 20 °C) with regional brain cooling has recently grown in popularity for several reasons including a perceived reduction in coagulopathy [19]. In a single institution retrospective study that evaluated bleeding risk in aortic operations with DHCA vs. MHCA there were no differences in transfused blood products, coagulation laboratory values, morbidity or mortality [20]. However, the extent of the operation influences the risk of bleeding. Dr. Svensson showed in his experience that the average type A dissection operation required 4 units of blood, while a total arch required 6 units [21]. As with all cardiac surgery, blood transfusion during aortic surgery has been associated with worse short and long-term outcomes [4, 22]. There have been no randomized trials evaluating bleeding with different techniques in hypothermic arrest.

Several techniques may be utilized to reduce bleeding during urgent aortic surgery (Table 2). A reliable surgical plan and meticulous surgical technique are paramount. A number of leaders in the field of aortic surgery have described safe and effective approaches to acute aortic syndromes [23–26]. The aphorism, "Go in dry, come out dry" is good reminder to maintain hemostasis throughout the operation. If axillary cannulation is performed, it is important to make sure the access site is hemostatic and a sump cardiotomy suction may be strategically utilized to avoid unnecessary blood loss during the operation. There are a number of hemostatic agents available [27] as adjuncts to hemostasis, and good surgical techniques such as choosing the correct graft size, mandating incorporation of aortic adventitia in the anastomosis, using felt or other material to buttress the suture line, and avoiding undue tension are critical [28]. Transfusion guided by standard coagulation laboratory values or viscoelastic hemostatic assays such as thromboelastography (TEG) and rotational thromboelastometry (ROTEM) are currently the best means to correct coagulopathy. As in trauma massive transfusion, balanced ratios of 1:1:1 of blood, FFP and platelets are important to avoid dilutional coagulopathy. Similarly, intraoperative blood salvage with Cell Saver provides great value, but also washes out coagulation factors as part of saving red blood cells and its judicious use will help prevent coagulopathy. Recombinant Factor VII may also be used to attempt to reduce significant post-operative bleeding. It has been shown to reduce bleeding without a significant increase in stroke, renal failure or mortality [29]. Postoperative bleeding may be formidable and efforts to minimize bleeding are vital to the survival of the patient.

Table 2 Strategies to minimize bleeding after repair of Type A aortic dissection

Strategies to minimize bleeding after repair of Type A aortic dissection
"Go in dry, come out dry"
Avoid blood loss from axillary and other cannulation sites
Warm core body temperature to at least 35.5 °C prior to weaning from CPB
Pack mediastinum during heparin reversal
Use of Bioglue or other hemostatic agents
Avoid acidosis
Judicious use of cell saver
Directed transfusion based on coagulation studies
1:1:1 RBC: FFP: platelet for massive transfusion
TEG/ROTEM to guide blood product transfusion
Consider use of Factor VII

Strategies discussed in this chapter are listed. CPB is cardiopulmonary bypass, RBC is red blood cells, FFP is fresh frozen plasma, TEG is thromboelastogram, ROTEM is rotational thromboelastometry

Malperfusion

Malperfusion in patients with TAD results in end organ ischemia and is secondary to limited perfusion of a false lumen, flap coverage or sheering of the ostia (Fig. 2). The obstruction of blood flow may be static, resulting in persistent ischemia or dynamic, leading to intermittent ischemia. Malperfusion syndrome occurs when the ischemia leads to end organ dysfunction and infarction [30]. Malperfusion is present in 10–30% of patients on initial evaluation for acute aortic dissection and is the second leading cause of death after aortic rupture [31]. In the treatment of patients with TAD, the traditional approach is repair of the proximal aorta with the goal of preventing death, restoring distal flow, and re-establishing the true lumen [32]. In patients who present with malperfusion and a significant lactic acidosis the prognosis is poor [33]. Mortality has been demonstrated to increase with increasing base deficit (BD) at presentation in one study and all patients with BD > −10 with abdominal malperfusion died. Similarly, the International Registry of Acute Aortic Dissection (IRAD) data have demonstrated increased mortality rates in patients with mesenteric or limb ischemia [34].

Recently, there has been interest in the management of malperfusion prior to aortic repair [35] (Fig. 3). If there are no high risk features of the TAD such as impending rupture, pericardial/pleural effusion or myocardial ischemia, this approach can be considered. This approach involves the use of endovascular techniques to fenestrate the dissection flap, stent the true lumen, or stent an obstructed visceral branch. The results of this approach in retrospective reports have shown improvement in survival in this complicated group of patients [36]. If malperfusion is recognized in the operating room after aortic repair, expeditious treatment to relieve the ischemia or manage tissue at risk is needed. This may involve percutaneous intervention to restore flow to visceral arterial branches or the lower extremities. Exploratory laparotomy to examine intra-abdominal end organs may be helpful and is generally low risk [37]. Additionally, femoral to femoral bypass can restore flow to an ischemic limb.

In the immediate post-operative setting the diagnosis of intra-abdominal malperfusion can be challenging. Patients are often sedated and on mechanical ventilation which makes symptom assessment and physical exam difficult. On physical exam the abdomen may be distended, although this is non-specific. The lactate may be elevated as the metabolic byproducts of cardiopulmonary bypass and hypothermic circulatory arrest wash out. The patient may be hemodynamically unstable and unable to be safely transported for CT scan. In cases in which the patient is critically ill and suspicion of intra-abdominal catastrophe is high, the best course may be exploratory laparoscopy or laparotomy. Often these procedures can be performed in the ICU if transport is considered too risky. One study utilizing the IRAD database noted that the incidence of mesenteric ischemia was 4% and mortality in mesenteric ischemia was significantly higher (up to 95% in patients managed medically vs. 42% in patients managed surgically or with a hybrid approach) [38].

Diagnosing limb ischemia is often more straightforward. There will usually be a pulse deficit in one or both limbs which are cool and mottled. Knowing the

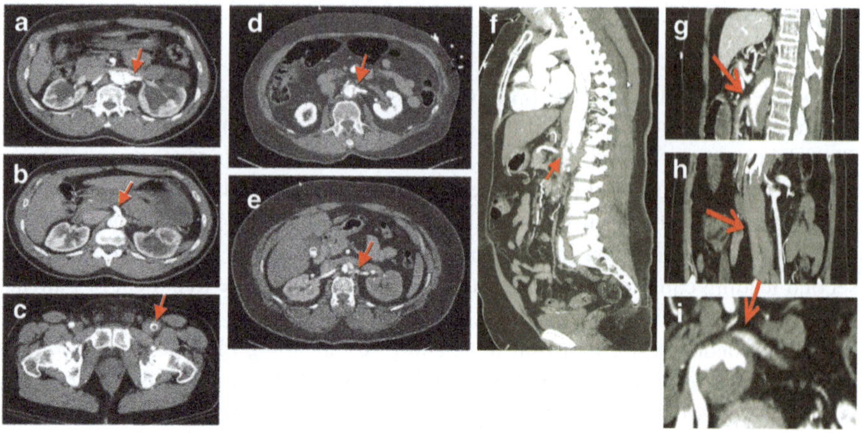

Fig. 2 Representative computed tomography images demonstrating malperfusion in type A aortic dissection patients. First panel top (**a**) Axial view with right renal artery supplied by the true lumen and left renal artery (red arrow) supplied by the false lumen (Previously published in Lawton et al., The profound impact of combined severe acidosis and malperfusion on operative mortality in the surgical treatment of type A aortic dissection. J Thorac Cardiovasc Surg 2018;155:897–904.). First panel middle (**b**) Axial view with superior mesenteric artery (red arrow) supplied by the false lumen (Previously published in Lawton et al., The profound impact of combined severe acidosis and malperfusion on operative mortality in the surgical treatment of type A aortic dissection. J Thorac Cardiovasc Surg 2018;155:897–904.). First panel bottom (**c**) Axial view with malperfusion of the left femoral artery (red arrow). (Previously published in Lawton et al., The profound impact of combined severe acidosis and malperfusion on operative mortality in the surgical treatment of type A aortic dissection. J Thorac Cardiovasc Surg 2018;155:897–904.). Second panel top (**d**) Axial view with malperfusion of the left renal artery (red arrow). Second panel bottom (**e**) Axial view with malperfusion of the left renal artery (red arrow) with multiple areas of intimal flap noted. Third panel (**f**) Sagittal view with extensive disease of the dissected thoracic and abdominal aorta and malperfusion of the celiac artery (red arrow). Fourth panel (**g**) Magnified sagittal view with malperfusion of the superior mesenteric artery (red arrow) due to intramural hematoma. (Previously published in Ong, C, Lawton JS, et al., The strongest risk factor for operative mortality in Acute Type A aortic dissection is acidosis: validation of risk model. Seminars in thoracic and Cardiovascular Surgery https://doi.org/10.1053/j.semtcvs.2020.02.023). Fourth panel (**h**) Magnified coronal view with malperfusion of the abdominal aorta due to intramural hematoma (red arrow). (Previously published in Ong, C, Lawton JS, et al., The strongest risk factor for operative mortality in Acute Type A aortic dissection is acidosis: validation of risk model. Seminars in thoracic and Cardiovascular Surgery https://doi.org/10.1053/j.semtcvs.2020.02.023). Fourth panel (**i**) Magnified axial view with malperfusion of the left renal artery (red arrow). (Previously published in Ong, C, Lawton JS, et al., The strongest risk factor for operative mortality in Acute Type A aortic dissection is acidosis: validation of risk model. Seminars in thoracic and Cardiovascular Surgery https://doi.org/10.1053/j.semtcvs.2020.02.023)

pre-operative pulse exam will help identify a change following aortic repair. Open or percutaneous techniques can be used to revascularize the limb. There should be a low threshold to perform a concomitant fasciotomy following significant malperfusion. In the IRAD database, 10% of patients presented with limb ischemia. The mortality rate for those with limb ischemia was 15% as compared to 7% in those without [34]. Over 90% were treated by endovascular means (fenestration or aorto-iliac stenting), and limb salvage rate was 93% [38].

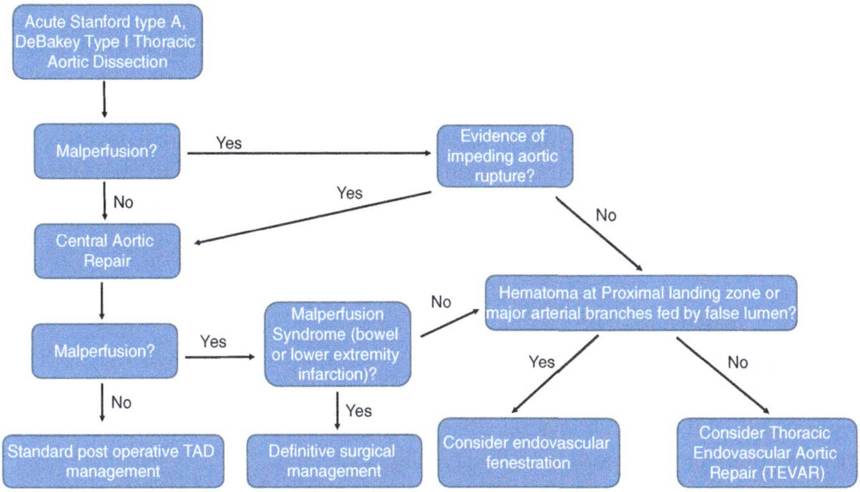

Fig. 3 Algorithm for management of acute type A aortic dissection with visceral or lower extremity malperfusion. In patients who are considered candidates for aortic intervention, the presence of visceral or lower extremity malperfusion may direct the initial strategy for management. This may include ischemia of the digestive tract, kidneys or lower extremities. Malperfusion on presentation can be assessed by history, physical exam, and/or laboratory or imaging findings. If after central aortic repair, malperfusion syndrome (infarction of intraabdominal organs or lower extremity muscle) is present, definitive management is warranted. This may include exploratory laparoscopy/laparotomy or open/endovascular treatment to restore flow to the ischemic organ with possible resection of necrotic tissue or fasciotomy

Myocardial Ischemia/Infarction

Aortic dissection presenting with myocardial ischemia is rare, occurs in approximately 3% of TAD patients, and carries a poor prognosis [34]. The presentation of myocardial ischemia is usually in the right coronary artery territory. The etiology may be coverage of the ostia by the dissection flap, extension of the dissection into the coronary artery or thrombosis of the vessel [39]. In a Japanese series, 6% of patients presented with myocardial ischemia, and the mortality rate was 33% (as compared to 8% in patients without ischemia) [40]. Postoperative myocardial ischemia can have several causes including poor myocardial protection, unrecognized coronary artery disease, aortic root dissection leading to ostial coronary occlusion, coronary dissection, embolism, obstruction from an aortic valve prosthesis or complications from coronary button implantation in root replacement. Recalcitrant malignant arrhythmias (VT/VF) that occur after aortic cross clamp release and reperfusion of the myocardium that do not abate should raise suspicion for myocardial ischemia. If myocardial ischemia is recognized in the operating room or in the early post-operative period, revision of the offending process can be undertaken. Often the simplest solution is to perform coronary artery bypass grafting to the ischemic territory as defined by wall motion abnormality on the echocardiogram. Revascularization should be prompt and within 3–6 h to avoid significant myocardial infarction. Coronary angiography can be used, however, the lesion may not be amenable to percutaneous intervention and may delay definitive management. If the injury is global, multi vessel CABG or veno-arterial extracorporeal membrane oxygenation (VA-ECMO) with a vent to decompress the left ventricle [41] and may be considered to facilitate potential recovery [42]. Finally, total artificial heart or transplant may be considered in the event of unrecoverable, devastating myocardial damage in appropriate candidates [43].

Aortic Complications

Complications of the aortic root and descending thoracic aorta may occur following replacement of the ascending aorta alone for the treatment of TAD. Early rupture of the unrepaired thoracic aorta after TAD repair occurs in in 1–2% of patients [44]. In a series of 324 patients who had TAD repair there were 7 patients (2%) with early aortic rupture and 100% mortality [45]. Two of the patients had aortic root rupture. Both patients had aortic insufficiency pre-operatively, intra-operative bleeding from the aortic root and high blood pressures prior to the rupture. The aortic roots of these patients were described as "fragile". In retrospect, the authors report that these patients should have had root replacement at the initial operation. Five patients in the series had rupture of the descending thoracic aorta. The authors conclude that meticulous blood pressure management should be maintained post-operatively.

TAD presenting with aortic insufficiency may be a marker of more extensive aortic root involvement, and root replacement may be considered in these patients. Data from the IRAD database indicate that 59% of patients had a supracoronary ascending aortic graft utilized alone in the treatment of TAD. Thirty-four percent had root procedures including aortic valve-sparing procedure (6%) or composite root replacement (16%) [46]. Patients with moderately-severe aortic insufficiency pre-operatively and those with more than mild aortic insufficiency after surgery were at significantly higher risk of severe aortic insufficiency 10 years after the index operation [47]. Additionally, some authors have advocated for aortic root replacement instead of repair to decrease the need for reoperation [48].

Neurologic Complications

Following repair of TAD, patients may have neurologic injury ranging from delirium to overt stroke. Approximately 10% of patients with TAD initially present with a brain injury, and approximately 70% of those patients also have aortic arch vessel dissection. Interestingly, 85% of patients in one study had improvement in stroke symptoms following surgery, suggesting that pre-operative stroke should not be a contraindication to TAD repair [46]. In one retrospective study of 102 TAD patients, 30% of patients presented with some neurologic symptom [49]. Mortality was 23% and the authors found that 50% of patients had post-operative neurologic symptoms. These included ischemic stroke (14%), spinal cord ischemia (4%), ischemic neuropathy (3%), hypoxic encephalopathy (8%), nerve compression (7%), and postoperative delirium (15%).

Stroke after repair of acute type A aortic dissection is a devastating complication. In one study of TAD patients, post-operative stroke occurred in 16% [50]. Risk factors for stroke included: bovine aortic arch, pre-operative CPR, and malperfusion. Patients with peri-operative stroke were more likely to have complications and longer hospital stay, but did not have an increased risk of in-hospital mortality. Treatment of post-operative stroke is usually supportive as these patients are not candidates for systemic lytic therapy and embolectomy is often not fruitful. A rare complication of TAD can occur when the aortic tear is circumferential and the false lumen telescopes proximally and distally simultaneously causing neurologic symptoms and myocardial ischemia and/or aortic sufficiency (Fig. 4).

Seizure at presentation is rare (about 3%) and post-operative seizure is also uncommon and reported to be approximately 0.4%. A study in which all patients underwent EEG monitoring during surgery showed an intra-operative seizure rate of 1.8% when DHCA was employed [51]. Patients with pre-operative neurologic symptoms appear to be at higher risk of seizure. Patients who remain in coma after cessation of all sedation will often require EEG to assess for seizure or other types of brain injury.

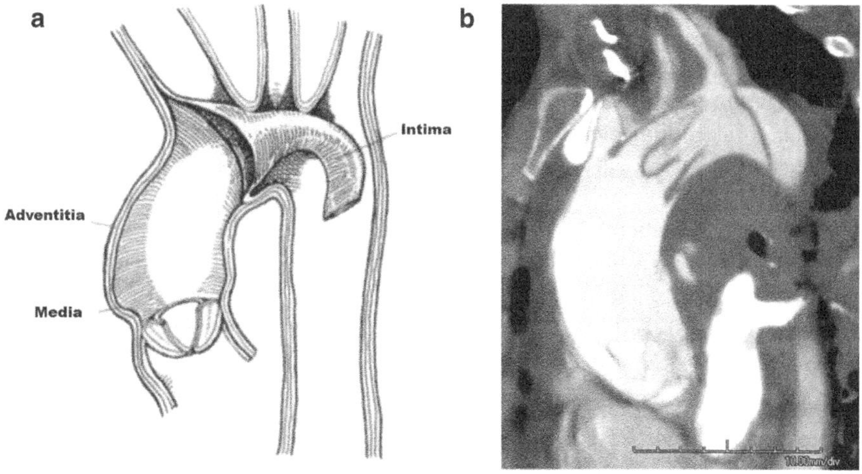

Fig. 4 Schematic demonstrating a complete circumferential tear of the ascending aortic false lumen with intussusception proximally and distally (**a**). Representative sagittal view from a contrasted enhanced CT scan showing a complete circumferential tear and intimal intussusception (**b**). This rare presentation can lead to simultaneous myocardial ischemia and/or aortic insufficiency and neurologic symptoms

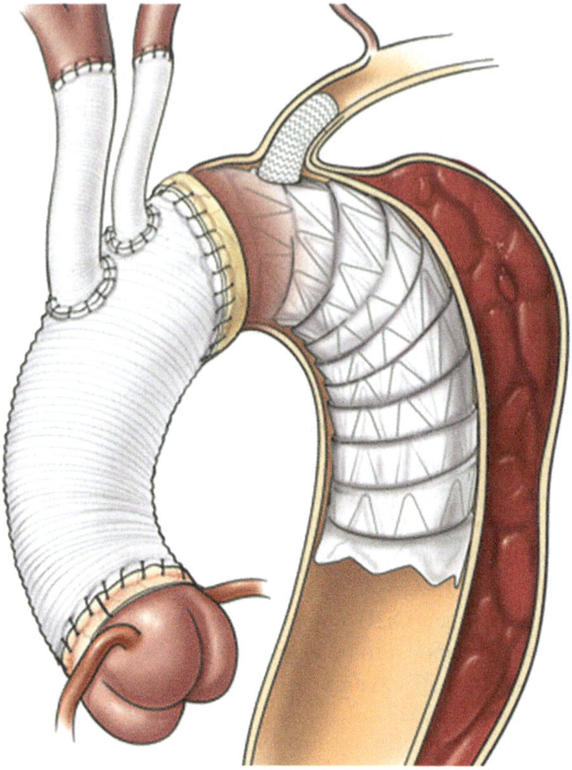

Fig. 5 Illustration of the frozen elephant aortic repair technique. There are several permutations of this approach, but the major goal is to treat the proximal aorta as well as the aortic arch and proximal descending thoracic aorta. This may lead to treatment of the entire diseased aorta or prepare for a later stage intervention on the remaining diseased aorta by open or endovascular approach. This example depicts an ascending aortic replacement with hybrid aortic arch management including Zone 2 replacement and frozen elephant trunk with physician modification of the thoracic endograft to allow for insertion of a branch stent into the left subclavian artery

Paraplegia can be a presenting symptom and has been reported to occur in approximately 3% of patients. It can be transient or permanent in nature and may resolve with restoration of the true lumen. For surgeons who employ the frozen elephant trunk the paraplegia rate is approximately 5% and is based on the length of the stent graft (12% for 150 mm stents vs. 2.5% for 100 mm stents) [52] (Fig. 5). In a meta-analysis of patients undergoing frozen elephant trunk the rate of paraplegia was twice that of patients having standard aortic arch operations [53]. Most authors have recommended using a 100 mm stent graft and avoiding 150 mm length stents or covering distal to the T8 level.

Other Complications

Patients with TAD are often critically ill, and like other cardiac surgery patients, are at risk for the usual maladies of the intensive care unit. Reported incidences of post-operative complications include: respiratory failure requiring prolonged mechanical ventilation (>72 h and/or tracheostomy) 6%, renal failure with oliguria in 3%, and mediastinitis in 2% [44]. Ventilator associated pneumonia, catheter associated bloodstream infections and catheter associated urinary tract infections can also occur in patients in the intensive care unit long-term.

Summary

TAD patients are complex and require expeditious, thoughtful, and competent medical and operative management by the entire surgical team with a constant high index of suspicion for complications. Complications of operative management of TAD can be substantial and life-threatening and include: bleeding, malperfusion, myocardial ischemia, aortic complications, and neurologic events. Careful operative planning, meticulous surgical technique and thorough post-operative management can help improve patient outcomes.

References

1. Crawford ES, Kirklin JW, Naftel DC, Svensson LG, Coselli JS, Safi HJ. Surgery for acute dissection of ascending aorta. Should the arch be included? J Thorac Cardiovasc Surg. 1992;104(1):46–59.
2. Fann JI, Smith JA, Miller DC, Mitchell RS, Moore KA, Grunkemeier G, et al. Surgical management of aortic dissection during a 30-year period. Circulation. 1995;92(9 Suppl):II113–21.
3. Kazui T, Washiyama N, Bashar AH, Terada H, Suzuki T, Ohkura K, et al. Surgical outcome of acute type A aortic dissection: analysis of risk factors. Ann Thorac Surg. 2002;74(1):75–81.
4. Robich MP, Koch CG, Johnston DR, Schiltz N, Chandran Pillai A, Hussain ST, et al. Trends in blood utilization in United States cardiac surgical patients. Transfusion. 2015;55(4):805–14.
5. Mora Mangano CT, Neville MJ, Hsu PH, Mignea I, King J, Miller DC. Aprotinin, blood loss, and renal dysfunction in deep hypothermic circulatory arrest. Circulation. 2001;104(12 Suppl 1):I276–81.
6. Zindovic I, Sjogren J, Bjursten H, Bjorklund E, Herou E, Ingemansson R, et al. Predictors and impact of massive bleeding in acute type A aortic dissection. Interact Cardiovasc Thorac Surg. 2017;24(4):498–505.
7. Cabasa A, Pochettino A. Surgical management and outcomes of type A dissection—the Mayo Clinic experience. Ann Cardiothorac Surg. 2016;5(4):296–309.
8. Fine NL, Applebaum J, Elguezabal A, Castleman L. Multiple coagulation defects in association with dissecting aneurysm. Arch Intern Med. 1967;119(5):522–6.
9. Paparella D, Rotunno C, Guida P, Malvindi PG, Scrascia G, De Palo M, et al. Hemostasis alterations in patients with acute aortic dissection. Ann Thorac Surg. 2011;91(5):1364–9.
10. ten Cate JW, Timmers H, Becker AE. Coagulopathy in ruptured or dissecting aortic aneurysms. Am J Med. 1975;59(2):171–6.
11. Gelb AB, Roth RI, Levin J, London MJ, Noall RA, Hauck WW, et al. Changes in blood coagulation during and following cardiopulmonary bypass: lack of correlation with clinical bleeding. Am J Clin Pathol. 1996;106(1):87–99.
12. Huang B, Tian L, Fan X, Zhu J, Liang Y, Yang Y. Low admission platelet counts predicts increased risk of in-hospital mortality in patients with type A acute aortic dissection. Int J Cardiol. 2014;172(3):e484–6.
13. Tanaka M, Kawahito K, Adachi H, Ino T. Platelet dysfunction in acute type A aortic dissection evaluated by the laser light-scattering method. J Thorac Cardiovasc Surg. 2003;126(3):837–41.
14. Coselli JS, Crawford ES, Beall AC Jr, Mizrahi EM, Hess KR, Patel VM. Determination of brain temperatures for safe circulatory arrest during cardiovascular operation. Ann Thorac Surg. 1988;45(6):638–42.
15. Mezrow CK, Midulla PS, Sadeghi AM, Gandsas A, Wang W, Dapunt OE, et al. Evaluation of cerebral metabolism and quantitative electroencephalography after hypothermic circulatory arrest and low-flow cardiopulmonary bypass at different temperatures. J Thorac Cardiovasc Surg. 1994;107(4):1006–19.

16. Polderman KH. Mechanisms of action, physiological effects, and complications of hypothermia. Crit Care Med. 2009;37(7 Suppl):S186–202.
17. Ferrara A, MacArthur JD, Wright HK, Modlin IM, McMillen MA. Hypothermia and acidosis worsen coagulopathy in the patient requiring massive transfusion. Am J Surg. 1990;160(5):515–8.
18. Hanke AA, Dellweg C, Kienbaum P, Weber CF, Gorlinger K, Rahe-Meyer N. Effects of desmopressin on platelet function under conditions of hypothermia and acidosis: an in vitro study using multiple electrode aggregometry*. Anaesthesia. 2010;65(7):688–91.
19. Leshnower BG, Myung RJ, Thourani VH, Halkos ME, Kilgo PD, Puskas JD, et al. Hemiarch replacement at 28°C: an analysis of mild and moderate hypothermia in 500 patients. Ann Thorac Surg. 2012;93(6):1910–5. discussion 5-6
20. Keenan JE, Wang H, Gulack BC, Ganapathi AM, Andersen ND, Englum BR, et al. Does moderate hypothermia really carry less bleeding risk than deep hypothermia for circulatory arrest? A propensity-matched comparison in hemiarch replacement. J Thorac Cardiovasc Surg. 2016;152(6):1559–69. e2
21. Svensson LG. Hemostasis for aortic surgery. J Card Surg. 1997;12(2 Suppl):229–31.
22. Vivacqua A, Koch CG, Yousuf AM, Nowicki ER, Houghtaling PL, Blackstone EH, et al. Morbidity of bleeding after cardiac surgery: is it blood transfusion, reoperation for bleeding, or both? Ann Thorac Surg. 2011;91(6):1780–90.
23. David TE, Armstrong S, Ivanov J, Barnard S. Surgery for acute type A aortic dissection. Ann Thorac Surg. 1999;67(6):1999–2001. discussion 14-9
24. Lawton JS, Liu J, Kulshrestha K, Moon MR, Damiano RJ Jr, Maniar H, et al. The impact of surgical strategy on survival after repair of type A aortic dissection. J Thorac Cardiovasc Surg. 2015;150(2):294–301. e1
25. Roselli EE, Idrees JJ, Bakaeen FG, Tong MZ, Soltesz EG, Mick S, et al. Evolution of simplified frozen elephant trunk repair for acute DeBakey Type I dissection: midterm outcomes. Ann Thorac Surg. 2018;105(3):749–55.
26. Rylski B, Urbanski PP, Siepe M, Beyersdorf F, Bachet J, Gleason TG, et al. Operative techniques in patients with type A dissection complicated by cerebral malperfusion. Eur J Cardiothorac Surg. 2014;46(2):156–66.
27. Spotnitz WD. Active and mechanical hemostatic agents. Surgery. 2007;142(4 Suppl):S34–8.
28. Strauch JT, Spielvogel D, Lansman SL, Lauten AL, Bodian C, Griepp RB. Long-term integrity of Teflon felt-supported suture lines in aortic surgery. Ann Thorac Surg. 2005;79(3):796–800.
29. Zindovic I, Sjogren J, Ahlsson A, Bjursten H, Fuglsang S, Geirsson A, et al. Recombinant factor VIIa use in acute type A aortic dissection repair: a multicenter propensity-score-matched report from the Nordic Consortium for Acute Type A Aortic Dissection. J Thorac Cardiovasc Surg. 2017;154(6):1852–9. e2
30. Yang B, Patel HJ, Williams DM, Dasika NL, Deeb GM. Management of type A dissection with malperfusion. Ann Cardiothorac Surg. 2016;5(4):265–74.
31. Geirsson A, Szeto WY, Pochettino A, McGarvey ML, Keane MG, Woo YJ, et al. Significance of malperfusion syndromes prior to contemporary surgical repair for acute type A dissection: outcomes and need for additional revascularizations. Eur J Cardiothorac Surg. 2007;32(2):255–62.
32. Lawton JS. Acute type A aortic dissection 101. J Thorac Cardiovasc Surg. 2015;150(4):769–70.
33. Lawton JS, Moon MR, Liu J, Koerner DJ, Kulshrestha K, Damiano RJ Jr, et al. The profound impact of combined severe acidosis and malperfusion on operative mortality in the surgical treatment of type A aortic dissection. J Thorac Cardiovasc Surg. 2018;155(3):897–904.
34. Mehta RH, Suzuki T, Hagan PG, Bossone E, Gilon D, Llovet A, et al. Predicting death in patients with acute type A aortic dissection. Circulation. 2002;105(2):200–6.
35. Deeb GM, Williams DM, Bolling SF, Quint LE, Monaghan H, Sievers J, et al. Surgical delay for acute type A dissection with malperfusion. Ann Thorac Surg. 1997;64(6):1669–75. discussion 75-7

36. Kamman AV, Yang B, Kim KM, Williams DM, Michael Deeb G, Patel HJ. Visceral malperfusion in aortic dissection: the Michigan experience. Semin Thorac Cardiovasc Surg. 2017;29(2):173–8.
37. Rodriguez R, Robich MP, Plate JF, Trooskin SZ, Sellke FW. Gastrointestinal complications following cardiac surgery: a comprehensive review. J Card Surg. 2010;25(2):188–97.
38. Henke PK, Williams DM, Upchurch GR Jr, Proctor M, Cooper JV, Fang J, et al. Acute limb ischemia associated with type B aortic dissection: clinical relevance and therapy. Surgery. 2006;140(4):532–9. discussion 9-40
39. Spittell PC, Spittell JA Jr, Joyce JW, Tajik AJ, Edwards WD, Schaff HV, et al. Clinical features and differential diagnosis of aortic dissection: experience with 236 cases (1980 through 1990). Mayo Clin Proc. 1993;68(7):642–51.
40. Kawahito K, Adachi H, Murata S, Yamaguchi A, Ino T. Coronary malperfusion due to type A aortic dissection: mechanism and surgical management. Ann Thorac Surg. 2003;76(5):1471–6. discussion 6
41. Donker DW, Brodie D, Henriques JPS, Broome M. Left ventricular unloading during veno-arterial ECMO: a review of percutaneous and surgical unloading interventions. Perfusion. 2019;34(2):98–105.
42. Lorusso R, Centofanti P, Gelsomino S, Barili F, Di Mauro M, Orlando P, et al. Venoarterial extracorporeal membrane oxygenation for acute fulminant myocarditis in adult patients: a 5-year multi-institutional experience. Ann Thorac Surg. 2016;101(3):919–26.
43. Attia T, Robich M, Lincoff AM, Shishehbor MH, Svensson L, Smedira NG. Successful treatment of aortic root dissection complicated with extensive myocardial infarction using the total artificial heart. J Surg Case Rep. 2017;2017(8):rjx123.
44. Chiappini B, Schepens M, Tan E, Dell' Amore A, Morshuis W, Dossche K, et al. Early and late outcomes of acute type A aortic dissection: analysis of risk factors in 487 consecutive patients. Eur Heart J. 2005;26(2):180–6.
45. Kimura N, Tanaka M, Kawahito K, Yamaguchi A, Ino T, Adachi H. Early postoperative aortic rupture following surgery for acute type A aortic dissection. Interact Cardiovasc Thorac Surg. 2009;8(4):431–4.
46. Evangelista A, Isselbacher EM, Bossone E, Gleason TG, Eusanio MD, Sechtem U, et al. Insights from the International Registry of acute aortic dissection: a 20-year experience of collaborative clinical research. Circulation. 2018;137(17):1846–60.
47. Kim DJ, Lee S, Lee SH, Youn YN, Chang BC, Yoo KJ, et al. The fate of residual aortic regurgitation after ascending aorta replacement in type A aortic dissection. J Thorac Cardiovasc Surg. 2020;160(6):1421–1430.e5.
48. Halstead JC, Spielvogel D, Meier DM, Rinke S, Bodian C, Malekan R, et al. Composite aortic root replacement in acute type A dissection: time to rethink the indications? Eur J Cardiothorac Surg. 2005;27(4):626–32. discussion 32-3
49. Gaul C, Dietrich W, Friedrich I, Sirch J, Erbguth FJ. Neurological symptoms in type A aortic dissections. Stroke. 2007;38(2):292–7.
50. Dumfarth J, Kofler M, Stastny L, Plaikner M, Krapf C, Semsroth S, et al. Stroke after emergent surgery for acute type A aortic dissection: predictors, outcome and neurological recovery. Eur J Cardiothorac Surg. 2018;53(5):1013–20.
51. Cheung AT, Weiss SJ, Kent G, Pochettino A, Bavaria JE, Stecker MM. Intraoperative seizures in cardiac surgical patients undergoing deep hypothermic circulatory arrest monitored with EEG. Anesthesiology. 2001;94(6):1143–7.
52. Preventza O, Liao JL, Olive JK, Simpson K, Critsinelis AC, Price MD, et al. Neurologic complications after the frozen elephant trunk procedure: a meta-analysis of more than 3000 patients. J Thorac Cardiovasc Surg. 2020;160(1):20–33. e4
53. Hanif H, Dubois L, Ouzounian M, Peterson MD, El-Hamamsy I, Dagenais F, et al. Aortic arch reconstructive surgery with conventional techniques vs frozen elephant trunk: a systematic review and meta-analysis. Can J Cardiol. 2018;34(3):262–73.

Neuroprotection During Dissection Repair

Christian V. Ghincea, Yuki Ikeno, Andrew L. Mesher, Muhammad Aftab, and T. Brett Reece

Introduction

The care of acute aortic syndrome patients can be incredibly complicated based on the anatomic divergences in perfusion that can occur to any end organ. Essentially, any tissue bed can be compromised due to loss of perfusion from either lack of cardiac output or loss of peripheral branch perfusion by true lumen compression or branch avulsion. The brain and spinal cord, of course, have the least tolerance to interruption of blood flow; therefore, preservation of flow is paramount. This chapter discusses the approaches to optimizing neurological outcomes when presented with acute aortic syndrome. As these approaches are not linear, the discussion addresses different problems that may present at varying times for varying patients. However, thoughtful consideration of an evolving picture is required for securing optimal outcomes, including neurological.

Presentation

Optimizing neurological outcomes begins as soon as the patient is identified by addressing the specific patients' condition at presentation and operative planning based on specific patients' unique dissection anatomy. This is paramount as both systemic and regional malperfusion can lead to neurological complications. Indeed, intraoperative neuroprotection approaches must not only align with, but to some extent, they will dictate the conduct of the operation. However, a myriad ofbackup plans must be engrained with some flexibility to evolve to alternate techniques

C. V. Ghincea · Y. Ikeno · A. L. Mesher · M. Aftab · T. Brett Reece (✉)
University of Colorado Anschutz Medical Campus, Aurora, CO, USA
e-mail: brett.reece@cuanschutz.edu

J. S. Coselli et al. (eds.), *Aortic Dissection and Acute Aortic Syndromes*,
https://doi.org/10.1007/978-3-030-66668-2_35

fluidly as patients' physiology and anatomy can be different than the imaging suggests or even change with dissection progression.

Mitigation of Prior Injury and Restoration of Cerebral Perfusion

Intraoperative neuroprotection strategy begins with mitigation of antecedent neurological injury followed by the prompt correction of central nervous system ischemia, or "neuromalperfusion." For patients presenting with stroke symptoms or spinal malperfusion, the injury must be deemed to benefit from an operation. In most situations, the patient will be better served by an operation than medical management. The exceptions may be dense coma, the extremes of age, extensive malperfusion of the gut, or loss of hemodynamics prior to arriving in the operating room, among others. Once surgical intervention is decided upon, the initial objective is to improve blood flow to the ischemic territory by optimizing cerebral and spinal perfusion and minimizing systemic hypotension. In the preoperative period, management revolves around medical therapy to balance perfusion and risk of dissection propagation or rupture. In almost all cases, the patient should undergo impulse control therapy, to reduce the blood pressure and heart rate resulting in a lesser pulse pressure. Careful coordination with the anesthesia team is necessary, in particular during anesthetic induction to prevent hemodynamic collapse. Significant aortic insufficiency or the presence of a pericardial effusion should prompt complete readiness of the surgical team at the time of induction. While this statement may seem obvious to the experienced team, subsequent intraoperative neuroprotection strategies may be nullified by the cumulative effects of multiple episodes of neuromalperfusion in the perioperative period.

Following induction, the subsequent, and nearly synonymous, neuroprotective strategy at the initiation of the operation requires prompt restoration of adequate cerebral and spinal perfusion. Malperfusion to the central nervous system can result from systemic or regional malperfusion. In cases of hemodynamically significant pericardial effusion, relief of tamponade is the logical first step to restore cardiac output. If a patient arrests on induction, the authors advocate immediate median sternotomy and pericardiotomy. This approach stands in contrast to common approaches of peripheral cannulation and immediate institution of cardiopulmonary bypass prior to sternotomy. We favor urgent sternotomy up front for a number of reasons. Pericardial tamponade frequently contributes to hemodynamic collapse and decompression can rapidly restore perfusion, at the same time relieving venous obstruction and hypotension contributing to decreased cerebral perfusion pressure. Aortic rupture can be controlled manually or with packing while cannulating for cardiopulmonary bypass. In the case of severe aortic insufficiency, there is the opportunity to decompress the left ventricle immediately after institution of CPB and prevent periods of ventricular distention. Of course, if enough team members are available simultaneous peripheral cannulation may be helpful with the caveat that the retrograde aortic perfusion can be complicated further by the dissection characteristics. Cannulation of the true lumen may not be straightforward from the femorals without intravascular ultrasound (IVUS) and/or transesophageal echo to guide cannula placement emergently.

In cases of complex dissection involving the brachiocephalic vessels, an extensive compressive dissection flap, with or without luminal thrombosis, may contribute to ongoing cerebral malperfusion despite pericardial drainage and initiation of bypass. Although patients presenting with neurological deficits have historically had a worse post-operative prognosis, earlier cerebral reperfusion may promote recovery, especially if less than 5 h [1]. These cases should be identified on preoperative imaging with development of a repair strategy to restore cerebral perfusion early in the conduct of the operation. At centers with specialization in aortic surgery, these patients will undergo full arch replacement with specific early bypass beyond the dissected head vessel such as the distal common carotid during systemic cooling. In fact, results from the University of Pittsburgh suggests an incredibly low stroke rate with early bypass to exclude proximal dissection in the brachiocephalic vessels [2]. While this approach does require planning and a split arterial line, it also removes the risk of cerebral embolization from the proximal perfusion vessels. The risk of dissection-related malperfusion in these vessels, both in the short and long term, will be essentially eliminated after bypass and reperfusion of the vessel.

Cannulation

Significant variation in practice continues among aortic surgeons with regards to cannulation strategies for repair of acute aortic dissection. Figure 1 illustrates the most common arterial cannulation sites utilized by our institution. While benefits of various sites of cannulation can be taken advantage of for specific dissection characteristics, the main principle remains restoration of flow to the true lumen of the aorta. In rare, and what might be considered salvage cases, the aorta can be transected and true lumencannulated directly, or cannulation can be achieved through the apex of the heart. The advantages and disadvantages of our most commonly utilized cannulation options are discussed here.

Right Axillary Cannulation

Theoretical benefits of peripheral right axillary cannulation include avoidance of atherosclerotic disease burden, intramural hematoma, or proximal dissection in the ascending aorta, and the ability to perform selective antegrade cerebral perfusion by occluding the innominate artery at the aortic arch. Arguments against the axillary stem from either the size of the vessel, leading to high arterial line pressures, or involvement of the innominate artery with the dissection, complicating the retrograde flow though this artery back to the true lumen systemically. The authors would argue that the axillary can be used safely in almost all dissections as true lumen flow is almost always preserved with true lumen flow distally.

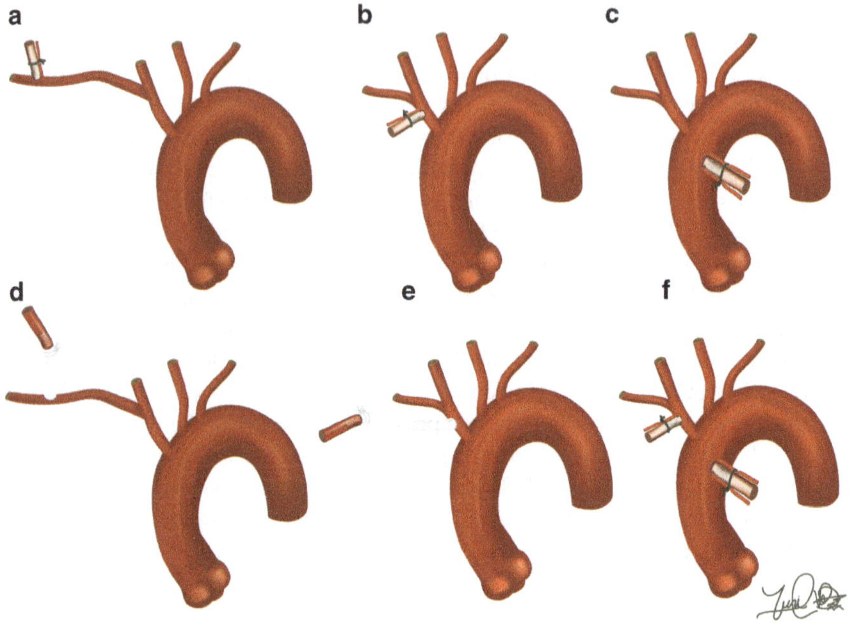

Fig. 1 Common routes of arterial cannulation for the initiation of cardiopulmonary bypass on acute aortic syndrome. (**a**) Right axillary cannulation using a tube graft sewn end-to-side. (**b**) Innominate artery cannulation using a tube graft sewn end to side. (**c**) Direct aortic cannulation using the Seldinger technique and epiaortic ultrasound/transesophageal echo to verify true lumen access (**d**) Right axillary cannulation using the Seldinger technique. (**e**) Right common carotid cannulation using a tube graft sewn end-to-side. (**f**) Left common carotid cannulation using a tube graft sewn end-to-side. Due to potentially complex dissection anatomy multiple arterial cannulation options must be considered with the goal perfusing the true lumen via the most feasible and expeditious route. In addition to the routes depicted in this figure, femoral artery and left subclavian cannulation are other options which can be utilized. In rare and what ought to be considered salvage cases, the aorta can be transected and cannulated directly, or cannulation can be achieved through the apex of the heart

Femoral Cannulation

Femoral cannulation has been traditionally preferred for rapid access and early cooling. Differential neurological outcomes have not been demonstrated for femoral cannulation versus other sites [3]. Femoral cannulation, especially using a percutaneous approach, is a safe strategy. The pitfalls of femoral cannulation include potential difficulty with accessing the true lumen and the need for separate cannulation to provide cerebral perfusion during circulatory arrest.

Evolving Cannulation Complexity and Strategy

As comfort with circulatory arrest has grown, our institution has become bolder with cannulation choices. In cases where the innominate artery is spared of dissection, free of significant atherosclerosis, and a hemiarch replacement is planned, the authors will frequently cannulate via 10 mm graft sewn end-to-side to the innominate artery with a partial occlusion clamp. However, this takes more time than routinely stated, so it has become less utilized institutionally. As more aggressive total arch replacement has become more commonplace, the authors favor central aortic cannulation (into the true lumen) when possible using transesophageal and epiaortic ultrasound guidance and a modified Seldinger technique (Fig. 1c) [4]. Simultaneous imaging is critical to confirm true lumen perfusion. While cooling, we proceed to split arterial perfusion and bypass the brachiocephalic vessels using a multibranch graft, as shown in Fig. 2, that is later connected to a branch of the arch graft.

The experience from Emory has shown the benefit of washout from retrograde cerebral perfusion (RCP) washout of debris from arterial manipulation during the cooling period. When using RCP, a 24 French cannula is placed in the superior vena cava immediately prior to circulatory arrest period with a Rummel tourniquet above the Azygous vein take off. This will be removed immediately after circulatory arrest so as not to obstruct venous return from the upper half of the body. The authors have used the SVC cannula for drainage in the context of bicaval cannulation and RCP but this configuration requires multiple connections to the cardiopulmonary bypass circuit. Institutionally we have begun to take advantage of both retrograde and antegrade perfusion during circulatory arrest. Specifics of perfusion management during the circulatory arrest period will be discussed later in the chapter.

Neuromonitoring/Neurophysiological Intraoperative Monitoring

Collectively termed neurophysiological intraoperative monitoring (NIOM), the most commonly employed modalities for monitoring neurologic function during aortic arch surgery include EEG, somatosensory evoked potentials (SSEP), motor evoked potentials (MEP), and cerebral oximetry by near-infrared spectroscopy (NIRS), as depicted in Fig. 3. The argument for overall NIOM use is early detection of neuromalperfusion. Measures can be instituted at this early point to reverse or minimize effects of the malperfusion such as suction embolectomy, adding arterial cannulation sites to watershed areas, or even simple measures like hemodynamic augmentation with increased central blood pressure. Opponents to NIOM suggest this monitoring leads to a lot of noise with false positive signals. The authors have found that while there is some noise, when the neuromonitoring is combined with clinical perspective, the information can be valuable for preserving neurologic patient outcomes [5].

Electroencephalography

Continuous EEG monitoring remains the primary NIOM modality utilized by the authors for all cases involving the aortic arch or hypothermic circulatory arrest, including hemiarch replacement. Although requiring specialized equipment,

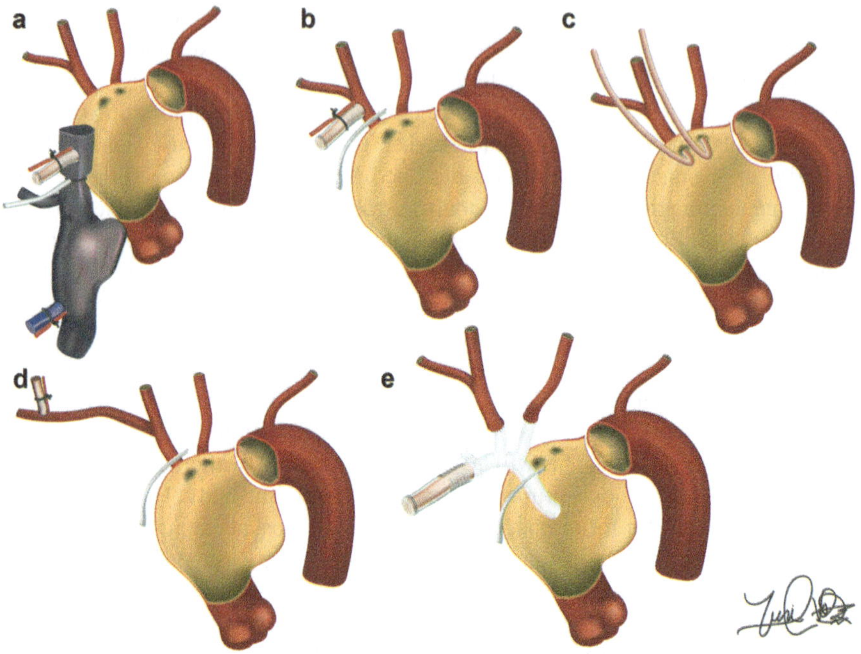

Fig. 2 Common routes of cannulation for cerebral perfusion during circulatory arrest. (**a**) For retrograde cerebral perfusion a right-angle cannula is placed into the superior vena cava above the insertion of the azygous vein. (**b**) The innominate artery can be cannulated either percutaneously (as shown in the figure) or using a graft sewn end-to-side to the vessel. (**c**) Upon initiation of circulatory arrest, once the aorta has been transected, the ostia of the innominate and left common carotid arteries can be directly cannulated with balloon tipped catheters. (**d**) The right axillary artery can be cannulated either percutaneously (as shown in the figure) or using a graft sewn end-to-side to the vessel. (**e**) With an already established alternate route of arterial cannulation for cardiopulmonary bypass, the innominate and left common carotid arteries can be sequentially debranched from the arch and sewn to a multibranch graft that is also connected to the bypass circuit, allowing for split arterial perfusion between the upper and lower body, and bilateral antegrade cerebral perfusion during circulatory arrest. In addition to the options depicted in this figure, right or left common carotid artery cannulation remain available for establishing unilateral antegrade cerebral perfusion, as shown in Fig. 1

additional set-up, and a dedicated neuromonitoring team intraoperatively, EEG can provide useful information especially in the case of acute aortic syndrome repair. When possible, without causing delay in definitive repair, the authors advocate its use routinely.

A reference EEG following induction of anesthesia but before cooling during CPB is obtained as a baseline. Anesthetic agents can dramatically influence electrocerebral activity, however it is important to establish the reference prior to the effects of hypothermia or any surgical manipulation. These objective data may be particularly important in the case of acute aortic syndrome with antecedent neurological injury or an imperfect or unreliable clinical neurological exam. Continuous EEG monitoring is maintained throughout the period of cardiopulmonary bypass.

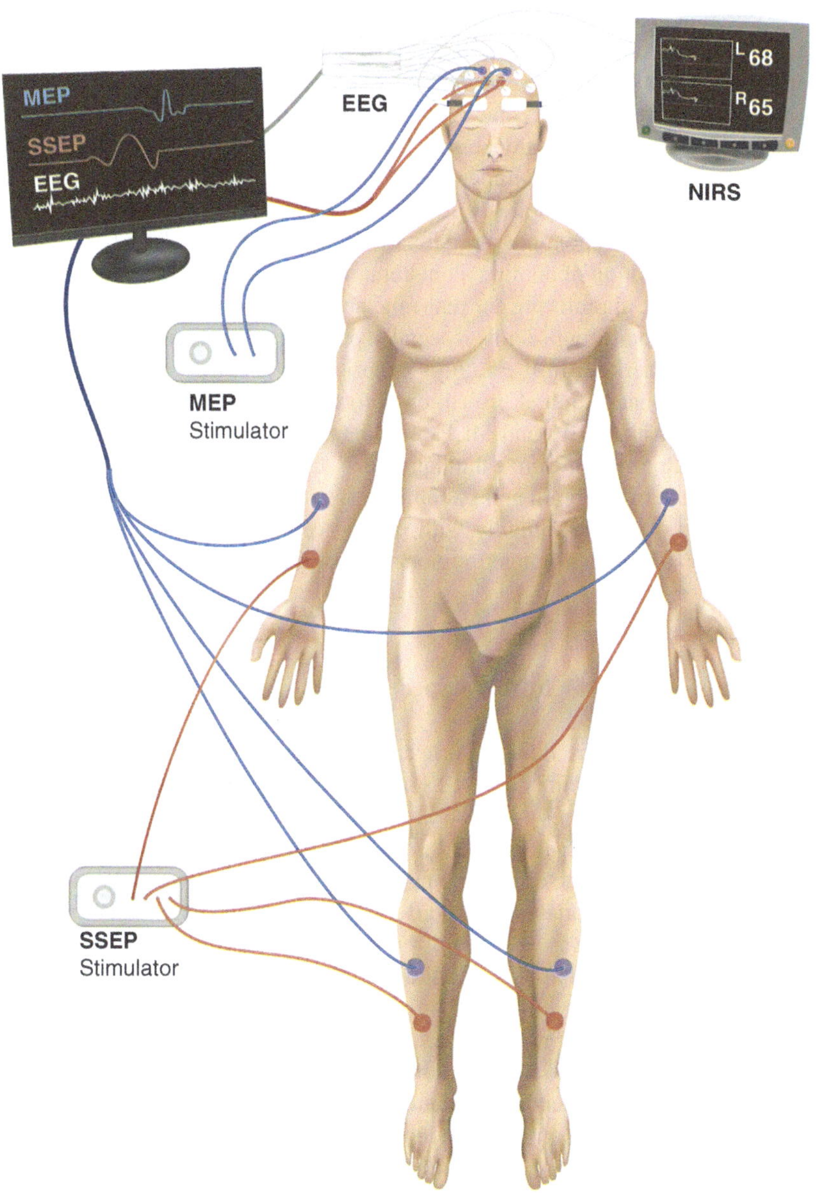

Fig. 3 Neurophysiological intraoperative monitoring (NIOM) is a term that refers to multiple modalities that are employed to actively monitor neurological function and perfusion during surgery for aortic dissection. These modalities include electroencephalography (EEG), motor evoked potentials (MEPs), somatosensory evoked potentials (SSEPs), and near infrared spectroscopy (NIRS). EEG utilizes multiple detector electrodes placed on the patient's scalp to monitor cerebral electrical activity. MEPs are produced by transcranial stimulation of the motor cortex with peripherally placed detectors to read a response. SSEPs are produced by peripheral electrical stimulation with transcranial detection of somatosensory cortical response. NIRS use scalp monitors to determine regional cerebral oxygen saturation

Electrocerebral activity follows a predictable pattern as cerebral hypothermia deepens and serves as surrogate for cerebral metabolism and energy consumption. Burst suppression typically develops between 15.7 °C and 33.0 °C [6, 7] with progression to complete electrocerebral inactivity (ECI) occurring between 12.5 °C and 27.2 °C. Surface and body temperature measurements have been demonstrated to poorly correlate with brain temperature. There also exists significant individual variability between temperature and electrocerebral activity [8]. Therefore, for a particular patient, extrapolating a prediction of cerebral metabolism based on core temperature or duration of cooling alone remains unreliable, highlighting the utility of continuous EEG monitoring for real-time acquisition of electrocerebral activity. This degree of monitoring seems especially pertinent when using more moderate degrees of hypothermia. In the authors experience, EEG has been very useful to determining adequate cerebral protection before circulatory arrest, and when used in combination with SSEPs and MEPs, has identified intraoperative stroke including areas of malperfusion from cannulation/dissection mismatch, when differential pressures exist between brain and systemic perfusion, or embolization. All of these instances were dealt with quickly with prompt reversal of the malperfusion, but would have resulted in prolonged regional ischemia without the neuromonitoring in place.

Cerebral Oximetry/Near Infrared Spectroscopy

While more commonly used in pediatric cardiac surgery, there is increased adoption of cerebral oximetry monitory by NIRS in adult cardiac [9] and aortic arch surgery [10, 11]. Attractive features of cerebral oximetry include its relative ease-of-use, ubiquity, simplified read-out, and real-time feedback. Regional ScO_2 levels generally increase from baseline during the period of cooling reaching a plateau prior to initiation of cerebral circulatory arrest after which they decline until cerebral perfusion is restored. Non-invasive cerebral oximetry historically has poor correlation with jugular bulb saturation [12] and limited data exist to suggest absolute saturation values to correlate with development or prevention of clinical neurological injury. Therefore, cerebral neuroprotection or perfusion strategies based on NIRS data alone remain nebulous. However, the reference to baseline and changes in symmetry may be helpful to identify problems intraoperatively that are related to altered perfusion. The identification of a sudden decreased in left sided cerebral regional saturation with initiation of selective antegrade cerebral perfusion through the innominate artery prompting subsequent conversion to a bilateral antegrade cerebral perfusion strategy is an example of directly actionable feedback that may be provided by NIRS monitoring. This has been exceeding helpful in the development of a protocol for selective arterial perfusion during hypothermic circulatory arrest with moderate hypothermia. Balanced oximetry suggests selective perfusion through one carotid is sufficient, but a drop in the contralateral saturations suggests a need for bilateral perfusion. While this may add nothing for short circulatory arrest times below 15–20 min, prolonged circulatory arrest times may benefit from increasing unilateral flow and pressure or even from adding a perfusion cannula to the opposite carotid.

Prevention of Further Neurological Injury

Temperature Management

Hypothermia remains the cornerstone of any cerebral protection strategy when periods of altered cerebral perfusion are anticipated during repair of acute aortic dissection. Analogous to other systemic tissue beds, neuronal cellular metabolic rate and oxygen consumption are dependent on tissue temperature via reductions in enzymatic activity. Experimentally, cerebral metabolic activity has been shown to decrease initially by 6–7% per degree Celsius below 37 degrees [13]. This roughly correlates to a separate descriptor of temperature modulated tissue metabolism, the *Q*10 rule, which describes an approximately 50% reduction in metabolic rate for every 10 degree decrease in temperature [14]. The effects of tissue temperature on neuronal survival have be exploited by aortic surgeons for the purpose of circulatory arrest for decades, however recommended temperature nadirs and adjunctive strategies continue to evolve.

In order to more accurately classify temperature strategies in aortic arch surgery, a consensus definition of hypothermia stratified into 4 categories has been devised [15], as shown in Table 1 [16]. Profound hypothermia (≤14 °C) is sufficient without adjuncts to induce electrocerebral inactivity (ECI) in approximately 80% of patients. Whereas deep hypothermia (14.1–20 °C) falls within a steeper section of Temperature-ECI curve and produces ECI with more individual variability, roughly 20–80% predicted. Moderate and mild categories of hypothermia are less likely to yield ECI and correspond to shorter predicted protection times during hypothermic circulatory arrest [6, 15]. The safety of deep hypothermic circulatory arrest (DHCA) strategies whereby the patient is systemically cooled until ECI prior to "straight" circulatory arrest for periods up to 30 min have been demonstrated during aortic arch surgery in a number of large series [8, 17–19]. A large study of 394 patients who underwent

Table 1 Temperature and predicted circulatory arrest protection time

Category	Temperature (°C)	HCA time (min)
Profound	≤14	30–40
Deep	14.1–20	20–30
Moderate	20.1–28	10–20
Mild	28.1–34	<10

HCA hypothermic circulatory arrest

arch repairs with this strategy showed no diminished cognitive function and a hypoperfusion-specific stroke rate of 1.8%, with an overall stroke rate less than 5% [20].

Despite both historical evidence and contemporary outcomes from Yale supporting the safety of a DHCA strategy, there are drawbacks to deep hypothermia that provide vigor for alternate methods using more moderate degrees of hypothermia. The main disadvantages to lower temperatures include longer durations of cardiopulmonary bypass needed for systemic cooling/rewarming and associated consequences. However, temperature specific issues such as hypothermia induced coaguloapathy may increase perioperative blood loss and the need for transfusion as well as the rate of reoperation for bleeding [21–23].

In order to achieve similar or superior neurological outcomes with warmer systemic and cerebral temperatures, adjunctive perfusion strategies and more efficient operative techniques are aimed at reducing time spent with relative cerebral hypoperfusion. It is the author's position that there is no truly "safe" duration of circulatory arrest regardless of temperature nadir or adjunctive measures that can ensure cerebral protection for all patients. Minimizing, ideally eliminating, time spent in sub-physiological cerebral perfusion remains our goal for all aortic procedures. Compared with elective aortic arch repair, acute dissection with or without antecedent injury remains a risk factor for neurological injury, further highlighting the need for speed in this particular patient group.

Adjunctive Cerebral Perfusion During Systemic Circulatory Arrest

Retrograde Cerebral Perfusion

The technique of retrograde cerebral perfusion exploits the anatomical lack of valves between the superior vena cava and the cerebral venous vasculature allowing perfusate to flow retrograde to the brain. A 24 french or similar cannula connected to the arterial limb of the CPB circuit is placed into the SVC within the chest and the SVC encircled by a snare above the azygous insertion (Fig. 4a). With the tourniquet cinched, the cerebral venous system can be selectively pressurized though the SVC cannula. RCP Flow has traditionally been targeted in the range of 100–300 ml/min at 10–12 °C. The authors transduce venous pressure through the side-arm of an introducer placed by anesthesia in the right internal jugular vein and increase flow to the achieve a venous pressure of 25 mmHg. Frequently RCP flows >500 ml/min are required to achieve pressure target of 25 mmHg and to observe retrograde flow from the innominate and left common carotid ostia. Significant oxygen and glucose delivery to the brain have not been demonstrated during RCP [24], so this technique in isolation is frequently coupled with deeper levels of hypothermia or shorter circulatory arrest periods. However, RCP does provide ongoing regional cooling, lowering cerebral metabolic demands even further. Additionally, RCP may "flush" out the arterial system of both air and possibly particulate emboli. Proponents of RCP cite the avoidance of additional arterial manipulation to minimize both local arterial injury and propagation of emboli [25].

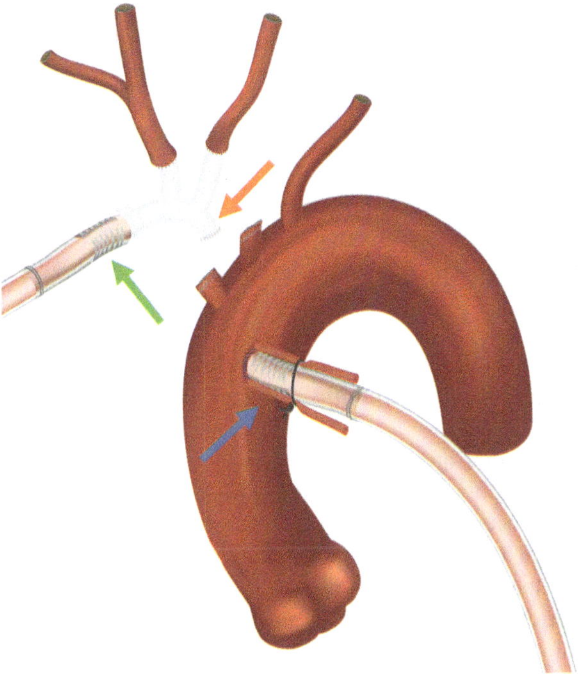

Fig. 4 In patients undergoing total arch replacement, the authors' preference is central aortic cannulation into the true lumen using the Seldinger technique and epiaortic ultrasound/transesophageal echo verification. During cooling, the innominate and left common carotid arteries are debranched from the aortic arch using a vascular stapler and sewn to a multibranch graft connected to a separate arterial line from the bypass circuit. In this way, unilateral cerebral perfusion is maintained during the relatively brief time it takes to sew the contralateral anastomosis, with bilateral cerebral perfusion maintained once both anastomoses are complete. This provides split upper and lower body perfusion prior to initiation of circulatory arrest

Antegrade Cerebral Perfusion

In order to precisely mimic natural cerebral blood flow during systemic circulatory arrest, antegrade perfusion must be established to all three arch vessels to supply both carotid arteries and both vertebral arteries. However, a number of ACP techniques with more limited antegrade access have been successfully described [26]. Most commonly, especially in the case of hemiarch replacement, is selective antegrade cerebral (sACP) perfusion via the innominate artery. Access for innominate sACP can be accomplished in a number of ways—percutaneous innominate cannulation (Fig. 4b), a graft conduit anastomosed end-to-side to the innominate, ostial balloon-tipped cannulation through an open arch (Fig. 4c), or axillary cannulation (Fig. 4d) with occlusion of the proximal innominate artery. The Circle of Willis is incomplete in up to 70% of the population (LF), however sufficient extracranial collaterals exist in the vast majority of patients allowing antegrade perfusion through the innominate artery to supply both cerebral hemispheres. Similar collaterals allow clamping of the innominate artery or the common carotid proximal to the bifurcation without regional malperfusion. However, a known incomplete Circle of Willis or significant ipsilateral carotid stenosis may represent relative contraindications to this technique. During innominate sACP, perfusate flow is established around 6–10 ml/kg/min and increased or decreased to maintain a mean arterial pressure of 40–60 mmHg as measured in a right upper extremity arterial line [3]. Bilateral ACP strategies require access to both the left common carotid as well as the innominate and are more typically employed during total arch replacement (Fig. 4e). Despite the intuitive sense that bilateral ACP would be more physiological than sACP, studies have failed to demonstrate superior neurological outcomes or decreased mortality with this technique [27].

Neuroprotection as a Function of Repair Technique and Perfusion Strategies: Buffalo Trunk Technique—Shaggy Aorta Protocol (RCP/ACP)

The technique for total arch replacement with frozen elephant practiced at the University of Colorado is a modification of the FET utilizing a separate branched graft for the brachiocephalic vessels and a branched graft–stent graft construct for arch and proximal descending aortic reconstruction. Longer durations of deep hypothermic circulatory arrest have been associated with worse postoperative neurologic dysfunction including stroke in patients undergoing arch replacement [28, 29]. The Buffalo Trunk technique [30] represents the authors efforts to minimize (ideally to eliminate) the period of cerebral, spinal, and systemic ischemia through operative and technical efficiency. Combined with optimizing cerebral perfusion by replacing dissected arch vessels, the Buffalo trunk procedure and other similar operations represent a method of neuroprotection as a function of the dissection repair strategy and technique.

In cases of dissection extending into the head vessels, our practice is to identify the extent of dissection and replaced the portion of the involved common carotid arteries up to the level of the internal and external bifurcation through an extended or separate cervical incision if necessary. The more severely affected side is typically debranched first in an end-to-end fashion to a separate trifurcated branched graft which is connected to a "Y'd" arterial limb of the cardiopulmonary bypass circuit. The contralateral side is subsequently debranched while perfusion is continued from the previously repaired side. A separate branched graft for the supraaortic vessels allows an independent connection to the cardiopulmonary bypass circuit and enables bilateral antegrade cerebral perfusion independent from body perfusion (Fig. 2). Central or peripheral cannulation is performed and CPB instituted prior to brachiocephalic debranching in order to begin the process of systemic cooling and creates some mild cerebral hypothermia during clamping of head vessels. A shunt during either carotid or innominate artery anastomosis is not typically needed due to contralateral perfusion through an intact circle of Willis and other arterial collaterals. Electroencephalography, cerebral oximetry by near-infrared spectroscopy, and other non-invasive neuromonitoring are used continuously to monitor for changes during a test occlusion of the head vessel and while proximally occluded for debranching. Early separation of the innominate and left common carotid arteries from the aorta in this technique may theoretically reduce the risk of anterior circulation emboli. However, with an anomalous left vertebral artery originating from the arch, the posterior circulation remains at risk, highlighting the importance of minimizing excessive aortic manipulation.

Patients are systemically cooled to moderate levels of hypothermia (20–28 °C) as the arch vessels are debranched. Following separation of the innominate and left common carotid from the aortic arch, a guidewire is advanced from the groin into the proximal transverse arch. Intravascular ultrasound is performed to identify the dissection anatomy and confirm true-lumen wire placement. Exchange for a stiff guidewire will serve as a rail for FET deployment into the true lumen. Transesophageal echo and fluoroscopy may be used as adjuncts to assess wire positioning, but do not supplant the need for IVUS to prevent a wire path that could traverse multiple fenestrations.

In acute aortic dissection, the authors will employ a "shaggy aorta" protocol for cerebral perfusion consisting of a 3-min period of RCP followed by subsequent ACP for the remaining duration of systemic circulatory arrest. The sequential combination of both cerebral perfusion adjuncts aims to optimize cerebral hypothermia, provide a short period of deairing and flushing of potential emboli, and sufficient oxygen and metabolite delivery. Arterial line management for both hemiarch and total arch operations utilizing the "shaggy aorta" protocol are shown in Fig. 5.

During systemic circulatory arrest, the aortic arch is transected and the Buffalo trunk graft-stent graft construct is advanced into the proximal descending thoracic aorta antegrade over the guidewire. The stent graft is released from the construct and further advanced until the proximal edge is flush with the cut edge of the divided aorta. An external felt strip, the aortic wall, the surgical graft, and the proximal end of the stent graft are incorporated in a single running external suture line comprising the distal anastomosis. Systemic circulation is recommenced though the perfusion limb of the aortic graft. The left subclavian artery and the separate branched graft to the innominate artery and LCCA are anastomosed to the aortic graft after completion of additional procedures to the aortic root and myocardial reperfusion. The completed arch replacement is shown in Fig. 6.

Pharmacological Neuroprotection

Various pharmacologic agents have been evaluated for their neuroprotective properties with regard to aortic surgery. These drugs act through a range of mechanisms which include the following categories: cardiovascular modulators, anti-inflammatories and immunomodulators, antioxidants, anti-apoptotic agents, drugs reducing neuronal excitotoxicity, drugs that reduce metabolic demand, and osmotic agents or diuretics to reduce tissue swelling. The literature on pharmacological neuroprotection is vast resulting in significant confusion as both agonists and inhibitors of certain receptors, or pathways, have demonstrated efficacy in different studies. For example, modulators of vascular tone can improve cerebral or spinal cord

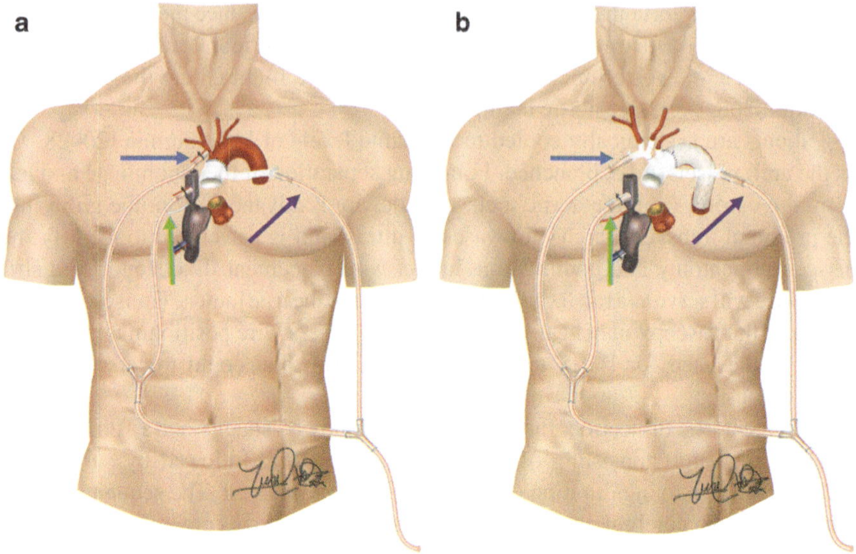

Fig. 5 Arterial line management for "Shaggy Aorta" protocol in hemiarch and total arch repair incorporating both the benefits of retrograde and antegrade cerebral pefusion. (**a**) For hemiarch replacement the ascending aorta is cannulated for institution of bypass. During cooling, the innominate artery is cannulated percutaneously, and the superior vena cava is cannulated with a right-angle cannula—each subsequently connected to an arterial line from the bypass circuit. At the start of hypothermic circulatory arrest, a 3-min period of retrograde cerebral perfusion is administered through the superior vena cava with maintenance of antegrade cerebral perfusion through the innominate artery for the remainder of circulatory arrest. After completion of the distal anastomosis, a side-arm on the hemiarch graft is used for reperfusion. (**b**) For total arch replacement the ascending aorta is cannulated for bypass. During cooling, innominate and left common carotid arteries are debranched and sewn to a multibranch graft as described in Figs. 3 and 4, and the superior vena cava is cannulated with a right-angle cannula—each subsequently connected to an arterial line from the bypass circuit. At the start of hypothermic circulatory arrest, a 3-min period of retrograde cerebral perfusion is administered through the superior vena cava with maintenance of bilateral antegrade cerebral perfusion through the branched graft sewn to the cranial vessels. After completion of the distal anastomosis, a side-arm on the arch graft is used for lower body reperfusion

perfusion by not only increasing the systemic arterial pressure, but also by decreasing vascular resistance through regional collaterals. Table 2 lists several agents that were favored in the past, are currently applied in the clinical setting, or have demonstrated neurological improvement in animal models of ischemia reperfusion injury [3, 31–41]. Although many agents have theoretical or anecdotal clinical potential, or have shown compelling results in animal models, a majority have not been validated by clinical trials.

In terms of cerebral pharmacological protection, modern practice has trended away from historically utilized agents proposed to decrease metabolic demand such as barbiturates or other coma-inducing agents. The contemporary goal has evolved

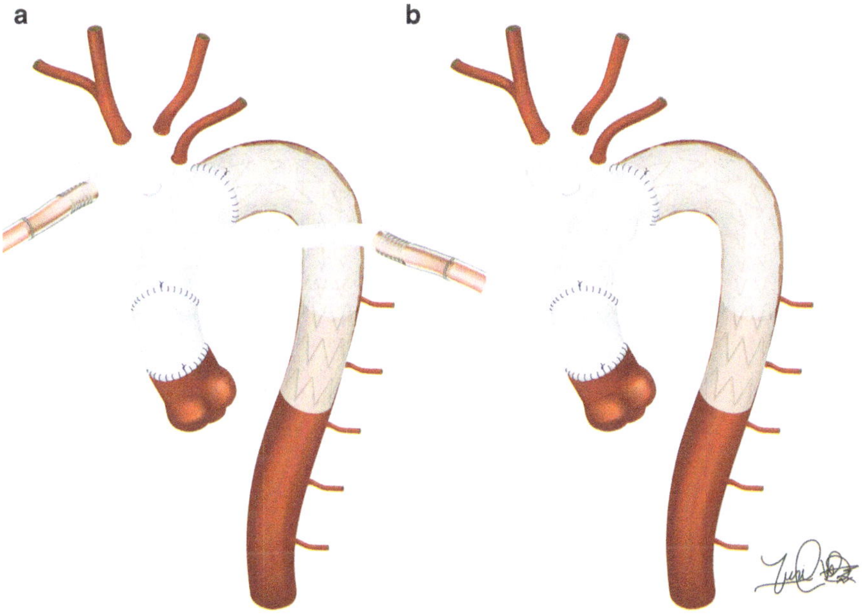

Fig. 6 Total arch replacement using a multibranch graft sewn to the innominate and left common carotid arteries and the Buffalo trunk technique for frozen elephant trunk deployment and distal anastomotic reconstruction. (**a**) Here the separate arterial lines connected to the multibranch graft and the arch graft perfusion side-arm respectively are shown. (**b**) Once the patient is weaned from bypass, the perfusion branches are ligated with a vascular stapler

toward expeditious emergence from anesthesia to obtain a reliable neurological exam. With the longer acting potent sedatives, patients could potentially take days to rouse sufficiently to be extubated. For spinal cord protection, while institutional practices may vary, the clinical standard of care for both prevention and treatment of spinal malperfusion remains vasopressor use to increase the driving mean arterial pressure to improve watershed perfusion [42]. But some institutions do rely on intrathecal papaverine to promote local vasodilatation with potential development of a longer-term collateral network.

Our institutional approach to pharmacological cerebral protection for circulatory arrest cases includes administration of methylprednisolone 500 mg upon induction, followed by lidocaine 100 mg and magnesium 2 g once the patient has reached the target nadir temperature before initiating circulatory arrest [3, 34]. As per the table, the steroid limits inflammation but also acts as a free radical scavenger, while the lidocaine and magnesium stabilize neuronal membrane potential and reduce metabolic demand. When temperature reduction alone does not sufficiently promote EEG silence, Propofol is bolused to reach EEG silence immediately prior to initiating HCA. The necessity of EEG silence to optimize metabolic reduction remains debated but it makes sense for cardiac surgeons who routinely use EKG activity as a marker of metabolic protection during cardiac arrest.

Table 2 Pharmacologic agents for neuroprotection

Drug category	Agent	Target effect	Evidence	Used clinically?
Cardiovascular modulators	Calcium channel blockers	Cerebral/ spinal	Theoretical	Yes
	Beta blockers	Cerebral/ spinal	Retrospective	Yes
	Vasopressors	Cerebral/ spinal	Retrospective	Yes
	Papaverine	Spinal	Retrospective	Yes
Anti-inflammatory/ immunomodulatory	Steroids	Cerebral/ spinal	Retrospective	Yes
	Cyclosporine A	Cerebral/ spinal	Experimental	No
	Aprotonin	Cerebral/ spinal	Retrospective	Yes
	Parecoxib	Cerebral/ spinal	Experimental	No
	Resveratrol	Cerebral/ spinal	Experimental	No
	Adenosine	Cerebral/ spinal	Experimental	No
Antioxidant	Superoxide dismutase	Cerebral/ spinal	Experimental	No
	Deferoxamine	Cerebral/ spinal	Experimental	No
	Allopurinol	Cerebral/ spinal	Experimental	No
	Naloxone	Cerebral/ spinal	Experimental	No
	Ulinastatin	Cerebral/ spinal	Experimental	No
Anti-apoptotic	Erythropoietin	Cerebral/ spinal	Experimental	No
	Acadesine	Cerebral/ spinal	Theoretical	Yes
	Gabapentin	Cerebral/ spinal	Experimental	Yes
	Minocycline	Cerebral/ spinal	Experimental	No
	Nitric oxide	Cerebral/ spinal	Theoretical	No
	Penehyclidine	Cerebral/ spinal	Experimental	No

(continued)

Table 2 (continued)

Drug category	Agent	Target effect	Evidence	Used clinically?
Anti-excitotoxic	Magnesium	Cerebral/ spinal	Retrospective	Yes
	Lidocaine	Cerebral/ spinal	Retrospective	Yes
	Ketamine	Cerebral/ spinal	Experimental	Yes
	Remacemide	Cerebral/ spinal	Retrospective	Yes
	Alpha 2-adrenergic agonists (Dexmedetomidine)	Cerebral/ spinal	Experimental	Yes
	Riluzole	Cerebral/ spinal	Experimental	No
	Fructose-1,6-bisphosphonate	Cerebral/ spinal	Experimental	No
Preconditioning	Anesthetic gases (Isofluorane, Sevofluorane)	Cerebral/ spinal	Experimental	Yes
	Diazoxide	Cerebral/ spinal	Experimental	No
Anti-metabolic	Barbiturates	Cerebral/ spinal	Retrospective	Yes
	Phenytoin	Cerebral/ spinal	Theoretical	Yes
	Narcotics	Cerebral/ spinal	Theoretical	Yes
	Propofol	Cerebral/ spinal	Theoretical	Yes
	Midazolam	Cerebral/ spinal	Theoretical	Yes
Anti-hyperglycemic	Insulin	Cerebral/ spinal	Theoretical	Yes
Diuretic	Mannitol	Cerebral/ spinal	Retrospective	Yes
	Furosemide	Cerebral/ spinal	Experimental	Yes

Coagulopathy Management

As hypotension and anemia significantly increase the risk of neurological injury, appropriate management of bleeding from complex aortic intervention remains paramount. Unfortunately, hemostasis can be a formidable challenge in the operating room, especially with redo operations, emergencies, and in the setting of the wide array of potent, irreversible anticoagulants. Potential large volume blood loss, hypothermia, fluid shifts, dilution from crystalloid and colloid infusions, cardiopulmonary bypass, and hypothermia all contribute to aberrations in the coagulation system. These abnormalities include consumption and dilution of coagulation factors and fibrinogen, consumption and malfunction of platelets, and hyperfibrinolysis [34]. Hematological and coagulation lab parameters monitored throughout the case are hemoglobin, platelets, INR, PTT, fibrinogen, and thromboelastometry (TEM) or thromboelastography (TEG) [43–46]. Particularly at the termination of cardiopulmonary bypass, once protamine [44–47] is administered for heparin reversal, aggressive correction of coagulopathy is undertaken. At our institution, all patients receive tranexamic or aminocaproic acid for hyperfibrinolysis [45]. Patients receive packed red blood cells for hemoglobin <7, platelets for thrombocytopenia <100, and fresh frozen plasma for INR >1.6 [45]. While there is a desire to limit coagulation resuscitation only response to abnormal lab results, this is not possible in many aortic cases, which require preemptive correction of blood and coagulation deficits. For coagulation factor replacement, in addition to fresh frozen plasma, prothrombin complex concentrate and recombinant factor 7a can be administered, though these may increase the risk of thrombosis [44]. Fibrinogen can be replaced with fresh frozen plasma, cryoprecipitate, or fibrinogen concentrate [34].

If patients continue with diffuse, nonsurgical bleeding despite appropriate resuscitation, our institutional preference is to temporarily close the chest with a vacuum device and complete their resuscitation in the cardiothoracic intensive care unit rather than prolonging their time with an open chest in the operating room. The field is usually packed with sponges—white sponges are placed over the heart, and the black vaccum sponge and dressing over the top. Vacuum at 125 mmHg is applied and adjusted if the RV appears affected by the pressure. Once the patient has been adequately resuscitated in the intensive care unit, they are returned to the operating room in 12–24 h for formal closure or washout. Opponents of delayed sternal closure argue that the technique increases the risk of infectious complications, however, in our experience, patients temporarily left open after complex aortic operations have not developed any mediastinal or sternal infections. The safety of this technique has also been demonstrated in large retrospective series [48].

Postoperative Care

In the immediate postoperative period after aortic dissection repair, patients should be monitored in the intensive care unit. Ongoing coagulopathy should be corrected, normal hemoglobin maintained, and high-normal oxygen saturation targeted. Appropriate volume resuscitation, preservation of adequate cardiac output with ionotropic support if needed, and use of vasopressors to achieve target blood pressure are additional management factors in maintaining hemodynamic stability to prevent secondary neurological injury from inadequate perfusion. We target a systolic blood pressure of 110–140 in all patients post-dissection repair. If patients are at high risk for spinal malperfusion due to their dissection anatomy or from the extent of thoracic aortic coverage, a mean arterial pressure of 80–100 is targeted [42].

Hourly neurologic exams should be performed postoperatively. If a patient demonstrates new stroke symptoms in the immediate postoperative period, we obtain contrasted brain imaging as soon as the patient's hemodynamic condition allows to identify embolic sources of stroke that may be amenable to catheter-based interventions. Concerns for spinal cord injury should prompt lumbar drain placement if not done preoperatively, more aggressive cerebrospinal fluid drainage as allowed by protocol, increased blood pressure goals (MAP 90–100) [49], and consideration of spinal imaging studies. Imaging studies are not helpful in the early diagnosis of spinal cord injury from malperfusion, but can demonstrate complications of lumbar drain placement. A bloody tap on insertion or unilateral symptoms should raise suspicion for possible epidural hematoma, rather than the bilateral motor symptoms seen with ischemic spinal cord injury.

Conclusion

Neurological optimization in acute aortic syndrome can be as complex as the anatomic derangements at presentation. Further, the anatomic derangements can evolve requiring attention to changes in both the neuromonitoring and the laboratory markers of tissue ischemia. While this requires incredible attention to detail, the reduction of neurological complications may be the most important factor in improving patient outcomes.

References

1. Erbel R, Aboyans V, Boileau C, et al. 2014 ESC guidelines on the diagnosis and treatment of aortic diseases. Eur Heart J. 2014;35(41):2873–926. https://doi.org/10.1093/eurheartj/ehu281.
2. Trivedi D, Navid F, Balzer JR, et al. Aggressive aortic arch and carotid replacement strategy for type a aortic dissection improves neurologic outcomes presented at the fifty-first annual meeting of the society of thoracic surgeons, San Diego, CA, Jan 24-28, 2015. Ann Thorac Surg. 2016;101(3):896–905. https://doi.org/10.1016/j.athoracsur.2015.08.073.
3. Bergeron EJ, Mosca MS, Aftab M, Justison G, Reece TB. Neuroprotection strategies in aortic surgery. Cardiol Clin. 2017;35(3):453–65. https://doi.org/10.1016/j.ccl.2017.03.011.
4. Reece TB, Tribble CG, Smith RL, et al. Central cannulation is safe in acute aortic dissection repair. J Thorac Cardiovasc Surg. 2007;133(2):428–34. https://doi.org/10.1016/j.jtcvs.2006.09.059.
5. Ghincea CV, Anderson DA, Ikeno Y, et al. Utility of neuromonitoring in hypothermic circulatory arrest cases for early detection of stroke: listening through the noise. J Thorac Cardiovasc Surg. 2020; https://doi.org/10.1016/j.jtcvs.2020.01.090.
6. Stecker MM, Cheung AT, Pochettino A, et al. Deep hypothermic circulatory arrest: I. Effects of cooling on electroencephalogram and evoked potentials. Ann Thorac Surg. 2001;71(1):14–21. https://doi.org/10.1016/S0003-4975(00)01592-7.

7. Stecker MM, Cheung AT, Pochettino A, et al. Deep hypothermic circulatory arrest: II. Changes in electroencephalogram and evoked potentials during rewarming. Ann Thorac Surg. 2001;71(1):22–8. https://doi.org/10.1016/S0003-4975(00)02021-X.
8. Coselli JS, Crawford ES, Beall AC, Mizrahi EM, Hess KR, Patel VM. Determination of brain temperatures for safe circulatory arrest during cardiovascular operation. Ann Thorac Surg. 1988;45(6):638–42. https://doi.org/10.1016/S0003-4975(10)64766-2.
9. Murkin JM. NIRS: a standard of care for CPB vs. an evolving standard for selective cerebral perfusion? J Extra Corpor Technol. 2009;41(1):12–5.
10. Olsson C, Thelin S. Regional cerebral saturation monitoring with near-infrared spectroscopy during selective antegrade cerebral perfusion: diagnostic performance and relationship to postoperative stroke. J Thorac Cardiovasc Surg. 2006;131(2):6–8. https://doi.org/10.1016/j.jtcvs.2005.08.068.
11. Urbanski PP, Lenos A, Kolowca M, et al. Near-infrared spectroscopy for neuromonitoring of unilateral cerebral perfusion. Eur J Cardiothorac Surg. 2013;43(6):1140–4. https://doi.org/10.1093/ejcts/ezs557.
12. Leyvi G, Bello R, Wasnick JD, Plestis K. Assessment of cerebral oxygen balance during deep hypothermic circulatory arrest by continuous jugular bulb venous saturation and near-infrared spectroscopy. J Cardiothorac Vasc Anesth. 2006;20(6):826–33. https://doi.org/10.1053/j.jvca.2006.01.001.
13. Wong KC. Physiology and pharmacology of hypothermia. West J Med. 1983;138(2):227–32.
14. Michenfelder JD, Milde JH. The relationship among canine brain temperature, metabolism, and function during hypothermia. Anesthesiology. 1991;75(1):130–6. https://doi.org/10.1097/00000542-199107000-00021.
15. Yan TD, Bannon PG, Bavaria J, et al. Consensus on hypothermia clasisfication. Ann Cardiothorac Surg. 2013;2(2):163–8. https://doi.org/10.3978/j.issn.2225-319X.2013.03.03.
16. Foley LS, Yamanaka K, Reece TB. Arterial cannulation and cerebral perfusion strategies for aortic arch operations. Semin Cardiothorac Vasc Anesth. 2016;20(4):298–302. https://doi.org/10.1177/1089253216672850.
17. Bavaria JE, Pochettino A, Brinster DR, et al. New paradigms and improved results for the surgical treatment of acute type A dissection. Ann Surg. 2001;234(3):336–43. https://doi.org/10.1097/00000658-200109000-00007.
18. Svensson LG, Crawford ES, Hess KR, et al. Deep hypothermia with circulatory arrest: determinants of stroke and early mortality in 656 patients. J Thorac Cardiovasc Surg. 1993;106(1):19–31. https://doi.org/10.1016/S0022-5223(19)33737-7.
19. Lima B, Williams JB, Bhattacharya SD, et al. Results of proximal arch replacement using deep hypothermia for circulatory arrest: is moderate hypothermia really justifiable? Am Surg. 2011;77(11):1438–44.
20. Gega A, Rizzo JA, Johnson MH, Tranquilli M, Farkas EA, Elefteriades JA. Straight deep hypothermic arrest: experience in 394 patients supports its effectiveness as a sole means of brain preservation. Ann Thorac Surg. 2007;84(3):759–67. https://doi.org/10.1016/j.athoracsur.2007.04.107.
21. Kamiya H, Hagl C, Kropivnitskaya I, et al. The safety of moderate hypothermic lower body circulatory arrest with selective cerebral perfusion: a propensity score analysis. J Thorac Cardiovasc Surg. 2007;133(2) https://doi.org/10.1016/j.jtcvs.2006.09.045.
22. Kazui T, Bashar AHM. The safety of moderate hypothermic circulatory arrest with selective cerebral perfusion. J Thorac Cardiovasc Surg. 2008;135(3):715. https://doi.org/10.1016/j.jtcvs.2007.03.070.
23. Leshnower BG, Thourani VH, Halkos ME, et al. Moderate versus deep hypothermia with unilateral selective antegrade cerebral perfusion for acute type A dissection. Ann Thorac Surg. 2015;100(5):1563–9. https://doi.org/10.1016/j.athoracsur.2015.05.032.
24. Bavaria JE, Pochettino A. Retrograde cerebral perfusion (RCP) in aortic arch surgery: efficacy and possible mechanisms of brain protection. Semin Thorac Cardiovasc Surg. 1997;9(3):222–32.

25. Appoo JJ, Augoustides JG, Pochettino A, et al. Perioperative outcome in adults undergoing elective deep hypothermic circulatory arrest with retrograde cerebral perfusion in proximal aortic arch repair: evaluation of protocol-based care. J Cardiothorac Vasc Anesth. 2006;20(1):3–7. https://doi.org/10.1053/j.jvca.2005.08.005.
26. Milewski RK, Pacini D, Moser GW, et al. Retrograde and antegrade cerebral perfusion: results in short elective arch reconstructive times. Ann Thorac Surg. 2010; https://doi.org/10.1016/j.athoracsur.2010.01.056.
27. Angeloni E, Benedetto U, Takkenberg JJM, et al. Unilateral versus bilateral antegrade cerebral protection during circulatory arrest in aortic surgery: a meta-analysis of 5100 patients. J Thorac Cardiovasc Surg. 2014;147(1):60–7. https://doi.org/10.1016/j.jtcvs.2012.10.029.
28. Reich DL, Kahn RA, Konstadt SN, et al. Neuropsychologic outcome after deep hypothermic circulatory arrest in adults. J Thorac Cardiovasc Surg. 1999;117(1):156–63.
29. Di Eusanio M, Wesselink RMJ, Morshuis WJ, Dossche KM, Schepens MAAM. Deep hypothermic circulatory arrest and antegrade selective cerebral perfusion during ascending aorta-hemiarch replacement: a retrospective comparative study. J Thorac Cardiovasc Surg. 2003;125(4):849–54. https://doi.org/10.1067/mtc.2003.8.
30. Eldeiry M, Aftab M, Bergeron E, et al. The buffalo trunk technique for aortic arch reconstruction. Ann Thorac Surg. 2019;108(3):680–6. https://doi.org/10.1016/j.athoracsur.2019.03.034.
31. De Haan P, Kalkman CJ, Jacobs MJHM. Pharmacologic neuroprotection in experimental spinal cord ischemia: a systematic review. J Neurosurg Anesthesiol. 2001;13(1):3–12. https://doi.org/10.1097/00008506-200101000-00002.
32. Tanaka A, Safi HJ, Estrera AL. Current strategies of spinal cord protection during thoracoabdominal aortic surgery. Gen Thorac Cardiovasc Surg. 2018;66(6):307–14. https://doi.org/10.1007/s11748-018-0906-1.
33. Kaplan S, Bisleri G, Morgan JA, Cheema FH, Oz MC. Resveratrol, a natural red wine polyphenol, reduces ischemia-reperfusion-induced spinal cord injury. Ann Thorac Surg. 2005;80(6):2242–9. https://doi.org/10.1016/j.athoracsur.2005.05.016.
34. Wilkey BJ, Weitzel NS. Anesthetic considerations for surgery on the aortic arch. Semin Cardiothorac Vasc Anesth. 2016;20(4):265–72. https://doi.org/10.1177/1089253216672853.
35. Krüger T, Hoffmann I, Blettner M, Borger MA, Schlensak C, Weigang E. Intraoperative neuroprotective drugs without beneficial effects? Results of the German registry for acute aortic dissection type a (GERAADA). Eur J Cardiothorac Surg. 2013;44(5):939–46. https://doi.org/10.1093/ejcts/ezt182.
36. Svyatets M, Tolani K, Zhang M, Tulman G, Charchaflieh J. Perioperative management of deep hypothermic circulatory arrest. J Cardiothorac Vasc Anesth. 2010;24(4):644–55. https://doi.org/10.1053/j.jvca.2010.02.010.
37. Van Der Starre PJA. Deep hypothermia and circulatory arrest. Thorac Aortic Dis. 2006;2006:101–8. https://doi.org/10.1007/3-540-38309-3_8.
38. Al-Hashimi S, Zaman M, Waterworth P, Bilal H. Does the use of thiopental provide added cerebral protection during deep hypothermic circulatory arrest? Interact Cardiovasc Thorac Surg. 2013;17(2):392–7. https://doi.org/10.1093/icvts/ivt184.
39. Salameh A, Dhein S, Dähnert I, Klein N. Neuroprotective strategies during cardiac surgery with cardiopulmonary bypass. Int J Mol Sci. 2016;17(11) https://doi.org/10.3390/ijms17111945.
40. Reece TB, Kern JA, Tribble CG, Cassada DC. The role of pharmacology in spinal cord protection during thoracic aortic reconstruction. Semin Thorac Cardiovasc Surg. 2003;15(4):365–77. https://doi.org/10.1053/S1043-0679(03)00088-1.
41. Scott JW. Spinal cord protection during thoracoabdominal aortic intervention: now and in the future-it's not all about hypothermia. J Cardiothorac Vasc Anesth. 2016;30(2):275–9. https://doi.org/10.1053/j.jvca.2016.01.006.
42. Lindsay H, Srinivas C, Djaiani G. Neuroprotection during aortic surgery. Best Pract Res Clin Anaesthesiol. 2016;30(3):283–303. https://doi.org/10.1016/j.bpa.2016.05.002.
43. Zaky A. Thromboelastometry versus rotational thromboelastography in cardiac surgery. Semin Cardiothorac Vasc Anesth. 2017;21(3):206–11. https://doi.org/10.1177/1089253217697146.

44. Sniecinski RM, Levy JH. Bleeding and management of coagulopathy. J Thorac Cardiovasc Surg. 2011;142(3):662–7. https://doi.org/10.1016/j.jtcvs.2011.03.015.
45. Ghadimi K, Levy JH, Welsby IJ. Perioperative management of the bleeding patient. Br J Anaesth. 2016;117:iii18–30. https://doi.org/10.1093/bja/aew358.
46. Meesters MI, von Heymann C. Optimizing perioperative blood and coagulation management during cardiac surgery. Anesthesiol Clin. 2019;37(4):713–28. https://doi.org/10.1016/j.anclin.2019.08.006.
47. Weber CF, Klages M, Zacharowski K. Perioperative coagulation management during cardiac surgery. Curr Opin Anaesthesiol. 2013;26(1):60–4. https://doi.org/10.1097/ACO.0b013e32835afd28.
48. Bakaeen FG, Haddad O, Ibrahim M, et al. Advances in managing the noninfected open chest after cardiac surgery: negative-pressure wound therapy. J Thorac Cardiovasc Surg. 2019;157(5):1891–1903.e9. https://doi.org/10.1016/j.jtcvs.2018.10.152.
49. Parotto M, Ouzounian M, Djaiani G. Spinal cord protection in elective thoracoabdominal aortic procedures. J Cardiothorac Vasc Anesth. 2019;33(1):200–8. https://doi.org/10.1053/j.jvca.2018.05.044.

Acute Type A Aortic Dissection: When Not to Operate

Ashraf A. Sabe, Ryan P. Plichta, and G. Chad Hughes

Introduction

Acute type A aortic dissection (ATAAD) is a surgical emergency. If left untreated, the mortality rate increases by 1–2% per hour after initial onset of symptoms, with up to a 90% 30-day mortality in the absence of surgical intervention [1–3]. In patients successfully treated with surgery, late survival rates are as high as 90% at 1 and 3 years. Rapid diagnosis and early surgical treatment after initial risk assessment is the standard of care for these patients. However, despite emphasis on early diagnosis and intervention, advancements in surgical technique, and refined perioperative care, surgery for ATAAD still carries an operative mortality of 10–30% in multiple series [4–7]. The International Registry of Aortic Dissection (IRAD) reports an overall surgical mortality of 25% in ATAAD, despite representing larger tertiary centers with expertise in aortic disease [6]. Recent data from the Society of Thoracic Surgeons Adult Cardiac Surgery Database (STS-ACSD) examining outcomes for ATAAD repair in North America from 2004 to 2016 in >25,000 patients, which is the largest report of ATAAD repairs to date [8], found no meaningful improvement in 30-day/in-hospital mortality over the time interval of the study (19% in 2004 to 18% in 2016) [9] (Fig. 1). This lack of improvement in outcomes

A. A. Sabe
Division of Cardiac Surgery, Brigham and Women's Hospital, Harvard Medical School, Boston, MA, USA

R. P. Plichta
Division of Cardiovascular and Thoracic Surgery, Duke University Medical Center, Durham, NC, USA

G. C. Hughes (✉)
Center for Aortic Disease, Division of Cardiovascular and Thoracic Surgery, Duke University Medical Center, Durham, NC, USA
e-mail: gchad.hughes@duke.edu

J. S. Coselli et al. (eds.), *Aortic Dissection and Acute Aortic Syndromes*,
https://doi.org/10.1007/978-3-030-66668-2_36

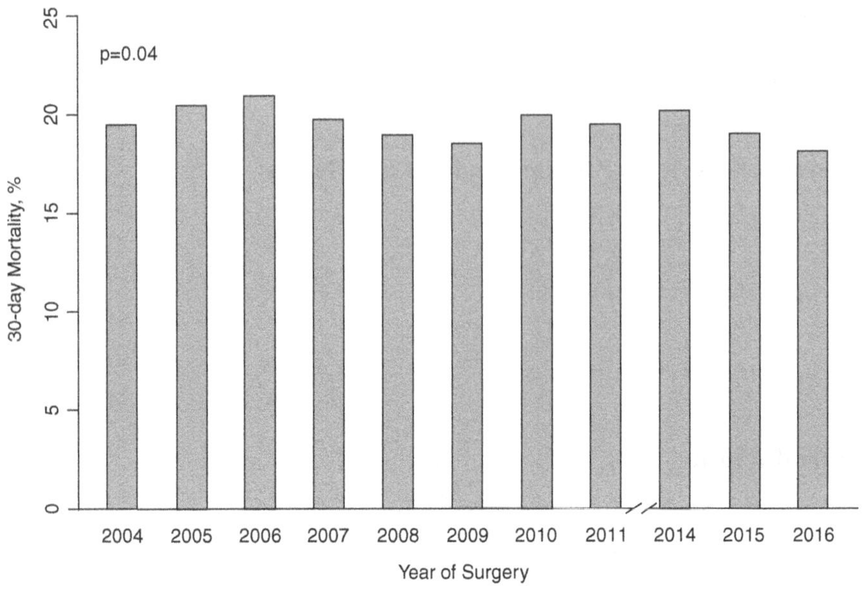

Fig. 1 Data from the Society of Thoracic Surgeons Adult Cardiac Surgery Database examining outcomes for ATAAD repair in North America demonstrates no meaningful improvement in 30-day mortality over time [8]

over time has prompted increasing investigation into identification of risks of mortality in ATAAD with and without repair.

Studies from IRAD have identified independent predictors of in-hospital mortality after ATAAD. These include advanced age (≥70), coma and/or cerebrovascular accident, hypotension/shock at presentation, prior aortic valve surgery, preoperative left or right ventricular dysfunction, and cardiac tamponade [10, 11]. Evidence of malperfusion syndromes, whether neurovascular, myocardial, mesenteric or limb ischemia, have all been associated with increased mortality in patients after ATAAD repair [11, 12]. Several groups have attempted to risk stratify patients with ATAAD to determine whether surgery would be overwhelmingly futile, or whether delaying surgery for other intervention may improve outcomes [7, 11, 13–15]. In this chapter, we review contemporary approaches to risk stratification of ATAAD patients with a focus on when to delay or defer central aortic repair (Table 1).

Patient Age, Functional Status and Co-morbid Conditions

With an aging population, several studies have investigated the increased risk of cardiac surgery in elderly patients [1, 16, 17]. Many of these patients have significant functional limitations and co-morbid conditions. In the acute setting, like with ATAAD, full assessment of frailty may be quite limited. Though age has been

Table 1 Considerations for potential delay or deferment of emergent type A aortic dissection repair

Advanced Age
Functional Status including Frailty and Dementia
Co-morbid Conditions
Patient Directed Goals of Care
Visceral and Extremity Malperfusion and Malperfusion syndromes
Cerebral Malperfusion and Major Brain Injury
Prior Cardiac Surgery and Redo Sternotomy
Direct Oral Anticoagulants
Patients Refusing Blood Products
Type A Intramural Hematoma (IMH)

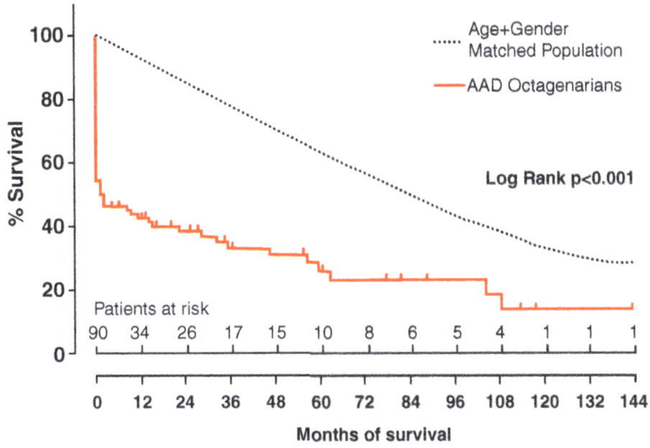

Fig. 2 Actuarial survival of octogenarians suffering from ATAAD compared with age and gender matched population [22]

shown to increase the risk of aortic surgery, there is no convincing evidence that an age-based cutoff should be used for ATAAD repair. Many relatively healthy octogenarians and nonagenarians have been reported to do very well after ATAAD repair [18, 19]. However, frailty and non-elective cardiac surgery have been demonstrated to be independent predictors of risk in proximal aortic surgery [20, 21].

Elderly patients frequently have comorbid conditions that increase their risk of elective surgery and, in the emergent setting, may make their surgical risk prohibitive. Octogenarians, in particular, carry a high morbidity and mortality rate when undergoing surgical treatment of ATAAD [22] (Fig. 2). It is especially important to evaluate the overall functional status and comorbid conditions of these patients when making the decision whether to operate. Several comorbid conditions including prior cerebrovascular disease, cardiac disease, and severe chronic lung disease have been shown to be independent predictors for 30-day mortality after ATAAD repair [8, 23]. An elderly patient on hemodialysis, or who is wheelchair bound, or who suffers from dementia, or who is living in a skilled nursing facility, poses a significant mortality risk in the setting of surgery for ATAAD. It is very reasonable to medically manage selected geriatric patients as the overall long term survival between surgery and medical management does not differ [22] (Fig. 3). Whether or not surgery is undertaken in this high-risk population, the patient and their family

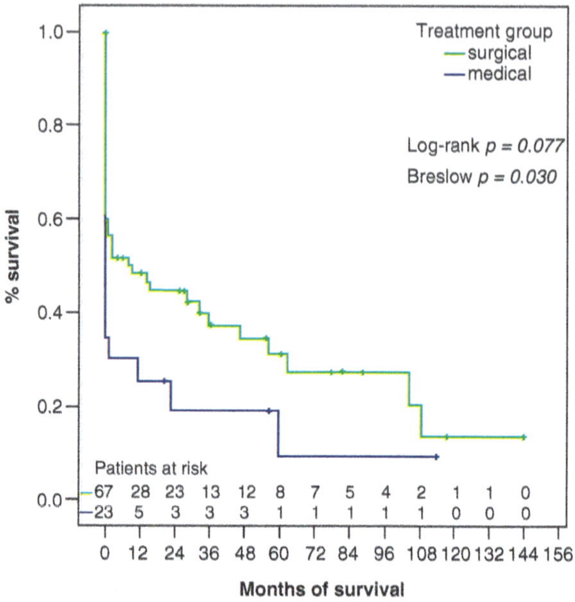

Fig. 3 Overall survival of octogenarians suffering from ATAAD undergoing surgical or medical management [22]

should be clearly counseled on "best-case" and "worst-case" scenarios. In a VA study evaluating 95,204 patients who underwent high risk surgery, only 770 (0.8%) received a palliative care consultation before surgery. Of all the patients who died within 90 days, 29.9% had received a palliative care consultation, with 5.6% having received consultation before surgery. Families of the decedents reported an overall significant increased satisfaction with end-of-life care, communication and support [24]. While challenging in the acute care setting, goals of care should always be carefully considered, particularly in geriatric patients.

Malperfusion and Malperfusion Syndromes

Malperfusion is commonly seen in ATAAD, occurring in 16–33% of patients [1]. Although one of the goals of proximal aortic replacement in the setting of ATAAD is to restore perfusion to the true lumen, success is variable as distal re-entry tears in the arch or thoracoabdominal aorta may result in persistent dynamic or static malperfusion despite resection of the proximal entry primary tear. Though the mechanisms and locations are variable, clinically apparent malperfusion of any kind is associated with a higher mortality rate. Mesenteric malperfusion syndrome in the setting of acute aortic dissection is particularly lethal and has a reported mortality rate of 60% or higher in multiple series. Even with early intervention, the mortality rate in these patients is still up to 42% [25]. In a retrospective review, Lawton et al. demonstrated that patients with malperfusion and severe acidosis (base deficit ≥10) had an operative mortality of 92%. There were no survivors when this acidosis was secondary to abdominal organ malperfusion [13].

Many groups have adopted treatment algorithms which delay operative repair of the proximal aorta in the setting of malperfusion with end-organ dysfunction [7, 13, 26]. Clearly defining and differentiating malperfusion alone from a "malperfusion syndrome" (MPS) is critical in optimizing treatment. Malperfusion is defined as "*inadequate blood flow to the end organs because of dissection related obstruction of the aorta and its branches*" whereas MPS is defined as "*tissue necrosis and failure of vital organs (such as viscera or lower extremity) secondary to late-stage malperfusion*" [26, 27]. As such, the diagnosis of MPS requires both clinical features (e.g., abdominal pain, tenderness, oliguria or anuria, extremity motor or sensory neurovascular deficits, focal neurologic deficits) and laboratory features (e.g., elevated lactate, serum creatinine, liver or pancreatic enzymes, creatinine kinase) [27] indicative of end-organ ischemia.

In 1997, Deeb et al. at the University of Michigan described their novel and highly controversial (at the time) strategy of operative delay for patients with MPS from ATAAD. This landmark study compared an historic cohort managed with immediate proximal aortic repair with a cohort managed with initial selective percutaneous intervention, primarily transcatheter fenestration of the dissection membrane to restore true lumen perfusion with or without branch vessel stenting, for MPS followed by delayed operative repair after resolution of malperfusion injury. The historic cohort managed with initial central aortic repair had an in-hospital mortality rate of 89% compared to a mortality rate of 25% for the group managed with delayed repair after restoring end-organ perfusion ($P = 0.003$). These results helped inform their group and others to adopt a consistent strategy, referred to as the "complication-specific approach", of correcting "significant end-organ malperfusion" prior to definitive surgical repair of ATAAD. Using this prospectively applied protocol over the next decade, Deeb et al demonstrated a 95% success rate in reperfusing malperfused vascular beds percutaneously [28]. Addressing significant MPS in a staged fashion, with a TEVAR first strategy to re-expand a compressed distal true lumen followed by delayed type A repair, has been successful in select patients and likely is superior to fenestration-based strategies for restoring true lumen flow [29, 30].

Over the years, this complication-specific approach has been refined and the University of Michigan group, along with others, have developed an algorithm for endovascular revascularization followed by delayed open repair in patients with MPS and no aortic rupture or cardiac tamponade (Fig. 4). A more recent study from the Michigan group evaluated outcomes over two decades using the aforementioned algorithm of endovascular reperfusion with delayed open repair compared with expected outcomes of an "upfront OR for every patient approach" using prognostic models from the literature [27]. In patients with MPS initially treated with fenestration/stenting, mortality from aortic rupture decreased from the first to second decades from 16 to 4% ($P = 0.05$). Notably, the risk of dying from organ failure was 6.6 times higher than the risk of death from aortic rupture (hazard ratio = 6.63; 95% CI, 1.5–29; $P = 0.01$) [27].

MPS presents a particular challenge and carries a high risk of morbidity and mortality. We emphasize the importance of careful patient selection when determining operative intervention in ATAAD with associated MPS. It is critical to highlight the difference between a dissection resulting in malperfusion based on imaging

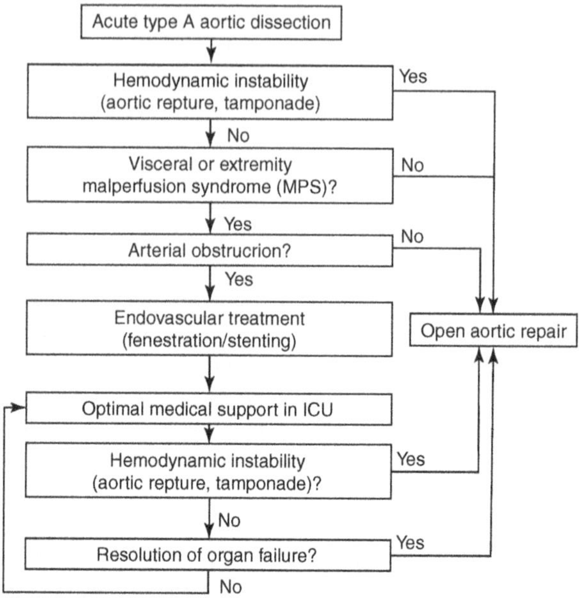

Fig. 4 Algorithm for clinical decision making in patients with ATAAD. MPS, malperfusion syndrome; ICU, intensive care unit [27]

findings alone (so-called "radiographic only" malperfusion), and MPS where there is additional clinical and laboratory evidence of end-organ ischemia [31]. Importantly, otherwise operative patients presenting with ATAAD and radiographic concern for malperfusion, but without clear evidence of resultant end-organ dysfunction, are still best treated with immediate repair of the ATAAD. In patients with true MPS who are otherwise operative candidates, we recommend delayed repair of the ATAAD after reversing clinically apparent mesenteric or limb MPS. These recommendations assume institutional capability to provide early endovascular reperfusion as necessary. Otherwise, in these high-risk patients with MPS and no evidence of tamponade, immediate transfer to another institution may be the best approach [32].

Cerebral Malperfusion

Cerebral malperfusion (CM) occurs in up to 15% of patients with ATAAD [33, 34] and poses a significant challenge in the emergent treatment of these patients. Hemorrhagic conversion of an ischemic insult while on cardiopulmonary bypass is of real concern and determining the appropriate patients for immediate surgery is a dilemma [35, 36]. Patients with CM have high rates of short-term mortality, reportedly as high as 50%, and very poor survival rates at 10 years [37]. Despite this, several studies have demonstrated that early intervention in patients with CM resulted in improved hospital mortality and significant neurologic recovery [14, 33, 38, 39]. An IRAD study evaluating 2402 patients who underwent surgery for ATAAD found 362 (15.1%) presented with CM. Patients with CM who underwent surgery for ATAAD had a higher incidence of postoperative cerebrovascular accident (17.5% vs. 7.2%, $P < 0.001$), higher incidence of acute kidney injury (28.3% vs 18.1%, $P < 0.001$), and higher in-hospital mortality than those without CM undergoing surgery (25.7% vs. 12%, $P < 0.001$) [34]. Although this study lacks data on long-term outcomes, the authors concluded that select patients with ATAAD and CM can undergo surgery with a hospital survival rate as high as 75% [34, 40]. An earlier observational study demonstrated select patients with CM and either CVA or coma who underwent surgery for ATAAD had 5-year mortality of 27% and 44%, respectively, as compared with a 76 and 100% mortality with medical management for either cohort. Moreover, 84% of patients with CVA and 79% of patients presenting with coma had reversal of brain injury after undergoing surgery [41] (Fig. 5). A more recent report combining data from three centers identified 1600 patients who underwent ATAAD repair, of which 150 had presented with a preoperative neurologic deficit. Of these patients, 62% had no to moderate postoperative neurologic deficits. Notably, patient age (odds ratio 1.041; $P = 0.02$) and history of prior stroke (odds ratio 2.651; $P = 0.03$) were predictive of poor clinical outcome, while presenting with coma was not. Hemorrhagic conversion occurred in only seven patients and no independent predictors were identified [42].

Similar to other cases of ATAAD, patients with ATAAD and CM who undergo surgery should be carefully selected by an experienced team based on age, frailty, comorbidities, tamponade, and extent of other malperfusion syndromes. In addition, patients with CM require special consideration with evaluation of extent and location of stroke, hemorrhagic conversion/risk for hemorrhagic conversion, symptom duration, and coma. Preoperative cerebral imaging can aid clinical prognostication, as demonstration of a large infarct or occluded internal carotid artery may predict a worse neurologic outcome [42, 43]. When experienced clinical evaluation otherwise portends a favorable prognosis in ATAAD with CM, early surgery may be performed with reasonable rates of survival and reversal of cerebral ischemia, including patients presenting with coma. Ultimately, this is an evolving realm and given recent data, including case reports describing potential advances in percutaneous intervention prior to surgery, cases should be considered a case-by-case basis [42, 44].

ATAAD in Patients with Prior Cardiac Surgery

Several studies have investigated operative risk for ATAAD repair after prior cardiac surgery [45–48]. A single center review from the University of Michigan of 545 patients who underwent ATAAD repair between July, 1996 and January, 2017 found no significant difference in 30-day major morbidity or mortality in the 50 patients who had previous cardiac surgery as compared to the other 495 patients [49]. A recent review of the STS-ACSD identified 1332 patients who underwent surgery for ATAAD, of whom 138 (10.4%) had a prior sternotomy. Patients who underwent redo-sternotomy for ATAAD repair had a significantly higher operative mortality (28% vs. 15%, $P < 0.01$) with a longer length of stay (13 vs. 10 days, $P < 0.02$) than

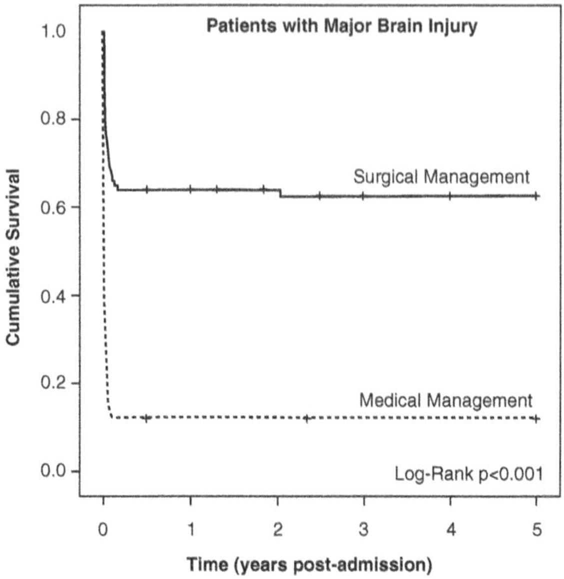

Survival Estimate	1-Year	2-Year	3-Year	4-Year	5-Year
Medical Management	12.2 ± 5.1%	12.2 ± 5.1%	12.2 ± 5.1%	12.2 ± 5.1%	12.2 ± 5.1%
Total Events	36	36	36	36	36
At Risk	4	4	3	3	2
Surgical Management	64.0 ± 4.8%	64.0 ± 4.8%	62.6 ± 4.9%	62.6 ± 4.9%	62.6 ± 4.9%
Total Events	36	36	37	37	37
At Risk	62	47	44	39	35

Fig. 5 Kaplan-Meier survival curves of patients with ATAAD presenting with major brain injury stratified by therapeutic management [41]

primary sternotomy patients. Although not reaching statistical significance, there was a trend towards decreased operative mortality for redo patients at high-volume centers (25.7% vs. 37.9%, $P = 0.19$). These studies suggest that patients with ATAAD and prior cardiac surgery should be carefully selected for operative repair, and perhaps centralized to higher volume centers [50].

Direct Oral Anticoagulants (DOACs)

Increased use of DOACs without a rapid, sustained reversal agent poses a particular challenge in patients with ATAAD [51]. There is a paucity of literature on patients with ATAAD on DOACs, and no consensus on how to manage these patients.

Antidotes for specific DOAC's have been approved in recent years. Idarucizumab is approved as a reversal agent for dabigitran, and andexenat alfa is approved as a reversal agent for rivaroxaban and apixaban. Idarucizumab, a monoclonal antibody fragment, has been given prior to heart transplant with good effect in a small case series [52]. Andexanet alfa acts as a factor Xa decoy, thus significantly reducing (but not eliminating) anticoagulant activity by binding and sequestering apixaban and rivaroxaban. Its use in the setting of emergent cardiac surgery, particularly with cardiopulmonary bypass, has been described in case reports but requires further investigation [53]. It is important to note that andexanet alfa reverses factor Xa inhibitor levels for ~2–3 h, after which levels return back to baseline [54, 55].

We recommend a multimodal approach in select patients requiring emergent surgery for ATAAD on DOACs. The patient's other risk factors for surgery and planned extent of operation (i.e. root versus supracoronary ascending replacement and hemi-versus total arch) should be carefully considered, as should other known risk factors for bleeding in proximal aortic repair (Table 2) [56]. Depending on institutional capability, initial options include delayed surgical repair until half-life clearance of the agent based on timing alone, global coagulation assay, thromboelastometry assays, or preferably direct measurements of anti-factor Xa levels. Post cardiopulmonary bypass options to treat coagulopathy include use of antifibrinolytics, standard blood products such as platelets, fresh frozen plasma, and cryoprecipitate, as well as recombinant hemostatic factors such as prothrombin complex concentrate [57], activated factor VIIa [58], human fibrinogen concentrate [59], and thoughtful administration of anti Xa antidotes as discussed earlier [60, 61].

Patients Refusing Blood Products

A patient's refusal to receive transfusion of blood and/or blood products may present a rare but difficult dilemma in patients with ATAAD. In particular, many members of the Jehovah's Witness community will not accept transfusion. Favorable outcomes have been demonstrated in studies of Jehovah's Witness patients undergoing elective cardiac surgery with appropriate preoperative planning [62, 63]. Unfortunately, the emergent nature of ATAAD, frequent need for circulatory arrest with systemic hypothermia, as well as near universal need for blood products presents a rare and difficult dilemma. For example, STS-ACSD data on 2982 patients undergoing surgical repair of ATAAD between 7/2011 and 9/2012 demonstrated a

Table 2 Predictors of massive transfusion in thoracic aortic procedures requiring hypothermic circulatory arrest (logistic regression model) [56]

Variable	Odds ratio	95% Wald confidence interval	Predictor *P* value
Preoperative hemoglobin (per 1-g/dL increment)	0.543	0.428–0.688	<0.0001
Cardiopulmonary bypass time (per 10-min increase)	1.15	1.05–1.26	0.0026
Emergency case status	4.02	1.532–10.553	0.0047

median blood product requirement of 5 units packed red blood cells, 4 units fresh frozen plasma, 1 unit of cryoprecipitate, and 3 units of platelets following surgical repair [64]. It is paramount, therefore, to have a clear, detailed discussion with the individual patient and/or their health care proxy. One must not assume that any individual will uniformly refuse transfusion of any blood products until properly counseled on the gravity of their refusal. Furthermore, treatment with purified proteins derived from plasma is acceptable to many patients [65]. Options which may be acceptable to patients include treatment with albumin, activated factor VIIa, factor eight inhibitor bypass activity (FEIBA), prothrombin complex concentrate, and human fibrinogen concentrate as detailed above [66]. Though minimal data exists regarding patients refusing blood transfusion with ATAAD, for select patients who do undergo surgery consideration should be given to limiting the scope of operation to the extent possible with avoidance of prolonged cardiopulmonary bypass times and deep cooling, strict attention to surgical hemostasis, liberal use of recombinant hemostatic factors to facilitate clotting, and vigilant postoperative blood pressure control with early return to the operating room for surgical control of bleeding [67].

Intramural Hematoma

Intramural hematoma (IMH) and acute aortic dissection present similarly and are often indistinguishable based on clinical findings alone. Differentiating the two requires contrasted and non-contrasted imaging of the aorta. IMH is relatively less common when compared with true aortic dissection with patent false lumen. An IRAD review of 1010 patients with acute aortic syndrome identified only 58 patients (5.7%) with IMH [68], although IMH appears to be more common in series from the Far East as compared to the West [69].

Given the lack of data, treatment strategies for acute Type A aortic IMH have been controversial. Traditionally, acute Type A aortic IMH was treated similarly to ATAAD, with early operative intervention. This is based on early experience in small patient populations demonstrating poor outcomes in patients with ascending aortic IMH [70]. More recently, larger studies have challenged this approach, and the treatment paradigm has evolved. Several centers have demonstrated success with medical management of select patients with acute ascending aortic IMH [71]. Though further studies are needed, based on current data, high risk patients with acute ascending IMH can be initially treated medically if hemodynamically stable, without refractory pain, with no evidence of tamponade or periaortic hematoma, and an aortic diameter < 5 cm [72]. A review of the IRAD database, although the patient numbers were small, demonstrated more favorable outcomes with medical management of IMH involving the aortic arch as compared with the more proximal ascending aorta [68]. High risk patients treated expectantly should undergo standard interval imaging and follow-up to evaluate for progression or resolution.

Alternative Management

It is important to underscore variable approaches to ATAAD repair. Clinical judgement is paramount in determining the extent of surgical repair. For instance, alternative strategies to cooling have been employed with excellent success. Patients in general may benefit from moderate hypothermia as opposed to deep hypothermic arrest. As discussed earlier, this may be particularly important in patients refusing transfusion of blood products, although data regarding the impact of the degree of hypothermia on bleeding outcomes has been mixed with several studies showing no difference in transfusion outcomes between deep and moderate hypothermia strategies [73]. Hemiarch replacement without circulatory arrest has also been described with favorable results [74], although larger studies are needed to evaluate the benefit of this method. Less aggressive surgical approaches, like an ascending aortic replacement instead of a hemiarch or partial/total arch replacement, have also been performed. However, a recent STS database study found patients who underwent ascending aortic replacement alone had a significantly higher 30-day mortality rate compared with those who underwent hemiarch replacement (19.1% vs. 16.3%, $P = 0.001$), but a lower 30-day mortality when compared with patients who had a total arch replacement (19.1% vs. 26.9%, $P < 0.001$) [8]. These subgroup analyses must be interpreted carefully as institutional and individual experience and surgical technique, including use of circulatory arrest and cannulation strategies, vary widely and may affect outcomes. Aortic dissection involving the arch branch vessels does not necessitate a zone 1/2/3 arch replacement, and a hemiarch alone is frequently sufficient [75]. Similarly, in dissections involving the aortic root, surgeons should use their judgement and experience prior to attempting a valve-sparing root surgery. Further, in a large proportion of patients with ATAAD, valve resuspension with neomedia sinus of Valsalva repair provides a durable long-term option [76]. Root replacement may be a better alternative compared with valve-sparing root surgery, particularly in patients who may not tolerate a prolonged cross clamp time and potential need to re-arrest the heart in the event of failure of a valve-preserving approach.

As discussed, clinical determination of patient operability is multifactorial. In patients who are at extreme or prohibitive risk for surgery, investigational and off-label use of thoracic endovascular aortic repair (TEVAR) in the ascending aorta has been applied. Despite being a higher risk patient population, small studies have demonstrated promising results in select patients [77, 78]. Studies have demonstrated good technical success, early mortality rates below 15%, and relatively low aorta-related mortality rates in the long term [79–81]. Finally, recent data from the IRAD database demonstrates that definitive medical management may be a reasonable option in certain high-risk patients, with 30-day survival rates of nearly 40% with medical management alone [69]. Predictors of success with medical management in ATAAD included prior cardiac surgery and most proximal dissection extent limited to the ascending aorta without root involvement, among several others (Fig. 6) [69].

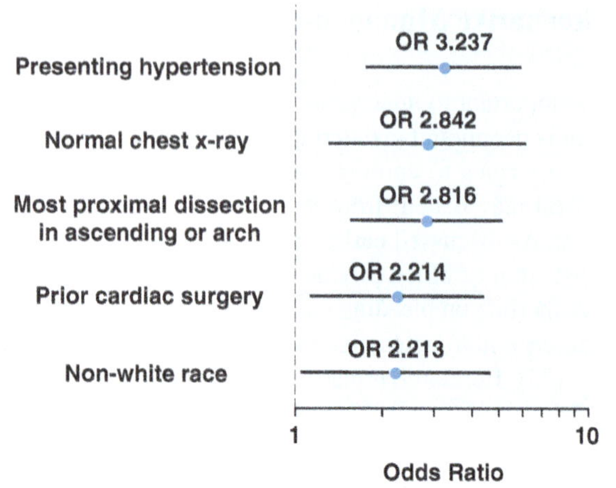

The figure depicts odds ratios (ORs) for survival with 95% confidence intervals for the OR.

Fig. 6 Variables associated with in-hospital survival after medical management of type A acute aortic dissection [69]

Conclusion

Despite advances in diagnostic imaging and surgical technique, the early morbidity and mortality after ATAAD remains high. Optimizing surgical outcomes requires thoughtful patient selection informed by predicted survival postoperatively, as well as patient goals of care. Timing of surgery requires a nuanced characterization of the severity and extent of dissection and potential reversibility of malperfusion syndromes. As with other procedures in cardiac surgery, age, frailty, comorbid conditions, prior surgical intervention or chest radiation, baseline functional status, extent of organ injury and predictive reversibility, and individual goals of care may deem a patient inoperable and are some of the most important predictors of outcome [23].

References

1. Bonser RS, Ranasinghe AM, Loubani M, Evans JD, Thalji NMA, Bachet JE, et al. Evidence, lack of evidence, controversy, and debate in the provision and performance of the surgery of acute type A aortic dissection. J Am Coll Cardiol. 2011;58:2455–74.
2. Olsson C, Thelin S, Stahle E. Thoracic aortic aneurysm and dissection: Increasing prevalence and improved outcomes reported in a nationwide population-based study of more than 14,000 cases from 1987 to 2002. J Vasc Surg. 2007;609. https://doi.org/10.1016/j.jvs.2007.07.017.
3. Ehrlich MP, Ergin MA, McCullough JN, Lansman SL, Galla JD, Bodian CA, et al. Results of immediate surgical treatment of all acute type A dissections. Circulation. 2000;III–248. https://doi.org/10.1161/01.cir.102.suppl_3.iii-248.
4. Kawahito K, Adachi H, Yamaguchi A, Ino T. Preoperative risk factors for hospital mortality in acute type A aortic dissection. Ann Thorac Surg. 2001;1239–43. https://doi.org/10.1016/s0003-4975(00)02654-0.

5. Olsson C. Modifiable risk factors for early mortality in low-risk Penn class Aa acute type A aortic dissection patients—a descriptive study. Aorta. 2017;117–23. https://doi.org/10.12945/j.aorta.2017.17.045.
6. Trimarchi S, Nienaber CA, Rampoldi V. Contemporary results of surgery in acute type A aortic dissection: The International Registry of Acute Aortic Dissection Experience. ACC Curr J Rev. 2005;45–6. https://doi.org/10.1016/j.accreview.2005.04.039.
7. Ghoreishi M, Wise ES, Croal-Abrahams L, Tran D, Pasrija C, Drucker CB, et al. A novel risk score predicts operative mortality after acute type A aortic dissection repair. Ann Thorac Surg. 2018;106:1759–66.
8. Helder MRK, Schaff HV, Day CN, Pochettino A, Bagameri G, Greason KL, et al. Regional and temporal trends in the outcomes of repairs for acute type A aortic dissections. Ann Thorac Surg. 2020;109:26–33.
9. Hughes GC. Invited commentary. Ann Thorac Surg. 2020;109:33–5.
10. Trimarchi S, Eagle KA, Nienaber CA, Rampoldi V, Jonker FHW, De Vincentiis C, et al. Role of age in acute type A aortic dissection outcome: report from the International Registry of Acute Aortic Dissection (IRAD). J Thorac Cardiovasc Surg. 2010;140:784–9.
11. Mehta RH, Suzuki T, Hagan PG. Predicting death in patients with acute type A aortic dissection. ACC Curr J Rev. 2002;11:14.
12. Yang B, Norton EL, Rosati CM, Wu X, Kim KM, Khaja MS, et al. Managing patients with acute type A aortic dissection and mesenteric malperfusion syndrome: A 20-year experience. J Thorac Cardiovasc Surg. 2018; https://doi.org/10.1016/j.jtcvs.2018.11.127.
13. Lawton JS, Moon MR, Liu J, Koerner DJ, Kulshrestha K, Damiano RJ Jr, et al. The profound impact of combined severe acidosis and malperfusion on operative mortality in the surgical treatment of type A aortic dissection. J Thorac Cardiovasc Surg. 2018;155:897–904.
14. Leontyev S, Légaré J-F, Borger MA, Buth KJ, Funkat AK, Gerhard J, et al. Creation of a scorecard to predict in-hospital death in patients undergoing operations for acute type A aortic dissection. Ann Thorac Surg. 2016;101:1700–6.
15. Patel HJ, Williams DM, Dasika NL, Suzuki Y, Michael Deeb G. Operative delay for peripheral malperfusion syndrome in acute type A aortic dissection: A long-term analysis. J Thorac Cardiovasc Surg. 2008;1288–96. https://doi.org/10.1016/j.jtcvs.2008.01.026.
16. Ullery BW, Peterson JC, Milla F, Wells MT, Briggs W, Girardi LN, et al. Cardiac surgery in select nonagenarians: should we or shouldn't we? Ann Thorac Surg. 2008;854–60. https://doi.org/10.1016/j.athoracsur.2007.10.074.
17. Santini F, Montalbano G, Messina A, Donofrio A, Casali G, Viscardi F, et al. Survival and quality of life after repair of acute type A aortic dissection in patients aged 75 years and older justify intervention. Eur J Cardio-Thorac Surg. 2006;386–91. https://doi.org/10.1016/j.ejcts.2005.12.016.
18. Kawahito K, Adachi H, Yamaguchi A, Ino T. Early and late surgical outcomes of acute type a aortic dissection in patients aged 75 years and older. Ann Thorac Surg. 2000;1455–9. https://doi.org/10.1016/s0003-4975(00)01934-2.
19. Augoustides J. Faculty of 1000 evaluation for early and late surgical outcomes of acute type A aortic dissection in octogenarians. F1000 - Post-publication peer review of the biomedical literature. 2017. https://doi.org/10.3410/f.732019021.793538243.
20. Ganapathi AM, Englum BR, Hanna JM, Schechter MA, Gaca JG, Hurwitz LM, et al. Frailty and risk in proximal aortic surgery. J Thorac Cardiovasc Surg. 2014;147:186–91.e1.
21. Williams JB, Peterson ED, Zhao Y, O'Brien SM, Andersen ND, Craig Miller D, et al. Contemporary results for proximal aortic replacement in North America. J Am Coll Cardiol. 2012;60:1156–62.
22. Dumfarth J, Peterss S, Luehr M, Etz CD, Schachner T, Kofler M, et al. Acute type A dissection in octogenarians: does emergency surgery impact in-hospital outcome or long-term survival? Eur J Cardiothorac Surg. 2017;51:472–7.
23. Chiappini B, Schepens M, Tan E, Dell'Amore A, Morshuis W, Dossche K, et al. Early and late outcomes of acute type A aortic dissection: analysis of risk factors in 487 consecutive patients. Eur Heart J. 2005;26:180–6.

24. Yefimova M, Aslakson RA, Yang L, Garcia A, Boothroyd D, Gale RC, et al. Palliative care and end-of-life outcomes following high-risk surgery. JAMA Surg. 2020; https://doi.org/10.1001/jamasurg.2019.5083.
25. Eusanio MD, Di Eusanio M, Trimarchi S, Patel HJ, Hutchison S, Suzuki T, et al. Clinical presentation, management, and short-term outcome of patients with type A acute dissection complicated by mesenteric malperfusion: Observations from the International Registry of Acute Aortic Dissection. J Thorac Cardiovasc Surg. 2013;385–90.e1. https://doi.org/10.1016/j.jtcvs.2012.01.042.
26. Deeb GM, Michael Deeb G, Williams DM, Bolling SF, Quint LE, Monaghan H, et al. Surgical delay for acute type A dissection with malperfusion. Ann Thorac Surg. 1997;64:1669–77.
27. Yang B, Rosati CM, Norton EL, Kim KM, Khaja MS, Dasika N, et al. Endovascular fenestration/stenting first followed by delayed open aortic repair for acute type A aortic dissection with malperfusion syndrome. Circulation. 2018;138:2091–103.
28. Deeb GM, Michael Deeb G, Patel HJ, Williams DM. Treatment for malperfusion syndrome in acute type A and B aortic dissection: A long-term analysis. J Thorac Cardiovasc Surg. 2010;S98–100. https://doi.org/10.1016/j.jtcvs.2010.07.036.
29. Parsa CJ, McCann RL, Chad HG. A novel approach to the treatment of distal malperfusion secondary to ascending aortic dissection. J Card Surg. 2010;25:220–2.
30. Leshnower BG, Veeraswamy RK, Duwayri YM, Chen EP. The "TEVAR-First" approach to DeBakey I aortic dissection with mesenteric malperfusion. Ann Thorac Surg. 2014;97:693–6.
31. Lombardi JV, Hughes GC, Appoo JJ, Bavaria JE, Beck AW, Cambria RP, et al. Society for Vascular Surgery (SVS) and Society of Thoracic Surgeons (STS) reporting standards for type B aortic dissections. Ann Thorac Surg. 2020;109:959–81.
32. Goldstone AB, Chiu P, Baiocchi M, Lingala B, Lee J, Rigdon J, et al. Interfacility transfer of medicare beneficiaries with acute type A aortic dissection and regionalization of care in the United States. Circulation. 2019;140:1239–50.
33. Eusanio MD, Di Eusanio M, Patel HJ, Nienaber CA, Montgomery DM, Korach A, et al. Patients with type A acute aortic dissection presenting with major brain injury: Should we operate on them? J Thorac Cardiovasc Surg. 2013;S213–21.e1. https://doi.org/10.1016/j.jtcvs.2012.11.054.
34. Sultan I, Bianco V, Patel HJ, Arnaoutakis GJ, Di Eusanio M, Chen EP, et al. Surgery for type A aortic dissection in patients with cerebral malperfusion: Results from the International Registry of Acute Aortic Dissection. J Thorac Cardiovasc Surg. 2019; https://doi.org/10.1016/j.jtcvs.2019.11.003.
35. Estrera AL, Garami Z, Miller CC, Porat EE, Achouh PE, Dhareshwar J, et al. Acute type A aortic dissection complicated by stroke: can immediate repair be performed safely? J Thorac Cardiovasc Surg. 2006;132:1404–8.
36. Estol CJ, Pessin MS. Anticoagulation: is there still a role in atherothrombotic stroke? Stroke. 1990;21:820–4.
37. Geirsson A, Szeto WY, Pochettino A, McGarvey ML, Keane MG, Woo YJ, et al. Significance of malperfusion syndromes prior to contemporary surgical repair for acute type A dissection: outcomes and need for additional revascularizations. Eur J Cardiothorac Surg. 2007;32:255–62.
38. Conzelmann LO, Hoffmann I, Blettner M, Kallenbach K, Karck M, Dapunt O, et al. Analysis of risk factors for neurological dysfunction in patients with acute aortic dissection type A: data from the German Registry for Acute Aortic Dissection type A (GERAADA). Eur J Cardiothorac Surg. 2012;42:557–65.
39. Estrera AL, Huynh TTT, Porat EE, Miller CC 3rd, Smith JJ, Safi HJ. Is acute type A aortic dissection a true surgical emergency? Semin Vasc Surg. 2002;15:75–82.
40. Zenati MA. Commentary: The conundrum of cerebral malperfusion in aortic dissection. J Thorac Cardiovasc Surg. 2019; https://doi.org/10.1016/j.jtcvs.2019.11.103.
41. Di Eusanio M, Patel HJ, Nienaber CA, Montgomery DM, Korach A, Sundt TM, et al. Patients with type A acute aortic dissection presenting with major brain injury: should we operate on them? J Thorac Cardiovasc Surg. 2013;145:S213–21.e1.

42. Kreibich M, Desai ND, Bavaria JE, Szeto WY, Vallabhajosyula P, Itagaki R, et al. Preoperative neurological deficit in acute type A aortic dissection. Interact Cardiovasc Thorac Surg. 2020; https://doi.org/10.1093/icvts/ivz311.
43. Matsubara S, Koga M, Ohara T, Iguchi Y, Minatoya K, Tahara Y, et al. Cerebrovascular imaging of cerebral ischemia in acute type A aortic dissection. J Neurol Sci. 2018;388:23–7.
44. Heran MKS, Balaji N, Cook RC. Novel percutaneous treatment of cerebral malperfusion before surgery for acute type A dissection. Ann Thorac Surg. 2019;108:e15–7.
45. Teman NR, Peterson MD, Russo MJ, Ehrlich MP, Myrmel T, Upchurch GR, et al. Outcomes of patients presenting with acute type A aortic dissection in the setting of prior cardiac surgery: an analysis from the International Registry of Acute Aortic Dissection. Circulation. 2013;S180–5. https://doi.org/10.1161/circulationaha.112.000342.
46. Collins JS. Differences in clinical presentation, management, and outcomes of acute type A aortic dissection in patients with and without previous cardiac surgery. Circulation. 2004;II–237. https://doi.org/10.1161/01.cir.0000138219.67028.2a
47. Hassan M, Carvalho EMF, Macedo FIB, Gologorsky E, Salerno TA. Paradigm change in the management of patients with acute type A aortic dissection who had prior cardiac surgery. J Card Surg. 2010;387–389. https://doi.org/10.1111/j.1540-8191.2010.01061.x.
48. Estrera AL, Miller CC, Kaneko T, Lee T-Y, Walkes J-C, Kaiser LR, et al. Outcomes of acute type a aortic dissection after previous cardiac surgery. Ann Thorac Surg. 2010;89:1467–74.
49. Norton EL, Rosati CM, Kim KM, Wu X, Patel HJ, Deeb GM, et al. Is previous cardiac surgery a risk factor for open repair of acute type A aortic dissection? J Thorac Cardiovasc Surg. 2019; https://doi.org/10.1016/j.jtcvs.2019.07.093.
50. Krebs ED, Mehaffey JH, Hawkins RB, Beller JP, Fonner CE, Kiser AC, et al. Outcomes after acute type A aortic dissection in patients with prior cardiac surgery. Ann Thorac Surg. 2019;108:708–13.
51. Hamad R, Amr G, Demers P. Delayed surgery in patients with acute type A aortic dissection who are receiving novel oral anticoagulants. J Thorac Cardiovasc Surg. 2018;155:e1–4.
52. Tralhão A, Aguiar C, Ferreira J, Rebocho MJ, Santos E, Martins D, et al. Dabigatran reversal with idarucizumab in a patient undergoing heart transplantation: first European report. Thromb J. 2017;15:23.
53. Flaherty D, Connors JM, Singh S, Sylvester KW, Rimsans J, Cornella L. Andexanet alfa for urgent reversal of apixaban before aortic surgery requiring cardiopulmonary bypass. A & A Pract. 2019;271–3. https://doi.org/10.1213/xaa.0000000000001052.
54. Levy JH, Welsby I. Andexanet alfa use in patients requiring cardiopulmonary bypass. A & A Pract. 2019;477. https://doi.org/10.1213/xaa.0000000000001115.
55. Levy JH, Douketis J, Weitz JI. Reversal agents for non-vitamin K antagonist oral anticoagulants. Nat Rev Cardiol. 2018;15:273–81.
56. Williams JB, Phillips-Bute B, Bhattacharya SD, Shah AA, Andersen ND, Altintas B, et al. Predictors of massive transfusion with thoracic aortic procedures involving deep hypothermic circulatory arrest. J Thorac Cardiovasc Surg. 2011;141:1283–8.
57. Wagner MA, Wang H, Benrashid E, Keenan JE, Krishnamurthy Y, Levy JH, et al. Protocolized hemostatic factor use in major thoracic aortic surgery. J Cardiovasc Surg. 2019. https://doi.org/10.23736/s0021-9509.19.10819-1.
58. Andersen ND, Bhattacharya SD, Williams JB, Fosbol EL, Lockhart EL, Patel MB, et al. Intraoperative use of low-dose recombinant activated factor VII during thoracic aortic operations. Ann Thorac Surg. 2012;93:1921–8. Discussion 1928–9
59. Hanna JM, Keenan JE, Wang H, Andersen ND, Gaca JG, Lombard FW, et al. Use of human fibrinogen concentrate during proximal aortic reconstruction with deep hypothermic circulatory arrest. J Thorac Cardiovasc Surg. 2016;151:376–82.
60. Schultz NH, Lundblad R, Holme PA. Activated prothrombin complex concentrate to reverse the factor Xa inhibitor (apixaban) effect before emergency surgery: a case series. J Med Case Rep. 2018;12:138.
61. Preventza O, Bracey A. Surgery for acute type A aortic dissection on oral anticoagulants: Being the dispatcher of a 911 call. J Thorac Cardiovasc Surg. 2018;e5–6.

62. Juraszek A, Kołsut P, Szymański J, Kuriata J, Kuśmierski K, Sitkowska-Rysiak E, et al. Results of open heart surgery in Jehovah's Witness patients. Single centre experience. Pol J Cardio-Thorac Surg. 2017;164–9. https://doi.org/10.5114/kitp.2017.70529.
63. Jassar AS, Ford PA, Haber HL, Isidro A, Swain JD, Bavaria JE, et al. Cardiac surgery in Jehovah's Witness patients: ten-year experience. Ann Thorac Surg. 2012;93:19–25.
64. Lee TC, Kon Z, Cheema FH, Grau-Sepulveda MV, Englum B, Kim S, et al. Contemporary management and outcomes of acute type A aortic dissection: An analysis of the STS adult cardiac surgery database. J Card Surg. 2018;33:7–18.
65. Hughes DB, Ullery BW, Barie PS. The contemporary approach to the care of Jehovah's witnesses. J Trauma. 2008;65:237–47.
66. Harris JE, Varnado S, Herrera E, Salazar E, Colavecchia AC. Evaluation of postoperative clinical outcomes in Jehovah's Witness patients who receive prothrombin complex concentrate during cardiac surgery. J Card Surg. 2020; https://doi.org/10.1111/jocs.14463.
67. Pasic M, Ruisz W, Koster A, Hetzer R. Bloodless surgery of acute type A aortic dissection in a Jehovah's Witness patient. Ann Thorac Surg. 2005;80:1507–10.
68. Evangelista A, Mukherjee D, Mehta RH, O'Gara PT, Fattori R, Cooper JV, et al. Acute intramural hematoma of the aorta. Circulation. 2005;1063–70. https://doi.org/10.1161/01.cir.0000156444.26393.80.
69. Wang A, Montgomery D, Brinster DR, Gilon D, Upchurch GR Jr, Gleason TG, et al. Predicting in-hospital survival in acute type A aortic dissection medically treated. J Am Coll Cardiol. 2020;75:1360–1.
70. Sundt TM. Management of intramural hematoma of the ascending aorta: still room for debate. J Thorac Cardiovasc Surg. 2002;894–5.
71. Song J-K, Yim JH, Ahn J-M, Kim D-H, Kang J-W, Lee TY, et al. Outcomes of patients with acute type a aortic intramural hematoma. Circulation. 2009;120:2046–52.
72. Evangelista A, Eagle KA. Is the optimal management of acute type a aortic intramural hematoma evolving? Circulation. 2009;2029–32.
73. Keenan JE, Wang H, Gulack BC, Ganapathi AM, Andersen ND, Englum BR, et al. Does moderate hypothermia really carry less bleeding risk than deep hypothermia for circulatory arrest? A propensity-matched comparison in hemiarch replacement. J Thorac Cardiovasc Surg. 2016;152:1559–69.e2.
74. Halbreiner MS, Yamashita M, Plichta R, Svensson LG. An alternative technique for hemiarch replacement without using deep hypothermic circulatory arrest. Semin Thorac Cardiovasc Surg. 2017;29:47–8.
75. Norton EL, Wu X, Farhat L, Kim KM, Patel HJ, Deeb GM, et al. Dissection of arch branches alone: an indication for aggressive arch management in type A dissection? Ann Thorac Surg. 2020;109:487–94.
76. Rylski B, Bavaria JE, Milewski RK, Vallabhajosyula P, Moser W, Kremens E, et al. Long-term results of neomedia sinus valsalva repair in 489 patients with type A aortic dissection. Ann Thorac Surg. 2014;98:582–8. Discussion 588–9
77. Muetterties CE, Menon R, Wheatley GH. A systematic review of primary endovascular repair of the ascending aorta. J Vasc Surg. 2018;332–42. https://doi.org/10.1016/j.jvs.2017.06.099.
78. Plichta RP, Hughes GC. Thoracic endovascular aortic repair for the ascending aorta: experience and pitfalls. J Visc Surg. 2018;4:92.
79. Roselli EE, Idrees J, Greenberg RK, Johnston DR, Lytle BW. Endovascular stent grafting for ascending aorta repair in high-risk patients. J Thorac Cardiovasc Surg. 2015;149:144–51.
80. Vallabhajosyula P, Gottret J-P, Bavaria JE, Desai ND, Szeto WY. Endovascular repair of the ascending aorta in patients at high risk for open repair. J Thorac Cardiovasc Surg. 2015;S144–50. https://doi.org/10.1016/j.jtcvs.2014.07.063.
81. Li Z, Lu Q, Feng R, Zhou J, Zhao Z, Bao J, et al. Outcomes of endovascular repair of ascending aortic dissection in patients unsuitable for direct surgical repair. J Am Coll Cardiol. 2016;68:1944–54.

Delayed Surgery for Acute Aortic Dissection

Polina Pinkhasova, Mohammad A. Zafar, Bulat A. Ziganshin, and John A. Elefteriades

Introduction

Acute Type A aortic dissection (ATAAD) has long been accepted as a surgical emergency. However, a semi-elective approach has successfully been explored for the late-presenting aortic dissector. Additionally, patients with severe comorbidities, advanced age, prior aortic valve replacement (AVR), and those with a completed stroke can benefit from intentional delay or even sole medical therapy. This chapter will explore appropriate deviations from the "emergent surgery" rule in very selected patient circumstances.

Outline

- Definition of Delay
- Natural History of Acute Aortic Dissection from Acute to Chronic

P. Pinkhasova
Aortic Institute at Yale-New Haven Hospital, Yale University School of Medicine, New Haven, CT, USA

Department of Internal Medicine, Danbury Hospital, Nuvance Health, Danbury, CT, USA

M. A. Zafar · J. A. Elefteriades (✉)
Aortic Institute at Yale-New Haven Hospital, Yale University School of Medicine, New Haven, CT, USA
e-mail: john.elefteriades@yale.edu

B. A. Ziganshin
Aortic Institute at Yale-New Haven Hospital, Yale University School of Medicine, New Haven, CT, USA

Department of Cardiovascular and Endovascular Surgery, Kazan State Medical University, Kazan, Russia

J. S. Coselli et al. (eds.), *Aortic Dissection and Acute Aortic Syndromes*,
https://doi.org/10.1007/978-3-030-66668-2_37

- Reasons for Delay
- Theory Behind Delay (transfer to high-volume center, multidisciplinary approach, daytime procedure)
- Outcomes of Delayed Approach (mortality data)

Definitions

While a large amount of data exists on emergent surgery for acute Type A aortic dissection itself, there is only minimal data available regarding delayed surgery for this condition. Operative delay, with interval medical management, is appropriate only for specific patient populations.

The prime patient example is a late-presenting dissector, arriving after surviving the initial 48 h of dissection symptoms [1]. These patients are either diagnosed late or transferred late to a referral center, having already successfully surmounted the initial "eye of the storm" [2]. These patients have remained hemodynamically stable under medical management. In other cases, surgeon experience may dictate intentional delay in management, as in patients with powerful morbidities or previous AVR (aortic valve replacement) or CABG (coronary artery bypass grafting). Other situations where surgical delay may be warranted will be discussed in the following sections.

It is also important to define the temporal phases of aortic dissection, which are generally subdivided into three categories. An "acute aortic dissection" extends up to 2 weeks from the onset of symptoms, "subacute" from 2 weeks to 3 months, and "chronic" beyond 3 months. The high mortality of acute aortic dissection during the first 24–72 h is well known, running about 1–2% per hour. However, little is known about the natural history and clinical implications of dissection beyond this time mark [3–5].

Natural History of Acute Aortic Dissection

In order to understand the clinical implications of a delayed surgical approach, it is important to understand the physiology of waiting. Up until very recently, almost no data existed on subacute or chronic dissections, given that some 90% of patients with Type A dissection are treated surgically. Following surgical delay for a variety of reasons, aortic dissectors who have evolved to the chronic stage do reach a durable state of stability. One study showed that about 60% of those who have become chronic-stage survivors of Type A dissection do require surgery during follow-up; their surgical results are significantly better compared with the acutely operated cohort [6].

To review, aortic dissection occurs when an intimomedial tear allows blood to enter the aortic wall, subsequently creating a false lumen [3]. The false lumen then propagates proximally or distally and often impairs or collapses the true lumen. Rapid propagation often causes rupture into the pericardial or pleural spaces. Lumen collapse can lead to malperfusion of organs and limbs. Most of the natural complications, such as rupture, aortic insufficiency, and organ ischemia, are expected during the very early period.

The acute to chronic transition involves all three layers of the aortic wall, including the tunica intima, media, and adventitia (see Table 1 and Fig. 1) [7, 8]. In the chronic state, the intima can become atherosclerotic and hyperplastic. The media can atrophy and also undergo fragmentation of elastic fibers, reducing tensile strength and elasticity. Medionecrosis and cystic medial necrosis progress as well. The adventitia is subject to inflammation and fibrosis. The fibrosis can impair the vasa vasorum, which are responsible for gas exchange. Mobility of the dissected septum tends to decrease over time, through fibrosis and gradually increasing tissue stiffness [9]. Some argue that this factor can adversely impact late endograft repair, as theoretically the less mobile septum accommodates the endograft less favorably. If the septum is stiff and fibrotic, the compressed true lumen is less likely to re-expand and obliterate the false lumen. Histologic changes correlate with imaging findings of thickened dissection flaps (see Table 2) [8].

Table 1 Histologic aortic grading, according to Schlatmann and Becker

	Grade I	Grade II	Grade III
Cystic medial necrosis	Minute cyst present within a single lamellar unit	Increased cyst size and number in total width of one lamellar unit	Large cyst extending over more than one lamellar unit
Elastin fragmentation	Fewer than 5 foci in one micro field (×200), smooth muscle orientation preserved	5 or more foci fragmented in one field (×200), confluent or scattered media, smooth muscle orientation preserved	Foci with elastin fragmentation in 5+ elastic lamellae, regardless of micro field, smooth muscle cells altered in orientation
Fibrosis (increased collagen)	Increase in collagen in area compromising less than 1/3rd of total width of media	Increase in collagen between 1/3rd and 2/3rds of total width of media	Increase collagen in area compromising > 2/3rd total width of media
Medionecrosis (focal loss of nuclei in the media)	Area compromising less than 1/3rd of total width of media	Area compromising between 1/3rd and 2/3rds of total width of media	Area compromising greater than 2/3rd of total width of media
Atheroma	Atheroma present		
Vasa vasorum fibrosis	Fibrosis present		
Inflammation	Inflammation present		
Intimal hyperplasia	Hyperplasia present		
Medial atrophy	Measured in mm		

Reprinted with permission from [7]

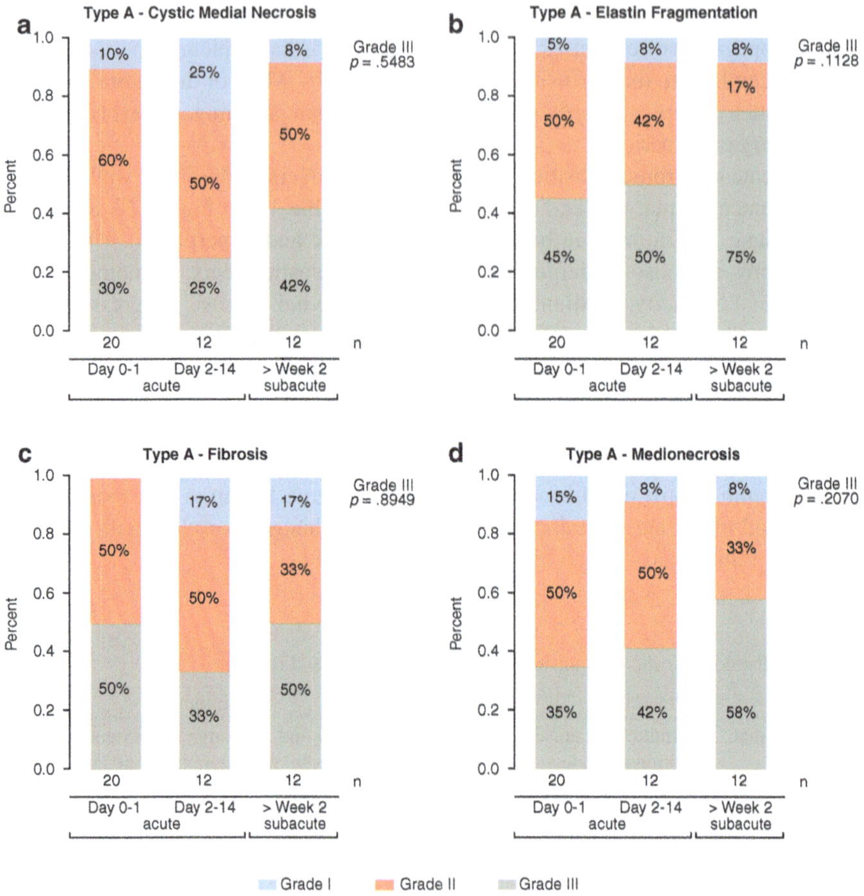

Fig. 1 Histopathology changes in type A dissection over time (**a**) cystic medial necrosis. (**b**) Elastin fragmentation. (**c**) Fibrosis. (**d**) Medionecrosis. Note: no significant differences were seen in grading of cystic medial necrosis, medionecrosis, elastin fragmentation, or fibrosis between acute, subacute, and chronic type A dissections, with the restriction of the admittedly (and expectedly) low numbers of late operated type A dissection patients. Despite the lack of statistical significance, a gradually increasing trend is grossly discernible in elastin fragmentation and medionecrosis over time. Refer to Table 1 for details on grading (reproduced with permission from [8])

Reasons for Surgical Delay

This chapter is in no way intended to suggest deviating from the standard of routine immediate surgery for acute Type A aortic dissection, which we agree constitutes a surgical emergency. This chapter merely means to clarify that for certain selected unusual patients, surgical delay may be appropriate. We cannot overemphasize the need for fast diagnosis and surgical repair in the early stages of dissection. Our knowledge of the selected role of delayed surgical therapy is based on experiences

Table 2 The changes in aortic morphology and histopathology as acute dissection transitions over time to chronic aortic dissection

Changes in aortic morphology and histopathology from acute to chronic dissection
• Aortic diameter increases remarkably rapidly early after dissection, with a later plateau
• The dissection flap thickens early and then plateaus, straightens, and becomes less mobile
• The false lumen patency has an adverse effect on the outcome, and mild progression of false lumen thrombosis is seen over time
• Longitudinal extension of dissection or new branch vessel involvement is rare
• The aortic wall is markedly abnormal in its histological pathology initially, and becomes increasingly more so over time
• Fibrosis of the aortic wall progresses over time; thus, flap thickness and stiffness (immobility) increase during the remodeling process

Reprinted with permission from [8]

with both intentional and unintentional delay. For instance, much of our data extrapolates from patients who experienced delay in recognition of the diagnosis of acute aortic dissection or delay in surgical referral.

Data from the International Registry of Acute Aortic Dissection (IRAD) published in 2011 provides an important timeline perspective. Time from hospital arrival to diagnosis of aortic dissection averaged 4.5 h. Time from diagnosis to surgery averaged 4.8 h. This makes for a total door-to-operating room time of just over 8 h. Longer delay from diagnosis to surgery occurred in nonwhites, those with prior cardiac surgery, and those without ongoing shock or hypotension [10]. These categories, in the IRAD report, are identified as needing improvement in diagnosis and triage. Delays were noted especially in non-tertiary centers, sites unfamiliar with aortic dissection [11, 12].

Several studies also note that patients hospitalized with acute aortic dissection on weekends may have delayed diagnosis of acute Type A dissection and its complications, leading to delay in management [12]. This is associated with short-staffing and absence of staff experienced with aortic dissection patients during the weekend time.

Aside from the issues of late diagnosis and late referral to surgical centers, some experience has been accumulated regarding *deliberate* delay of surgical therapy. A retrospective study performed at Duke University explored the outcomes of acute Type A aortic dissection before and after initiation of a multidisciplinary thoracic aortic surgery program (TASP) [13]. The program consists of CT surgery, vascular surgery, cardiac anesthesia, cardiovascular medicine, cardiac critical care, radiology, neurology, pathology, medical genetics, blood bank, nursing, and perfusionists. The CT surgeons themselves had subspecialized in thoracic aortic surgery. While unstable patients and those presenting within 48 h of symptom onset were taken to the OR emergently, patients who were stable, asymptomatic, and had crossed the 48 h mark underwent preoperative evaluation. Operative mortality after TASP decreased dramatically, from 33.9 to 2.8%. Survival benefit extended to late follow-up, with survival at 5 years of 85% after TASP, versus 55% before.

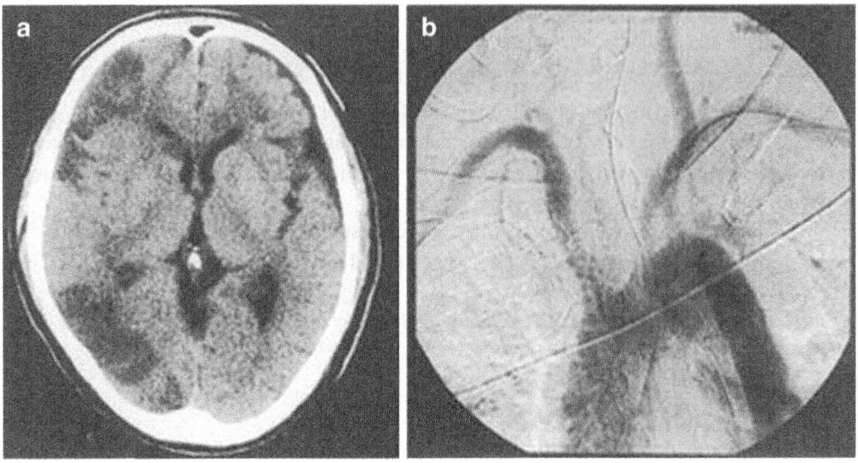

Fig. 2 (**a**) Brain CT scan demonstrating multiple low-density infarctions in the right hemisphere, with moderate cerebral edema. (**b**) Arch angiogram of the same patient, demonstrating impaired flow through the right carotid artery as a result of the dissection process. It was thought that immediate surgical intervention was not appropriate in the acute phase of the dissection. Interval medical management was undertaken, with eventual aortic replacement 3 months after initial presentation (reproduced with permission [15])

TASP chooses to defer surgery until daylight hours in late-presenters based on some literature that notes a low rate of acute decompensation or rupture in stable patients who present after 48 h from onset of symptoms [13, 14]. The proportion of cases initiated at night decreased from 48 to 29% after the onset of TASP. Emergent cases decreased from 89 to 75%. Despite these observations, clinically emergent cases are performed immediately.

Several groups have demonstrated superior outcomes with intentional delay for acute strokes complicating acute Type A aortic dissection. Acute stroke serves as another reason intentional delay may be elected. A completed stroke may be noted at presentation or at arrival to the referral center. A case series out of Japan concluded that intentional surgical delay and medical observation are useful for patients who present with both aortic dissection and cerebral infarct [15] (See Fig. 2). Blood flow reestablishment in the area of infarct or administration of anticoagulation during cardiopulmonary bypass may worsen the clinical picture due to hemorrhagic conversion and possible brain edema and/or herniation. This topic of stroke and acute Type A dissection remains controversial, as Estrera and colleagues have advocated for immediate repair of acute Type A aortic dissection in the setting of stroke. They have not noted neurological devastation due to early surgery in the face of acute stroke. However, they do note that patient approach should be individualized, with surgeon-dependent decision making [16]. While we advise for the standard emergent approach for an evolving stroke, delay should be considered for a completed acute cerebral event [2, 17].

Intentional delay of surgery may also appropriately be made due to acute dissection while on anticoagulation. Good clinical outcomes have been demonstrated with delay to permit dissipation of novel direct-acting anticoagulants (DOACs) [18].

Table 3 Subset analysis of reason for delay or avoidance of surgery in "group A"—cohort of patients with surgical delay of >48 h after initial symptom onset or sole medical therapy. "Group A" consisted of 93 patients which was further subdivided into 53 patients who ultimately underwent operative repair and 40 who did not. Percentages may not sum to 100, as some patients had multiple reasons for delay

	Group A > 48 h to surgery (all patients)		
Variable	Eventual surgery, n (%)	Medical management, n (%)	*p* Value
Unknown	1 (1.9)	11 (28.2)	0.0002
Delay in diagnosis	27 (50.9)	7 (18.0)	0.0012
Overall medical condition	16 (29.4)	7 (18.0)	0.7374
Subacute dissection	6 (11.3)	2 (5.1)	0.2975
Chronic obstructive pulmonary disease	2 (3.8)	3 (7.7)	0.4126
Acute renal failure	0 (0.0)	1 (2.6)	0.2411
Congestive heart failure	3 (5.7)	2 (5.1)	0.9114
Cerebrovascular accident	1 (1.9)	3 (7.7)	0.1772
Patient refusal	4 (7.6)	2 (5.1)	0.6424
Other	10 (18.9)	4 (10.3)	0.2558

Reprinted with permission from [6]

Although numerous groups including ours have demonstrated positive outcomes with surgical delay of surgery for acute Type A dissection in selected patients, some groups argue against this approach. A group out of Japan notes that, as opposed to a medical management mortality of about 59%, operative mortality was about 49% even in the high-risk patients with potential reasons for surgical delay. Higher mortality in the medical group was attributed directly to operative delay. Notably, patients in the medical group were somewhat older (62 vs. 58 years old), with over 70% history of hypertension (often longstanding), and more common incidence of left ventricular hypertrophy compared to those who underwent surgical management [19]. Another Japanese study indicates poor long-term survival in those undergoing a delayed operative approach, with cause of death attributed to rupture of aneurysms [20].

Table 3 lists reasons for pursuing intentional surgical delay in acute Type A aortic dissection [6].

Experience with Intentional Surgical Delay

Importance of Medical Management with Anti-impulse Therapy Medical management involves the well-known anti-impulse therapy, which is instituted immediately and continued during the interval of non-operative therapy. The concept of anti-impulse therapy is to decrease the strength of each cardiac contraction, to inhibit and discourage propagation of the dissection and aortic rupture. The impact of anti-impulse therapy is indicated in Fig. 3 [21]. Please note that afterload reduction alone actually increases the dp/dt (change in pressure over time), exacerbating

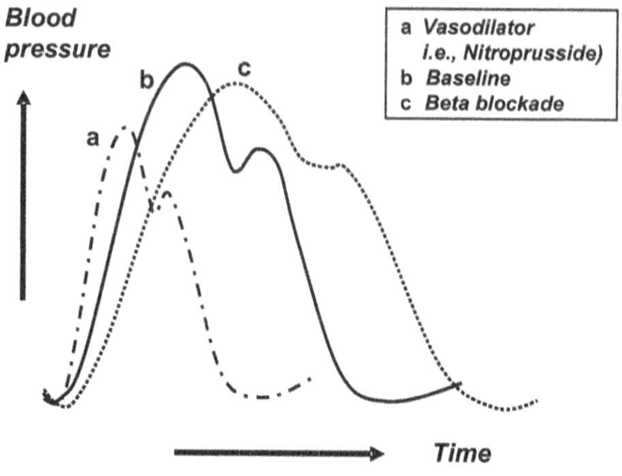

Fig. 3 Aortic pressure curves under various conditions. Curve (a) demonstrates administration of a vasodilator agent such as nitroprusside, curve (b) baseline state, and curve (c) Beta-blocker administration. Curves (a, b) show significant decrease in blood pressure and acceleration in heart rate at the expense of the steeper portion of the ascending curve (increased dp/dt). Curve (c) shows that although the degree of pressure lowering is usually smaller, the characteristic negative chronotropy and inotropy result in a blunted upstroke of the blood pressure curve, representing decreased impulse and dp/dt (reproduced with permission from [29])

the adverse impact on the aorta. A β-blocker is essential, in addition to afterload reducers, to blunt the aortic pressure wave. So, anti-impulse therapy involves both afterload reducers and B-blockers. Table 4 shows drugs that can be utilized in anti-impulse therapy [21].

Delay Until Morning in Stable Patients Presenting Beyond 48 h Multiple groups have documented the relative benefit of not taking the patient to the OR in the middle of the night if they are late-presenters (beyond 48 h) [6]. Theoretical benefits to support the practice of waiting until AM include having a rested surgical and anesthetic team, completion of thorough pre-operative evaluation, and presence of a full, high-quality ancillary operating room team. As these patients have survived the "eye of the storm" it has been found unlikely that they will rupture before the first morning surgical timeslot [2, 6]. We have published this data to provide a modicum of legal protection for surgeons waiting until morning.

Non-operative Therapy for Octogenarians Advanced age and severe comorbidities can certainly impact the decision of many surgeons. We have shown that late-presenters in this group can have acceptable outcomes if surgery is delayed to address comorbidities or not performed at all. For instance, data demonstrates that emergent Type A aortic dissection surgery in octogenarians is associated with relatively high intraoperative and perioperative mortality. Even though immediate post-surgical survival may be better, long-term survival does not differ between medical and surgical patients in this advanced age group [2, 22].

Table 4 Intravenous agents for treatment of acute type A aortic dissection

Name	Category	Loading dose	Maintenance dose	Adverse effects	Caution
Sodium nitroprusside	Vasodialator	0.3–3 mcg/kg/min, max limit for adult is 10 mcg/kg/min for 10 min	1–3 mcg/kg/min	Nausea, vomiting, agitation, muscle twitching, sweating, cutis anserina, thyocyanate and cyanide toxicity, tachycardia	In patients with hepatic or renal dysfunction
Propranolol	Beta-Blocker	1–3 mg (given at 1 mg intervals over 1 min). Can be repeated in not less than every 4 h	1–3 mg every 4 h	Hypotension, nausea, dizziness, cold extremities, reversible hair loss, bradycardia	In patients with bradycardia or history of CHF and bronchospasm. Max initial dose should not exceed 0.15 mg/h (approx. 10 mg)
Esmolol	Beta-Blocker	500 mcg/kg bolus	Continuous 50 mcg/kg/min up to 200 μg/kg/min	Hypotension, nausea, dizziness, bronchospasm, dyspepsia, constipation, increases digoxin level	In patients with CHF, asthma, on concomitant CCB therapy
Labetalol	Alpha and Beta Blocker	20 mg over 2 min then 40–80 mg every 10–15 min (max 300)	continuous IV at 2 mg/min and titrate upto 5–10 mg/min	Vomiting, nausea, scalp, tingling, burning in throat, dizziness, heart block, orthostatic hypotension	In patients with lung disease, concomitant CCB therapy
Diltiazem	CCB	0.25 mg/kg IV bolus (upto 25 mg)	5–10 mg/h by continuous infusion	Peripheral edema, nausea, vomiting	In patients on concomitant beta blockers
Enalapril	Vasodialator ACE Inhibiter	0.625–1.25 mg Bolus	0.625–5 mg every 6 h	Precipitates fall in BP in high renin states, variable response, renal failure	In patients with high possibility of MI, renal dysfunction
Fenoldopam	Dopamine D1 receptor agonist	0.03–0.1 mcg/kg/min initially	0.1–0.3 mcg/kg/min max. 1.6 mcg/kg/min	Tachycardia, hypotension, headache, nausea, flushing, hypokalemia, elevation of IOP	In patients with Glaucoma

(continued)

Table 4 (continued)

Name	Category	Loading dose	Maintenance dose	Adverse effects	Caution
Nicardipine	CCB	5 mg/h; may increase by 2.5 mg/h every 5 min (for rapid titration) to every 15 min (for gradual titration) up to a maximum of 15 mg/h	For rapidly titrated patients, consider reduction to 3 mg/h after response is achieved	Flushing, pedal edema, exacerbation of angina pectoris, hypotension, palpitations, tachycardia, headache, dizziness, nausea, vomiting, dyspepsia	In patients with mild to moderate aortic stenosis, severe left ventricular dysfunction (particularly with concomitant beta-blockade), hepatic impairment, hypertrophic cardiomyopathy, renal impairment
Clevidipine	CCB	Initial 1–2 mg/h; dose may be doubled at 90-s intervals toward blood pressure goal. As blood pressure approaches goal, dose may be increased by less than double every 5–10 min. For every 1–2 mg/h increase in dose, an approximate reduction of 2–4 mmHg in systolic blood pressure may occur	4–6 mg/h; maximum: 21 mg/h	Atrial fibrillation, fever, insomnia, nausea, headache, vomiting, postprocedural hemorrhage, acute renal failure, pneumonia, respiratory failure	In patients with heart failure and pheochromocytoma. Avoid abrupt withdrawal of concomitant beta-blocker therapy

Modified with permission from [21]

Table 5 List of reasons for intentional surgical delay of acute type A aortic dissection

Reasons for intentional surgical delay of acute type A aortic dissection
• Presentation beyond 48-h mark
• Optimization of comorbidities
• Completed stroke
• Transfer to a multidisciplinary center
• Prior AVR

Reprinted with permission from [2]

Table 5 presents a list of reasons for delay or avoidance of surgery in a cohort of patients from a Yale study. Patients divided into one group with definitive operative management post the 48-h mark or another group with sole medical management shared similar postoperative outcomes [6].

Delay in Surgery in Cases with Prior AVR In prior years, many patients who underwent aortic valve replacement (AVR) did not undergo concomitant resection of a dilated aorta. More recently, with the recognition of the relationship between bicuspid aortic valve and ascending aortopathy, aortic resection is recommended for anyone undergoing elective aortic valve replacement with a moderately dilated aorta (greater than 4.5 cm) [23]. Given this fact, we believe that patients who present with acute Type A aortic dissection late after prior AVR can be operated in a delayed fashion, waiting for morning in most cases [2]. The prior AVR provides a certain degree of protection due to the prosthetic valve, as the biologic or mechanical replacement valve is not vulnerable to dissection-related aortic insufficiency. The prior surgery itself produces dense periaortic adhesions, which likely discourage free rupture. Also, the dissection process cannot cross the aortotomy suture line, thereby protecting the right coronary artery (RCA) from dissection. These mitigating anatomic factors are schematized in Fig. 4. The behavior of these post-AVR patients resembles those with a Type B aortic dissection, often permitting a conveniently timed or even semi-elective surgical approach [2].

Delay in Surgery in Cases with Prior CABG Type A aortic dissection in patients with prior remote coronary artery bypass (CABG) represents a very serious situation. We sometimes cautiously delay surgery for a high-quality computerized tomographic scan (CT) to delineate the anatomy of the grafts. It is quite important to know which veins are open and to note the exact position of the internal mammary artery (IMA) graft. Some of the mitigating anatomic factors mentioned above for the post-AVR setting apply to the post-CABG setting and are diagrammed in Fig. 5. The adhesions from the prior surgery may provide a modicum of protection from free rupture of the ascending aorta. The proximal anastomoses may "tether" the dissections somewhat, inhibiting completely free propagation [24].

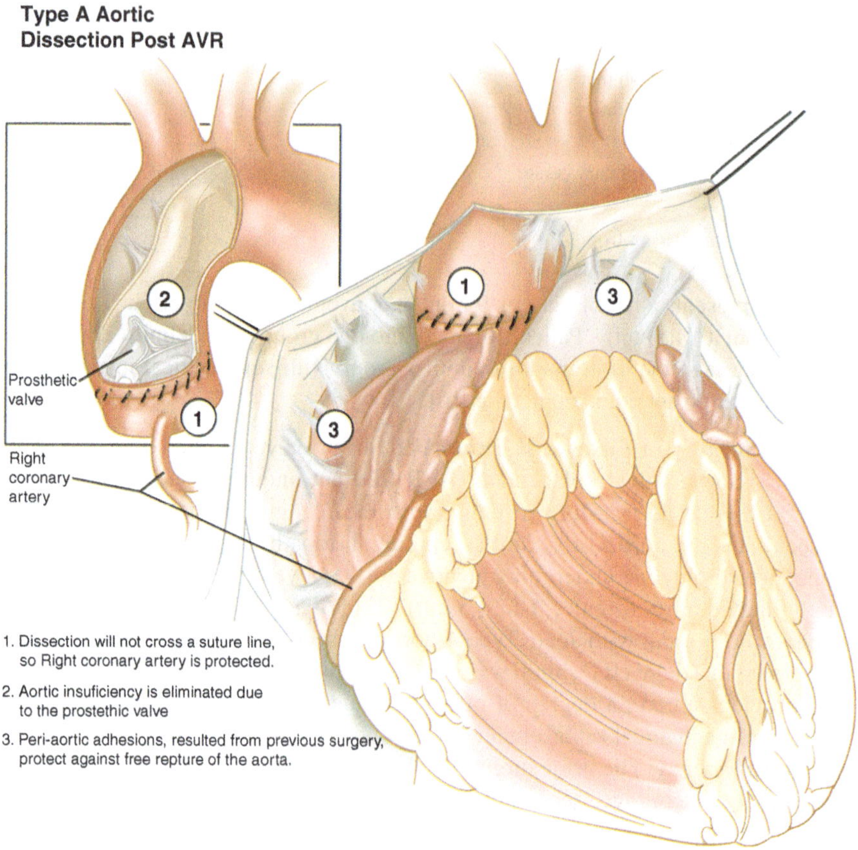

Fig. 4 The prior AVR provides a degree of protection due to the prosthetic valve, as the biologic or mechanical replacement valve is not vulnerable to dissection-related aortic insufficiency. The prior surgery itself produces dense periaortic adhesions, which likely discourage free rupture. The dissection process cannot cross the aortotomy suture line, thereby protecting the right coronary artery (RCA) from dissection (reproduced with permission from [2])

Outcomes of a Delayed Surgical Approach

Permanent Non-operative Management In terms of permanent non-operative management, IRAD data estimates surgically managed acute Type A aortic dissection mortality to be about 26%, compared to medically managed patients whose early mortality is 58% [14]. We recommend early operative management as a general policy, with short-interval non-operative management reserved for patients presenting more than 48 h after onset of pain. We recommend permanent non-operative therapy only for select patients groups with extremely advanced age or profound comorbidities.

Short-Interval Delayed Surgical Therapy Several studies demonstrated satisfactory survival for patients undergoing short-interval delayed surgical treatment for

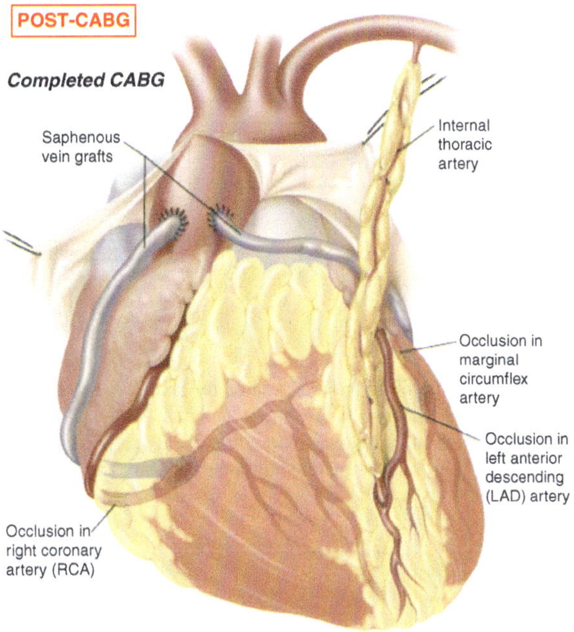

Fig. 5 Type A aortic dissection patients with prior remote coronary artery bypass (CABG) present a serious challenge. Surgery is at times delayed in pursuit of a high-quality computerized tomographic scan (CT) to delineate the anatomy of the grafts to know which veins are open and to note the exact position of the internal mammary artery (IMA) graft. Some of the mitigating anatomic factors mentioned above for the post-AVR setting apply to the post-CABG setting

acute Type A aortic dissection. One of our studies of high-risk patients with substantial comorbidities had a mean time period between dissection and surgical intervention of about 11 days (see Fig. 6) [25]. All who had a delay in treatment with interval medical therapy survived to reach definitive operation. There was no significant difference in short-term survival between the group undergoing delayed surgery and early operation [3, 25].

Another one of our patient series included 42 patients who underwent surgical repair of Type A dissection after the 48-h mark with 1-year survival of over 88%; 5-year survival was over 70%, which was significantly higher compared to patients who did not undergo eventual repair [1]. We underscore that this management strategy is pertinent only to select patients who survived the first 48-h from dissection onset and presented substantial comorbidities that required optimization. These select patients can potentially be managed via semi-elective operation. Patients who underwent this operative strategy generally had more comorbidities (which is one of reasons some of these patients undergo intentional delay) without significant difference in survival rates compared to emergent cases. Patients undergoing semi-elective operation also tended toward improved long-term survival despite higher rates of comorbidities. Figures 7 and 8 illustrate survival comparisons for groups with immediate vs. delayed surgical approach as well as comparison with medical treatment.

Malperfusion Malperfusion (usually of legs or viscera) is a very serious presenting symptom and essentially rules out any delay in surgery. In our recent experience, although there was no significant difference in early or midterm outcomes for

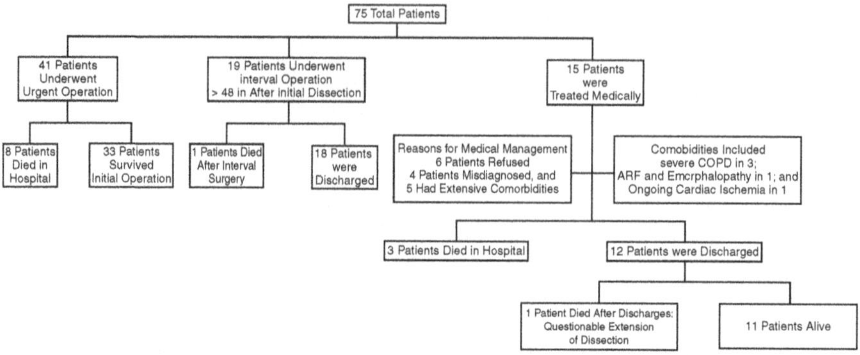

Fig. 6 Outcome of all patients treated for acute type A aortic dissection. The three main branch points represent, respectively, those patients treated with urgent surgery, patients undergoing delayed operation, and those undergoing exclusively medical management. ARF, acute renal failure; COPD, chronic obstructive pulmonary disease (reproduced with permission from [25])

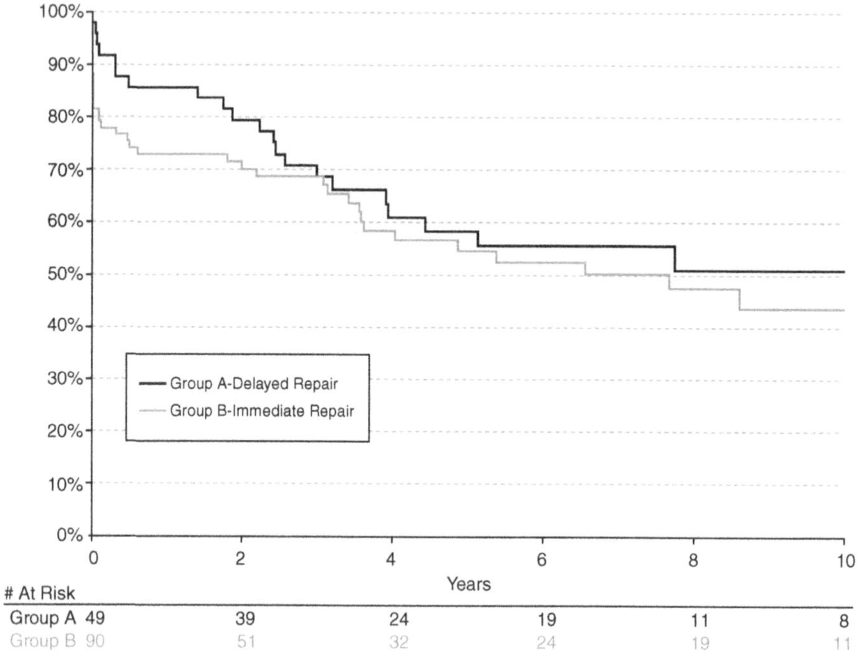

Fig. 7 Kaplan-Meier cumulative survival after operative repair. Ten-year survival is illustrated for patients undergoing operation as a function of the timing of repair. Survival is equivalent between Group A (delayed repair, dark line) and group B (immediate repair, gray line; $p = 0.3669$) (reproduced with permission from [6])

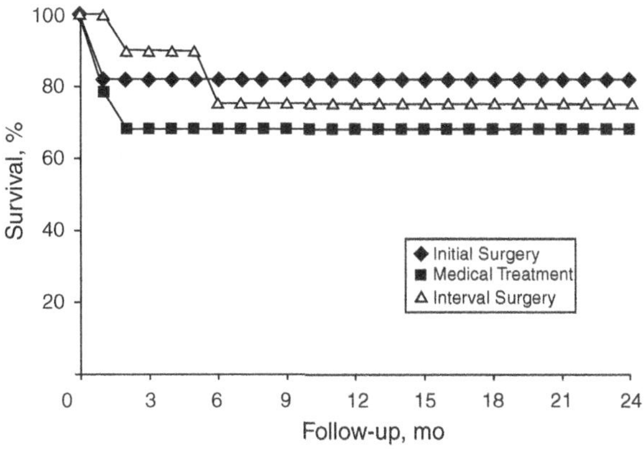

Fig. 8 Kaplan-Meier actuarial survival curve from date of initial presentation and treatment. Note that survivals over the first 2 years are equivalent. Comparison made using log-rank test ($p = 0.44$) (reproduced with permission from [25])

patients with and without malperfusion, those with malperfusion were taken to the OR more rapidly [26]. The Michigan group (and others) have recently argued that patients with Acute Type A dissection and malperfusion should first undergo percutaneous reperfusion, with surgery delayed until reperfusion injury resolves [10, 27, 28]. This is a controversial approach, with most teams arguing for immediate direct aortic surgery in the malperfusion setting. Proper replacement of the ascending aorta and undersurface of the aortic arch, directing blood back into the true aortic lumen, usually reverses malperfusion immediately. Of course, already completed injury at patient presentation, due to the malperfusion, cannot be reversed even by ideal ascending aortic surgery. Such patients have a poor outcome regardless of approach.

Conclusion

Interval non-operative therapy has a role in acute Type A dissection. Specifically, patients presenting in the middle of the night stable for more than 48 h after pain onset can generally safely be delayed until the first morning operating room slot. Patients with anticoagulants on board may need to be delayed to prevent perioperative hemorrhage. Patients with prior AVR are partially protected by adhesions from the prior surgery, by the prosthetic valve, and by the aortotomy itself; they can usually be operated semi-electively. Patients in extreme advanced age or with profound comorbidities may be treated with permanent non-operative therapy, in highly selected cases, with a reasonable chance of survival.

References

1. Gallo A, Davies RR, Coe MP, Elefteriades JA, Coady MA. Indications, timing, and prognosis of operative repair of aortic dissections. Semin Thorac Cardiovasc Surg. 2005;17:224–35.
2. Elefteriades JA, Feldman M. Acute type A aortic dissection: surgical intervention for all: CON. Cardiol Clin. 2010;28:325–31.
3. Coady MA, Rizzo JA, Goldstein LJ, Elefteriades JA. Natural history, pathogenesis, and etiology of thoracic aortic aneurysms and dissections. Cardiol Clin. 1999;17:615–35. vii
4. Hagan PG, Nienaber CA, Isselbacher EM, et al. The International Registry of Acute Aortic Dissection (IRAD): new insights into an old disease. JAMA. 2000;283:897–903.
5. Weigang E, Nienaber CA, Rehders TC, Ince H, Vahl CF, Beyersdorf F. Management of patients with aortic dissection. Dtsch Arztebl Int. 2008;105:639–45.
6. Davies RR, Coe MP, Mandapati D, et al. What is the optimal management of late-presenting survivors of acute type A aortic dissection? Ann Thorac Surg. 2007;83:1593–601. Discussion 1601–2
7. Schlatmann TJ, Becker AE. Histologic changes in the normal aging aorta: implications for dissecting aortic aneurysm. Am J Cardiol. 1977;39:13–20.
8. Peterss S, Mansour AM, Ross JA, et al. Changing pathology of the thoracic aorta from acute to chronic dissection: literature review and insights. J Am Coll Cardiol. 2016;68:1054–65.
9. Criado FJ. Aortic dissection: a 250-year perspective. Tex Heart Inst J. 2011;38:694–700.
10. Froehlich W, Tolenaar JL, Harris KM, et al. Delay from diagnosis to surgery in transferred type A aortic dissection. Am J Med. 2018;131:300–6.
11. Harris KM, Strauss CE, Eagle KA, et al. Correlates of delayed recognition and treatment of acute type A aortic dissection: the International Registry of Acute Aortic Dissection (IRAD). Circulation. 2011;124:1911–8.
12. Kumar N, Venkatraman A, Pandey A, Khera R, Garg N. Weekend hospitalizations for acute aortic dissection have a higher risk of in-hospital mortality compared to weekday hospitalizations. Int J Cardiol. 2016;214:448–50.
13. Andersen ND, Ganapathi AM, Hanna JM, Williams JB, Gaca JG, Hughes GC. Outcomes of acute type a dissection repair before and after implementation of a multidisciplinary thoracic aortic surgery program. J Am Coll Cardiol. 2014;63:1796–803.
14. Bonser RS, Ranasinghe AM, Loubani M, et al. Evidence, lack of evidence, controversy, and debate in the provision and performance of the surgery of acute type A aortic dissection. J Am Coll Cardiol. 2011;58:2455–74.
15. Fukuda I, Imazuru T. Intentional delay of surgery for acute type A dissection with stroke. J Thorac Cardiovasc Surg. 2003;126:290–1.
16. Estrera AL, Safi HJ. Acute type A aortic dissection: surgical intervention for all: PRO. Cardiol Clin. 2010;28:317–23.
17. Bavaria JE, Brinster DR, Gorman RC, Woo YJ, Gleason T, Pochettino A. Advances in the treatment of acute type A dissection: an integrated approach. Ann Thorac Surg. 2002;74:S1848–52; Discussion S1857–63.
18. Hamad R, Amr G, Demers P. Delayed surgery in patients with acute type A aortic dissection who are receiving novel oral anticoagulants. J Thorac Cardiovasc Surg. 2018;155:e1–4.
19. Tanaka K, Teruo T, Sasaki K, et al. Medical vs surgical treatment of acute aortic dissection in an intensive care unit. Jpn Circ J. 1991;55:815–20.
20. Hashimoto A, Kimata S, Hosoda S. Acute aortic dissection. A comparison between the results of medical and surgical treatments. Jpn Circ J. 1991;55:821–3.
21. Feldman M, Shah M, Elefteriades JA. Medical management of acute type A aortic dissection. Ann Thorac Cardiovasc Surg. 2009;15:286–93.
22. Dumfarth J, Peterss S, Luehr M, et al. Acute type A dissection in octogenarians: does emergency surgery impact in-hospital outcome or long-term survival? Eur J Cardiothorac Surg. 2017;51:472–7.

23. Borger MA, Fedak PWM, Stephens EH, et al. The American Association for Thoracic Surgery consensus guidelines on bicuspid aortic valve-related aortopathy: Full online-only version. J Thorac Cardiovasc Surg. 2018;156:e41–74.
24. Myrmel T, Lai DT, Miller DC. Can the principles of evidence-based medicine be applied to the treatment of aortic dissections? Eur J Cardiothorac Surg. 2004;25:236–42. Discussion 242–35
25. Scholl FG, Coady MA, Davies R, et al. Interval or permanent nonoperative management of acute type A aortic dissection. Arch Surg. 1999;134:402–5. Discussion 405–6
26. Bin Mahmood SU, Mori M, Luo J, et al. Rapid diagnosis and treatment of patients with acute type A aortic dissection and malperfusion syndrome may normalize survival to that of patients with uncomplicated type A aortic dissection. AORTA (Stamford). 2019;7:42–8.
27. Deeb GM, Williams DM, Bolling SF, et al. Surgical delay for acute type A dissection with malperfusion. Ann Thorac Surg. 1997;64:1669–75. Discussion 1675–7
28. Yagdi T, Atay Y, Engin C, et al. Impact of organ malperfusion on mortality and morbidity in acute type A aortic dissections. J Card Surg. 2006;21:363–9.
29. Sanz J, Einstein AJ, Fuster V. Acute aortic dissection: anti-impulse therapy. In: Elefteriades JA, editor. Acute aortic disease. New York: Informa Healthcare; 2007. p. 229–48.

Anesthetic Management of Acute Aortic Dissection

Michael Tien and Albert T. Cheung

Introduction

Acute aortic dissection is a life-threatening condition associated with mortality rates that approach 30% depending on the location, extent, and complications of the dissection [1]. Recent advances in disease awareness, diagnosis, surgical and endovascular repair technique, anesthetic management, perioperative care, and risk stratification have reduced mortality rates to 20% or less [2, 3]. Emergency surgical repair of acute dissections involving the ascending aorta is necessary to prevent acute life-threatening complications that include branch-vessel malperfusion, cardiac tamponade, and aortic regurgitation. Acute dissections involving the descending thoracic aorta require emergent operation for rupture, end-organ malperfusion, or limb ischemia. The perioperative and anesthetic management of patients with aortic dissection is important for improving outcomes by detecting complications related to the dissection, pharmacologically controlling arterial blood pressure and heart rate, expediting transport to the operating room, using intraoperative transesophageal echocardiography (TEE) to verify the diagnosis and characterize the dissection, ensuring end-organs are protected during circulatory arrest, treating blood loss and coagulopathies, and correcting the postoperative metabolic derangements as a consequence of the operation.

M. Tien · A. T. Cheung (✉)
Department of Anesthesiology, Perioperative and Pain Medicine, Stanford University School of Medicine, Stanford, CA, USA
e-mail: ATCheung@stanford.edu

J. S. Coselli et al. (eds.), *Aortic Dissection and Acute Aortic Syndromes*,
https://doi.org/10.1007/978-3-030-66668-2_38

Preoperative Management

Once the decision is made that a patient with a presumed or established acute aortic dissection requires open surgical or endovascular repair, the anesthesiologist and operating room staff should be immediately notified. Safely expediting transfer of the patient to the operating room or interventional suite has the potential to affect outcome because early mortality increases over time. Important information to convey to the accepting team includes an estimate of the timing of patient arrival, the likelihood that the diagnosis has been established, the planned surgical intervention upon verification of the diagnosis, the medical condition of the patient, the type and location of vascular access, and the medications being administered by intravenous infusion (Table 1).

Table 1 Preoperative information for direct admission to the operating room in acute aortic dissection

1. Presumed or Established Diagnosis of Aortic Dissection
(a) Pre-admission imaging studies: CTA, MRI, echocardiogram, CXR
(b) Need to verify diagnosis by TEE
(c) Planned surgical or endovascular intervention
2. Classification of Aortic Dissection
(a) Stanford Classification
I Type A: Involves the ascending aorta
II Type B: Confined to the descending aorta
3. Medical Condition of the Patient
(a) Spontaneously breathing
(b) Required endotracheal intubation and mechanical ventilatory support
(c) Laboratory test results
(d) Penn Classification
I Penn class a: No malperfusion or circulatory instability
II Penn class b: presence of malperfusion
III Penn Class c: Presence of circulatory shock
IV Penn Class b+c: Presence of both malperfusion and circulatory shock
4. Medical treatment
(a) Vascular access and sites
I Arterial catheter
II Peripheral venous catheters
III Central venous catheters
(b) Medications
I Vasopressor infusions
II Vasodilator infusions
III Beta-blockers
IV Sedatives
V Narcotic analgesics

Abbreviations: CTA, computed tomographic angiography; CXR, chest roentgenogram; MRI, magnetic resonance imaging; TEE, transesophageal echocardiography

History and Physical Exam

The history and physical examination can usually be performed simultaneously with the review of pre-admission medical records, imaging studies, and laboratory testing by assigning specific tasks to selected members of the admitting team. At the same time, transfer of care from the transport team is systematically accomplished by transitioning physiologic monitors, intravenous lines, and medications to equipment that will be used in the operating room. Consent for surgery and anesthesia can then be obtained once a decision is made to proceed with operation.

The focus of the history and physical is to confirm the diagnosis and to detect evidence of malperfusion or circulatory compromise. The classic signs and symptoms of acute aortic dissection include severe, sharp or tearing pain in the chest, back, or abdomen [1, 4]. Evidence of malperfusion may include the presence of variation in pulse amplitude or a pulse deficit in one extremity. New focal neurological deficits, altered mental status, or syncope may indicate cerebral malperfusion due to involvement of the aortic arch branch vessels or carotid arteries. Nausea, melena, or abdominal tenderness may indicate mesenteric ischemia. Spinal cord ischemia may manifest as new onset lower extremity weakness or paraplegia.

Circulatory compromise and the potential for cardiovascular collapse or circulatory shock should be suspected in patients with cardiac tamponade from rupture of the ascending aorta into the pericardium, acute aortic regurgitation from extension of the dissection into the aortic root, right or left ventricular failure from coronary artery malperfusion, or hypovolemia from rupture of the descending aorta into the pleural space [5, 6]. Venous congestion, dyspnea, tachypnea, tachycardia, ischemic changes in the electrocardiogram, hypoxemia, asymmetric breath sounds, rales, diastolic murmur, pulsus paradoxus, pulmonary edema on the chest roentgenogram, or the presence of hemothorax or significant pleural effusions may all indicate impending cardiovascular collapse. In these patients, beta-blocker therapy could worsen the condition and antihypertensive drugs should be discontinued upon the induction of general anesthesia to prevent severe hypotension.

The history and physical should also elicit the presence of coexisting diseases or conditions that may affect anesthetic and surgical management. For instance, atherosclerotic and peripheral vascular disease may increase the risk of thromboembolic complications. Clinically significant carotid artery disease increases the risk of stroke and cerebral malperfusion. Severe, longstanding hypertension in combination with occlusive vascular disease may alter cerebral and end-organ blood flow autoregulation and require maintaining a higher mean arterial blood pressure during cardiopulmonary bypass (CPB) to maintain cerebral and renal perfusion. The presence of pre-existing chronic renal disease, ischemic heart disease, cardiomyopathy, pulmonary disease, or liver disease also impacts outcome and convalescence after operative repair. Some patients presenting with acute aortic dissections may also have hereditary or genetic aortic syndromes such as bicuspid aortic valves, Loeys-Deitz syndrome, Ehlers-Danlos syndrome, or Marfan's syndrome and their corresponding medical problems.

Finally, large aortic aneurysms, dissections, or hematomas can compress the right ventricular outflow tract, right pulmonary artery, trachea, or left mainstem

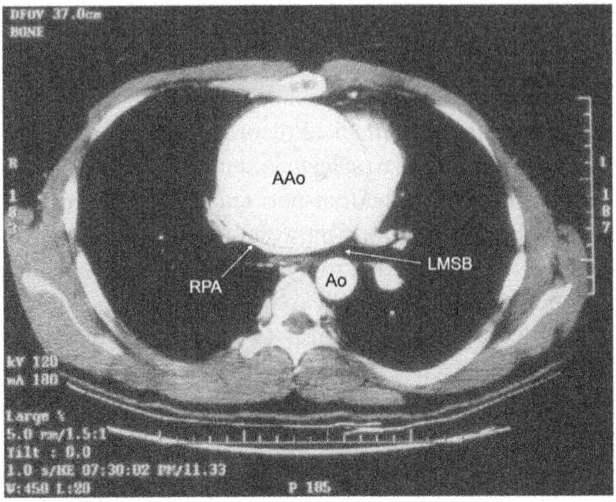

Fig. 1 Computed tomorgraphic angiography (CTA) axial cross section at the level of the tracheal carina in a patient with a dilated ascending aorta (AAo) causing simultaneous compression of the pulmonary artery and airway that places the patient at risk of respiratory failure from airway obstruction, hypoxemia from ventilation/perfusion mismatching from obstruction of the right pulmonary artery (RPA) together with the left mainstem bronchus (LMSB), and heart failure from right ventricular outflow tract obstruction in response to the induction of general anesthesia

bronchus, which may contribute to hemodynamic or airway compromise during the induction of general anesthesia (Fig. 1) [7–10]. These structural complications can be anticipated by careful review of the pre-admission imaging studies.

The Importance of Classification

There are three widely used classification schemes in the management of patients with acute aortic dissection. The DeBakey classification and the Stanford classification schemes characterize aortic dissections according to anatomic location and extent [11, 12]. The DeBakey classification was originally used to determine the surgical approach and operative repair: Type I (involving the ascending aorta, arch, and descending thoracic aorta), Type II (confined to the ascending aorta), Type IIIa (involving the descending thoracic aorta up to the celiac artery), and Type IIIb (involving the descending thoracic aorta and the abdominal aorta) [11]. The Stanford classification demonstrated that patients with Type A dissections involving the ascending aorta had better outcomes in response to emergency surgical repair, but that outcomes were similar between surgery and conservative medical management among patients with Type B dissections that were confined to the descending aorta [12]. The interim development and refinement of endovascular procedures has provided additional interventional options for the management of patients with Stanford type B aortic dissections, selected patients with Stanford Type A aortic dissections, and as an adjunct to open surgical repair [1].

The Penn classification for acute aortic dissection was originally developed to supplement the Stanford classification to explain the heterogeneity of surgical outcomes by risk-stratifying patients based on their ischemic pattern or circulatory condition at the time of presentation [13]. In patients undergoing surgical treatment for acute Stanford Type A aortic dissections, the Penn classification improved outcome prediction based on presence or absence of branch-vessel malperfusion, circulatory collapse, or both [13, 14]. Patients are classified as Penn class a if there is no evidence of malperfusion or circulatory collapse, Penn class b if there is branch-vessel malperfusion (i.e. stroke, paraplegia, pulse deficits, acute kidney injury, mesenteric ischemia, etc.), Penn class c if there is circulatory collapse (i.e., left or right ventricular dysfunction, pericardial tamponade, acute coronary ischemia, myocardial infarction, etc.), and Penn class b+c if there is both branch-vessel malperfusion and circulatory collapse [13]. A recent study demonstrated that the Penn classification was also effective for predicting outcome among patients with acute Stanford Type B aortic dissections [3]. Because the Penn classification identifies patients with life-threatening pathophysiological complications of acute aortic dissection that affects the surgical, intraoperative, and postoperative management, it is of particular importance to the anesthesiologist.

Diagnostic Imaging

The diagnosis of aortic dissection may be suspected based on the presence of high-risk clinical features, but confirmatory cardiovascular imaging is necessary to establish the diagnosis of aortic dissection and characterize its location and extent. Increased awareness for aortic dissection and the wide availability of computed tomographic (CT) imaging has increased the rate of detection of acute aortic dissections. Although different imaging modalities can be used to diagnose aortic dissection, the sensitivity, specificity, and information provided by the tests may vary depending on the quality of the study, the experience of the physician interpreting the study, and the presence of atypical features of aortic dissection [15–17]. CT and CT angiography (CTA) are the most common initial studies used to diagnose aortic dissection. If the CT scan is not diagnostic, or the diagnosis cannot be confirmed because of imaging artifacts, the patient can still be directly admitted to the operating room and the diagnosis verified using intraoperative TEE before proceeding with operation. Although TEE cannot completely image the distal ascending aorta and aortic arch, it can reliably diagnose Stanford Type A aortic dissection with involvement of the ascending aorta. In addition, TEE provides valuable information on the presence of aortic regurgitation, physiologic evidence of cardiac tamponade, and the presence or severity of right or left ventricular dysfunction. Ultrasound and Doppler imaging can also be applied in the operating room to detect extension of the aortic dissection into the carotid arteries (Fig. 2).

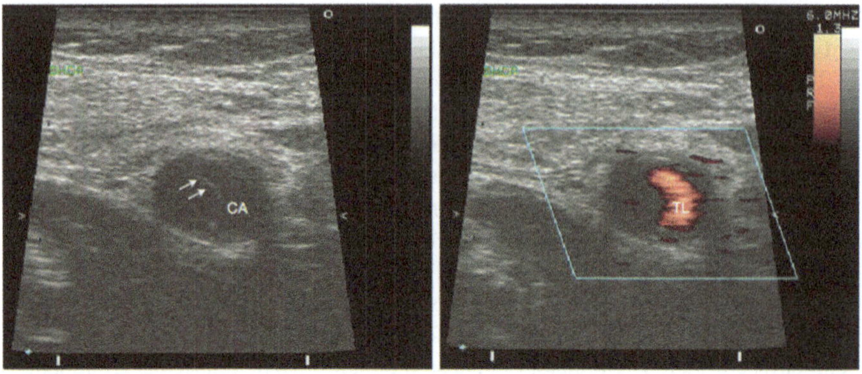

Fig. 2 Intraoperative Duplex imaging of the right common carotid artery (CA) in short-axis demonstrating extension of the dissection into the carotid artery in a patient with an acute Stanford type A aortic dissection. Two dimensional ultrasound imaging of the carotid artery (left panel) demonstrates the presence of an intimal flap (arrows) within the lumen of the artery. Color flow imaging (right panel) demonstrated blood flow in the true lumen (TL) with the onset of cardiopulmonary bypass

Intraoperative Management

Intraoperative Physiologic Monitoring and Setup

In addition to standard basic physiologic monitoring recommended by the American Society of Anesthesiologists (ASA), patients undergoing repair of aortic dissections benefit from a full spectrum of invasive and noninvasive physiologic monitors for intraoperative and postoperative management. This should ideally include an intra-arterial catheter, central venous catheter, pulmonary artery catheter, and TEE. However, if the patient is in extremis, the potential risks and benefits of spending additional time to secure central venous access or invasive monitoring modalities should be weighed against the need for emergent surgical intervention.

An intraarterial catheter is required for continuous blood pressure measurement, analysis of respiratory variation in the arterial pressure waveform, and frequent blood sampling for intraoperative laboratory testing. The arterial catheter should ideally be placed prior to induction of general anesthesia. The choice of site for arterial pressure monitoring is important in patients with aortic dissection. If there is a pulse deficit or limb ischemia, placement of the arterial catheter in an unaffected limb will provide the best estimate of central aortic pressures. If axillary artery cannulation or perfusion is planned, an intraarterial catheter in the ipsilateral arm will not provide measurements when the axillary artery is temporarily occluded while it is surgically accessed, and may overestimate systemic arterial blood pressures during cardiopulmonary bypass (CPB) when the axillary artery is perfused. An arterial catheter in the contralateral arm or femoral artery provides the best estimation of systemic arterial blood pressures during CPB with axillary artery perfusion, but cannot measure cerebral perfusion pressure during selective antegrade cerebral perfusion. For endovascular or open repair of Stanford Type B aortic dissections with involvement near the origin of the left subclavian artery, placement of the arterial catheter in the right arm will provide continuous arterial pressure monitoring in the event that the left subclavian artery has to be clamped or excluded. If feasible, the ability to secure intraarterial catheters in both upper extremities and a femoral artery provides useful information, vascular access, and redundancy if one of the arterial blood pressure monitoring sites fails to function or provide accurate measurements during operation.

A pulmonary artery catheter provides continuous measurements of the central venous pressure, pulmonary artery pressure, cardiac output, and mixed venous oxygen saturation throughout the operation and into the postoperative period. This information is valuable for guiding intraoperative resuscitation with fluids and blood products, and titrating inotropic and vasoactive medications, especially in the setting of acute aortic dissections when the condition of the patient can fluctuate quickly and unpredictably. The pulmonary artery catheter also provides critical information to guide postoperative management in the intensive care unit to enable precise fluid management and assist in the rapid diagnosis of complications such as postoperative bleeding, cardiac tamponade, pulmonary edema, or ventricular failure. In addition to physiologic measurements, the pulmonary artery catheter in combination with its vascular introducer sheath provides central intravenous access for the administration of vasoactive medications and infusions together with a site for the rapid administration of fluids and blood products to respond to hypovolemia or hemorrhage.

Temperature monitoring is important for the safe conduct of deliberate hypothermia, selective antegrade cerebral perfusion (SACP), and deep hypothermic circulatory arrest (DHCA). A temperature probe in the nasopharynx provides the most accurate reflection of brain temperature. Specially designed temperature probes placed in the ear canals can also be used to measure the temperature near the tympanic membranes and are also often used to estimate brain temperature. An esophageal temperature probe or thermistor at the tip of the pulmonary artery catheter accurately measures central blood temperature but is not accurate during CPB when there is no pulmonary blood flow or during cardioplegia when topical ice is applied to the pericardium adjacent to the esophagus. A temperature probe at the tip of the urinary catheter provides a measurement of the bladder temperature that correlates with blood temperature if urinary output is brisk, but values may lag behind changes in blood temperature if the patient is oliguric or anuric. A rectal temperature probe can also be used to estimate core temperature, but takes time to equilibrate. In addition, the temperature of the blood entering the CPB circuit through the venous cannula and the temperature of the blood exiting the membrane oxygenator and heat exchanger of the CPB circuit can be measured directly. Information from temperature monitoring at multiple sites is integrated to guide cooling for deliberate hypothermia, establish the target endpoint for the initiation of DHCA or SACP, guide the rate of active rewarming to prevent hyperthermia during reperfusion, and estimate the systemic temperature that will be achieved at equilibrium after rewarming on CPB to prevent hypothermia in the postoperative period.

Brain function monitors are available to indirectly evaluate and monitor brain activity and perfusion during general anesthesia and CPB. Full montage electroencephalography (EEG) monitoring can be used for the early detection of cerebral hypoperfusion. EEG can be used to detect the characteristic pattern in response to deliberate hypothermia, and the onset of electrocortical silence has been used as a physiologic endpoint for the safe initiation of DHCA [18]. Commercially available instruments to measure processed EEG and provide a value such as the bispectral index (BIS) or patient state index (PSI) are commonly used to quantify the depth of general anesthesia, but also reflect changes associated with hypothermia. These monitors are widely available, easy to use and interpret, performed using sensors applied as an adhesive patch onto the scalp, do not require specialized personnel, and can be quickly implemented in an emergency setting. However, no direct comparisons with full montage EEG have been performed to determine their sensitivity and specificity for the detection of hypoperfusion or electrocortical silence.

Near-infrared spectroscopy (NIRS) cerebral oximetry can be utilized to continuously monitor cerebral regional oxygen saturation (rSO_2) in the right and left bilateral frontal cortices to evaluate cerebral perfusion during CPB. In the setting of acute aortic dissection, NIRS may improve the ability to detect cerebral hypoperfusion. In addition to detecting global cerebral hypoperfusion, NIRS may detect contralateral cerebral hypoperfusion due to an incomplete Circle of Willis during unilateral SACP. Asymmetry in the NIRS values during unilateral SACP can be used to prompt surgical interventions to augment perfusion to the contralateral hemisphere or to cannulate and directly perfuse the contralateral carotid artery. In addition to cerebral perfusion, the rSO_2 values obtained by NIRS monitoring also provides an indirect indicator of the mixed venous oxygen saturation, and can indicate hypoxemia, hypovolemia, anemia, venous congestion, or low cardiac output. Simultaneous EEG and NIRS monitoring may be useful for determining the physiologic consequences of reductions in the rSO_2 values on brain electrical activity. This approach can be useful for hybrid open and endovascular aortic arch repairs that require temporary serial occlusion of the innominate and left carotid arteries.

Neurophysiologic monitoring of central nervous system and spinal cord function with somatosensory evoked potentials (SSEP) and motor evoked potentials (MEP) can be performed during operations under general anesthesia, but requires specialized equipment and personnel. Intraoperative SSEP and MEP monitoring has been used to detect spinal cord ischemia and stroke during cardiac and major thoracic aortic operations [19, 20].

Intraoperative TEE

The clinical application of intraoperative TEE together with increasing expertise in its use and refinements in the imaging platform have represented a major advancement in the perioperative management of acute aortic dissection. Guideline statements from the American Heart Association, American Society of Anesthesiology, and the Society of Cardiovascular Anesthesiologists recommend the routine use of intraoperative TEE for acute aortic dissection [15, 20]. The TEE probe can be inserted immediately after the induction of general anesthesia and images analyzed to confirm the diagnosis of acute aortic dissection and evaluate for evolution of the disease in comparison to pre-admission studies prior to the start of operation. TEE can provide useful information about the location of intimal tear, extent of the dissection, or the presence of aortic regurgitation to guide surgical repair. TEE also provides both structural and physiologic information on the presence and severity of pericardial effusions, right and left ventricular size and function, evidence of myocardial ischemia, and co-existing structural heart disease.

TEE is also useful in guiding the management of CPB. TEE can be used to guide central aortic cannulation for CPB, and establish that the true lumen is perfused during CPB (Fig. 3). The true lumen of the aorta is typically smaller in diameter, is in continuity with the aortic valve, expands during systole, and has rounded borders due to the continuity of the intimal layer. The false lumen of the aorta is typically larger, crescent-shaped, with sharp edges at the site where the intimal flap separates from the adventitia. The false lumen may contain thrombus or hematoma. The TEE examination can be combined with images from the CTA to verify and distinguish the true lumen from the false lumen of the aorta. After initiation of CPB, TEE can be used to detect left ventricular distention if there is aortic regurgitation. Prior to separation from CPB, TEE is used to guide the evacuation of intracardiac air in the left atrium, left ventricle, and aorta. After aortic valve repair or resuspension, TEE can detect and quantify the severity of any residual aortic regurgitation. TEE can also be used to evaluate left ventricular and right ventricular function to verify that coronary blood flow has been properly restored after aortic root replacement. Coronary artery insufficiency or malperfusion will appear immediately on the TEE examination as right ventricular failure or segmental left ventricular wall motion abnormalities corresponding to the territories supplied by the affected coronary arteries.

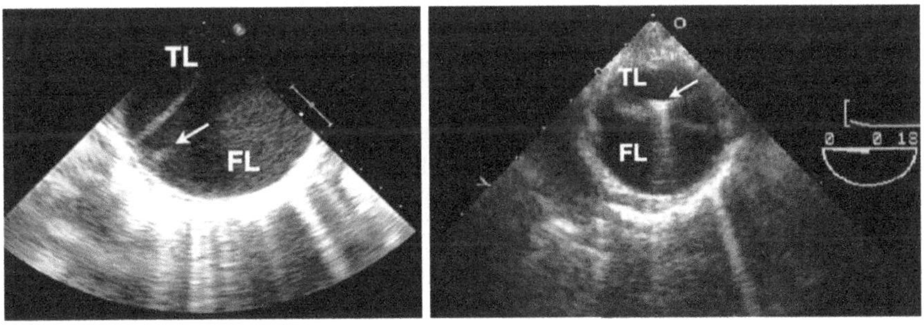

Fig. 3 During central aortic cannulation using the Seldinger technique in a patient with aortic dissection, intraoperative transesophageal echocardiography (TEE) imaging of the proximal descending thoracic aorta demonstrated that the guidewire was in the false lumen (FL) of the dissected aorta (left panel). TEE guidance was used to reposition the guidewire into the true lumen (TL) of the aorta (right panel) before insertion of the arterial cannula to prevent cerebral malperfusion upon initiation of cardiopulmonary bypass

General Anesthesia in Patients with Acute Aortic Dissection

Induction of general anesthesia for patients with acute aortic dissection requires attention to the usual concerns for emergency operations in addition to specific concerns related to the aortic dissection. Rapid sequence induction and tracheal intubation with cricoid pressure is normally performed for patients with a full stomach and increased risk of aspiration of gastric contents. However, the risks associated with hemodynamic instability as a consequence of a precipitous induction should be weighed against the risk of gastric aspiration. Increased blood pressure in response to tracheal intubation due to inadequate analgesia or failure to attenuate sympathetic nervous system response could increase the risk of aortic rupture or extension of the dissection. Anesthetic or narcotic analgesics administered in combination with intravenous antihypertensive agents may precipitate severe hypotension or circulatory shock upon induction of general anesthesia in patients with cardiac tamponade, acute aortic regurgitation, heart failure, or who are dependent on endogenous sympathetic tone to maintain hemodynamic function. For these reasons, it is important to anticipate the hemodynamic responses to the anesthetic drugs used to induce general anesthesia and be prepared to intervene immediately to maintain cardiovascular stability. Usual strategies include the discontinuation of intravenous vasodilator therapy prior to the induction of general anesthesia in anticipation of hypotension caused by the direct action of the anesthetic drugs and the attenuation of sympathetic nervous system tone. In patients with poorly controlled hypertension, anesthetic drugs and narcotics may need to be supplemented with beta-blockers or intravenous vasodilator therapy to attenuate the heightened sympathetic response to tracheal intubation. In patients at risk for circulatory shock due to cardiac tamponade, aortic regurgitation, or heart failure, anesthetic drugs that have minimal direct actions on the cardiovascular system and cause less attenuation of the sympathetic nervous system (i.e., ketamine or etomidate) can be administered together with the immediate availability of inotropes and vasopressors if necessary. In the case of cardiac tamponade, the anesthesiologist must also be prepared to immediately treat hypertension upon opening of the pericardium to prevent aortic rupture when the arterial pressure acutely increases. Although consensus guidelines recommend the early use of beta-blocker therapy to treat acute aortic dissection, tachycardia in a patient with acute aortic dissection may also indicate cardiovascular instability and impending shock due to cardiac tamponade, aortic regurgitation, or heart failure. In patients with tachycardia due to cardiovascular instability, beta-blockers should be used with caution or avoided altogether due to concerns for precipitating cardiogenic shock.

Maintenance of general anesthesia is achieved usually with a combination of inhaled anesthetic agents, narcotic analgesics, intravenous sedative hypnotic agents, and neuromuscular blocking agents. Processed EEG with anesthetic depth monitoring can be useful to maintain a consistent level of anesthetic depth for prolonged operations that involve the use of deliberate hypothermia. Continuous infusion of narcotic analgesics and sedative hypnotic agents may be useful to maintain therapeutic drug concentrations in prolonged operations that involve CPB. It is also important to note that anesthetic requirements decrease in response to deliberate hypothermia and that anesthetic drug-induced EEG suppression should not be considered equivalent to hypothermia-induced metabolic suppression of the brain when determining adequate conditions for brain protection for hypothermic circulatory arrest. When intraoperative neurophysiologic monitoring with SSEP is used, the dose of inhaled anesthetic agent is maintained constant by monitoring the concentration of the volatile anesthetic in the expired gases together with maintaining complete neuromuscular blockade to optimize the recording of the SSEPs and minimize anesthetic-induced changes in the amplitude or latency of the evoked potentials. In contrast, when intraoperative MEP monitoring is used, neuromuscular blocking agents and inhaled anesthetic agents are avoided altogether and anesthesia is maintained with intravenous narcotics and sedatives to maintain the fidelity of the MEPs.

The anesthetic regimen is also typically designed to last into the early postoperative period to permit a controlled and gradual emergence from anesthesia in the intensive care unit while the patient remains on mechanical ventilatory support. This can usually be accomplished with continuous infusions of sedative hypnotic agents or narcotic analgesics such as propofol, dexmedetomidine, or fentanyl. Dexmedetomidine has the advantage that it provides sedation and attenuates sympathetic nervous system tone without suppressing respiration. Contemporary practice favors the avoidance of long acting benzodiazepines, particularly among older patients, because they may contribute to postoperative confusion or delirium.

The surgical management of patients requiring open repair for Stanford Type B dissections involving the descending thoracic aorta that are not amenable to endovascular repair requires a left thoracotomy. For these cases, one-lung ventilation is required to facilitate surgical exposure. Lung isolation and selective ventilation of either the right or left lung can be achieved with placement of a double-lumen endotracheal or endobronchial tube. Alternatively, a bronchial blocker can be positioned in the left mainstem bronchus through a standard endotracheal tube to selectively ventilate only the right lung. The advantage of the double-lumen endotracheal tube is the ability to quickly deflate or re-expand the left lung as needed throughout the operation. However, it can sometimes be difficult to position correctly if the descending aorta distorts the left mainstem bronchus. Additionally, the double-lumen endotracheal tube must eventually be exchanged to a single-lumen endotracheal tube at the end of the operation to facilitate postoperative mechanical ventilatory support in the intensive care unit.

Cerebral Protection

Surgical repairs of the distal ascending aorta or aortic arch require temporary cessation of cerebral and systemic blood flow or a period of circulatory arrest. The primary technique that has been consistently demonstrated to provide ischemic protection to the brain and other organs during a period of circulatory arrest is deliberate hypothermia. In contemporary practice, deliberate hypothermia is often used alone or in combination with SACP or retrograde cerebral perfusion (RCP) depending on surgeon and institutional expertise or preferences [15]. The original physiologic rationale for the application of deliberate hypothermia for ischemic protection was that the ischemic tolerance of the brain could be increased proportionally to the reduction of the cerebral metabolic rate caused by hypothermia. In response to hypothermia, cerebral oxygen consumption decreases by a factor of 2.3 for every 10 °C decrease in body temperature [21, 22]. Assuming an ischemic tolerance of 4 to 5 minutes at normothermia, the reduction in metabolic rate achieved at a temperature between 14 and 18 °C would provide a safe ischemic time for circulatory arrest of between 20 and 30 min (Fig. 4) [21, 22]. In actual clinical practice, this approach has been successful, but the protective effects of hypothermia likely extend beyond its sole actions on the cerebral metabolic rate.

Despite being widely implemented, there is no consensus or definitive evidence to dictate the optimal temperature for the conduct of DHCA, the ideal site to estimate brain temperature as a target for the initiation of circulatory arrest, the safe duration of circulatory arrest, or the degree of hypothermia necessary for protection when SACP or RCP is used in conjunction with hypothermia. A meta-analysis performed on existing published studies did not demonstrate any differences in outcomes between the use of DHCA alone or in combination with RCP or SACP [23]. However, clinical practice consistently demonstrates that the risk of neurologic injury increases with increasing duration of circulatory arrest, particularly when extending beyond 30–45 min without perfusion. DHCA lasting longer than 45 min has been shown to be associated with increased incidence of postoperative neurological complications such as seizures, neurologic deficits, and stroke [24, 25]. If cerebral perfusion is supplemented by SACP, the duration of circulatory arrest can be safely extended even at temperatures in the range of 28 °C [23, 26, 27]. Deliberate hypothermia is primarily achieved by actively cooling the blood through the heat exchanger of the CPB circuit. Application of ice to the surface of the scalp has been commonly used as an adjunct to achieve and maintain cerebral hypothermia, but its effectiveness has not been proven. RCP may assist in maintaining cerebral hypothermia, provide some degree of

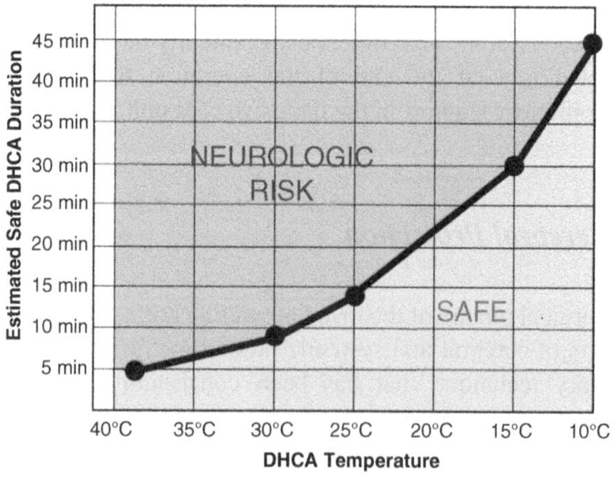

Fig. 4 Estimated "safe" duration of deep hypothermic circulatory arrest (DHCA) for operations on the aortic arch corresponding to brain temperature in adults based on clinical experience and a Q_{10} ratio of 2.3 (cerebral oxygen consumption ratio of 2.3 for a 10 °C difference in brain temperature)

metabolic substrate delivery during circulatory arrest and also serve to flush embolic material from the arterial circulation prior to the restoration of antegrade cerebral perfusion. In addition, adjuvant pharmacologic neuroprotective drugs such as glucocorticoids, barbiturates, propofol, ketamine, mannitol, furosemide, lidocaine, or magnesium are commonly administered in combination with hypothermia, but the effectiveness of pharmacologic adjuncts for neuroprotection have not been proven [15].

In addition to providing controlled deliberate hypothermia, consensus recommendations support a controlled and gradual rewarming rate with the avoidance of hyperthermia during reperfusion [15]. There may also be a protective benefit to a period of hypothermic reperfusion prior to initiation of rewarming [28]. Rewarming should be carried out gradually, with a temperature gradient no greater than 10 °C maintained between the venous inlet and arterial outlet of the CPB circuit. When the patient temperature reaches 30 °C, this gradient should be no more than 4 °C. It is important that the rewarming process occur slowly at ≤0.5 °C/min with the arterial outlet temperature less than 36.5 °C, and keeping the nasopharyngeal or tympanic membrane temperature less than 37 °C to decrease the risk of cerebral hyperthermia [29, 30]. Cerebral hyperthermia has been shown to have detrimental effects on postoperative neurocognitive outcomes by exacerbating ischemia-reperfusion neurologic injury [31, 32]. In addition, attention to maintain arterial perfusion pressure and ensure adequate venous drainage during CPB can prevent cerebral hypoperfusion caused by arterial hypotension or venous hypertension.

Because the temperature of the brain cannot be measured directly, a variety of approaches have been attempted to ensure the target conditions for brain hypothermia have been achieved prior to the initiation of circulatory arrest. In addition to estimating the brain temperature using nasopharyngeal, tympanic, blood, and bladder temperature probes, the EEG can also be used as a physiologic surrogate for the effects of hypothermia on the brain. The average nasopharyngeal temperature for electrocortical silence by EEG is 18 °C, but cooling to a target nasopharyngeal temperature of approximately 12.5 °C is necessary to ensure electrocortical silence in 99.5% of patients when EEG is not available [18, 33]. When using EEG changes as a target for the delivery of hypothermia, it is important to discontinue inhaled anesthetics and avoid the administration of propofol or barbiturates until conditions for circulatory arrest have been achieved since these drugs cause suppression of the EEG independently of the effects of hypothermia. Alternatively, one study has even reported the use of jugular bulb oxygen saturation measurements as a method to track the reduction of cerebral metabolic rate in response to deliberate hypothermia and employed a jugular bulb venous oxygen saturation of 90% as an target for the initiation of circulatory arrest [34].

Perfusion Management

Specific perfusion techniques have been developed and utilized to provide systemic perfusion and selective perfusion to the brain for operations on the aortic arch that are important for cerebral protection. A meta-analysis of published studies has indicated that central cannulation for CPB was superior to peripheral cannulation with regards to mortality and neurologic injury in aortic surgery [35]. Central cannulation and perfusion can be achieved by direct cannulation of the true lumen of the dissected aorta after sternotomy, direct cannulation of the innominate artery, or through a branched graft to an axillary artery. The advantages of central cannulation include decreasing the risk of cerebral thromboembolism by avoiding retrograde arterial blood flow to the brain through a diseased aorta, decreased risk of perfusing the aorta through the false lumen, and decreased risk of the intimal flap occluding the aortic arch branch vessels with the onset of extracorporeal circulation.

RCP was a technique developed to improve the safety of DHCA and potentially prolong the safe duration of circulatory arrest to the brain. To implement RCP, a venous cannula is inserted into the superior vena cava and snared between the right atrium and the azygous vein. Upon initiating circulatory arrest after achieving deliberate hypothermia, cold oxygenated blood can be perfused in a retrograde fashion into the superior vena cava cannula at a rate of 150–250 mL/min. During RCP, the patient is positioned in approximately 10° Trendelenburg to decrease the risk of cerebral arterial air embolism. Superior vena cava pressures should be continuously monitored via the side port of an introducer sheath in the internal jugular vein and maintained below 25–30 mm Hg to prevent cerebral edema. It is important to note that existing studies have demonstrated that RCP does not fulfill the metabolic demands of the brain even in the presence of deep hypothermia and cannot be used indefinitely to prevent neuronal ischemia [36, 37]. Proponents of RCP believe that the technique is simple to perform, avoids instrumentation of the aortic arch branch vessels, helps to maintain cerebral hypothermia after antegrade perfusion is discontinued, provides some degree of metabolic substrate delivery to the brain to prevent neuronal ischemia during circulatory arrest, and provides a mechanism to flush out thromboembolic material in the arterial circulation before resuming antegrade cerebral perfusion.

SACP is becoming the most widely used perfusion technique for brain protection during aortic arch operations. Advantages of SACP include the ability to provide complete metabolic substrate delivery to the brain to extend the safe duration of circulatory arrest necessary to complete complex aortic arch or extended arch reconstruction and the ability to selectively provide deep hypothermia to the brain while maintaining higher core systemic temperatures in the range of 22–28 °C to reduce the duration on CPB necessary to achieve hypothermia and the subsequent time required for rewarming. SACP is performed by perfusing the brain using oxygenated blood at 10–12 °C from the CPB circuit via cannulation of the axillary artery, innominate artery, or direct cannulation of the aortic arch branch vessels. In unilateral SACP through the right axillary artery, the base of the innominate artery is clamped to direct the oxygenated blood into the right carotid and vertebral arteries. Blood flow to the contralateral side of the brain is provided by collateral circulation via the Circle of Willis. Flow rates for selective antegrade cerebral perfusion are typically 5–7 mL/kg/min to achieve a mean arterial blood pressure of 60–70 mm Hg measured in the ipsilateral radial artery. The adequacy of cerebral perfusion and oxygenation can be monitored with continuous or processed EEG in combination with cerebral oximetry. Acute decreases in rSO_2 or the attenuation of EEG amplitude may indicate suboptimal positioning of perfusing cannula. Asymmetrical decreases in the EEG amplitude or rSO_2 values on the contralateral side of the brain may indicate inadequate collateral circulation. Perfusion to the contralateral side of the brain can be augmented during unilateral SACP by increasing blood flow, increasing the perfusion pressure, or clamping the base of the contralateral carotid and subclavian arteries. If these maneuvers are not effective, bilateral SACP may be necessary to ensure adequate global cerebral perfusion. Bilateral SACP can be accomplished by direct cannulation of the innominate, left carotid, and left subclavian arteries in the open aortic arch. Existing evidence and clinical experience has not demonstrated the superiority unilateral or bilateral SACP over RCP or DHCA alone for aortic arch operations [23, 38]. The choice of perfusion technique used for aortic operations is typically specific to the preferences and expertise of individual surgeons and institutions. Potential disadvantages of SACP include the added time necessary to expose and cannulate the axillary artery, increased surgical instrumentation of the aortic arch branch vessels, and the increased risk for cerebral thromboembolism.

Spinal Cord Protection

Spinal cord ischemia is well known complication of thoracoabdominal aortic aneurysm repair and can affect patients undergoing either open or endovascular operations. The risk of spinal cord ischemia and infarction depends on the extent of the descending thoracic and abdominal aorta that is replaced and the number of intercostal and segmental arteries that are sacrificed. In addition, injury or impaired blood flow to the vertebral arteries, inferior mesenteric artery, or branches off the iliac arteries that supply collateral blood flow to the spinal cord can potentiate the risk of spinal cord ischemia. Although spinal cord ischemia can manifest as a complication of acute aortic dissection in rare instances, it is not established whether patients with aortic dissection are at increased risk of spinal cord ischemia [39]. Spinal cord ischemia has also been reported as a complication in approximately 2% of patients with Stanford Type A aortic dissection undergoing extended aortic arch repair with frozen elephant trunk grafting into the proximal descending thoracic aorta [40].

Strategies to prevent spinal cord ischemia in patients undergoing open or endovascular thoracoabdominal aortic aneurysm repair include prophylactic lumbar cerebrospinal fluid drainage, arterial blood pressure augmentation, mild deliberate hypothermia, distal aortic perfusion, reimplantation of critical intercostal and segmental arteries, and the application of intraoperative SSEP or MEP monitoring for early detection of spinal cord ischemia [15, 39, 41]. In patients who initially have a normal postoperative neurologic examination but subsequently develop spinal cord ischemia, early detection combined with early intervention with lumbar cerebrospinal fluid drainage and arterial pressure augmentation has been shown to be effective for preventing or decreasing the severity of permanent paraplegia [42–44]. The physiologic rationale for lumbar cerebrospinal fluid drainage and blood pressure augmentation is to increase spinal cord perfusion pressure that is approximated by the difference between the mean arterial pressure and the cerebrospinal fluid pressure. In addition, hypotension caused by neurogenic shock as a consequence of spinal cord ischemia requires early and aggressive treatment [44]. Although case reports describe the use of lumbar cerebrospinal fluid drainage and blood pressure augmentation to treat spinal cord ischemia caused by acute aortic dissection, there is insufficient evidence or clinical experience to recommend this treatment for patients with spinal cord ischemia complicating Stanford Type A aortic dissections [45]. In these situations, the risks and benefits of increasing the arterial pressure or instrumenting the spinal canal must be carefully considered.

Mesenteric Organ Protection

Deliberate hypothermia not only serves to protect the brain, but also serves to protect other vital organs such as the liver and kidneys during the period of ischemia from circulatory arrest. The optimal temperature for systemic or mesenteric organ protection and the safe duration of circulatory arrest for organs outside the central nervous system is not completely understood, but existing clinical experience suggests that these organs can tolerate a longer period of DHCA without permanent damage. In operations on the thoracoabdominal aorta, mesenteric perfusion can also be provided by direct cannulation and perfusion of the renal, celiac, or superior mesenteric arteries. Alternatively, partial left heart bypass or partial CPB with distal aortic perfusion can be used to minimize the duration of mesenteric ischemia during thoracoabdominal aortic reconstruction. Perioperative renal injury is often multifactorial as a consequence of pre-existing chronic kidney disease, peripheral arterial disease, recent exposure to radiographic contrast agents, and ischemia during operative repair. There is insufficient evidence to support the efficacy of pharmacologic agents to protect against acute kidney injury for patients undergoing major aortic operations, but techniques commonly used in an effort to protect the kidneys and preserve renal function include preoperative intravenous hydration, intravenous mannitol, and diuretics to maintain urine output.

Blood Loss and Fluid Management

Operations on the thoracic aorta always pose a risk of serious hemorrhage and proper intraoperative preparation requires having the capability to rapidly replace blood and fluid losses and restore hemostatic function at the completion of the operation. Large-bore peripheral intravenous access as well as large-bore central venous access permits rapid administration of fluids or blood products. Apparatuses to rapidly infuse and warm intravenous fluids and blood products (i.e., Belmont or Level 1) are useful for responding to acute or ongoing hemorrhage. Packed red blood cells together with fresh frozen plasma is typically prepared and made readily available at the start of operation and at the conclusion of CPB. The volume of salvaged blood that is readministered should be tracked so that the equivalent volume of plasma, platelets, or cryoprecipitate can be replaced.

In addition to surgical blood loss, operations for acute aortic dissection are often complicated by diffuse microvascular bleeding. Antifibrinolytic agents such as tranexamic acid and aminocaproic acid are routinely used to decrease blood loss. Other prothrombotic agents such as recombinant factor VIIa, prothrombin complex concentrate (PCC), and anti-inhibitor coagulant complex (FEIBA) are commonly needed for the treatment of diffuse microvascular bleeding. Acute care laboratory studies and point-of-care testing are also useful for guiding the treatment of patients requiring massive transfusion and its associated metabolic consequences. Testing typically includes checking arterial and venous blood gas measurements of pH, partial pressure of oxygen, partial pressure of carbon dioxide, base deficit, complete blood count, electrolytes, calcium, glucose, lactate, and activated whole blood clotting time. Furthermore, tests of coagulation such as prothrombin time, activated partial thromboplastin time, International Normalized Ratio (INR), platelet count, or rotational thromboelastometry (ROTEM) and thromboelastography (TEG) can be used to guide the administration of blood products and factors in a bleeding and coagulopathic patient.

Postoperative Care

Virtually every physiologic organ system can be affected by acute aortic dissection and the operations performed to treat it. From a neurocognitive standpoint, patients undergoing these surgical repairs are often disoriented and confused upon emergence from anesthesia because of drug effects, metabolic disturbances, and pain from the operation. They may not fully understand what had just happened to them, where they are, or even what time of day it is. For these reasons, it is important to re-orient the patient, explain to them what had just happened to them, and what to expect during their recovery. The multimodal treatment of postoperative pain with acetaminophen, gabapentin, and narcotic analgesics is effective for reducing the total dose of any single agent and their corresponding side effects. If safe, early emergence from anesthesia and sedation is desirable to assess for evidence of stroke, spinal cord ischemia, seizures, encephalopathy, and to perform a complete physical examination.

The incidence of postoperative stroke ranges from 3% to 10% depending on patient comorbidities and risk factors, and whether the operation was elective or emergent [23, 27, 31]. If postoperative stroke is suspected, appropriate CT imaging can reveal the location and extent of infarct, hemorrhage, or cerebral edema. Global cerebral ischemia from shock or hypoperfusion during circulatory arrest may manifest as neurocognitive dysfunction, delirium, encephalopathy, or as a transient neurologic deficit. Encephalopathy and delirium both typically improve with time, but may require supportive care and management with antipsychotics or sedatives. If postoperative seizures are suspected, EEG can be diagnostic, and the patient should be appropriately treated with antiepileptics while determining the underlying etiology of the seizure.

Patients undergoing extended arch repair, frozen elephant trunk graft, thoracoabdominal aortic repair or TEVAR are at risk for spinal cord ischemia [15, 40]. Routine examination to test for proximal and distal lower extremity weakness or loss of sensation is important for the early detection of spinal cord ischemia. Clinical experience suggests that early detection and interventions to treat spinal cord ischemia can be effective for preventing or decreasing the severity of permanent paraplegia or paraparesis [42, 43].

Postoperative mechanical respiratory support is typically necessary after open surgical operations until pulmonary function returns. Perioperative lung injury or respiratory insufficiency may be sustained as a consequence of pulmonary edema from heart failure, transfusion related circulatory overload (TACO), transfusion related acute lung injury (TRALI), ventilation/perfusion mismatching from atelectasis and vasodilator therapy, or phrenic nerve injury. Postoperative dysphagia increases the risk of aspiration pneumonia. Spinal cord ischemia or infarction may impair the function of accessory muscles necessary for respiration and clearing of pulmonary secretions.

The hemodynamic condition of patients in the early postoperative period is often dynamic because of blood loss, fluid shifts, the effects of drugs or pain on autonomic nervous system function, the need for vasopressor or vasodilator therapy during operation, and the state of myocardial function after reperfusion. The risks of exacerbating surgical bleeding and the aortic dissection due to hypertension must also be weighed against the risk of cerebral, spinal, and renal hypoperfusion if blood pressure is too low. Pre-existing chronic hypertension may alter end-organ autoregulation of blood flow and a greater-than-normal mean arterial blood pressure may be necessary to ensure end-organ perfusion. Concentric left ventricular hypertrophy may also be a consequence of pre-existing hypertension and associated with diastolic dysfunction. Ongoing mediastinal bleeding in the postoperative period may cause cardiac tamponade. Avoiding venous hypertension and venous congestion is also important to optimize end-organ perfusion. Patients with aortic dissection are also at risk for occult peripheral, cerebral, or coronary vascular disease that may not be fully characterized because of the emergency nature of the operation. Once circulatory stability has been achieved and continuous vasoactive medications have been discontinued, treatment with beta-blockers, antihypertensive therapy, and a statin should be considered to reduce the risk of postoperative atrial fibrillation and attenuate disease progression.

Acute kidney injury is common after repair of aortic dissection because of preoperative exposure to radiographic contrast agents, pre-existing chronic renal disease, renal malperfusion from the aortic dissection, thromboembolism, temporary ischemia during operation, or hypoperfusion as a consequence of hypotension or antihypertensive therapy. Efforts to aid the recovery of renal function include optimizing arterial pressure, venous pressure, and cardiac output together with avoiding nephrotoxic agents. Renal malperfusion from dissection may be amenable to treatment with endovascular stenting. There are no proven pharmacologic agents effective for the prevention or treatment of acute kidney injury, but diuretic therapy can be useful in the management of volume overload in nonoliguric renal failure. In cases of oliguric renal failure, continuous renal replacement therapy or intermittent hemodialysis may be necessary.

Metabolic acidosis with elevated lactate is common in the postoperative period as a consequence of circulatory arrest. The nadir for arterial pH and peak of serum lactate levels occur approximately 6 h after circulatory arrest, and typically return to normal over 18–20 h [46]. Postoperative metabolic and lactic acidosis as a normal consequence of the operation must be distinguished from acidosis caused by new or unresolved mesenteric ischemia or circulatory shock. The efficacy of treating metabolic acidosis with sodium bicarbonate is controversial, and the administration of sodium bicarbonate correlates with the severity of postoperative hypernatremia [47]. Hypernatremia may contribute to agitation, confusion, and delirium. The subsequent need to treat hypernatremia with the administration of free water can contribute to volume overload. Hyperkalemia may manifest during reperfusion, though more commonly hypokalemia occurs as a consequence of hyperglycemia and treatment with insulin, diuretics, and beta-adrenergic agonists.

Intraoperative and postoperative bleeding requiring transfusion of blood products is common in aortic surgery [48]. The combination of tissue factor exposure in the false lumen of the dissection, CPB, deliberate hypothermia, blood loss with hemodilution, and renal dysfunction leads to complex dynamic changes in the coagulation and hemostatic pathways [49, 50]. Although the optimal approach is to have therapy guided by acute care laboratory studies of the coagulation profile and complete blood count, the time it takes to obtain laboratory results may cause delays in the management of life-threatening bleeding. Blood and coagulation factor replacement must sometimes be carried out empirically. Additionally, antifibrinolytic agents, and specific factor concentrates such as recombinant activated factor VIIa, PCC, or FEIBA may be necessary to treat microvascular bleeding, decrease blood product requirements, and achieve hemostasis [51]. Uncontrolled bleeding can lead to serious consequences such as cardiac tamponade, hemothorax, anemia, thrombocytopenia, hypovolemic or hemorrhagic shock, and dilutional coagulopathy. Surgical re-exploration for bleeding complications may be necessary if bleeding is refractory to conservative treatment. Once hemostasis has been achieved, prophylaxis for venous thromboembolism should be considered. The potential for heparin-induced thrombocytopenia and thrombosis should also be considered in patients with persistent thrombocytopenia or unexplained thrombotic complications.

Occasionally, branch vessel malperfusion as a result of the aortic dissection or the operative repair itself can cause mesenteric ischemia. Signs or symptoms of mesenteric ischemia range from subtle to overt depending on severity. Mesenteric ischemia should be suspected in patients with persistent or worsening metabolic or lactic acidosis, abnormal hepatic function, postoperative ileus, abdominal pain, food intolerance, or lower gastrointestinal bleeding. Dysphagia and the risk of gastric aspiration should be considered before resuming oral intake. Risk factors for dysphagia include prolonged endotracheal intubation, advanced age, use of TEE, delirium, encephalopathy, stroke, vocal cord injuries, or injury to the recurrent laryngeal nerve. In the absence of gastrointestinal complications, early initiation of enteral nutrition and stool softeners to prevent constipation will facilitate convalescence.

Acute limb ischemia from malperfusion is a common complication of acute aortic dissection. In severe cases, reperfusion after operative repair may cause compartment syndrome requiring fasciotomy. In addition, limb ischemia may also be caused by thromboembolism, occlusive peripheral vascular disease, or vascular access site complications. The routine assessment of peripheral pulses and perfusion is important for the early detection of limb ischemia or compartment syndrome.

Postoperative hypothermia can be expected after operations performed with deliberate hypothermia. The recommendation for gradual rewarming and the avoidance of hyperthermia in combination with surgical exposure, the administration of intravenous fluids, and blood products contributes to the risk of postoperative hypothermia. Attention to temperature monitoring and early application of external forced air warming in the postoperative period can prevent further temperature drift and restore normothermia. Although neuroprotective, hypothermia increases the risk of infection and potentially impairs hemostatic function and wound healing.

Conclusion

Success rates for operative outcomes for uncomplicated acute aortic dissections has improved over time and mortality has decreased from 20% to as low as 5% at centers of excellence [2, 3]. Improvements in the management of acute aortic dissection can be attributed to recent innovations in diagnosis, surgical techniques, anesthetic care, and postoperative management. Important advancements also include increased public awareness of the condition and rapid diagnosis with expedited surgical and anesthetic care at experienced medical centers. Endovascular repair techniques and the availability of hybrid operating room suites with intraoperative imaging capability have greatly expanded treatment options. The clinical application of intraoperative TEE for the surgical and anesthetic management has permitted real-time diagnosis and management of life-threatening complications of aortic dissection. The application of intraoperative neurophysiologic monitoring, cerebral oximetry and processed EEG has helped to refine techniques for neuroprotection during aortic arch repair. Routine attention to the prevention, detection, and treatment of spinal cord ischemia has decreased the risk of permanent paraplegia. Despite the many advances in the perioperative care of patients with acute aortic dissection, the comprehensive care of these patients is resource intensive, requires experienced teams, continues to remain challenging, and is always associated with a risk of complications that can lead to high mortality.

References

1. Hagan PG, Nienaber CA, Isselbacher EM, et al. The International Registry of Acute Aortic Dissection (IRAD): new insights into an old disease. JAMA. 2000;283:897–903.
2. Evangelista A, Isselbacher EM, Bossone E, et al. Insights from the International Registry of Acute Aortic Dissection: a 20-year experience of collaborative clinical research. Circulation. 2018;137:1846–60.
3. Tien M, Ku A, Martinez-Acero N, Zvara J, Sun EC, Cheung AT. The Penn classification predicts hospital mortality in acute Stanford type A and type B aortic dissections. J Cardiothorac Vasc Anesth. 2020;34:867–73.
4. Pape LA, Awais M, Woznicki EM, et al. Presentation, diagnosis, and outcomes of acute aortic dissection: 17-year trends from the International Registry of Acute Aortic Dissection. J Am Coll Cardiol. 2015;66:350–8.
5. Nienaber CA, Fattori R, Mehta RH, et al. Gender-related differences in acute aortic dissection. Circulation. 2004;109:3014–21.
6. Nallamothu BK, Mehta RH, Saint S, et al. Syncope in acute aortic dissection: diagnostic, prognostic, and clinical implications. Am J Med. 2002;113:468–71.
7. Nishiwaki K, Komatsu T, Shimada Y, Takeuchi E, Abe T. Severe tracheal compression caused by false aneurysm arising from the ascending aorta: successful airway management using induced hypotension and bronchoscopy. Anesthesiology. 1990;73:1047–9.
8. MacGillivray RG. Tracheal compression caused by aneurysms of the aortic arch. Implications for the anaesthetist. Anaesthesia. 1985;40:270–7.
9. Kutcher WL, Kaufman BS. Occlusion of the right pulmonary artery by an acute dissecting aortic aneurysm. Crit Care Med. 1988;16:564–5.
10. Downey RJ, Austin JH, Pepino P, Dickstein ML, Homma S, Rose EA. Right ventricular obstruction in aortic dissection: a mechanism of hemodynamic collapse. Ann Thorac Surg. 1996;61:988–90.
11. Debakey ME, Henly WS, Cooley DA, Morris GC, Crawford ES, Beall AC. Surgical management of dissecting aneurysms of the aorta. J Thorac Cardiovasc Surg. 1965;49:130–49.
12. Daily PO, Trueblood HW, Stinson EB, Wuerflein RD, Shumway NE. Management of acute aortic dissections. Ann Thorac Surg. 1970;10:237–47.
13. Augoustides JGT, Geirsson A, Szeto WY, Walsh EK, Cornelius B, Pochettino A, Bavaria JE. Observational study of mortality risk stratification by ischemic presentation in patients with acute type A aortic dissection: the Penn classification. Nat Clin Pract Cardiovasc Med. 2009;6:140–6.
14. Augoustides JGT, Szeto WY, Desai ND, Pochettino A, Cheung AT, Savino JS, Bavaria JE. Classification of acute type A dissection: focus on clinical presentation and extent. Eur J Cardio-Thorac Surg Off J Eur Assoc Cardio-Thorac Surg. 2011;39:519–22.
15. Hiratzka LF, Bakris GL, Beckman JA, et al. 2010 ACCF/AHA/AATS/ACR/ASA/SCA/SCAI/SIR/STS/SVM guidelines for the diagnosis and management of patients with Thoracic Aortic Disease: a report of the American College of Cardiology Foundation/American Heart Association Task Force on Practice Guidelines, American Association for Thoracic Surgery, American College of Radiology, American Stroke Association, Society of Cardiovascular Anesthesiologists, Society for Cardiovascular Angiography and Interventions, Society of Interventional Radiology, Society of Thoracic Surgeons, and Society for Vascular Medicine. Circulation. 2010;121:e266–369.
16. Erbel R, Aboyans V, Boileau C, et al. 2014 ESC Guidelines on the diagnosis and treatment of aortic diseases: Document covering acute and chronic aortic diseases of the thoracic and abdominal aorta of the adult. The Task Force for the Diagnosis and Treatment of Aortic Diseases of the European Society of Cardiology (ESC). Eur Heart J. 2014;35:2873–926.
17. Goldstein SA, Evangelista A, Abbara S, et al. Multimodality imaging of diseases of the thoracic aorta in adults: from the American Society of Echocardiography and the European Association of Cardiovascular Imaging: endorsed by the Society of Cardiovascular Computed

Tomography and Society for Cardiovascular Magnetic Resonance. J Am Soc Echocardiogr Off Publ Am Soc Echocardiogr. 2015;28:119–82.
18. Stecker MM, Cheung AT, Pochettino A, Kent GP, Patterson T, Weiss SJ, Bavaria JE. Deep hypothermic circulatory arrest: I. Effects of cooling on electroencephalogram and evoked potentials. Ann Thorac Surg. 2001;71:14–21.
19. Cheung AT, Savino JS, Weiss SJ, Patterson T, Richards RM, Gardner TJ, Stecker MM. Detection of acute embolic stroke during mitral valve replacement using somatosensory evoked potential monitoring. Anesthesiology. 1995;83:208–10.
20. American Society of Anesthesiologists and Society of Cardiovascular Anesthesiologists Task Force on Transesophageal Echocardiography. Practice guidelines for perioperative transesophageal echocardiography. An updated report by the American Society of Anesthesiologists and the Society of Cardiovascular Anesthesiologists Task Force on Transesophageal Echocardiography. Anesthesiology. 2010;112:1084–96.
21. Gordon AS, Meyer BW, Jones JC. Open-heart surgery using deep hypothermia without an oxygenator. J Thorac Cardiovasc Surg. 1960;40:787–99.
22. McCullough JN, Zhang N, Reich DL, Juvonen TS, Klein JJ, Spielvogel D, Ergin MA, Griepp RB. Cerebral metabolic suppression during hypothermic circulatory arrest in humans. Ann Thorac Surg. 1999;67:1895–9. Discussion 1919–21
23. Hu Z, Wang Z, Ren Z, Wu H, Zhang M, Zhang H, Hu X. Similar cerebral protective effectiveness of antegrade and retrograde cerebral perfusion combined with deep hypothermia circulatory arrest in aortic arch surgery: a meta-analysis and systematic review of 5060 patients. J Thorac Cardiovasc Surg. 2014;148:544–60.
24. Gaynor JW, Nicolson SC, Jarvik GP, Wernovsky G, Montenegro LM, Burnham NB, Hartman DM, Louie A, Spray TL, Clancy RR. Increasing duration of deep hypothermic circulatory arrest is associated with an increased incidence of postoperative electroencephalographic seizures. J Thorac Cardiovasc Surg. 2005;130:1278–86.
25. Fleck TM, Czerny M, Hutschala D, Koinig H, Wolner E, Grabenwoger M. The incidence of transient neurologic dysfunction after ascending aortic replacement with circulatory arrest. Ann Thorac Surg. 2003;76:1198–202.
26. Cook RC, Gao M, Macnab AJ, Fedoruk LM, Day N, Janusz MT. Aortic arch reconstruction: safety of moderate hypothermia and antegrade cerebral perfusion during systemic circulatory arrest. J Card Surg. 2006;21:158–64.
27. Preventza O, Coselli JS, Garcia A, et al. Moderate hypothermia at warmer temperatures is safe in elective proximal and total arch surgery: Results in 665 patients. J Thorac Cardiovasc Surg. 2017;153:1011–8.
28. Ehrlich MP, McCullough J, Wolfe D, Zhang N, Shiang H, Weisz D, Bodian C, Griepp RB. Cerebral effects of cold reperfusion after hypothermic circulatory arrest. J Thorac Cardiovasc Surg. 2001;121:923–31.
29. Engelman R, Baker RA, Likosky DS, Grigore A, Dickinson TA, Shore-Lesserson L, Hammon JW, Society of Thoracic Surgeons, Society of Cardiovascular Anesthesiologists, American Society of ExtraCorporeal Technology. The Society of Thoracic Surgeons, The Society of Cardiovascular Anesthesiologists, and The American Society of ExtraCorporeal Technology: clinical practice guidelines for cardiopulmonary bypass—temperature management during cardiopulmonary bypass. Ann Thorac Surg. 2015;100:748–57.
30. Nussmeier NA, Cheng W, Marino M, Spata T, Li S, Daniels G, Clark T, Vaughn WK. Temperature during cardiopulmonary bypass: the discrepancies between monitored sites. Anesth Analg. 2006;103:1373–9.
31. Grigore AM, Grocott HP, Mathew JP, et al. The rewarming rate and increased peak temperature alter neurocognitive outcome after cardiac surgery. Anesth Analg. 2002;94:4–10, table of contents.
32. Grocott HP, Mackensen GB, Grigore AM, Mathew J, Reves JG, Phillips-Bute B, Smith PK, Newman MF, Neurologic Outcome Research Group (NORG), Cardiothoracic Anesthesiology Research Endeavors (CARE) Investigators' of the Duke Heart Center. Postoperative hyper-

thermia is associated with cognitive dysfunction after coronary artery bypass graft surgery. Stroke. 2002;33:537–41.
33. James ML, Andersen ND, Swaminathan M, et al. Predictors of electrocerebral inactivity with deep hypothermia. J Thorac Cardiovasc Surg. 2014;147:1002–7.
34. Reich DL, Horn LM, Hossain S, Uysal S. Using jugular bulb oxyhemoglobin saturation to guide onset of deep hypothermic circulatory arrest does not affect post-operative neuropsychological function. Eur J Cardio-Thorac Surg Off J Eur Assoc Cardio-Thorac Surg. 2004;25:401–6. Discussion 406–8
35. Benedetto U, Raja SG, Amrani M, Pepper JR, Zeinah M, Tonelli E, Biondi-Zoccai G, Frati G. The impact of arterial cannulation strategy on operative outcomes in aortic surgery: evidence from a comprehensive meta-analysis of comparative studies on 4476 patients. J Thorac Cardiovasc Surg. 2014;148:2936–43.e1–4.
36. Cheung AT, Bavaria JE, Weiss SJ, Patterson T, Stecker MM. Neurophysiologic effects of retrograde cerebral perfusion used for aortic reconstruction. J Cardiothorac Vasc Anesth. 1998;12:252–9.
37. Cheung AT, Bavaria JE, Pochettino A, Weiss SJ, Barclay DK, Stecker MM. Oxygen delivery during retrograde cerebral perfusion in humans. Anesth Analg. 1999;88:8–15.
38. Angeloni E, Melina G, Refice SK, Roscitano A, Capuano F, Comito C, Sinatra R. Unilateral versus bilateral antegrade cerebral protection during aortic surgery: an updated meta-analysis. Ann Thorac Surg. 2015;99:2024–31.
39. Etz CD, Weigang E, Hartert M, et al. Contemporary spinal cord protection during thoracic and thoracoabdominal aortic surgery and endovascular aortic repair: a position paper of the vascular domain of the European Association for Cardio-Thoracic Surgery. Eur J Cardio-Thorac Surg Off J Eur Assoc Cardio-Thorac Surg. 2015;47:943–57.
40. Smith HN, Boodhwani M, Ouzounian M, Saczkowski R, Gregory AJ, Herget EJ, Appoo JJ. Classification and outcomes of extended arch repair for acute Type A aortic dissection: a systematic review and meta-analysis. Interact Cardiovasc Thorac Surg. 2017;24:450–9.
41. Sinha AC, Cheung AT. Spinal cord protection and thoracic aortic surgery. Curr Opin Anaesthesiol. 2010;23:95–102.
42. Cheung AT, Pochettino A, McGarvey ML, Appoo JJ, Fairman RM, Carpenter JP, Moser WG, Woo EY, Bavaria JE. Strategies to manage paraplegia risk after endovascular stent repair of descending thoracic aortic aneurysms. Ann Thorac Surg. 2005;80:1280–8. Discussion 1288–9
43. Keith CJ, Passman MA, Carignan MJ, Parmar GM, Nagre SB, Patterson MA, Taylor SM, Jordan WD. Protocol implementation of selective postoperative lumbar spinal drainage after thoracic aortic endograft. J Vasc Surg. 2012;55:1–8. Discussion 8
44. Cheung AT, Weiss SJ, McGarvey ML, Stecker MM, Hogan MS, Escherich A, Bavaria JE. Interventions for reversing delayed-onset postoperative paraplegia after thoracic aortic reconstruction. Ann Thorac Surg. 2002;74:413–9. Discussion 420–1
45. Ullery BW, Hobbs RD, Cheung AT. Reversible spinal cord ischemia as a complication of acute aortic intramural hematoma. Vascular. 2015;23:427–31.
46. Ghadimi K, Gutsche JT, Setegne SL, Jackson KR, Augoustides JGT, Ochroch EA, Bavaria JE, Cheung AT. Severity and duration of metabolic acidosis after deep hypothermic circulatory arrest for thoracic aortic surgery. J Cardiothorac Vasc Anesth. 2015;29:1432–40.
47. Ghadimi K, Gutsche JT, Ramakrishna H, Setegne SL, Jackson KR, Augoustides JG, Ochroch EA, Weiss SJ, Bavaria JE, Cheung AT. Sodium bicarbonate use and the risk of hypernatremia in thoracic aortic surgical patients with metabolic acidosis following deep hypothermic circulatory arrest. Ann Card Anaesth. 2016;19:454–62.
48. Trimarchi S, Nienaber CA, Rampoldi V, et al. Contemporary results of surgery in acute type A aortic dissection: The International Registry of Acute Aortic Dissection experience. J Thorac Cardiovasc Surg. 2005;129:112–22.
49. Paparella D, Galeone A, Venneri MT, Coviello M, Scrascia G, Marraudino N, Quaranta M, de Luca Tupputi Schinosa L, Brister SJ. Activation of the coagulation system during coro-

nary artery bypass grafting: comparison between on-pump and off-pump techniques. J Thorac Cardiovasc Surg. 2006;131:290–7.
50. Paparella D, Rotunno C, Guida P, Malvindi PG, Scrascia G, De Palo M, de Cillis E, Bortone AS, de Luca Tupputi Schinosa L. Hemostasis alterations in patients with acute aortic dissection. Ann Thorac Surg. 2011;91:1364–9.
51. Gregory SH, Yalamuri SM, Bishawi M, Swaminathan M. The perioperative management of ascending aortic dissection. Anesth Analg. 2018;127:1302–13.

Coagulopathy and Bleeding Management for Aortic Dissection Surgery

Jerrold H. Levy and Roman M. Sniecinski

Introduction

Patients who undergo surgical repair following aortic dissections have multiple hemostatic abnormalities due to numerous factors that contribute to coagulopathy and bleeding [1]. Anticoagulation and its reversal, exposure to extracorporeal circulation, tissue injury due to blood exposure in the false lumen, and further acquired defects [2] can all contribute to impaired hemostasis. Bleeding management in this patient population requires a multimodal approach [3, 4]. Developing specific bleeding management strategies and algorithms to guide transfusion decisions is an integral part of patient blood management which not only reduce allogeneic blood transfusions but optimize clinical care [5, 6]. Cardiac surgical patients undergoing aortic dissection repair are exposed to extensive surgery and often long cardiopulmonary bypass times, which place them at high risk for developing coagulopathy [7]. This chapter will review therapies focused on this patient population, including coagulation testing, blood product transfusion, and pharmacologic strategies to decrease bleeding.

J. H. Levy (✉)
Cardiothoracic Anesthesiology, Critical Care, and Surgery (Cardiothoracic), Duke University School of Medicine, Duke University Medical Center, Durham, NC, USA
e-mail: jerrold.levy@duke.edu

R. M. Sniecinski
Cardiothoracic Anesthesiology, Emory University School of Medicine, Atlanta, GA, USA

J. S. Coselli et al. (eds.), *Aortic Dissection and Acute Aortic Syndromes*,
https://doi.org/10.1007/978-3-030-66668-2_39

Coagulation Testing

In patients who are bleeding following aortic surgery, coagulation testing is important to help define contributing hemostatic defects. Although standard laboratory coagulation tests are typically available (i.e., prothrombin time, partial thromboplastin time, platelet counts, fibrinogen levels), these have limitations with regard to specificity and reporting time. As a result, viscoelastic testing with the use of thromboelastography (TEG) or thromboelastometry (ROTEM) is increasingly used in bleeding management as it examines multiple aspects of the hemostatic system. Since whole blood is used for these tests, their samples require reduced preparation compared to standard laboratory tests, and thus reduced time, before actionable information can be obtained.

In cardiac surgical patients, impaired platelet function, in addition to reduced numbers, is a significant cause of bleeding [8]. However, platelet specific function testing is not widely available despite the use of viscoelastic testing and other point-of-care (POC) analyzers such as VerifyNow® and PFA-100®. POC platelet tests have not been validated in acutely bleeding patients since thrombocytopenia and hematocrit significantly influences their reported values. Even with standard TEG and ROTEM, it is important to understand that results are also affected by platelet number, and not function, due to the activators within the test (e.g., kaolin, tissue factor). Until better platelet function testing for the post-CPB period is developed, platelet transfusions for assumed dysfunction will continue to be administered empirically or based on platelet numbers [9].

Despite the lack of studies supporting platelet function tests in the perioperative management of cardiac surgical patients, multiple studies have shown that using pre-determined algorithms can decrease bleeding and transfusion requirements after cardiac surgery. Transfusion algorithms based upon objective measurements decrease the empirical administration of hemostatic factors [10]. Furthermore, algorithms based upon POC viscoelastic testing have been shown to reduce bleeding, the need for allogeneic transfusions, returned to the operating room for bleeding, and overall cost of transfusional therapy in aortic dissection patients [11]. An example of a viscoelastic tracing is provided in Fig. 1.

While POC tests have gained widespread use, most institutions have internally developed their own algorithms using these devices. In many randomized studies, point-of-care testing and transfusion algorithms decrease transfusions and improve hemostasis [10, 12–15]. However, different POC platforms have been used in these studies, along with different transfusion triggers. This is why meta-analyses of viscoelastic POC devices tend to show minimal effects [16–18]. Therefore, it is not clear whether the actual testing devices or the algorithms, which guide transfusion and decrease empirical administration, have the largest impact on reducing blood product usage.

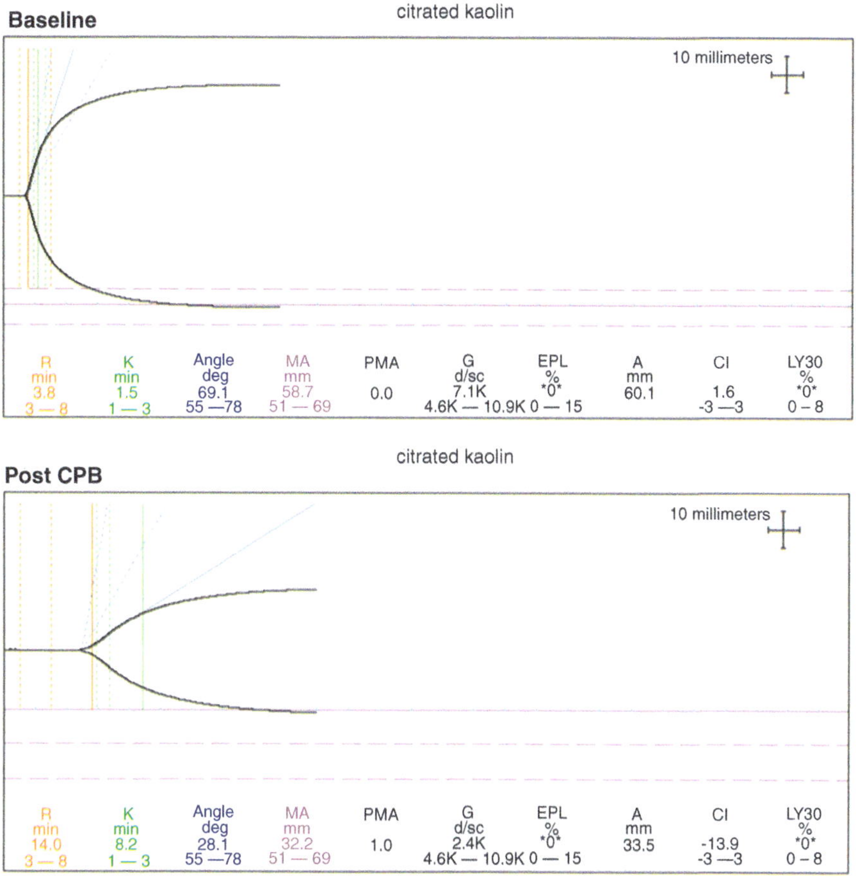

Fig. 1 Examples of normal and hypocoagulable viscoelastic tracings. These are 2 tracings from a TEG® 5000 machine (Haemonetics, Braintree, MA). Although this is a static image, it should be noted that the tracing develops over time and can be read in a dynamic fashion. The top tracing ("Baseline") depicts a normal coagulable state, while the bottom one ("Post CPB") shows hypocoagulability. Measured components are depicted in color with their solid lines depicting the final value and the dashed reference lines representing the normal range. The R time (orange) is measured in minutes and represents initial thrombin generation and fibrin formation. The K time (green) is the amount of time for the clot strength to reach 20 mm in amplitude and represents a measure of fibrin build-up. The angle (blue) is formed by a tangential line to the curve at the K time and provides information on the speed of fibrin cross-linking. MA (purple) is the maximum amplitude of the clot strength and reflects fibrin and platelet interactions. The black numbers are derived from the curve and calculated. A: clot amplitude at any given time along the curve. PMA: projected MA, with a value of '0.0' meaning the clot is likely to reach an MA in normal limits and a value of '1.0' indicating it is unlikely. G: shear elastic modulus strength of the clot which is derived from MA. CI: coagulation index, which is a TEG® value calculated from the measured values to provide a summary of coagulability; CI >3.0 is indicative of hypercoagulability and a CI< –3.0 indicative of hypocoagulability. Fibrinolysis is not depicted on these curves (tracings were each stopped after ~50 min) since the patient was already receiving antifibrinolytic therapy, which is typical in cardiac surgery. EPL: estimated percent lysis at 30 min after MA reached and is continually updated until LY30 point is reached. LY30: percent lysis at 30 min after MA reached

Transfusion Therapy and Transfusion Guidelines

Multiple studies continue to define the role of transfusional therapies in acute bleeding in cardiac surgery. Unfortunately, most of the studies to date have focused on red blood cell (RBC) transfusions and defining the ideal hemoglobin as a transfusion trigger. There is less objective data available that evaluates the role of hemostatic blood components, which include fresh frozen plasma (FFP), platelets, and cryoprecipitate. Despite few controlled trials, there are an increasing number of guidelines and practice documents for bleeding management in cardiac surgical patients [19, 20]. Although these guidelines are reported as generally applicable recommendations, there are also other important considerations regarding the use of specific blood products in cardiac surgical patients that need to be considered. The rationale for the transfusion of individual blood components will be addressed in the following sections.

Red Blood Cells

Although many studies have focused on a specific hemoglobin trigger in cardiac surgery, multiple factors should be assessed when deciding on RBC transfusions in aortic dissection surgery. With acute hemorrhage, the rate of bleeding, which can be quite high in these situations, much be taken into account [21]. Transfusion decisions when hemoglobin concentrations are approximately 7–10 g/dL should be based on any potential or continuing bleeding rate and magnitude, and the intravascular volume status [21].

In general, the number of patients being transfused RBCs during cardiac surgery has significantly decreased over the past decade [22]. In a large, multi-center, randomized study, the TRICS III trial demonstrated a 'restrictive' (Hgb <7.5 g/dL) transfusion trigger was non-inferior to a 'liberal' trigger (Hgb <9.5 g/dL in the ICU) with respect to important patient outcomes [23]. It should be noted, however, that few patients in transfusion trials are undergoing aortic surgery, which is often an emergency and may be complicated by other undiagnosed patient co-morbidities and underlying coagulopathies. Hemoglobin triggers for RBC transfusion are not to be taken as absolute indications, and patients undergoing aortic dissection repair should be transfused if signs of inadequate perfusion are present.

Fresh Frozen Plasma (FFP)

FFP is overused in most surgical patients, often because of empirical therapy or to treat abnormal prothrombin times (PT) and/or partial thromboplastin times (PTT). Although these standard coagulation tests are used clinically to evaluate bleeding, they do not reflect bleeding in surgical patients and can be abnormal in patients who are not bleeding. Despite the extensive use of FFP, there is no data supporting its efficacy outside of trauma patients requiring massive transfusion [24]. Analyses of randomized controlled trials have been unable to demonstrate consistent evidence of benefit for plasma in most clinical scenarios [25]. The use of plasma to treat elevated international normalized ratios (INRs), especially when the INR is less than 1.7, is problematic since the INR of the FFP itself is about 1.5 [26]. Paradoxically, the overuse of FFP is therefore more likely to result in dilution and exacerbation of coagulopathy. The use of PCCs is now preferred over FFP for reversal of vitamin K antagonists [27].

This is not to say that FFP has no role in the treatment of aortic dissection patients. It has been well demonstrated that multiple plasma proteins, including coagulation factors and anticoagulation factors, significantly fall during aortic surgery with prolonged CPB [28]. FFP has a role in restoring these important proteins, although its use should be judicious. In situations of massive transfusion (see below), FFP is recommended as part of a balanced resuscitation. Although rare, catastrophic thrombosis following cardiac surgery can happen when only procoagulant therapies are administered following prolonged CPB [29]. More research is needed to determine the role of FFP in preventing this deadly event.

Cryoprecipitate

Cryoprecipitate is obtained from thawing FFP. The proteins that precipitate in a small volume include fibrinogen, factors VIII, XIII, and von Willebrand factor. Prior to administration, individual units of cryoprecipitate from multiple donors are pooled in the blood bank and administered usually as 5–10 units. Although initially developed for treating hemophilia due to its high factor VIII levels, the primary use of cryoprecipitate currently is to replete fibrinogen levels when specific fibrinogen concentrates are not available, or for acquired Factor XIII deficiency [30].

In Europe and other countries, cryoprecipitate is not available, and specific purified fibrinogen concentrates are used to treat bleeding. In the current era, the target hemostatic level of fibrinogen is 150–200 mg/dL (1.5–2.0 g/L), but the normal fibrinogen levels in plasma range from approximately 200–400 mg/dL and higher. Fibrinogen is critical to clot strength, and fibrinogen repletion for aortic surgery has been extensively studied and will be discussed later in factor concentrates. The levels of fibrinogen less than 100 mg/dL (1 g/L) can a prolong the clot-based coagulation tests PTT and PTT, and FFP administration is unlikely to correct. Cryoprecipitate or other methods of fibrinogen repletion should be considered in patients following aortic surgery as part of a multimodal protocol to manage bleeding [31].

Platelets

One of the major causes of bleeding in aortic surgery is both platelet dysfunction due to activation and extracorporeal circulation, as well as thrombocytopenia due to dilution and consumption. As previously stated, monitoring platelet function in acutely bleeding patients is problematic. As a result, platelets are administered based on a platelet count, as well as empirically administered when patients are bleeding. Most platelets transfused are obtained from single donors by apheresis or, alternatively, pooled multi-donor concentrates.

Following cardiac surgery, including aortic surgery, most transfusion algorithms suggest a threshold for platelet administration to be less than 100,000/μL, which is similar to neurosurgical procedures. As a reminder, normal platelet counts are 150,000–400,000 platelets/μL. Although viscoelastic testing is thought to assess platelet function, this is highly dependent on what activators are used, as well as fibrinogen levels.

Massive Transfusion

In aortic surgical patients, extensive bleeding may occur that requires large volume transfusions. This is often referred to as 'massive transfusion,' which is defined as the acute replacement of more than one blood volume or more than 10 units of PRBC within several hours [32, 33]. Treatment of the coagulopathy should include volume replacement, normothermia, resolution of acid-base abnormalities, and blood component therapy.

Most aortic surgical centers who routinely perform these procedures have protocols and facilities that are capable of providing allogeneic blood products as well as factor concentrates in a timely manner. However, in patients who have major bleeding, using fixed ratios of 1:1:1 for RBCs, plasma, and platelets, is standard management and part of damage control resuscitation [34]. Additionally, because of fibrinolysis, an antifibrinolytic should be considered in the bleeding cardiac surgical patient. Further management strategies include targeting fibrinogen levels in the form of cryoprecipitate or fibrinogen concentrates [34]. However, point-of-care monitoring and other goal-directed therapy can follow with fibrinogen levels and facilitate additional potential therapeutic approaches. The role of off-label use of factor concentrates to manage bleeding that cannot be controlled by conventional measures is still evolving (see below).

Adverse Effects of Transfusions

Allogeneic blood product transfusions are extensively used in aortic surgical patients, of which potential acute adverse effects include hypersensitivity reactions, sepsis, acute respiratory failure defined as transfusion-related acute lung injury (TRALI), and even volume overload describe is transfusion associated circulatory overload (TACO) [35–37]. In general, the higher the quantity of blood products transfused, the greater probability of developing acute respiratory distress syndrome (ARDS) [38].

Pharmacologic Therapies

Multiple systemic and topical pro-hemostatic agents are used during cardiac surgery. One of the unique aspects in this patient population is the ability to preemptively treat patients for potential bleeding problems, specifically with antifibrinolytic agents. The multiple agents used will be reviewed in this section.

Antifibrinolytic Agents

One of the mainstay therapies for both preventing and treating hemorrhage in patients following aortic surgery is the use of antifibrinolytic agents. There are multiple causes and initiation of fibrinolysis, both due to cardiopulmonary bypass as well as the activation that occurs following aortic dissection [39–43]. Efficacy in decreasing bleeding and transfusion is well established, as noted by the guidelines published by the Society of Thoracic Surgeons and The Society of Cardiovascular Anesthesiologists [44].

The current antifibrinolytic agents used are the lysine analogues: epsilon aminocaproic acid (EACA) and tranexamic acid (TXA). Both occupy the lysine binding site of plasminogen, preventing it from interacting with fibrin [45]. An extensive database supports the efficacy of antifibrinolytic agents in cardiac surgery to decrease bleeding and transfusion [46]. Although TXA is the primary agent used worldwide, it does come with potential for causing seizures, which is likely a dose-dependent effect [47]. Large scale clinical trials in CABG patients have suggested that cumulative doses above 50 mg/kg should be avoided [48]. Given that the risk of seizures may be increased when circulatory arrest is used, many clinicians often use EACA in this setting despite its potential to have an increased risk of renal failure and fewer studies in cardiac surgical patients [49, 50].

Protamine

One of the benefits of heparin anticoagulation is that it is acutely reversible with protamine, a highly basic peptide isolated from salmon sperm that binds heparin by forming a simple acid-base interaction [51]. Protamine rapidly reverses heparin to allow clot formation. Protamine can cause adverse reactions, including anaphylaxis, acute pulmonary vasoconstriction, and right ventricular failure, and hypotension [51]. Different reactions to protamine have been reported ranging from minimal cardiovascular effects to life-threatening cardiovascular collapse. Risk factors for protamine reactions have been reported to be allergies to NPH insulin and men who have had vasectomies, while aspirin administration may be protective [52].

Protamine administration for heparin reversal after cardiac surgery is often highly empirical administering large doses of protamine for persistent bleeding when bleeding is related to multiple other factors. What should be remembered is that protamine itself can inhibit platelet aggregation and prolong the ACT. Multiple studies report that excess protamine beyond what is needed for actual reversal decreases clot strength. Clinicians' routine administration of additional protamine to treat a prolonged activated clotting time may actually further increase clotting time and contribute to excess bleeding [53]. Therefore, approaches to avoid excess protamine using heparin protamine titrations or fixed protamine doses based on time and duration of cardiopulmonary bypass are important as part of a multimodal strategy [54].

Desmopressin

Desmopressin (also called DDAVP) is an analog of vasopressin that releases large von Willebrand factor multimers from their storage site in endothelial cells [55–58]. Rapid administration can cause hypotension, and as a result, it should be given slowly using doses of 0.3 mcg/kg to avoid vasodilation [59, 60]. despite its extensive use in cardiac surgical patients, 18 trials of desmopressin in 1295 patients undergoing cardiac surgery only demonstrated small reductions on blood loss with ~115 mL median volume reduction), and little data supporting any efficacy [60, 61]. The best use for DDAVP in cardiac surgery may be in patients with impaired renal function.

Fibrinogen Concentrate

Fibrinogen is a critical coagulation factor that has been extensively studied in aortic surgical patients for repletion using fibrinogen concentrates. Fibrinogen levels also have been reported to be predictors of perioperative bleeding [62, 63]. As previously discussed, both cryoprecipitate and purified fibrinogen concentrates are the two major methods of repeating fibrinogen levels. However, fibrinogen concentrate has been the focus of most trials to date.

In one of the first prospective, randomized, and blinded studies of patients undergoing elective aortic replacement surgery, 61 patients were randomized to receive either fibrinogen concentrate or placebo [64]. Fibrinogen levels were determined using viscoelastic monitoring with FIBTEM testing following separation from cardiopulmonary bypass and protamine reversal. Fibrinogen concentrate administration reduced transfusions compared to placebo (2 units versus 13 units), and transfusion avoidance occurred in 13 of 29 patients receiving fibrinogen concentrates compared to none of the placebo-treated patients. Of note, the FIBTEM test is a point of care viscoelastic testing method that removes the platelet contribution for clot formation by inhibiting platelet activation to evaluate fibrinogen levels or abnormalities in clot formation, and generally correlates with laboratory-based fibrinogen assays (Clauss assays).

Other retrospective studies and prospective studies have reported fibrinogen concentrate administration and aortic surgery reduces bleeding and the need for transfusions both intraoperatively and postoperatively [65–69]. In another study of patients undergoing elective aortic valve and ascending aorta replacement, fibrinogen concentrate reduced 24-h postoperative bleeding and blood product administration [66]. Bleeding and transfusion were also reduced in a similar retrospective evaluation of fibrinogen repletion using purified concentrates and guided by of-care fibrinogen measurements using FIBTEM for post-bypass bleeding following thoracoabdominal aortic aneurysm repair [67]. The need for subsequent blood product transfusion was reduced in these patients, as was 24-h chest tube drainage volume.

Because of the success of reducing both bleeding and allogeneic blood transfusion using fibrinogen concentrates, the concept was expanded to a worldwide multicenter randomized clinical trial that evaluated 519 patients from 34 different medical centers to fibrinogen replacement using a five-minute bleeding mass to determine whether patients would be treated. A total of 152 patients met inclusion criteria for fibrinogen repletion with similar median and interquartile ranges of pretreatment 5 min bleeding masses of 107 (76–138) grams in the fibrinogen group compared to placebo with 91 (71–112) grams. In the fibrinogen concentrate and placebo groups, respectively ($P = 0.13$). Of note is that patients who received fibrinogen concentrates received more allogeneic blood products in the first 24 h postoperatively: 5.0 units (2.0–11.0), when compared with placebo, 3.0 (0.0–7.0). Most of the prior studies that showed marked efficacy of fibrinogen concentrates reducing bleeding were from a single European center with a large active aortic surgical program. In the large multicenter study, low bleeding rates and normal fibrinogen levels, along with the inability to follow a complex transfusion algorithm, likely influenced the results. The overall message for the clinician is that preemptively raising fibrinogen levels alone without treating the underlying coagulopathy is not likely beneficial and levels should be targeted as discussed above.

Recombinant Factor VIIa (rFVIIa)

Recombinant activated factor VII (rFVIIa) is approved in most countries for the treatment of bleeding episodes and perioperative management in adults and children with hemophilia A or B with inhibitors, congenital Factor VII (FVII) deficiency, and Glanzmann's thrombasthenia with refractoriness to platelet transfusions, with or without antibodies to platelets. However, clinicians have used it off label for intractable bleeding, including in cardiac surgical patients.

In one of the first prospective trials, Gill et al. enrolled patients following cardiac surgery who were bleeding more than 200 mL/h and had not been otherwise treated [70]. In this phase II, dose-escalation study, 35 patients were randomized to receive rFVIIa at doses of 40 mcg/kg rFVIIa, 69 patients received 80 mcg/kg rFVIIa, and 68 patients received placebo. Although the primary endpoint was serious adverse events, secondary end points included rates of re-exploration, additional transfusions, and amount of blood loss. There were no statistically significant differences in adverse events among the groups however, significantly fewer patients treated with rFVIIa group underwent re-exploration for bleeding (P = 0.03) or required allogeneic transfusions (P = 0.01) [70].

A more extensive safety study of 4468 subjects that included 4119 patients and 349 healthy volunteers reported a higher rate of arterial thromboembolic events among those subjects who received rFVIIa compared to placebo (5.5% vs. 3.2%) [71]. Interestingly, venous thromboembolic events were similar (5.3% vs. 5.7%). It should be noted that major bleeding in cardiac surgical patients increases the risk of serious adverse events, including operative mortality, as does increased transfusion of blood products [72]. Therefore, when evaluating 'rescue therapies' such as rFVIIa, these risks must be weighed against potential complications of the therapy. In patients major aortic surgery with refractory bleeding, rFVIIa as salvage therapy has been reported and recommended [73].

Prothrombin Complex Concentrates

Prothrombin complex concentrates (PCCs) are purified, freeze-dried coagulation factors derived from pools of plasma that include factors II, VII, IX, and X in concentrations that depend on the manufacturer [74]. In the United States, both three factor and four factor PCCs are available. The three factor PCCs were originally for hemophilia therapy and included factor IX products that include Profilnine SD [Grifols, Barcelona, Spain], Bebulin VH [Baxter], and Factor Eight Inhibitory Bypassing Activity(FEIBA) VH [Baxter] [75]. Bebulin and Profilnine contain low levels of factor VII, while FEIBA contains the activated form of VII (VIIa). Four-Factor PCCs are approved for warfarin and other vitamin K antagonist reversal. Three-factor PCCs are often administered for bleeding rather than vitamin K antagonist reversal and used for off-label indications, including bleeding in surgical patients. Kcentra (CSL Behring) is the only four component PCC available in the United States but is called Beriplex P/N in other countries. Other four component PCCs available in most countries and include Octaplex (Octapharma, Vienna, Austria) [75–79]. While PCCs have been around for decades, modern agents differ in that most also include low levels of anticoagulants including Protein C and Protein S, as well as antithrombin.

In Europe, viscoelastic monitoring is used extensively for goal-directed bleeding management, and algorithms for bleeding in cardiac surgical patients routinely include the use of four component PCCs, although the body of evidence for this is currently small. Retrospective evaluation of a large database reported that initial treatment using POC testing with PCCs, decreased bleeding as well as thrombotic complications [80]. There was also a reduced need for allogeneic transfusion with FFP, but platelet transfusions were increased [80].

Much like rVIIa, PCCs have also been reported as rescue therapy for life-threatening bleeding refractory to conventional treatment. One report of 25 patients who received FEIBA as rescue therapy included aortic root replacement and heart transplants. Following a mean FEIBA doses of 2154 units, FFP and platelet transfusions decreased without need for re-exploration [81]. One Canadian multicenter phase II study is underway, the Factor Replacement in Surgery Trial (NCT04114643), to better evaluate the role of factor concentrates versus FFP in cardiac surgical bleeding.

Topical Hemostatic Agents

In aortic surgical patients, hemostatic agents are often applied as adjunctive measures to promote hemostasis. Multiple agents have been reported in cardiac surgical patients, and commonly encountered ones are summarized in Table 1. They are typically applied directly to the site of oozing within the surgical field. In patients with active bleeding, the application of such agents can be challenging, which may limit their efficacy. Although much of the data evaluating these agents is from retrospective analyses, there are some randomized clinical trials that have been previously reviewed [82]. Topical agents can be broadly classified into those that provide a mechanical barrier, those that contain an active hemostatic agent, or those that combine both of these elements.

Table 1 Topical hemostatic agents commonly used in aortic surgery

Class of agent	Brand name (manufacturer)	Major component
Mechanical agents	Avitene (Bard Davol Inc, Warwick, RI)	Bovine collagen
	Gelfoam (Baxter, Deerfield, IL)	Porcine gelatin
	Surgicel (Ethicon/J&J, New Brunswick, NJ)	Cellulose
Non-active sealants	Bioglue (Cryolife, Kennesaw, GA)	Bovine albumin + glutaraldehyde
	Coseal (Baxter, Deerfield, IL)	Polyethylene glycol
Active agents	Thrombin JMI (Pzifer, New York, NY)	Bovine thrombin
	Evithrom (Ethicon/J&J, New Brunswick, NJ)	Pooled human thrombin
	Recothrom (Baxter, Deerfield, IL)	Recombinant human thrombin
Combination agents	Floseal (Baxter, Deerfield, IL)	Human thrombin + bovine gelatin
	Surgiflo (Ethicon/J&J, New Brunswick, NJ)	Human thrombin + porcine gelatin
	Evicel (Ethicon/J&J, New Brunswick, NJ)	Human thrombin + human fibrinogen
	Tisseal (Baxter, Deerfield, IL)	Human thrombin + human fibrinogen

Mechanical hemostatic agents are used to provide a barrier at the site of bleeding to allow for potential hemostatic activation and provide a scaffold for the accumulation of critical hemostatic factors. Because they rely on the patient's coagulation system, they should be left in place until clot forms. The most widely used agent of this type is simply bone wax, whose application is almost ubiquitous with sternal closure. Other agents are mainly derived from porcine gelatin or bovine collagen, which in its anhydrous form, can bind bleeding surfaces. Collagen sponges are similar to microfibrillar collagen but obtained from bovine tendon or skin.

Synthetic sealants are also applied to reduce bleeding in a mechanical fashion. A synthetic polyethylene glycol has been extensively used in Bentall thoracic aortic surgery [83]. For major aortic and other cardiac surgical patients, Coselli et al. examined the use a "bioglue" that contains bovine albumin with glutaraldehyde and reported improved hemostasis at anastomotic sites [84]. Despite the potential efficacy, glutaraldehyde may have the potential for tissue injury compared to other potential topical hemostatic products [85].

The compound for most active topical agents is thrombin, used either as a single therapy or combined by the surgeon with a mechanical agent (e.g., a gelatin sponge). The concept of topical thrombin is to locally activate the clotting cascade. Early topical thrombin preparations were bovine derived. Unfortunately, the xenogenic source induced antibody formation against human thrombin and factor V, causing potential hypersensitivity reactions as well as complex coagulopathic bleeding states. As a result, bovine thrombin is seldom used in the current era. The development of both purified and recombinant human thrombin has reduced these adverse reactions.

Therapeutic agents that combine both mechanical properties and have an active hemostatic agent fall into two categories: gelatin plus thrombin (often termed 'flowable' agents), and fibrin sealants. The gelatin used for flowable agents is either porcine or bovine derived and then combined with human thrombin. The product must be reconstituted when ready to use and is typically delivered via a specialized applicator. Fibrin sealants contain two critical hemostatic factors, thrombin, and fibrinogen. They can be administered as either a patch or in liquid form to provide local hemostasis, but require a relatively dry field to be effective. For these different agents, different sources of hemostatic factors are used in individual preparations and include human, bovine collagen and thrombin, and equine collagen. Fibrin sealants can also be mixtures of human fibrinogen, thrombin, and an antifibrinolytic agent to prevent clot lysis, traditionally aprotinin [86].

Summary

Coagulopathy and bleeding management requires a multimodal approach that includes fibrinogen repletion, providing appropriate procoagulants, and antifibrinolytic agents. When patients bleed, surgical sources of bleeding should also be considered, especially in an ICU setting. In addition to allogeneic blood transfusions, factor concentrates are increasingly management strategies to consider in treatment algorithms. With major hemorrhage, specific protocols for massive transfusion should be considered. Bleeding management algorithms in cardiac surgical patients are increasingly used that include this multimodal therapy along with as well as goal-directed management with point-of-care viscoelastic testing.

References

1. Despotis GJ, Avidan MS, Hogue CW Jr. Mechanisms and attenuation of hemostatic activation during extracorporeal circulation. Ann Thorac Surg. 2001;72(5):S1821–31.
2. Levy JH, Tanaka KA, Steiner ME. Evaluation and management of bleeding during cardiac surgery. Curr Hematol Rep. 2005;4(5):368–72.
3. Levy JH, Despotis GJ. Transfusion and hemostasis in cardiac surgery. Transfusion. 2008;48(1 Suppl):1S.
4. Levy JH. Pharmacologic methods to reduce perioperative bleeding. Transfusion. 2008;48(1 Suppl):31S–8S.
5. Goodnough LT, Levy JH, Murphy MF. Concepts of blood transfusion in adults. Lancet. 2013;381(9880):1845–54.
6. Steiner ME, Despotis GJ. Transfusion algorithms and how they apply to blood conservation: the high-risk cardiac surgical patient. Hematol Oncol Clin North Am. 2007;21(1):177–84.
7. Levy JH, Dutton RP, Hemphill JC 3rd, Shander A, Cooper D, Paidas MJ, et al. Multidisciplinary approach to the challenge of hemostasis. Anesth Analg. 2010;110(2):354–64.
8. Ortmann E, Klein AA, Sharples LD, Walsh R, Jenkins DP, Luddington RJ, et al. Point-of-care assessment of hypothermia and protamine-induced platelet dysfunction with multiple electrode aggregometry (Multiplate(R)) in patients undergoing cardiopulmonary bypass. Anesth Analg. 2013;116(3):533–40.
9. Despotis GJ, Skubas NJ, Goodnough LT. Optimal management of bleeding and transfusion in patients undergoing cardiac surgery. Semin Thorac Cardiovasc Surg. 1999;11(2):84–104.
10. Avidan MS, Alcock EL, Da Fonseca J, Ponte J, Desai JB, Despotis GJ, et al. Comparison of structured use of routine laboratory tests or near-patient assessment with clinical judgement in the management of bleeding after cardiac surgery. Br J Anaesth. 2004;92(2):178–86.
11. Hanke AA, Herold U, Dirkmann D, Tsagakis K, Jakob H, Gorlinger K. Thromboelastometry based early goal-directed coagulation management reduces blood transfusion requirements, adverse events, and costs in acute type A aortic dissection: a pilot study. Transfus Med Hemother. 2012;39(2):121–8.
12. Nuttall GA, Oliver WC, Santrach PJ, Bryant S, Dearani JA, Schaff HV, et al. Efficacy of a simple intraoperative transfusion algorithm for nonerythrocyte component utilization after cardiopulmonary bypass. Anesthesiology. 2001;94(5):773–81; Discussion 5A–6A.
13. Despotis GJ, Grishaber JE, Goodnough LT. The effect of an intraoperative treatment algorithm on physicians' transfusion practice in cardiac surgery. Transfusion. 1994;34(4):290–6.
14. Shore-Lesserson L, Manspeizer HE, DePerio M, Francis S, Vela-Cantos F, Ergin MA. Thromboelastography-guided transfusion algorithm reduces transfusions in complex cardiac surgery. Anesth Analg. 1999;88(2):312–9.
15. Karkouti K, Callum J, Wijeysundera DN, Rao V, Crowther M, Grocott HP, et al. Point-of-care hemostatic testing in cardiac surgery: a stepped-wedge clustered randomized controlled trial. Circulation. 2016;134(16):1152–62.
16. Lodewyks C, Heinrichs J, Grocott HP, Karkouti K, Romund G, Arora RC, et al. Point-of-care viscoelastic hemostatic testing in cardiac surgery patients: a systematic review and meta-analysis. Can J Anaesth. 2018;65(12):1333–47.

17. Serraino GF, Murphy GJ. Routine use of viscoelastic blood tests for diagnosis and treatment of coagulopathic bleeding in cardiac surgery: updated systematic review and meta-analysis. Br J Anaesth. 2017;118(6):823–33.
18. Deppe AC, Weber C, Zimmermann J, Kuhn EW, Slottosch I, Liakopoulos OJ, et al. Point-of-care thromboelastography/thromboelastometry-based coagulation management in cardiac surgery: a meta-analysis of 8332 patients. J Surg Res. 2016;203(2):424–33.
19. Goodnough LT, Despotis GJ, Hogue CW Jr, Ferguson TB Jr. On the need for improved transfusion indicators in cardiac surgery. Ann Thorac Surg. 1995;60(2):473–80.
20. Karkouti K, Cohen MM, McCluskey SA, Sher GD. A multivariable model for predicting the need for blood transfusion in patients undergoing first-time elective coronary bypass graft surgery. Transfusion. 2001;41(10):1193–203.
21. Practice guidelines for perioperative blood transfusion and adjuvant therapies: an updated report by the American Society of Anesthesiologists Task Force on Perioperative Blood Transfusion and Adjuvant Therapies. Anesthesiology. 2006;105:198–208.
22. D'Agostino RS, Jacobs JP, Badhwar V, Fernandez FG, Paone G, Wormuth DW, et al. The Society of Thoracic Surgeons Adult Cardiac Surgery Database: 2019 update on outcomes and quality. Ann Thorac Surg. 2019;107(1):24–32.
23. Mazer CD, Whitlock RP, Fergusson DA, Hall J, Belley-Cote E, Connolly K, et al. Restrictive or liberal red-cell transfusion for cardiac surgery. N Engl J Med. 2017;377(22):2133–44.
24. Gonzalez EA, Moore FA, Holcomb JB, Miller CC, Kozar RA, Todd SR, et al. Fresh frozen plasma should be given earlier to patients requiring massive transfusion. J Trauma. 2007;62(1):112–9.
25. Muller MC, Straat M, Meijers JC, Klinkspoor JH, de Jonge E, Arbous MS, et al. Fresh frozen plasma transfusion fails to influence the hemostatic balance in critically ill patients with a coagulopathy. J Thromb Haemost. 2015;13(6):989–97.
26. Holland LL, Brooks JP. Toward rational fresh frozen plasma transfusion: The effect of plasma transfusion on coagulation test results. Am J Clin Pathol. 2006;126(1):133–9.
27. Witt DM, Nieuwlaat R, Clark NP, Ansell J, Holbrook A, Skov J, et al. American Society of Hematology 2018 guidelines for management of venous thromboembolism: optimal management of anticoagulation therapy. Blood Adv. 2018;2(22):3257–91.
28. Okita Y, Takamoto S, Ando M, Morota T, Yamaki F, Matsukawa R, et al. Coagulation and fibrinolysis system in aortic surgery under deep hypothermic circulatory arrest with aprotinin: the importance of adequate heparinization. Circulation. 1997;96(9 Suppl):II-376–81.
29. Williams B, Wehman B, Mazzeffi MA, Odonkor P, Harris RL, Kon Z, et al. Acute intracardiac thrombosis and pulmonary thromboembolism after cardiopulmonary bypass: a systematic review of reported cases. Anesth Analg. 2018;126(2):425–34.
30. Leslie SD, Toy PT. Laboratory hemostatic abnormalities in massively transfused patients given red blood cells and crystalloid. Am J Clin Pathol. 1991;96(6):770–3.
31. Nascimento B, Goodnough LT, Levy JH. Cryoprecipitate therapy. Br J Anaesth. 2014;113(6):922–34.
32. Hardy JF, de Moerloose P, Samama CM. Massive transfusion and coagulopathy: pathophysiology and implications for clinical management. Can J Anaesth. 2006;53(6 Suppl): S40–58.
33. Karkouti K, O'Farrell R, Yau TM, Beattie WS. Prediction of massive blood transfusion in cardiac surgery. Can J Anaesth. 2006;53(8):781–94.
34. Cap AP, Pidcoke HF, Spinella P, Strandenes G, Borgman MA, Schreiber M, et al. Damage control resuscitation. Mil Med. 2018;183(suppl_2):36–43.
35. Sheppard CA, Logdberg LE, Zimring JC, Hillyer CD. Transfusion-related Acute Lung Injury. Hematol Oncol Clin North Am. 2007;21(1):163–76.
36. Spiess BD. Risks of transfusion: outcome focus. Transfusion. 2004;44(12 Suppl):4S–14S.
37. Despotis GJ, Zhang L, Lublin DM. Transfusion risks and transfusion-related pro-inflammatory responses. Hematol Oncol Clin North Am. 2007;21(1):147–61.
38. Alam A, Huang M, Yi QL, Lin Y, Hannach B. Perioperative transfusion-related acute lung injury: the Canadian Blood Services experience. Transfus Apher Sci. 2014;50(3):392–8.

39. Levy JH, Tanaka KA. Inflammatory response to cardiopulmonary bypass. Ann Thorac Surg. 2003;75(2):S715–20.
40. Paparella D, Brister SJ, Buchanan MR. Coagulation disorders of cardiopulmonary bypass: a review. Intensive Care Med. 2004;30(10):1873–81.
41. Eaton MP. Antifibrinolytic therapy in surgery for congenital heart disease. Anesth Analg. 2008;106(4):1087–100.
42. Munoz JJ, Birkmeyer NJ, Birkmeyer JD, O'Connor GT, Dacey LJ. Is epsilon-aminocaproic acid as effective as aprotinin in reducing bleeding with cardiac surgery?: a meta-analysis. Circulation. 1999;99(1):81–9.
43. Sedrakyan A, Treasure T, Elefteriades JA. Effect of aprotinin on clinical outcomes in coronary artery bypass graft surgery: a systematic review and meta-analysis of randomized clinical trials. J Thorac Cardiovasc Surg. 2004;128(3):442–8.
44. Ferraris VA, Ferraris SP, Saha SP, Hessel EA 2nd, Haan CK, Royston BD, et al. Perioperative blood transfusion and blood conservation in cardiac surgery: the Society of Thoracic Surgeons and The Society of Cardiovascular Anesthesiologists clinical practice guideline. Ann Thorac Surg. 2007;83(5 Suppl):S27–86.
45. Levy JH. Pharmacologic preservation of the hemostatic system during cardiac surgery. Ann Thorac Surg. 2001;72(5):S1814–20.
46. Koster A, Faraoni D, Levy JH. Antifibrinolytic therapy for cardiac surgery: an update. Anesthesiology. 2015;123(1):214–21.
47. Murkin JM, Falter F, Granton J, Young B, Burt C, Chu M. High-dose tranexamic acid is associated with nonischemic clinical seizures in cardiac surgical patients. Anesth Analg. 2009;110(2):350–3.
48. Myles PS, Smith JA, Forbes A, Silbert B, Jayarajah M, Painter T, et al. Tranexamic acid in patients undergoing coronary-artery surgery. N Engl J Med. 2017;376(2):136–48.
49. Makhija N, Sarupria A, Kumar Choudhary S, Das S, Lakshmy R, Kiran U. Comparison of epsilon aminocaproic acid and tranexamic Acid in thoracic aortic surgery: clinical efficacy and safety. J Cardiothorac Vasc Anesth. 2013;27(6):1201–7.
50. Martin K, Wiesner G, Breuer T, Lange R, Tassani P. The risks of aprotinin and tranexamic acid in cardiac surgery: a one-year follow-up of 1188 consecutive patients. Anesth Analg. 2008;107(6):1783–90.
51. Levy JH, Adkinson NF. Anaphylaxis during cardiac surgery: implications for clinicans. Anesth Analg. 106(2):392–403.
52. Kimmel SE, Sekeres M, Berlin JA, Ellison N. Mortality and adverse events after protamine administration in patients undergoing cardiopulmonary bypass. Anesth Analg. 2002;94(6):1402–8, table of contents.
53. Mochizuki T, Olson PJ, Szlam F, Ramsay JG, Levy JH. Protamine reversal of heparin affects platelet aggregation and activated clotting time after cardiopulmonary bypass. Anesth Analg. 1998;87(4):781–5.
54. Sniecinski RM, Levy JH. Bleeding and management of coagulopathy. J Thorac Cardiovasc Surg. 2011;142(662-7):662–7.
55. Mannucci PM, Levi M. Prevention and treatment of major blood loss. N Engl J Med. 2007;356(22):2301–11.
56. Mannucci PM. Treatment of von Willebrand's disease. N Engl J Med. 2004;351(7):683–94.
57. Mannucci PM. Hemostatic drugs. N Engl J Med. 1998;339(4):245–53.
58. Mannucci PM. Desmopressin (DDAVP) in the treatment of bleeding disorders: the first 20 years. Blood. 1997;90(7):2515–21.
59. Frankville DD, Harper GB, Lake CL, Johns RA. Hemodynamic consequences of desmopressin administration after cardiopulmonary bypass. Anesthesiology. 1991;74(6):988–96.
60. Rocha E, Llorens R, Paramo JA, Arcas R, Cuesta B, Trenor AM. Does desmopressin acetate reduce blood loss after surgery in patients on cardiopulmonary bypass? Circulation. 1988;77(6):1319–23.
61. de Prost D, Barbier-Boehm G, Hazebroucq J, Ibrahim H, Bielsky MC, Hvass U, et al. Desmopressin has no beneficial effect on excessive postoperative bleeding or blood prod-

uct requirements associated with cardiopulmonary bypass. Thromb Haemost. 1992;68(2): 106–10.
62. Nielsen VG, Levy JH. Fibrinogen and bleeding: old molecule—new ideas. Anesth Analg. 2007;105(4):902–3.
63. Levy JH. Massive transfusion coagulopathy. Semin Hematol. 2006;43(1 Suppl 1):S59–63.
64. Rahe-Meyer N, Solomon C, Hanke A, Schmidt DS, Knoerzer D, Hochleitner G, et al. Effects of fibrinogen concentrate as first-line therapy during major aortic replacement surgery: a randomized, placebo-controlled Trial. Anesthesiology. 2013;118(1):40–50.
65. Karlsson M, Ternstrom L, Hyllner M, Baghaei F, Flinck A, Skrtic S, et al. Prophylactic fibrinogen infusion reduces bleeding after coronary artery bypass surgery. A prospective randomised pilot study. Thromb Haemost. 2009;102(1):137–44.
66. Rahe-Meyer N, Pichlmaier M, Haverich A, Solomon C, Winterhalter M, Piepenbrock S, et al. Bleeding management with fibrinogen concentrate targeting a high-normal plasma fibrinogen level: a pilot study. Br J Anaesth. 2009;102(6):785–92.
67. Rahe-Meyer N, Solomon C, Winterhalter M, Piepenbrock S, Tanaka K, Haverich A, et al. Thromboelastometry-guided administration of fibrinogen concentrate for the treatment of excessive intraoperative bleeding in thoracoabdominal aortic aneurysm surgery. J Thorac Cardiovasc Surg. 2009;138(3):694–702.
68. Solomon C, Pichlmaier U, Schoechl H, Hagl C, Raymondos K, Scheinichen D, et al. Recovery of fibrinogen after administration of fibrinogen concentrate to patients with severe bleeding after cardiopulmonary bypass surgery. Br J Anaesth. 2010;104(5):555–62.
69. Solomon C, Schochl H, Hanke A, Calatzis A, Hagl C, Tanaka K, et al. Haemostatic therapy in coronary artery bypass graft patients with decreased platelet function: comparison of fibrinogen concentrate with allogeneic blood products. Scand J Clin Lab Invest. 2012;72(2):121–8.
70. Gill R, Herbertson M, Vuylsteke A, Olsen PS, von Heymann C, Mythen M, et al. Safety and efficacy of recombinant activated factor VII: a randomized placebo-controlled trial in the setting of bleeding after cardiac surgery. Circulation. 2009;120(1):21–7.
71. Levi M, Levy JH, Andersen HF, Truloff D. Safety of recombinant activated factor VII in randomized clinical trials. N Engl J Med. 2010;363(19):1791–800.
72. Ranucci M, Baryshnikova E, Castelvecchio S, Pelissero G, Surgical and Clinical Outcome Research (SCORE) Group. Major bleeding, transfusions, and anemia: the deadly triad of cardiac surgery. Ann Thorac Surg. 2013;96(2):478–85.
73. Pagano D, Milojevic M, Meesters MI, Benedetto U, Bolliger D, von Heymann C, et al. 2017 EACTS/EACTA Guidelines on patient blood management for adult cardiac surgery. Eur J Cardiothorac Surg. 2018;53(1):79–111.
74. Levy JH, Douketis J, Steiner T, Goldstein JN, Milling TJ. Prothrombin complex concentrates for perioperative vitamin K antagonist and non-vitamin K anticoagulant reversal. Anesthesiology. 2018;129(6):1171–84.
75. Levy JH, Tanaka KA, Dietrich W. Perioperative hemostatic management of patients treated with vitamin K antagonists. Anesthesiology. 2008;109(5):918–26.
76. Brown KS, Zahir H, Grosso MA, Lanz HJ, Mercuri MF, Levy JH. Nonvitamin K antagonist oral anticoagulant activity: challenges in measurement and reversal. Crit Care. 2016;20(1):273.
77. Ghadimi K, Levy JH, Welsby IJ. Prothrombin complex concentrates for bleeding in the perioperative setting. Anesth Analg. 2016;122(5):1287–300.
78. Bershad EM, Suarez JI. Prothrombin complex concentrates for oral anticoagulant therapy-related intracranial hemorrhage: a review of the literature. Neurocrit Care. 2010;12(3):403–13.
79. Levy JH, Douketis J, Weitz JI. Reversal agents for non-vitamin K antagonist oral anticoagulants. Nat Rev Cardiol. 2018;15(5):273–81.
80. Gorlinger K, Dirkmann D, Hanke AA, Kamler M, Kottenberg E, Thielmann M, et al. First-line therapy with coagulation factor concentrates combined with point-of-care coagulation testing is associated with decreased allogeneic blood transfusion in cardiovascular surgery: a retrospective, single-center cohort study. Anesthesiology. 2011;115(6):1179–91.

81. Song HK, Tibayan FA, Kahl EA, Sera VA, Slater MS, Deloughery TG, et al. Safety and efficacy of prothrombin complex concentrates for the treatment of coagulopathy after cardiac surgery. J Thorac Cardiovasc Surg. 2014;147(3):1036–40.
82. Bracey A, Shander A, Aronson S, Boucher BA, Calcaterra D, Chu MWA, et al. The use of topical hemostatic agents in cardiothoracic surgery. Ann Thorac Surg. 2017;104(1):353–60.
83. Natour E, Suedkamp M, Dapunt OE. Assessment of the effect on blood loss and transfusion requirements when adding a polyethylene glycol sealant to the anastomotic closure of aortic procedures: a case-control analysis of 102 patients undergoing Bentall procedures. J Cardiothorac Surg. 2012;7:105.
84. Coselli JS, Bavaria JE, Fehrenbacher J, Stowe CL, Macheers SK, Gundry SR. Prospective randomized study of a protein-based tissue adhesive used as a hemostatic and structural adjunct in cardiac and vascular anastomotic repair procedures. J Am Coll Surg. 2003;197(2):243–52; Discussion 52–3.
85. Furst W, Banerjee A. Release of glutaraldehyde from an albumin-glutaraldehyde tissue adhesive causes significant in vitro and in vivo toxicity. Ann Thorac Surg. 2005;79(5):1522–8. Discussion 9
86. Schenk WG 3rd, Burks SG, Gagne PJ, Kagan SA, Lawson JH, Spotnitz WD. Fibrin sealant improves hemostasis in peripheral vascular surgery: a randomized prospective trial. Ann Surg. 2003;237(6):871–6. Discussion 6

Part IV
Postoperative Monitoring and Medical Management

Monitoring After Surgery for Acute Aortic Syndromes

Andrew M. Vekstein and Adam R. Williams

Immediate Post-operative Monitoring

After Type A Dissection Repair

Management of Hemodynamics

While patients presenting with Type A Aortic Dissection require aggressive anti-impulse therapy initially, hemodynamics after surgical repair are highly variable. In general, the fragile nature of aortic suture lines requires very close monitoring of blood pressure, with systolic blood pressure (SBP) less than 120 mmHg and diastolic blood pressure (DBP) less than 80 mmHg [1]. We recommend placement of bilateral radial artery lines and treatment based off of the line with higher pressures. If there is concern for differential perfusion pressures in patients with complex true versus false luminal flow, then a femoral artery line should also be inserted. Due to often long periods of cardiopulmonary bypass and hypothermic circulatory arrest, patients are often severely vasodilated post-operatively requiring vasopressors and ongoing volume resuscitation upon arrival in the intensive care unit [2]. If the dissection involved the aortic root and replacement of the sinuses of Valsalva is required, myocardial protection intra-operatively becomes critical to optimizing the early recovery period. If patients develop low cardiac output syndrome, inotropic agents such as epinephrine may be utilized cautiously.

A. M. Vekstein · A. R. Williams (✉)
Division of Thoracic and Cardiovascular Surgery, Department of Surgery, Duke University Medical Center, Durham, NC, USA
e-mail: adam.r.williams@duke.edu

J. S. Coselli et al. (eds.), *Aortic Dissection and Acute Aortic Syndromes*,
https://doi.org/10.1007/978-3-030-66668-2_40

Coagulopathy

Surgical repair for acute aortic syndromes is associated with profound derangements in the coagulation cascade. The etiology of coagulopathy is multifactorial and includes factor and platelet dysfunction after hypothermic circulatory arrest and the exposure of blood to the aortic media, which results in cascade activation and consumptive coagulopathy, with both clotting factor and fibrinogen levels continuing to drop even after ascending aortic repair [3]. A systematic and aggressive approach to transfusion is needed to obtain hemostasis intra-operatively and prevent ongoing bleeding post-operatively. At our institution, all patients undergoing hypothermic circulatory arrest have platelet and fibrinogen levels, as well as thromboelastography, checked before weaning from cardiopulmonary bypass, and receive prophylactic transfusion of four units of pooled platelet concentrate before separating from bypass. Once off bypass, protamine and ε-aminocaproic acid infusions are initiated, along with single dose of desmopressin, two units of platelets, and two units of cryoprecipitate. After management of any surgical bleeding sources, laboratory values are again checked and transfusion dictated by international normalized ratio, platelet, fibrinogen, activated clotting time and hematocrit levels (Fig. 1). In patients with ongoing medical bleeding, defined by uncontrolled flow through needle holes and raw surfaces, one milligram dose of recombinant factor VIIa (rFVIIa) is given. If there is ongoing bleeding then prothrombin complex concentrate 10 units/kg is administered. This protocol is repeated for continued bleeding. Once hemostasis is achieved the sternum is closed. In cases of massive bleeding not responsive to blood products, the chest is packed with sponges and the patient transferred to the ICU for ongoing resuscitation with delayed sternal closure.

Post-operatively, close monitoring of chest tube output and thromboelastography guided transfusion is recommended. In patients presenting with DeBakey Type I aortic dissection, an ongoing consumptive coagulopathy is expected even after ascending and/or arch repair due to ongoing flow in the false lumen [2].

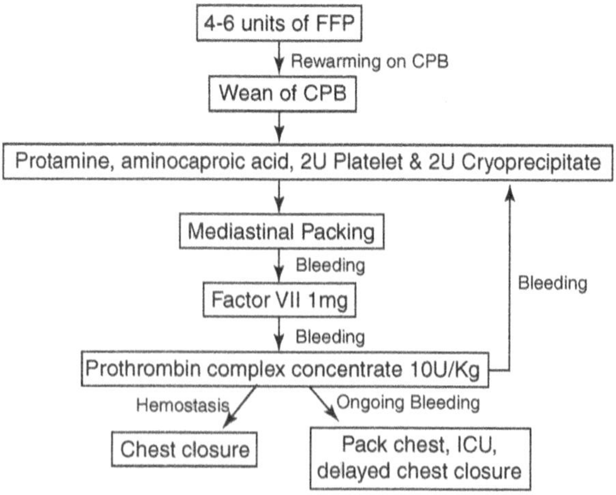

Fig. 1 Guidelines for transfusion for coagulopathic bleeding after type A dissection repair. Adapted from J Cardiovasc Surg 2019;60:633–6 [4]

Ongoing Malperfusion Syndromes

In general, reperfusion of the true lumen through ascending aortic repair is thought to improve malperfusion syndromes after Type A Dissection [5]. However, every dissection generates a different flap anatomy with variable re-entry tears. Furthermore, malperfusion may be a static or dynamic process. Static malperfusion refers to a process in which the dissection tear propagates into a branch vessel or the intimal flap herniates into a branch vessel. Static malperfusion quickly leads to branch vessel thrombosis, which may not improve with improved perfusion of the true lumen. By contrast, dynamic malperfusion refers to intermittent occlusion of a branch vessel by the dissection flap, and usually improves with improved true luminal flow [6].

Post-operatively, sedation should be weaned and neurologic examination performed as soon as is appropriate with patients' hemodynamic status to assess for new or worsening stroke. Renal replacement therapy may be required early after surgery for acute renal failure related to malperfusion and overall metabolic derangements. Abdominal pain post-operatively is an ominous sign as mesenteric malperfusion and bowel ischemia is associated with very poor outcomes (as high as 70% mortality) [7]. Many centers have shifted towards a TEVAR and/or intimal fenestration approach if mesenteric ischemia is suspected [5]. Concern for limb ischemia on initial presentation similarly may alter treatment algorithm and require delay in ascending aortic repair [8]. Peripheral pulse exam should be noted before ascending repair and before leaving the operating room. Any concern for worsening exam after initial operation should prompt Vascular Surgical consultation, as urgent bypass and/or fasciotomy may be required [9].

After Endovascular Repair for Type B Aortic Dissection

Management of Hemodynamics

Hemodynamic management after TEVAR differs greatly from the initial management for with Type B dissection. On initial presentation, aggressive anti-impulse therapy should be initiated, typically with intravenous esmolol or labetalol. Second line agents include calcium channel blockers, such as nicardipine, and nitroprusside. After TEVAR, however, permissive hypertension (SBP > 140–160 mmHg) is often pursued to optimize spinal cord perfusion [10, 11]. There are competing interests, though, as the Vascular Surgery literature has suggested that perioperative hypertension may increase type II endoleak and inhibit shrinkage of abdominal aortic aneurysm sac [12].

Spinal Cord Protection

Although utilized frequently during open thoracoabdominal aortic aneurysm or dissection repair, the use of lumbar cerebrospinal fluid (CSF) drainage before TEVAR is highly variable among institutions. Common indications for CSF drainage include patients with prior open or endovascular repair of the thoracic, abdominal or thoracoabdominal aorta. At our institution, spinal drains are only placed if greater than 75% coverage of the descending thoracic aorta, including intercostals below vertebral level T6, is planned [10]. However, new data suggests that with high blood pressure goals post operatively (SBP > 160 mmHg), even extended length TEVAR (defined as endograft coverage of the entire descending thoracic aorta from the left subclavian artery to below the diaphragm to the level of the celiac artery) may be performed without spinal drain without adding significant risk of spinal cord ischemia [13]. However, there should be a low threshold to place drain post-operatively if patients develop any signs or symptoms of spinal cord ischemia, notably lower extremity weakness or urinary retention, which does not improve with augmentation of blood pressure. Although typically employed intra-operatively, motor and somatosensory evoked potential monitoring may be utilized post-operatively for early identification of potential spinal cord injury and adjust hemodynamic management accordingly when neurologic exam cannot yet be performed [14].

Retrograde Type A Dissection

One of the most feared complications of TEVAR is the propagation of Type B dissection retrotgrade into the ascending aorta. Although it only occurs in 2.5% of cases, retrograde Type A dissection (RTAD) is associated with high mortality (up to 40%). Some studies suggest that RTAD is associated with devices with bare metal proximal stents [15]. Ideally, RTAD should be identified in the hybrid operating room during completion aortogram. At our institution we also perform intraoperative TEE on all TEVAR patients to assess the ascending aorta after stent deployment. If the patient is a surgical candidate, RTAD is an indication for emergent sternotomy and ascending aortic repair.

Long Term Monitoring and Surveillance

Risk Factor Modification

Most patient's presenting with acute aortic syndromes have multiple risk factors, such as poorly controlled hypertension, hyperlipidemia and smoking [16]. After initial management, coordination with primary care providers and Cardiologists is crucial for risk factor modification. For patients with any thoracic aortic disease, AHA/AATS/STS Guidelines [17] recommend target blood pressure <140/90 mmHg for non-diabetic patients or <130/80 mmHg for patients with diabetes or chronic kidney disease. Although the exact post-dissection medication regimen is institution dependent, beta-blockers have been favored anti-hypertensive to prevent long-term aneurysmal degeneration in multiple studies [18]. A statin is recommended with

Low Density Lipoprotein (LDL) <70 and smoking cessation resources should be provided to all patients who currently use tobacco products. Medications should be reviewed at all subsequent surgical follow up appointments. If patients have features concerning for connective tissue disorder, a referral to Genetics is also warranted. Patient's diagnosed with Marfan's Syndrome should be started on an angiotensin II-receptor blocker, which has been demonstrated in animal and human studies to reduce the rate of aortic-root dilation [19].

Imaging Frequency and Modality

Consistent institutional imaging and follow-up guidelines after acute aortic syndromes are an important element of an aortic center. However, specific national and international guidelines lack strong evidence to guide frequency of imaging [17]. Our institutional protocol after Type A dissection repair (Fig. 2) is for repeat imaging 3 and 9 months after initial surgical repair, then annually henceforth. If imaging is stable after 5 years, imaging frequency is liberalized to every 18–24 months. If there is concern for dilated segment greater than 4 cm, additional imaging is obtained 6 months after initial operation.

Computed tomographic angiography has typically been the preferred examination to diagnose acute aortic syndrome and surveil patients after aortic repair. Specific thoraco-abdominal aortic and dissection protocols yield even more sensitive and specific results. However, magnetic resonance angiography (MRA) has been increasingly utilized in the acute and chronic settings. Potential benefits of MRA include assessment of ventricular and valvular function, advanced analysis with four dimensional protocols and computational fluid dynamics, in addition to reduced radiation exposure for patients who will require lifelong surveillance [17]. At our institution, we frequently alternate annually between CTA with Echocardiography versus MRA alone for annual monitoring.

After Type A Dissection Repair

Monitoring of Valvular and Ventricular Function

If aortic root replacement is indicated at the time of index operation, whether valve sparing or with valve replacement (Bentall Operation), STS/AHA guidelines recommend echocardiography before discharge and annually post-operatively [20]. Some centers advocate for more frequent echo in the first year, paired with CTA or MRA. Particular attention should be paid to stenotic or regurgitant changes in the native or prosthetic aortic valve, cardiomyopathy, ventricular dimensions, among other Echo findings [21].

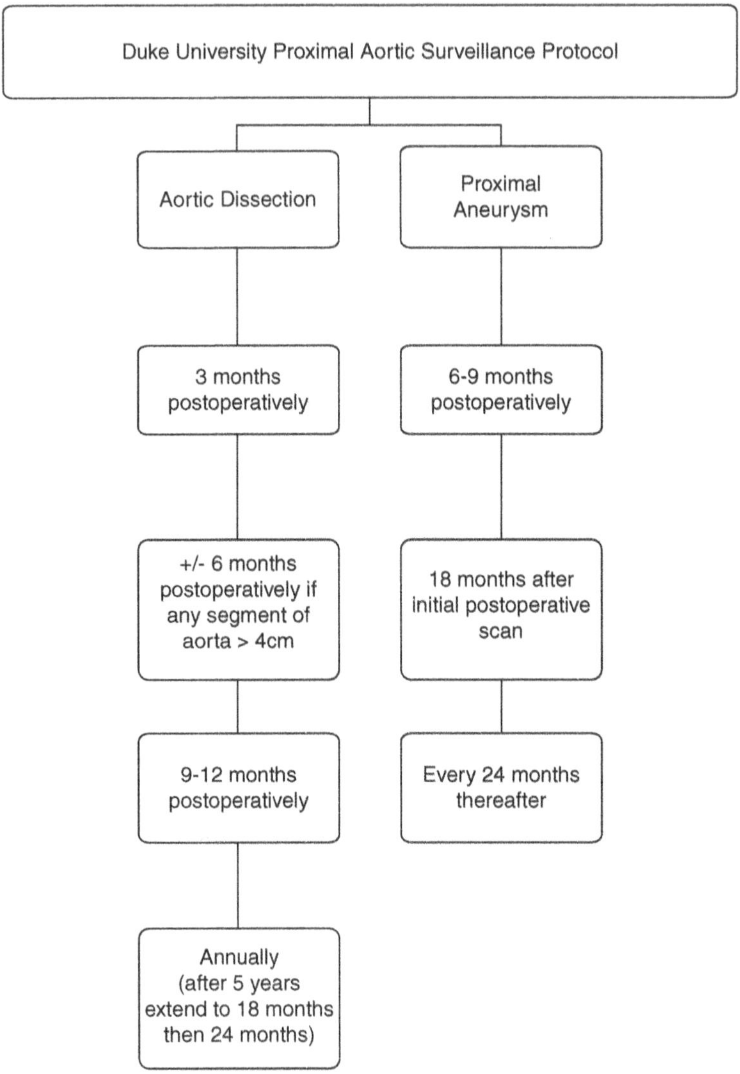

Fig. 2 Duke University Aortic Center protocol for aortic surveillance [18]

Fate of the Distal Aorta

The extent of repair of a Debakey Type I aortic dissection during initial surgery is a topic of disagreement among experts, with some centers advocating for ascending or hemi-arch repair alone and others pursuing a more aggressive total arch approach with or without elephant trunk extended into descending aorta [21]. Regardless of the initial repair, important considerations during follow up include suture line pseudoaneurysm (Fig. 3) and the downstream untreated aorta. Rate of re-intervention on the descending aorta after ascending/hemi-arch repair for Type A dissection is reported between 20 and 40% [22].

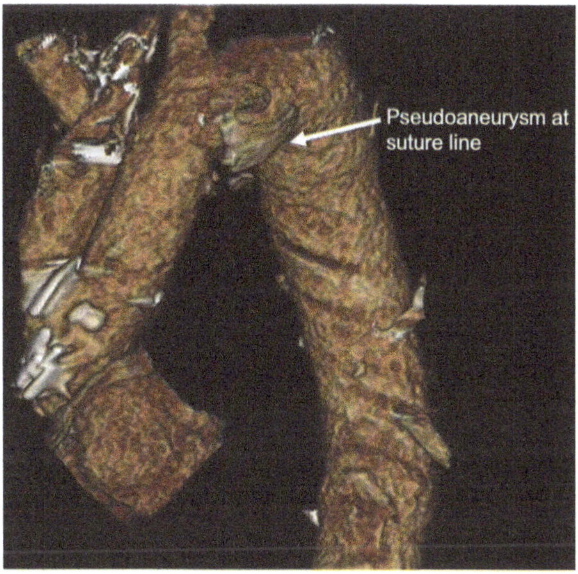

Fig. 3 Patient who developed a pseudoaneurysm at the distal suture line after zone 1 total arch replacement for type A dissection

Potential complications of residual Type B dissection after ascending/hemi-arch repair for Type A dissection include late malperfusion, aneurysmal degeneration and frank rupture. Indications for repair are the same as for Type B dissection in isolation, and include end-organ malperfusion (e.g. visceral, limb), refractory pain despite medical management, chronic dilation >5.5 cm or rapid dilation >0.5 cm in 6 months or 1.0 cm in a year. Approach to repair of residual type B dissection after ascending repair is dependent upon each patient and anatomy. If dissection involves the aortic arch with significant aneurysmal changes, total arch replacement with or without elephant trunk may be required. In patients with minimal arch involvement and degeneration of the descending thoracic aorta, TEVAR may be considered. Criteria for success with TEVAR in this context includes suitable landing zone >2 cm (with or without coverage of left subclavian artery), minimal distal fenestrations throughout descending aorta and ideally all four visceral branches coming off of the false lumen. In patients with visceral branches off the false lumen or multiple distal fenestrations, TEVAR and subsequent thrombosis of the false lumen may create malperfusion syndrome or lead to endoleak [22]. Open thoracoabdominal aortic repair may be required in appropriate surgical candidates in this scenario.

After Type B Dissection Repair

Aneurysmal Dilatation of Untreated Segments

Dilation and degeneration of the distal descending and visceral aortic segments after TEVAR represents a complex challenge requiring multi-disciplinary, patient-specific management. Unlike primary aneurysmal disease, which is frequently limited to the infra-renal abdominal aorta, post-dissection aneurysm involves all visceral vessels and is associated with significant aortic remodeling and tortuosity. Open thoraco-abdominal aortic replacement is an option in patients who are bridged through their initial acute dissection with TEVAR, but is associated with significant morbidity and mortality. Early feasibility studies for fenestrated/branched thoracic endovascular repair show promising results, but are limited by small numbers [23].

Endoleak

Thoracic endografts were initially designed and FDA approved for thoracic aortic aneurysm. When increasingly utilized for aortic dissection, the anatomy of landing zones becomes suboptimal, placing patients at higher risk for endoleak in the early and late settings. Endoleak is blood flow into the aneurysm sac after endovascular repair and can be characterized into five types: Type IA and IB represent perigraft leakage at proximal or distal graft attachment sites respectively. Type II is retrograde flow from branch vessels within aneurysm sac. Type III is leakage through defect in the graft or between two endoprostheses. Type IV is leakage through the graft due to the porosity of the fabric. Type V is expansion of the aneurysm sac without obvious source on imaging [24]. The most common indication for intervention after TEVAR is Type IA endoleak, which presents high risk for rupture [25].

Stent Graft Induced New Entry Tears

When utilized for aortic dissection, TEVAR involves landing a device within the true lumen against the intimal flap, which may be associated with new intimal injury at the proximal or distal ends of the graft. Stent graft-inducted new entry tear (SINE) has an incidence as high as 28% with the most significant risk factor being oversizing of prosthesis [26]. Assessment for SINE is a critical component of follow up imaging, as this may present early or late after initial TEVAR. The frozen elephant trunk technique for type A repair can also result in PAU at the distal landing site (Fig. 4). Proximal SINE presents high risk of retrograde dissection and requires urgent intervention, while distal SINE may result in visceral malperfusion or more rapid expansion of the false lumen, but can often be managed with staged extension of endograft [27]. Stent graft associated wall injury without new entry tear is an emerging entity that must also be observed on imaging, as it is associated with pseudoaneurysm formation.

Conclusion

As surgical and endovascular therapies for acute aortic syndromes continue to evolve, a systematic approach is required for patient monitoring post-operatively and surveillance in the long term. Perioperatively, an understanding of

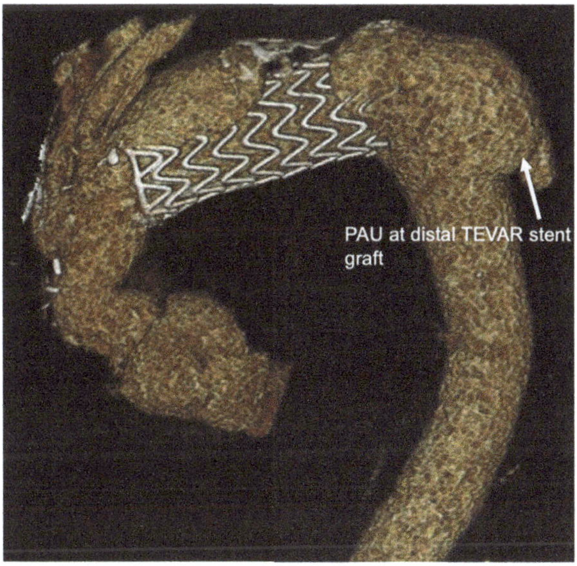

Fig. 4 Patient who developed a large penetrating aortic ulcer (PAU) at distal stent graft site following frozen elephant trunk for type A dissection

hemodynamics, spinal cord protection and the profound metabolic derangements associated with acute aortic syndromes leads to improved outcomes. In the long term, frequently monitoring with echocardiography, CT and MR imaging should focus on both common and more rare complications. As new technology and surgical approaches, such as the increased use of bare metal stents for endovascular repair of dissection, are utilized, further investigation into aortic remodeling and potential complications is warranted [28].

References

1. Melby SJ, Zierer A, Damiano RJ, Moon MR. Importance of Blood pressure control after repair of acute type A aortic dissection: 25-year follow-up in 252 patients. J Clin Hypertens. 2013;15(1):63–8.
2. Dayan V, Cal R, Giangrossi F. Risk factors for vasoplegia after cardiac surgery: a meta-analysis. Interact Cardiovasc Thorac Surg. 2019;28(6):838–44.
3. Liu Y, Han L, Li J, Gong M, Zhang H, Guan X. Consumption coagulopathy in acute aortic dissection: principles of management. J Cardiothorac Surg. 2017;12(1):50.
4. Wagner MA, Wang H, Benrashid E, Keenan JE, Krishnamurthy Y, Levy JH, et al. Protocolized hemostatic factor use in major thoracic aortic surgery. J Cardiovasc Surg (Torino). 2019 Oct;60(5):633–6.
5. Yang B, Patel HJ, Williams DM, Dasika NL, Deeb GM. Management of type A dissection with malperfusion. Ann Cardiothorac Surg. 2016;5(4):265–74.
6. Crawford TC, Beaulieu RJ, Ehlert BA, Ratchford EV, Black JH. Malperfusion syndromes in aortic dissection. Vasc Med. 2016;21(3):264–73.
7. Perera NK, Galvin SD, Seevanayagam S, Matalanis G. Optimal management of acute type A aortic dissection with mesenteric malperfusion. Interact Cardiovasc Thorac Surg. 2014;19(2):290–4.

8. Lawton JS. Commentary: A lethal disease begging for treatment consensus. J Thorac Cardiovasc Surg. 2019;158(6):1525–6.
9. Gargiulo M, Massoni CB, Gallitto E, Freyrie A, Trimarchi S, Faggioli G, et al. Lower limb malperfusion in type B aortic dissection: a systematic review. Ann Cardiothorac Surg. 2014;3(4):351–67.
10. Hanna JM, Andersen ND, Aziz H, Shah AA, McCann RL, Hughes GC. Results with selective preoperative lumbar drain placement for thoracic endovascular aortic repair. Ann Thorac Surg. 2013;95(6):1968–75.
11. Scali ST, Wang SK, Feezor RJ, Huber TS, Martin TD, Klodell CT, et al. Preoperative prediction of spinal cord ischemia after thoracic endovascular aortic repair. J Vasc Surg. 2014;60(6):1481–90.e1.
12. Miura S, Kurimoto Y, Ujihira K, Iba Y, Maruyama R, Yamada A, et al. Postoperative initial 2-day blood pressure management facilitates the shrinkage of abdominal aortic aneurysm after endovascular aneurysm repair by reducing the incidence of type II endoleak. J Vasc Surg. 2018;67(1):166–73.
13. Lou X, Duwayri YM, Jordan WD, Chen EP, Veeraswamy RK, Leshnower BG. The safety and efficacy of extended TEVAR in acute type B aortic dissection. Ann Thorac Surg [Internet]. 2020 [cited 2020 Apr 23]. Available from: https://www.annalsthoracicsurgery.org/article/S0003-4975(20)30091-6/abstract
14. Liu LY, Callahan B, Peterss S, Dumfarth J, Tranquilli M, Ziganshin BA, et al. Neuromonitoring using motor and somatosensory evoked potentials in aortic surgery. J Card Surg. 2016;31(6):383–9.
15. Chen Y, Zhang S, Liu L, Lu Q, Zhang T, Jing Z. Retrograde type A aortic dissection after thoracic endovascular aortic repair: a systematic review and meta-analysis. J Am Heart Assoc. 6(9):e004649.
16. Braverman AC. Acute aortic dissection. Circulation. 2010;122(2):184–8.
17. Hiratzka LF, Bakris GL, Beckman JA, Bersin RM, Carr VF, Casey DE, et al. 2010 ACCF/AHA/AATS/ACR/ASA/SCA/SCAI/SIR/STS/SVM guidelines for the diagnosis and management of patients with thoracic aortic disease. J Am Coll Cardiol. 2010;55(14):e27–129.
18. Zierer A, Voeller RK, Hill KE, Kouchoukos NT, Damiano RJ, Moon MR. Aortic enlargement and late reoperation after repair of acute type A aortic dissection. Ann Thorac Surg. 2007;84(2):479–87.
19. Brooke BS, Habashi JP, Judge DP, Patel N, Loeys B, Dietz HC. Angiotensin II blockade and aortic-root dilation in Marfan's syndrome. N Engl J Med. 2008;358(26):2787–95.
20. Iribarne A, Keenan J, Benrashid E, Wang H, Meza JM, Ganapathi A, et al. Imaging surveillance after proximal aortic operations: is it necessary? Ann Thorac Surg. 2017;103(3):734–41.
21. Svensson LG, Adams DH, Bonow RO, Kouchoukos NT, Miller DC, O'Gara PT, et al. Aortic valve and ascending aorta guidelines for management and quality measures. Ann Thorac Surg. 2013;95(6):S1–66.
22. Bavaria JE. Late aortic complications after type A dissection repair. Penn Physician VideoLink [Internet]. [cited 2020 Jun 9]. Available from http://videolink.pennmedicine.org/videos/late-aortic-complications-after-type-a-dissection-repair
23. Oikonomou K, Kopp R, Katsargyris A, Pfister K, Verhoeven EL, Kasprzak P. Outcomes of fenestrated/branched endografting in post-dissection thoracoabdominal aortic aneurysms. Eur J Vasc Endovasc Surg. 2014;48(6):641–8.
24. Baum RA, Stavropoulos SW, Fairman RM, Carpenter JP. Endoleaks after endovascular repair of abdominal aortic aneurysms. J Vasc Interv Radiol. 2003;14(9, Part 1):1111–7.
25. Svensson LG, Kouchoukos NT, Miller DC, et al. Expert consensus document on the treatment of descending thoracic aortic disease using endovascular stent-grafts. Ann Thorac Surg. 2008;85(1):A1.

26. Hughes GC. Stent graft-induced new entry tear (SINE): intentional and NOT. J Thorac Cardiovasc Surg. 2019;157(1):101–6.e3.
27. Pantaleo A, Jafrancesco G, Buia F, Leone A, Lovato L, Russo V, et al. Distal stent graft-induced new entry: an emerging complication of endovascular treatment in aortic dissection. Ann Thorac Surg. 2016;102(2):527–32.
28. Kazimierczak A, Rynio P, Jędrzejczak T, Samad R, Rybicka A, Gutowski P. Aortic remodeling after extended PETTICOAT technique in acute aortic dissection type III B. Ann Vasc Surg. 2020;66:183–92.

Medical Management of Uncomplicated Type B Acute Aortic Syndromes

Arvind K. Pandey, Umberto Campia, and Patrick T. O'Gara

Introduction

Medical management is the primary treatment approach to type B acute aortic syndromes (AAS). While immediate surgical intervention has been shown to improve outcomes, including mortality, in patients with type A dissection, similar benefit has not been demonstrated for type B patients. Endovascular aortic repair (EVAR), when anatomically appropriate, has become increasingly utilized in preference to surgery for management of complicated type B AAS. The effects of EVAR on outcomes in patients with uncomplicated type B AAS is the focus of ongoing research. This chapter reviews the evaluation, monitoring and medical treatment of patients with uncomplicated type B AAS with emphasis on imaging, heart rate/blood pressure (impulse) control, and long-term surveillance.

Clinical Outcomes

Since the development of effective surgical approaches nearly 70 years ago by DeBakey and colleagues, acute aortic dissection (AAD) isolated to the descending aorta (Stanford Type B, DeBakey Type III) has been recognized as having a natural history and outcomes distinct from AAD involving the ascending aorta (Stanford Type A, DeBakey Type I, II) [1, 2]. Studies from contemporary cohorts have confirmed these prior observations. Data from the International Registry of Aortic Dissection (IRAD) and the Spanish Acute Aortic Syndrome Study (SAAS) have demonstrated a more than two-fold higher in-hospital mortality for patients with type A versus type B

A. K. Pandey · U. Campia · P. T. O'Gara (✉)
Division of Cardiovascular Medicine, Department of Medicine, Brigham and Women's Hospital, Harvard Medical School, Boston, MA, USA
e-mail: pogara@bwh.harvard.edu

J. S. Coselli et al. (eds.), *Aortic Dissection and Acute Aortic Syndromes*,
https://doi.org/10.1007/978-3-030-66668-2_41

AAD [3, 4]. For patients who survive to hospital discharge, mortality curves flatten for both type A and type B AAD. In an analysis of IRAD data, type A AAD patients had 88% and 68% survival at 1 and 3 years, respectively, and type B AAD patients had 90% and 79%, respectively, over the same time frames [5, 6]. In the Oxford Vascular Study, 5-year survival rates of 85% for type A AAD and 83% for type B AAD were observed in patients surviving to hospital discharge [7]. Patients with type A and B intra-mural hematoma (IMH) demonstrate natural histories that are similar to those for patients with AAD [8]. Outcomes in penetrating aortic ulcers (PAUs) have been difficult to define due to differences in patient selection and inclusion across studies. PAUs that are found incidentally on imaging studies performed for another indication may often be followed conservatively and may not be associated with excess mortality. PAUs requiring intervention for high-risk features or early complications, however, may be associated with 30-day mortality rates approaching 15% [9].

Despite the comparatively lower mortality with type B AAD and the favorable outcomes associated with medical therapy alone for uncomplicated disease, lower survival rates have been observed in the setting of high-risk clinical features, including threatened or demonstrable rupture [10], malperfusion syndromes [11], hemodynamic instability and/or persistent pain with difficult to control hypertension [12] (Table 1). These clinical features should prompt consideration of an interventional approach. Reflecting the high-risk nature of these patients, type B AAD patients undergoing surgical intervention have a nearly three-fold higher in-hospital mortality rate than those treated medically (31.4% versus 10.7%) [4], largely due to established complications from the dissection, patient co-morbidities, and the need for urgent intervention prompted by clinical decline. Short-term survival is higher with EVAR than with acute surgical intervention as reported in observational studies [13] and could offer an alternative approach for appropriately selected patients. Conservative medical management alone in type B AAD patients with early complications is associated with in-hospital mortality rates of up to 50% [11].

Initial Diagnostic Approach

History and Laboratory Testing

Patient history can provide clues to the diagnosis of type B AAD. However, presenting symptoms have limited sensitivity and specificity. Indeed, nearly one-third of patients with AAS are initially suspected as having an alternative diagnosis [14]. In

Table 1 High-risk features in the first 48 h of type B AAD

End organ malperfusion
Impending aortic rupture
Rapid expansion of the false lumen
Refractory pain
Difficult to control hypertension

the IRAD registry, 98% of patients experienced some form of pain, typically of abrupt onset and severe in nature. While nearly three-fourths of type A AAD patients reported chest pain, the most frequent location of pain in type B AAD was reported to be in the back [4]. However, patients may describe abdominal and chest pain with similar frequency, and the character of the pain may not provide further diagnostic clarity. At presentation, type B AAD patients are more likely to be hypertensive, and less likely to exhibit hypotension, pulse deficit, neurological compromise, or a murmur of aortic regurgitation than their type A counterparts [3, 4]. Of note, absence of typical symptoms at presentation, including chest and back pain, is associated with increased in-hospital mortality, possibly due to delays in seeking medical care and in establishing a diagnosis [15].

Several genetic syndromes predisposing to aortic aneurysms and dissection have been identified, including Marfan syndrome (mutations in *FBN1* gene, which encodes for fibrillin-1), Type IV (vascular) Ehlers-Danlos syndrome (mutations in *COL3A1* gene, which encodes for type 3 collagen), Loeys-Dietz syndrome (mutations in genes associated with transforming growth factor [TGF-β] pathway), familial thoracic aortic aneurysm disease (mutations in *ACTA2* gene, which encodes for α-smooth muscle actin) and others [16]. These genetic syndromes are more commonly associated with ascending aortic disease, but descending aortic involvement can be observed. Whereas genetic testing in the acute phase is currently not useful at the point of care, elicitation of a three-generation family history and clinical recognition of a syndromic disorder can inform decisions regarding manipulation or instrumentation of the aorta. Marfan syndrome, for example, is usually considered a contraindication to EVAR [17, 18].

Biomarkers have a very limited role in establishing the diagnosis of AAD but may be useful in evaluating alternative diagnoses. D-dimer has the most extensive evidence base in AAD. Data from IRAD, other registries, and observational series suggest that d-dimer levels have a sensitivity for AAD of >95% but a relatively poor specificity of <50%, indicating that its role may be best suited to exclude the diagnosis [19, 20]. Inflammatory markers such as C-reactive protein (CRP) correlate with the presence of dissection but are non-specific [21]. Other biomarkers that have been investigated include smooth muscle myosin heavy chain [22], the BB isozyme of creatine kinase [23], calponin [24], elastin degradation products [25], and TGF-β [26] (Table 2). Further studies in large cohorts of patients will be needed to better understand the pattern and timing of release of these markers, determine whether biomarkers may correlate with progression of dissection or complications, and establish appropriate cut-off values [27, 28].

Imaging of the Aorta

Accurate and rapid diagnosis of acute type B AAS relies on non-invasive imaging, usually with computed tomographic angiography (CTA). Chest x-ray abnormalities are only present in about half of type B patients [15]. Nearly three-fourths of patients with type B dissections undergo CT imaging as their initial diagnostic study,

Table 2 Biomarkers investigated in the diagnosis AAD

Biomarker	References
D-dimer	[19, 20]
CRP	[21]
Smooth muscle myosin heavy chain	[22]
BB isozyme of creatine kinase	[23]
Calponin	[24]
Elastin degradation products	[25]
TGF-β	[26]

CRP C-reactive protein, *TGF-β* Transforming growth factor beta

although a majority will eventually receive other imaging as well [15]. CTA, magnetic resonance angiography (MRA), and transesophageal echocardiography (TEE) all have similarly high (>95%) sensitivity and specificity [29], so the use of a specific modality often depends on availability, local expertise and patient-specific factors. Advantages of CTA include excellent spatial resolution, rapid imaging protocols, and widespread availability. Protocols for CT studies that include non-contrast imaging to evaluate for intramural hematoma, arterial phase images to evaluate characteristics of the dissection flap, and venous phase images to examine the false lumen, are routinely utilized. TEE provides excellent temporal resolution and visualization of portions of the aorta without exposing patients to ionizing radiation; however, it may not provide full anatomic interrogation in type B patients, particularly of the abdominal aorta and its vascular branches. Moreover, its semi-invasive nature and the need for sedation limit its applicability. MRA does not involve the use of ionizing radiation but has several disadvantages in the acute setting, given its relatively limited availability, longer scan times, the distance between the scanner and emergency clinical personnel, and potential issues arising from metallic patient-support devices. However, it does offer similar anatomic resolution and the possibility of enhanced functional assessment over CT. Additionally, contrast-enhanced scanning with MRA may provide better evaluation for underlying inflammatory and vasculitic conditions than other imaging modalities.

Features on initial imaging can be helpful in predicting potential adverse events in uncomplicated type B AAD patients. These include both positive and negative predictors of aortic enlargement [30] that may help guide initial management strategies. Multiple studies have demonstrated that an aortic diameter of 40 mm or greater on initial imaging is associated with further growth and increased risk of intervention [31–40]. However, some studies, including one from the IRAD cohort, have observed the opposite relationship, namely faster aortic growth rates with smaller initial aortic diameters [41, 42]. The cause for this discrepancy is not fully understood but may be due to selection bias (patients with larger aortic sizes may be directed towards intervention) or the presence of undiagnosed connective tissue disorders, which would have a greater propensity towards adverse remodeling. Patency or partial thrombosis of the false lumen has also been associated with aortic growth on subsequent imaging as well as worse clinical outcomes, whereas complete thrombosis of the false lumen is a negative predictor of growth [32, 33, 36, 39, 43–45]. Other morphological characteristics that may signal worse long-term outcomes in type B patients include dissection/false lumen situated along the inner curvature of the aorta, rounded configuration of the false lumen with elliptical true lumen, and a single or large entry tear [30, 46].

Initial Medical Therapy in Type B AAS

Hemodynamic Principles

Medical therapy has been recognized as an important component of the management of acute aortic syndromes since the 1960s. Studies on cardiac work in the early twentieth century related forces impacting the aorta to changes in the momentum of systolic blood flow. Reducing the velocity of ejected blood over time, and hence the force transmitted onto the aorta, as well as diminishing the pressure differential of each systolic blood wave, were identified as the major targets for medical intervention [10]. This recognition led to the use of anti-adrenergic drugs as the primary agents for medical management of AAD [47–49], with heart rate and blood pressure (and the rate of rise of blood pressure, dP/dt) as the key markers for the desired decrease in myocardial kinetic work. DeBakey recognized the key contribution of blood pressure control in aortic dissection patients. In his observational cohort, patients with blood pressure less than 150/90 had no mortality, whereas those with higher blood pressures had a 36% mortality [1]. In the initial description of the anti-adrenergic medical regimen by Wheat, decreased slope and amplitude of the myocardial contractility curve created by the combination therapy of reserpine, propranolol, and guanethidine resulted in better survival in AAD patients [47]. Due to the extra-cardiac side effects of non-beta-blocker anti-adrenergic agents, and animal studies showing that beta-blocker therapy in particular reduced myocardial contractility without lowering perfusion pressure [48, 49], medical therapy has been refined and simplified to include beta blockers as the foundational approach.

Pharmacotherapy

The therapeutic targets for medical management focus on heart rate and blood pressure. Heart rate is targeted to less than 60–65 beats per minute, and systolic blood pressure is reduced to 120 mmHg. Intravenous (IV) medications are prioritized to rapidly reduce heart rate and blood pressure to these goals in order to halt dissection propagation. However, therapy must be individualized to maintain adequate cerebral and visceral perfusion; in patients with chronically and severely elevated blood pressures, a higher, intermediate target for initial blood pressure control may be more appropriate in order to compensate for altered autoregulatory mechanisms.

Table 3 Therapeutic agents for treatment of type B AAD[a]

Acute/In-hospital drugs		Long-term medication classes
Beta blockers	Esmolol (IV)	Beta blockers
	Labetalol (IV)	Calcium channel blockers
	Metoprolol (IV)	ACE inhibitors
Calcium channel blockers	Diltiazem (IV)	Angiotensin receptor blockers
	Nicardipine (IV)	Diuretics
Nitric oxide donors	Nitroprusside (IV)	Aldosterone antagonists
	Nitroglycerin (IV)	Direct vascular smooth muscle relaxants

[a]Initial in-hospital therapy should be provided in an intensive care unit setting. Intravenous medications are advised for the first 48 h with transition to an oral program thereafter and further titration over the course of the hospitalization. An individualized approach is necessary

Historical experience and contemporary data have demonstrated favorable outcomes associated with beta blocker therapy [50–52]. In patients intolerant to beta blockers, non-dihydropyridine calcium channel blockers are a suitable alternative, and they are the second-most common agent to be used in AAD therapy after beta blockers [51]. Indeed, one study from IRAD suggests that calcium channel blockers may have particular benefit in type B AAD patients [53]. In this study, although beta blockers were associated with improved mortality in all patients with dissections, type B patients in particular had significantly improved survival when on a calcium channel blocker at the time of discharge. The cause for this discrepancy is not known; however, non-dihydropyridine calcium channel blockers would be expected to have similar benefits as beta blocker therapy on reducing myocardial contractile force. Tighter heart rate control has been shown to improve outcomes and reduce aortic complications over a strategy with less-stringent control [54].

Pure afterload reduction is delayed until after adequate control of myocardial contractile force and heart rate are achieved. This is done to avoid reflex tachycardia from vasodilators that may augment cardiac contractility and hence increase, rather than reduce, the exposure of the aorta to deleterious cardiac kinetic forces. Once adequate heart rate control is established, vasodilators may be added to provide enhanced blood pressure control. One protocol for initial pharmacotherapy is to achieve heart rate control with IV bolus doses of metoprolol as an intravenous drip of esmolol is being started. The non-selective beta blocker labetalol (given intravenously), is also an option for initial therapy. If the patient cannot tolerate beta blocker therapy, IV diltiazem is a suitable alternative. Next, IV vasodilators can be added for blood pressure control as needed; options usually include sodium nitroprusside or nicardipine (Table 3).

In-Hospital Course

Patients are optimally monitored in an intensive care unit setting to allow for close hemodynamic assessment and medication adjustment, in addition to regular assessment of end-organ perfusion and the development of complications [55] (Fig. 1).

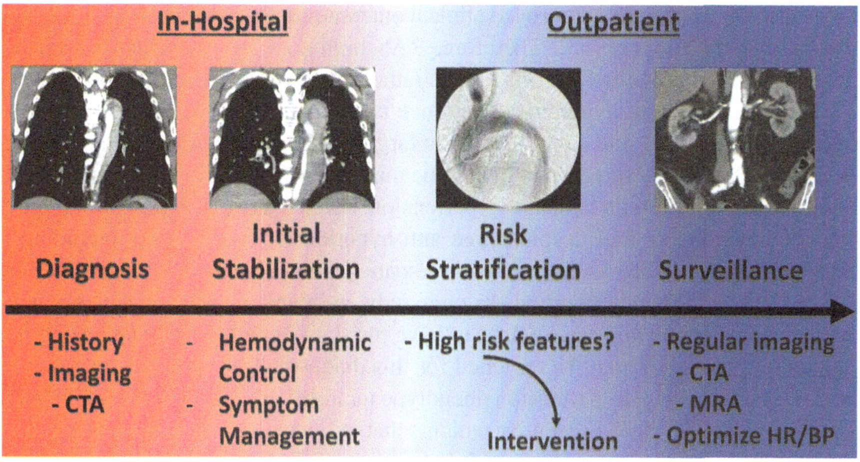

Fig. 1 Care paradigm for medical management of type B acute aortic syndromes. Initial care of type B acute aortic syndromes centers on diagnosis and hemodynamic stabilization. High-risk phenotypes that may benefit from intervention should be recognized. As patients transition from the hospital to the outpatient setting, regular follow-up with surveillance imaging and optimal heart rate (HR) and blood pressure (BP) control are crucial to prevent complications. *CTA* computed tomographic angiography, *MRA* magnetic resonance angiography

Short-term imaging, typically after the first 24–48 h, is important to ensure stability of the aorta and dissection flap. In patients who symptomatically improve and maintain stable anatomy, monitoring can be de-escalated and medications transitioned to oral regimens. For patients who develop high-risk features, including evidence of visceral or extremity malperfusion, resistant hypertension, or refractory pain, consideration should be given to interventional treatment. Worsening clinical course or recrudescence of symptoms should be paired with urgent or emergent imaging for rapid reassessment. Care should be coordinated among cardiovascular medicine, cardiac surgery, and vascular surgery. Several centers have created formal multidisciplinary teams across these specialties in order to effectively triage and manage patients not just for emergent surgical care of type A AAD, but for comprehensive treatment for all AAD patients from admission to discharge.

Long-term Therapy and Monitoring in Type B AAS

Intermediate- to long-term management of uncomplicated type B AAD includes strict heart rate and blood pressure control, periodic surveillance imaging, and vigilance for the development of aortic and cardiovascular complications (Fig. 1). Medical therapy that has been started at the time of diagnosis, including beta blockers and calcium channel blockers, is continued. Specific use of renin-angiotensin system (RAS) inhibitors was initially hoped to have particular benefit in patients with Marfan syndrome due to a favorable impact on pathologic TGF-β signaling [56]. However, this has not translated into improved clinical outcomes in this patient group [57] or in the larger IRAD cohort [53]. Therefore, RAS inhibitors are primarily utilized for additional blood pressure lowering effects rather than dissection-specific benefits.

Titration of the anti-hypertensive regimen is often necessary to achieve goal systolic blood pressures, and a more stringent target, typically 120/80 mmHg or less, is warranted. Heart rate should continue to be maintained optimally less than 65 beats per minute. Patients with resistant hypertension, defined as those whose blood pressure remains above goal despite three anti-hypertensive medications including a diuretic [58], should be identified, as these patients will require more intensive follow-up for medical optimization. In one study, as many as 40% of patients with chronic aortic dissection were found to have resistant hypertension, suggesting the dissection population may be enriched for this diagnosis [59]. Risk factors associated with the resistant hypertension phenotype included age and obesity, which may serve as additional clues to identify patients that will need close follow-up for blood pressure control. Additionally, imaging for these patients should be reviewed to ensure that residual dissection flap is not creating anatomic or functional renal artery stenosis, as this too may be an indication for intervention.

Physical activity following aortic syndromes needs to be balanced to promote cardiovascular fitness while not exposing patients to increased risk for further vascular injury. Patient fears regarding possible deleterious effects from physical exertion can be a significant impediment to maintaining or improving pre-dissection activity levels; more often, patients will have a decrease in physical activity and an increase in emotional stress following the dissection [60]. Exercise has several cardiovascular benefits, including aiding in blood pressure control, maintaining ideal body weight, decreasing the risk of atherosclerotic vascular disease, and improving stress and quality of life measures. Vigorous and isometric exercises are generally avoided due to adverse hemodynamic profiles that develop during these activities. Studies in healthy volunteers have demonstrated that static exercise can lead to large increases in mean arterial pressure without associated decrease in total peripheral resistance [61, 62], mimicking a pressor response and worsening aortic wall stress by Laplace's law. Additionally, resistance exercises to the point of exhaustion appear to exacerbate increases in blood pressure, particularly in patients who are hypertensive, compared to normotensive counterparts [63]. While similar studies are scarce in AAD patients, theoretical risks suggest this type and level of activity should be avoided. By contrast, mild to moderate physical activity is typically well-tolerated. Patients undergoing supervised exercise in a cardiac rehabilitation program at a moderate intensity level after surgical repair of type A AAD are able to achieve a significant increase in maximum workload following completion of the program without an increase in rates of post-surgical complications [64]. Moreover, patients experience improved physical and mental quality of life [65] and those who are able to maintain mild to moderate exercise activity long-term demonstrate reduced resting blood pressures [60]. Based on these findings and the known long-term cardiovascular benefits of exercise, light to moderate aerobic exercise appears safe and can be encouraged in AAD patients [66]. Weight training may also be considered on an individual basis if kept at a light load and the degree of exertion is maintained significantly below exhaustion.

Table 4 Long-term clinical predictors of vascular events in type B AAD

Age < 60 years
Hypertension
Intimal tear on the aortic inner curvature
Patent or partially thrombosed false lumen
Enlarged (> 40 mm) aortic diameter on presentation
Accelerated growth rate on surveillance scans (> 10 mm/year)
Absolute aortic diameter > 55 mm

Follow-up imaging is an important component of the long-term care plan for type B aortic syndromes. Since non-operative therapy is the mainstay of management of uncomplicated patients, monitoring for the development of malperfusion or adverse remodeling is essential. Short-term interval imaging is typically pursued at 1 month, 3 months, and 6 months post-discharge. If a patient's course remains stable and there are no new or concerning vascular changes, then a plan for semi-annual clinical follow-up with yearly imaging can be pursued. MRA is an attractive option for follow-up imaging due to the lack of radiation exposure. In younger patients who may require decades of follow-up, cumulative radiation dose should be considered among other clinical factors when deciding on the type of surveillance imaging. Key features on imaging include the size and contour of the aorta, any interim change in aortic size, and the development or worsening of branch vessel compromise. Predicting which patients will have a benign course and which may require intervention in this chronic phase is difficult. Similar to acute risk stratification, initial dissection characteristics can be utilized to help predict long-term vascular events. These include false lumen patency, initial aortic diameter, location of the intimal tear, age, and presence of elevated blood pressure [30, 46, 67, 68]. The presence of these risk factors may prompt closer follow-up or tighter hemodynamic control as an outpatient. Factors which should encourage consideration for intervention include aortic diameter growth of more than 10 mm in a year, an absolute aortic diameter greater than 55 mm, and/or development of malperfusion syndrome (Table 4).

Conclusions

The principles of management for type B AAD include prompt diagnosis and risk assessment followed by careful and intensive hemodynamic management with emphasis on decreasing myocardial work and contractility to reduce aortic wall stress. Although event rates are lower in uncomplicated versus complicated type B AAD, there remain opportunities to improve outcomes. Whether EVAR should be routinely expanded to the treatment of uncomplicated type B AAD remains to be determined. Improved identification of high-risk subgroups within type B dissections might allow for earlier targeting and delivery of this therapy. Medical therapy will remain critical for initial stabilization and long-term optimization to prevent adverse sequalae and promote favorable remodeling of the aorta.

References

1. DeBakey ME, Henly WS, Cooley DA, Crawford ES, Morris GC Jr. Surgical treatment of dissecting aneurysm of the aorta. Circulation. 1961;24:290–303.
2. Debakey ME, Henly WS, Cooley DA, Morris GC Jr, Crawford ES, Beall AC Jr. Surgical management of dissecting aneurysms of the aorta. J Thorac Cardiovasc Surg. 1965;49:130–49.
3. Evangelista A, Padilla F, Lopez-Ayerbe J, Calvo F, Lopez-Perez JM, Sanchez V, et al. Spanish Acute Aortic Syndrome Study (RESA). Better diagnosis is not reflected in reduced mortality. Rev Esp Cardiol. 2009;62(3):255–62. https://doi.org/10.1016/s1885-5857(09)71554-3.
4. Hagan PG, Nienaber CA, Isselbacher EM, Bruckman D, Karavite DJ, Russman PL, et al. The International Registry of Acute Aortic Dissection (IRAD): new insights into an old disease. JAMA. 2000;283(7):897–903. https://doi.org/10.1001/jama.283.7.897.
5. Tsai TT, Evangelista A, Nienaber CA, Trimarchi S, Sechtem U, Fattori R, et al. Long-term survival in patients presenting with type A acute aortic dissection: insights from the International Registry of Acute Aortic Dissection (IRAD). Circulation. 2006;114(1 Suppl):I350–6. https://doi.org/10.1161/CIRCULATIONAHA.105.000497.
6. Tsai TT, Fattori R, Trimarchi S, Isselbacher E, Myrmel T, Evangelista A, et al. Long-term survival in patients presenting with type B acute aortic dissection: insights from the International Registry of Acute Aortic Dissection. Circulation. 2006;114(21):2226–31. https://doi.org/10.1161/CIRCULATIONAHA.106.622340.
7. Howard DP, Banerjee A, Fairhead JF, Perkins J, Silver LE, Rothwell PM, et al. Population-based study of incidence and outcome of acute aortic dissection and premorbid risk factor control: 10-year results from the Oxford Vascular Study. Circulation. 2013;127(20):2031–7. https://doi.org/10.1161/CIRCULATIONAHA.112.000483.
8. Harris KM, Braverman AC, Eagle KA, Woznicki EM, Pyeritz RE, Myrmel T, et al. Acute aortic intramural hematoma: an analysis from the International Registry of Acute Aortic Dissection. Circulation. 2012;126(11 Suppl 1):S91–6. https://doi.org/10.1161/CIRCULATIONAHA.111.084541.
9. Evangelista A, Czerny M, Nienaber C, Schepens M, Rousseau H, Cao P, et al. Interdisciplinary expert consensus on management of type B intramural haematoma and penetrating aortic ulcer. Eur J Cardiothorac Surg. 2015;47(2):209–17. https://doi.org/10.1093/ejcts/ezu386.
10. Wheat MW Jr, Palmer RF. Dissecting aneurysms of the aorta: present status of drug versus surgical therapy. Prog Cardiovasc Dis. 1968;11(3):198–210. https://doi.org/10.1016/0033-0620(68)90010-8.
11. Jonker FH, Patel HJ, Upchurch GR, Williams DM, Montgomery DG, Gleason TG, et al. Acute type B aortic dissection complicated by visceral ischemia. J Thorac Cardiovasc Surg. 2015;149(4):1081–6 e1. https://doi.org/10.1016/j.jtcvs.2014.11.012.
12. Trimarchi S, Eagle KA, Nienaber CA, Pyeritz RE, Jonker FH, Suzuki T, et al. Importance of refractory pain and hypertension in acute type B aortic dissection: insights from the International Registry of Acute Aortic Dissection (IRAD). Circulation. 2010;122(13):1283–9. https://doi.org/10.1161/CIRCULATIONAHA.109.929422.
13. Fattori R, Tsai TT, Myrmel T, Evangelista A, Cooper JV, Trimarchi S, et al. Complicated acute type B dissection: is surgery still the best option?: a report from the International Registry of Acute Aortic Dissection. JACC Cardiovasc Interv. 2008;1(4):395–402. https://doi.org/10.1016/j.jcin.2008.04.009.
14. Hansen MS, Nogareda GJ, Hutchison SJ. Frequency of and inappropriate treatment of misdiagnosis of acute aortic dissection. Am J Cardiol. 2007;99(6):852–6. https://doi.org/10.1016/j.amjcard.2006.10.055.
15. Suzuki T, Mehta RH, Ince H, Nagai R, Sakomura Y, Weber F, et al. Clinical profiles and outcomes of acute type B aortic dissection in the current era: lessons from the International Registry of Aortic Dissection (IRAD). Circulation. 2003;108(Suppl 1):II312–7. https://doi.org/10.1161/01.cir.0000087386.07204.09.

16. Nienaber CA, Clough RE, Sakalihasan N, Suzuki T, Gibbs R, Mussa F, et al. Aortic dissection. Nat Rev Dis Primers. 2016;2:16053. https://doi.org/10.1038/nrdp.2016.53.
17. Waterman AL, Feezor RJ, Lee WA, Hess PJ, Beaver TM, Martin TD, et al. Endovascular treatment of acute and chronic aortic pathology in patients with Marfan syndrome. J Vasc Surg. 2012;55(5):1234–40.; disucssion 40-1. https://doi.org/10.1016/j.jvs.2011.11.089.
18. Bockler D, Meisenbacher K, Peters AS, Grond-Ginsbach C, Bischoff MS. Endovascular treatment of genetically linked aortic diseases. Gefasschirurgie. 2017;22(Suppl 1):1–7. https://doi.org/10.1007/s00772-016-0221-z.
19. Suzuki T, Distante A, Zizza A, Trimarchi S, Villani M, Salerno Uriarte JA, et al. Diagnosis of acute aortic dissection by D-dimer: the International Registry of Acute Aortic Dissection Substudy on Biomarkers (IRAD-Bio) experience. Circulation. 2009;119(20):2702–7. https://doi.org/10.1161/CIRCULATIONAHA.108.833004.
20. Sodeck G, Domanovits H, Schillinger M, Ehrlich MP, Endler G, Herkner H, et al. D-dimer in ruling out acute aortic dissection: a systematic review and prospective cohort study. Eur Heart J. 2007;28(24):3067–75. https://doi.org/10.1093/eurheartj/ehm484.
21. Sakakura K, Kubo N, Ako J, Wada H, Fujiwara N, Funayama H, et al. Peak C-reactive protein level predicts long-term outcomes in type B acute aortic dissection. Hypertension. 2010;55(2):422–9. https://doi.org/10.1161/HYPERTENSIONAHA.109.143131.
22. Suzuki T, Katoh H, Tsuchio Y, Hasegawa A, Kurabayashi M, Ohira A, et al. Diagnostic implications of elevated levels of smooth-muscle myosin heavy-chain protein in acute aortic dissection. The smooth muscle myosin heavy chain study. Ann Intern Med. 2000;133(7):537–41. https://doi.org/10.7326/0003-4819-133-7-200010030-00013.
23. Suzuki T, Katoh H, Kurabayashi M, Yazaki Y, Nagai R. Biochemical diagnosis of aortic dissection by raised concentrations of creatine kinase BB-isozyme. Lancet. 1997;350(9080):784–5. https://doi.org/10.1016/S0140-6736(05)62569-X.
24. Suzuki T, Distante A, Zizza A, Trimarchi S, Villani M, Salerno Uriarte JA, et al. Preliminary experience with the smooth muscle troponin-like protein, calponin, as a novel biomarker for diagnosing acute aortic dissection. Eur Heart J. 2008;29(11):1439–45. https://doi.org/10.1093/eurheartj/ehn162.
25. Shinohara T, Suzuki K, Okada M, Shiigai M, Shimizu M, Maehara T, et al. Soluble elastin fragments in serum are elevated in acute aortic dissection. Arterioscler Thromb Vasc Biol. 2003;23(10):1839–44. https://doi.org/10.1161/01.ATV.0000085016.02363.80.
26. Suzuki T, Trimarchi S, Sawaki D, Grassi V, Costa E, Rampoldi V, et al. Circulating transforming growth factor-beta levels in acute aortic dissection. J Am Coll Cardiol. 2011;58(7):775. https://doi.org/10.1016/j.jacc.2010.01.079.
27. Parolari A, Tremoli E, Songia P, Pilozzi A, Di Bartolomeo R, Alamanni F, et al. Biological features of thoracic aortic diseases. Where are we now, where are we heading to: established and emerging biomarkers and molecular pathways. Eur J Cardiothorac Surg. 2013;44(1):9–23. https://doi.org/10.1093/ejcts/ezs647.
28. Suzuki T, Bossone E, Sawaki D, Janosi RA, Erbel R, Eagle K, et al. Biomarkers of aortic diseases. Am Heart J. 2013;165(1):15–25. https://doi.org/10.1016/j.ahj.2012.10.006.
29. Shiga T, Wajima Z, Apfel CC, Inoue T, Ohe Y. Diagnostic accuracy of transesophageal echocardiography, helical computed tomography, and magnetic resonance imaging for suspected thoracic aortic dissection: systematic review and meta-analysis. Arch Intern Med. 2006;166(13):1350–6. https://doi.org/10.1001/archinte.166.13.1350.
30. van Bogerijen GH, Tolenaar JL, Rampoldi V, Moll FL, van Herwaarden JA, Jonker FH, et al. Predictors of aortic growth in uncomplicated type B aortic dissection. J Vasc Surg. 2014;59(4):1134–43. https://doi.org/10.1016/j.jvs.2014.01.042.
31. Kato M, Bai H, Sato K, Kawamoto S, Kaneko M, Ueda T, et al. Determining surgical indications for acute type B dissection based on enlargement of aortic diameter during the chronic phase. Circulation. 1995;92(9 Suppl):II107–12. https://doi.org/10.1161/01.cir.92.9.107.
32. Marui A, Mochizuki T, Koyama T, Mitsui N. Degree of fusiform dilatation of the proximal descending aorta in type B acute aortic dissection can predict late aortic events. J Thorac Cardiovasc Surg. 2007;134(5):1163–70. https://doi.org/10.1016/j.jtcvs.2007.07.037.

33. Onitsuka S, Akashi H, Tayama K, Okazaki T, Ishihara K, Hiromatsu S, et al. Long-term outcome and prognostic predictors of medically treated acute type B aortic dissections. Ann Thorac Surg. 2004;78(4):1268–73. https://doi.org/10.1016/j.athoracsur.2004.02.031.
34. Winnerkvist A, Lockowandt U, Rasmussen E, Radegran K. A prospective study of medically treated acute type B aortic dissection. Eur J Vasc Endovasc Surg. 2006;32(4):349–55. https://doi.org/10.1016/j.ejvs.2006.04.004.
35. Kunishige H, Myojin K, Ishibashi Y, Ishii K, Kawasaki M, Oka J. Predictors of surgical indications for acute type B aortic dissection based on enlargement of aortic diameter during the chronic phase. Jpn J Thorac Cardiovasc Surg. 2006;54(11):477–82. https://doi.org/10.1007/s11748-006-0039-9.
36. Marui A, Mochizuki T, Mitsui N, Koyama T, Kimura F, Horibe M. Toward the best treatment for uncomplicated patients with type B acute aortic dissection: a consideration for sound surgical indication. Circulation. 1999;100(19 Suppl):II275–80. https://doi.org/10.1161/01.cir.100.suppl_2.ii-275.
37. Ray HM, Besho JM, Au J, Charlton-Ouw KM, Estrera AL, Miller CC 3rd, et al. The role of ascending aortic size in outcomes of patients with uncomplicated acute type B aortic dissection. J Vasc Surg. 2019;69(4):1011–20. https://doi.org/10.1016/j.jvs.2018.07.048.
38. Spinelli D, Benedetto F, Donato R, Piffaretti G, Marrocco-Trischitta MM, Patel HJ, et al. Current evidence in predictors of aortic growth and events in acute type B aortic dissection. J Vasc Surg. 2018;68(6):1925–35 e8. https://doi.org/10.1016/j.jvs.2018.05.232.
39. Reutersberg B, Trenner M, Haller B, Geisbusch S, Reeps C, Eckstein HH. The incidence of delayed complications in acute type B aortic dissections is underestimated. J Vasc Surg. 2018;68(2):356–63. https://doi.org/10.1016/j.jvs.2017.11.089.
40. Lou X, Duwayri YM, Chen EP, Jordan WD Jr, Forcillo J, Zehner CA, et al. Predictors of failure of medical management in uncomplicated type B aortic dissection. Ann Thorac Surg. 2019;107(2):493–8. https://doi.org/10.1016/j.athoracsur.2018.08.012.
41. Jonker FH, Trimarchi S, Rampoldi V, Patel HJ, O'Gara P, Peterson MD, et al. Aortic expansion after acute type B aortic dissection. Ann Thorac Surg. 2012;94(4):1223–9. https://doi.org/10.1016/j.athoracsur.2012.05.040.
42. Kotelis D, Grebe G, Kraus P, Muller-Eschner M, Bischoff M, von Tengg-Kobligk H, et al. Morphologic predictors of aortic expansion in chronic type B aortic dissection. Vascular. 2016;24(2):187–93. https://doi.org/10.1177/1708538115591941.
43. Akutsu K, Nejima J, Kiuchi K, Sasaki K, Ochi M, Tanaka K, et al. Effects of the patent false lumen on the long-term outcome of type B acute aortic dissection. Eur J Cardiothorac Surg. 2004;26(2):359–66. https://doi.org/10.1016/j.ejcts.2004.03.026.
44. Kamman AV, Jonker FHW, Sechtem U, Harris KM, Evangelista A, Montgomery DG, et al. Predictors of stable aortic dimensions in medically managed acute aortic syndromes. Ann Vasc Surg. 2017;42:143–9. https://doi.org/10.1016/j.avsg.2017.01.012.
45. Tsai TT, Evangelista A, Nienaber CA, Myrmel T, Meinhardt G, Cooper JV, et al. Partial thrombosis of the false lumen in patients with acute type B aortic dissection. N Engl J Med. 2007;357(4):349–59. https://doi.org/10.1056/NEJMoa063232.
46. Tolenaar JL, van Keulen JW, Jonker FH, van Herwaarden JA, Verhagen HJ, Moll FL, et al. Morphologic predictors of aortic dilatation in type B aortic dissection. J Vasc Surg. 2013;58(5):1220–5. https://doi.org/10.1016/j.jvs.2013.05.031.
47. Wheat MW Jr, Palmer RF, Bartley TD, Seelman RC. Treatment of dissecting aneurysms of the aorta without surgery. J Thorac Cardiovasc Surg. 1965;50:364–73.
48. Palmer RF, Wheat MW Jr. Treatment of dissecting aneurysms of the aorta. Ann Thorac Surg. 1967;4(1):38–52. https://doi.org/10.1016/s0003-4975(10)66476-4.
49. Simpson CF, Boucek RJ, Noble NL. Influence of d-, l-, and dl-propranolol, and practolol on beta-amino-propionitrile-induced aortic ruptures of turkeys. Toxicol Appl Pharmacol. 1976;38(1):169–75. https://doi.org/10.1016/0041-008x(76)90170-8.
50. Genoni M, Paul M, Jenni R, Graves K, Seifert B, Turina M. Chronic beta-blocker therapy improves outcome and reduces treatment costs in chronic type B aortic dissection. Eur J Cardiothorac Surg. 2001;19(5):606–10. https://doi.org/10.1016/s1010-7940(01)00662-5.

51. Hiratzka LF, Bakris GL, Beckman JA, Bersin RM, Carr VF, Casey DE Jr, et al. 2010 ACCF/AHA/AATS/ACR/ASA/SCA/SCAI/SIR/STS/SVM guidelines for the diagnosis and management of patients with thoracic aortic disease: a report of the American College of Cardiology Foundation/American Heart Association Task Force on Practice Guidelines, American Association for Thoracic Surgery, American College of Radiology, American Stroke Association, Society of Cardiovascular Anesthesiologists, Society for Cardiovascular Angiography and Interventions, Society of Interventional Radiology, Society of Thoracic Surgeons, and Society for Vascular Medicine. Circulation. 2010;121(13):e266–369. https://doi.org/10.1161/CIR.0b013e3181d4739e.
52. Shores J, Berger KR, Murphy EA, Pyeritz RE. Progression of aortic dilatation and the benefit of long-term beta-adrenergic blockade in Marfan's syndrome. N Engl J Med. 1994;330(19):1335–41. https://doi.org/10.1056/NEJM199405123301902.
53. Suzuki T, Isselbacher EM, Nienaber CA, Pyeritz RE, Eagle KA, Tsai TT, et al. Type-selective benefits of medications in treatment of acute aortic dissection (from the International Registry of Acute Aortic Dissection [IRAD]). Am J Cardiol. 2012;109(1):122–7. https://doi.org/10.1016/j.amjcard.2011.08.012.
54. Kodama K, Nishigami K, Sakamoto T, Sawamura T, Hirayama T, Misumi H, et al. Tight heart rate control reduces secondary adverse events in patients with type B acute aortic dissection. Circulation. 2008;118(14 Suppl):S167–70. https://doi.org/10.1161/CIRCULATIONAHA.107.755801.
55. Wheat MW Jr. Treatment of dissecting aneurysms of the aorta: current status. Prog Cardiovasc Dis. 1973;16(1):87–101. https://doi.org/10.1016/0033-0620(73)90006-6.
56. Habashi JP, Judge DP, Holm TM, Cohn RD, Loeys BL, Cooper TK, et al. Losartan, an AT1 antagonist, prevents aortic aneurysm in a mouse model of Marfan syndrome. Science. 2006;312(5770):117–21. https://doi.org/10.1126/science.1124287.
57. Lacro RV, Dietz HC, Sleeper LA, Yetman AT, Bradley TJ, Colan SD, et al. Atenolol versus losartan in children and young adults with Marfan's syndrome. N Engl J Med. 2014;371(22):2061–71. https://doi.org/10.1056/NEJMoa1404731.
58. Whelton PK, Carey RM, Aronow WS, Casey DE Jr, Collins KJ, Dennison Himmelfarb C, et al. 2017 ACC/AHA/AAPA/ABC/ACPM/AGS/APhA/ASH/ASPC/NMA/PCNA Guideline for the prevention, detection, evaluation, and management of high blood pressure in adults: a report of the American College of Cardiology/American Heart Association Task Force on Clinical Practice Guidelines. Hypertension. 2018;71(6):e13–e115. https://doi.org/10.1161/HYP.0000000000000065.
59. Eggebrecht H, Schmermund A, von Birgelen C, Naber CK, Bartel T, Wenzel RR, et al. Resistant hypertension in patients with chronic aortic dissection. J Hum Hypertens. 2005;19(3):227–31. https://doi.org/10.1038/sj.jhh.1001800.
60. Chaddha A, Kline-Rogers E, Braverman AC, Erickson SR, Jackson EA, Franklin BA, et al. Survivors of aortic dissection: activity, mental health, and sexual function. Clin Cardiol. 2015;38(11):652–9. https://doi.org/10.1002/clc.22418.
61. Bezucha GR, Lenser MC, Hanson PG, Nagle FJ. Comparison of hemodynamic responses to static and dynamic exercise. J Appl Physiol Respir Environ Exerc Physiol. 1982;53(6):1589–93. https://doi.org/10.1152/jappl.1982.53.6.1589.
62. Lind AR, McNicol GW. Circulatory responses to sustained hand-grip contractions performed during other exercise, both rhythmic and static. J Physiol. 1967;192(3):595–607. https://doi.org/10.1113/jphysiol.1967.sp008319.
63. de Souza NS, Gomides RS, da Silva GV, de Moraes Forjaz CL, Mion D Jr, Tinucci T. Intra-arterial blood pressure response in hypertensive subjects during low- and high-intensity resistance exercise. Clinics (Sao Paulo). 2010;65(3):271–7. https://doi.org/10.1590/S1807-59322010000300006.
64. Corone S, Iliou MC, Pierre B, Feige JM, Odjinkem D, Farrokhi T, et al. French registry of cases of type I acute aortic dissection admitted to a cardiac rehabilitation center after surgery. Eur J Cardiovasc Prev Rehabil. 2009;16(1):91–5. https://doi.org/10.1097/HJR.0b013e32831fd6c8.

65. Fuglsang S, Heiberg J, Hjortdal VE, Laustsen S. Exercise-based cardiac rehabilitation in surgically treated type-A aortic dissection patients. Scand Cardiovasc J. 2017;51(2):99–105. https://doi.org/10.1080/14017431.2016.1257149.
66. Chaddha A, Eagle KA, Braverman AC, Kline-Rogers E, Hirsch AT, Brook R, et al. Exercise and physical activity for the post-aortic dissection patient: the clinician's conundrum. Clin Cardiol. 2015;38(11):647–51. https://doi.org/10.1002/clc.22481.
67. Juvonen T, Ergin MA, Galla JD, Lansman SL, McCullough JN, Nguyen K, et al. Risk factors for rupture of chronic type B dissections. J Thorac Cardiovasc Surg. 1999;117(4):776–86. https://doi.org/10.1016/S0022-5223(99)70299-0.
68. Augoustides JG, Szeto WY, Woo EY, Andritsos M, Fairman RM, Bavaria JE. The complications of uncomplicated acute type-B dissection: the introduction of the Penn classification. J Cardiothorac Vasc Anesth. 2012;26(6):1139–44. https://doi.org/10.1053/j.jvca.2012.06.024.

Symptomatic Thoracic Aortic Aneurysms

Rizwan Q. Attia, Arminder S. Jassar, and Duke E. Cameron

Introduction

The first clinical depiction of aneurysms is from the second century AD when Galen first provided accurate description, mentioning pulsatile quality, disappearance of the mass with pressure and the contents of bright blood warmer than venous blood. He cautioned that 'if an aneurysm be wounded, the blood is spouted out with so much violence that it can scarcely be arrested' [1]. Contributions to the understanding of aneurysms were gained only from autopsy studies till the nineteenth century. Swaine and Latham are credited for reporting the first antemortum diagnosis 1855 [2]. Peacock first published a comprehensive series of 80 cases in 1863 [3]. The importance of symptom onset was recognized early, along with increase in size, as the two most important variables that determine when to surgically treat aneurysms [4]. It can be argued that little has changed in determining when to intervene over the past 60 years on symptomatic aneurysm. Symptoms are a harbinger of rapid aortic expansion, rupture or dissection. This chapter details the significance of symptoms and how best to approach such patients clinical care.

Epidemiology

The true incidence aneurysmal disease is unknown as patients are usually asymptomatic till incidental discovery on imaging present with symptoms, the latter is estimated to be between 5–10%. Overall age and gender adjusted incidence rates are around 10.4 per 100, 000 person years [5, 6]. The incidence has increased over

R. Q. Attia · A. S. Jassar · D. E. Cameron (✉)
Division of Cardiac Surgery, Corrigan Minehan Heart Center, Massachusetts General Hospital, Boston, MA, USA
e-mail: rqattia@mgh.harvard.edu; ajassar@mgh.harvard.edu; decameron@mgh.harvard.edu

J. S. Coselli et al. (eds.), *Aortic Dissection and Acute Aortic Syndromes*,
https://doi.org/10.1007/978-3-030-66668-2_42

time likely due to better and increased frequency of imaging and an aging population. Median age of diagnosis is in the 69-years. Rupture is the most common cause of death. Of all aortic ruptures thoracic aneurysms account for 13.2% and thoracoabdominal 1.5%. Age specific mortality is 3.1 per million persons for thoracic and 0.4 per million for thoracoabdominal aneurysms [7].

Aneurysm Biology

Aortic wall inflammation and extracellular matrix remodeling are key events that occur in development, expansion and rupture of aneurysms [8–10]. Aneurysm formation is a genetic disease and the causal role of inflammation in its development is debated [11, 12]. Gene expression is modified by post-translational changes mediated through microRNA networks in aneurysm wall [13–16]. There is a complex interaction between genetic predisposition, vascular inflammation and extracellular matrix degradation leading to aortic wall expansion, altered wall shear stress and hemodynamics in the pathophysiology of aneurysmal disease [17, 18]. In the clinical management algorithm these key genetic, cellular and molecular changes are discounted; with decision making often based on aneurysm size, patient symptoms and aneurysm expansion rate [19, 20].

It is postulated that symptom onset informs us of biological events occurring in the aortic wall. It might signify increased inflammatory activity with leukocyte infiltration, degradation of extracellular matrix, vascular smooth muscle cell dysregulation leading to rapid expansion and potential rupture. Elastin breakdown in the tunica media caused by proteolysis through the action of matrix metalloproteinases [21, 22] other proteolytic enzymes such as cathepsins [23, 24], and increased levels of pro-inflammatory cytokines could provide the stimulation for a chronic inflammatory response in the aortic wall [25]. Certain patients with small aneurysms will develop expansion and rupture whilst others with large aneurysms will remain well. However symptomatic patients always go on to develop adverse outcomes.

Natural History

Successful surgical treatment depends on understanding the risks of surgery balanced against the natural history of the disease. Natural history data come from those aneurysm patients who did not have operative treatment. For thoracic aortic aneurysms overall, 74% of patients rupture and of these 94% of patients will subsequently die from this [26]. Complications such as aortic rupture and dissection are determined by aortic diameter and underlying aortic pathology.

The diameter of the aneurysm increases the wall tension ($T = PR$, Laplace's law); where tension is proportional to pressure x radius. Therefore, increased systemic blood pressure and increased aneurysm diameter markedly increase the risk of rupture. Logistic regression analysis has demonstrated over four fold increased rupture or dissection risk when aneurysm is 6.0–6.9 cm in diameter compared to 4.0–4.9 cm [27]. Aneurysm size and growth rate are important clinical predictors for treatment decisions as they are know to determine aortic outcome. A 5 cm thoracic aneurysm expands at an average rate of 0.08–0.12 cm/year; whereas larger aneurysms grow at a greater rate: 8 cm aneurysms grow at around 0.19–0.22 cm/ year [28–30]. The growth rate varies depending on the site of aortic aneurysm independent of size. Ascending aortic aneurysms grow at 0.1 cm annually compared to 0.29 for descending thoracic aneurysms. Mean growth rate is approximately 0.42 cm per year [31]. This rate is accelerated in patients who smoke. Although hypertension is a risk factor for aneurysm development, none of the measures of hypertension are associated with thoracic aortic disease [28]. However, there are indications that there is an association between diastolic blood pressure and the rate of aortic expansion [32].

Mechanical forces also contribute to aortic remodeling with three distinct influences on the aortic wall: i) pressure created by the hydrostatic forces ii) circumferential stretch exerting longitudinal forces and iii) shear stress caused by the blood flow [33]. The net resultant force comprises therefore of the pressure along the aortic wall, shear stress and the difference in the maximal pressure differences i.e. pulse pressure. Perturbation in the flow conditions leads to flow turbulence, contributing to aneurysm growth. Areas of oscillating flow and extremes in shear stress (high and low) correlate to sites of development of aneurysms [33, 34]. Clinical studies have shown conflicting data where flow in aortic aneurysms can be smooth and laminar or irregular and turbulent with little information on the effects of wall shear stress in aneurysms. The accelerated rate of aneurysm growth and deaths from rupture in patients with monogenetic causes of aneurysmal disease have provided the impetus for earlier aneurysm repair to be undertaken in these patients [35–38].

When lifetime risks of rupture and dissection are analyzed, there emerges a concept of aortic "hinge points", where there is a sharp increase in risk of complications due to an aneurysms size. These hinge points occur at 6 cm in the ascending aorta, 7 cm in the descending aorta and 6 cm in the abdominal aorta, in those without connective tissue disease [39, 40]. It is also widely recognized that symptomatic aneurysms should be treated regardless of size as symptoms herald rapid aortic expansion, potential rupture or dissection [41, 42]. However 5% of patients are symptomatic and the first presenting symptom in 95% of cases is death. The overall 5-year survival for thoracic aortic aneurysms is 60–64% [29, 43, 44]. Survival is lower in descending aortic aneurysms (39% at 5 years) with poor outcomes in patients who develop aortic dissection [45].

Symptom Etiology

Symptoms are rare in this disease and occur in only 5% of patents prior to an acute aortic event. Sixty percent of thoracic aortic aneurysms involve the aortic root (Fig. 1) and/or ascending aorta (Fig. 2), 40% involve the descending aorta (Fig. 3),

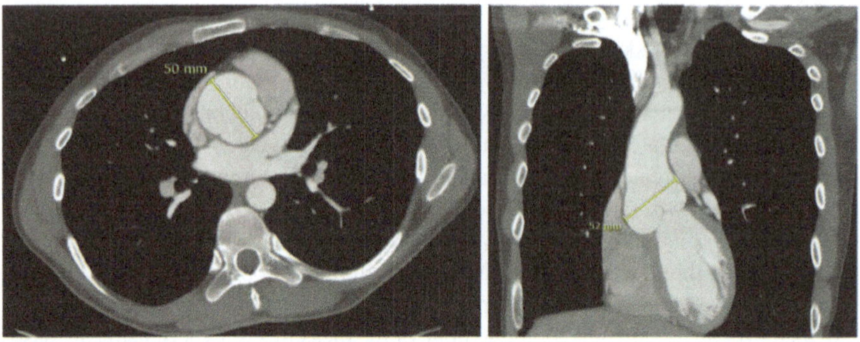

Fig. 1 Axial and sagittal contrast CT scan showing an isolated aortic root aneurysm

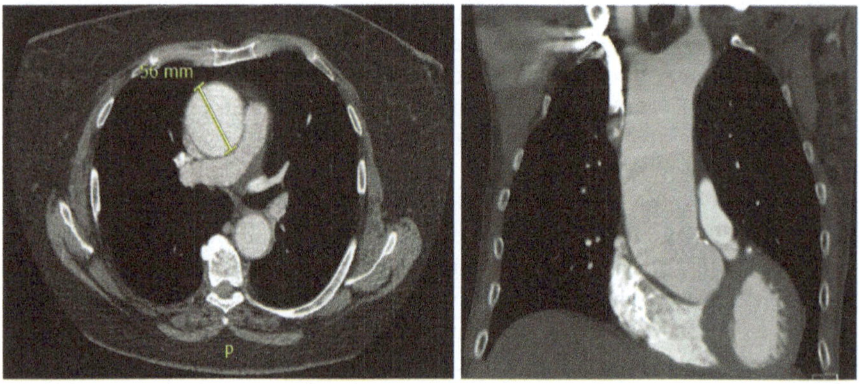

Fig. 2 Axial and sagittal contrast CT scan showing an isolated ascending aortic aneurysm

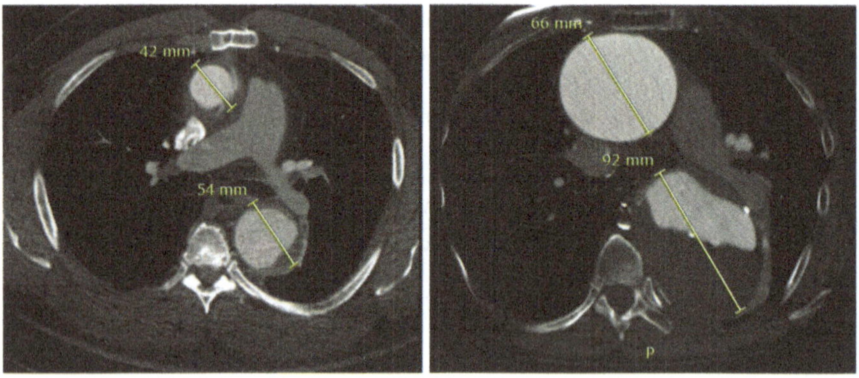

Fig. 3 Serial axial contrast CT scan demonstrating enlarging ascending and proximal descending thoracic aortic aneurysms

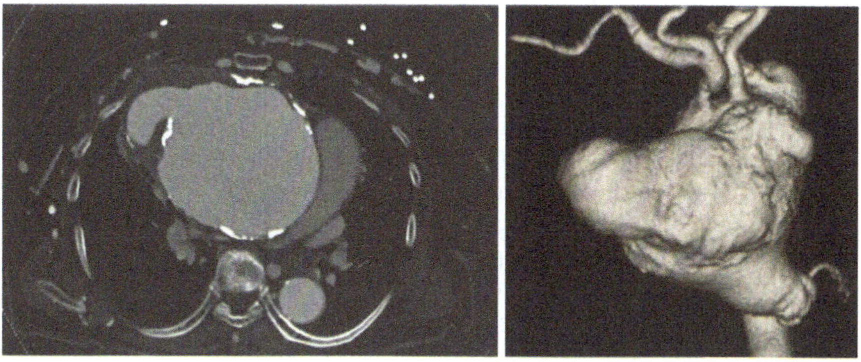

Fig. 4 Large ascending and aortic arch aneurysm eroding through the chest wall on axial contrast CT scan effacing the pulmonary artery. 3D reconstruction of scan shows a normal aortic root and dilated ascending aorta that was measured at 13 cm. The aneurysm involves the aortic arch with arch vessels arising from the aneurysmal aorta

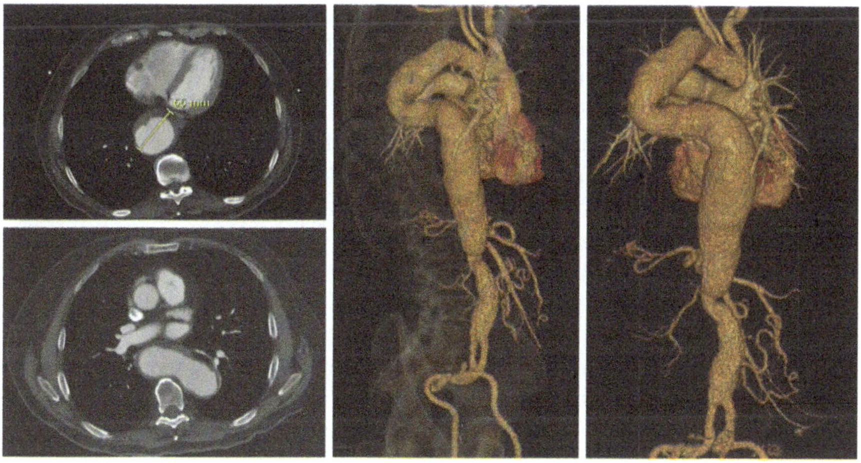

Fig. 5 Axial contrast CT scans and 3D reconstructions demonstrating degenerating elongating descending thoracic aortic aneurysm which dilates from the proximal descending portion down to the diaphragm

10% involve the arch (Fig. 4) and 10% involve the thoracoabdominal aorta (Fig. 5) [46]. Patients often overlapping with affected diseased aortic segments. Symptoms can be attributed to the neural activation due to aneurysm expansion leading to pain, compression of surrounding structures, disruption to distal flow or embolization and disruption of aortic valve function.

Pain

In general, ascending aneurysms produce retrosternal pain that is usually non-exertional in nature and descending aneurysms produce interscapular pain. The pain is usually described as severe, sharp in nature and radiating to the back or epigastrium. Patients may also describe a tearing or ripping sensation when there is either rapid expansion or dissection. Once present, the pain can be relentless and incompletely relived by analgesia. Such patients are usually hypertensive. It is imperative to achieve good blood pressure control with anti-impulse therapy. The recurrence of pain is generally ominous. Although the initial symptoms are sternal with progression to the back, the pain may begin at any location including the jaw, neck, shoulders and abdomen. Symptoms can be attributed to stretch of the aortic wall activating the cardiac and aortic plexus of nerves. The plexuses are formed from sympathetic postganglionic axons arising from the thoracic chain, parasympathetic preganglionic axons from the vagus, and segmental visceral sensory nerves travelling across the intercostal nerve bundles. The nerves in the plexus are close to each other but do not interact or synapse together. The superficial part of cardiac plexus lies under the aortic arch anterior to the right pulmonary artery. The cardiac plexus is formed by superior cardiac branch of left sympathetic trunk and lower superior cervical branch of the left vagus. Pain can also be due to compression of adjacent structures such as the descending thoracic aneurysm compressing the vertebrae. Large aneurysms may erode into the chest wall, vertebral column and lead to neurological symptoms.

Compression

Patients can present with difficult breathing and cough due to compression of the distal trachea by a large arch aneurysm and more commonly the left main bronchus from proximal descending thoracic aortic aneurysm. Rarely patients may present with signs of superior vena cava (SVC) syndrome with edema of upper limbs and face, plethora, distended veins of face, neck and chest wall, shortness of breath, cough and headache. Hoarseness may occur due to compression or stretching of the left recurrent laryngeal nerve. Distal arch, descending thoracic aortic aneurysms, aberrant right subclavian, Kommerell diverticulum, Felson and Palayew type I and II right-sided aortic arch lesions may cause dysphagia (dysphagia lusoria) due to esophageal compression.

Rupture

Ascending or root aneurysms can present with signs of heart failure due to rupture into the right atrium or SVC or with hemoptysis due to bleeding into the lung.

Contained rupture of descending thoracic aortic aneurysms can lead to dyspnea and cough due to irritation of the pleural lining and compression of lung parenchyma along with hypotension and hemodynamic collapse.

Disruption to Distal Flow and Embolization

Certain aneurysms, especially in the descending thoracic aorta, can undergo atherosclerotic degeneration with embolic debris from plaque, including cholesterol embolism, platelet aggregates and micro thrombi. This material can embolize to the brain causing transient ischemic attacks and strokes. Emboli can cause limb ischemia, renal infarction and mesenteric ischemia. Clinical manifestations range from asymptomatic to severe multi-organ failure with high mortality rate.

Heart Failure

Patients with large root aneurysms that splay apart the aortic valve leaflets may present with symptoms and signs of aortic regurgitation. This may progress to symptoms of left ventricular failure with fatigue, dyspnea and orthopnea and characteristics signs of aortic insufficiency on clinical exam. Rarely, patients may develop angina that can be nocturnal or exertional in nature. This is due to decreased diastolic aortic pressure and increased left ventricular end-diastolic pressure reducing coronary artery diastolic flow. On examination, there is a diastolic murmur and widened pulse pressure. Additionally, patients should be examined for physical signs of Marfan and Loeys Dietz syndromes as part of an effort to identify syndromic etiology.

Nervous System

There are numerous neurological phenomena described in patients with thoracic aortic aneurysms, ranging from paraesthesias, weakness, paraplegia or hemiplegia. The etiology of these might be brain or spinal cord embolization. Blindness and transient scotomata have been reported as well as Horner's syndrome.

There is additionally an association between cerebral aneurysm and thoracic aneurysms which on imaging studies is as high as 20–25% [47, 48]. There is a case for extended CT scan to involve intracranial circulation when evaluating patients with thoracic aneurysms.

Systemic Symptoms

Inflammatory disease or mycotic aneurysms can occasionally lead to fever and constitutional symptoms of tiredness, lethargy and malaise.

Clinical Evaluation

This includes a detailed history of medical complaints, cardiovascular risk factors, family history of arterial disease or sudden death. A focused physical examination can be directed by the symptoms and includes auscultation of the heart and lungs, palpation and auscultation of the abdomen, flank for bruits and full peripheral vascular and neurological assessment.

Laboratory Testing

Laboratory blood tests are usually of limited value in diagnosis of the disease, however, as most patients will require surgical or endovascular treatment. This includes evaluation of complete blood count, assessment of renal function, coagulation, cross matching and in cases where inflammatory etiology is suspected serum proteins such as high-sensitivity C-reactive protein, D-Dimers and erythrocyte sedimentation rate.

Imaging

Once aneurysm is suspected, echocardiography, chest x-ray and contrast computer tomography is required to visualize the entire aorta [19, 49, 50]. Key decisions regarding management of aortic aneurysms depend on size, location, presence of co-existing pathologies such as intramural hematoma, penetrating aortic ulcers, rupture and branch vessel involvement of aneurysmal disease.

Computer Tomography

High-resolution ECG-gated protocols allow reduced motion artifact assessment of the aorta. Non-enhanced, followed by contrast enhanced angiography is performed to delineate aortic dimensions. Measurement of aortic diameter is undertaken at reproducible anatomic landmarks perpendicular to axis of blood flow. External diameter is measured at the widest point. For each imaging place diameters are measured at six levels;

1. The aortic annulus,
2. The sinotubular junction,
3. Mid ascending aorta, halfway between the sinotubular junction and aortic arch, at the level of the right pulmonary artery,
4. Transverse aortic arch,
5. Mid descending aorta at the level of the sinotubular junction and
6. Distal descending aorta at the diaphragmatic hiatus

In case of gated CT scan, cardiac image reconstruction protocols allow assessment of coronary anatomy and disease. Patients with atherosclerotic aneurysms of descending aorta are at higher risk of coronary artery disease as they share cardiovascular risk factors. Additionally patients with symptomatic thoracic aortic aneurysms with inflammatory etiology such as Takaysau and giant cell arteritis may have inflammatory coronary involvement with coronary stenosis or coronary aneurysms (less than 10%) [51–53]. If aortic root, ascending or arch surgery is being considered identification of coronary anatomy and underlying coronary artery disease is important for planning surgery.

It is recommended maximum aneurysm diameter is measured perpendicular to the centerline of the vessel. Three-dimensional reconstructions should be performed where possible. This approach allows accurate reproducible assessment of aortic dimension, compared to cross sectional diameters when the aorta might be tortuous or kinked and the aortic axis is not parallel to the patients' cranio-caudal axis. Compared to short-axis the maximum diameter measurements perpendicular to the centerline have greater reproducibility.

Echocardiography

This allows assessment of aortic root and ascending aortic dimensions, aortic valve morphology and function. Aortic regurgitation can be graded and the mechanism evaluated to provide information for aortic valve repair. Associated important findings in symptomatic aortic aneurysms include identification of pericardial effusion; exclude myocardial ischemia based on assessment of ventricular function and segmental wall motion anomalies. Transthoracic echocardiography (TTE) has lower sensitivity and specificity for proximal aortic imaging compared to transesophgeal (TEE) studies. As part of pre-operative patient evaluation TTE usually suffices to provide required information for pre-operative planning. TEE is reserved for intra-operative open and endovascular repairs when it most useful for procedural guidance and detection of endovascular graft leak detection.

Coronary Angiography

Invasive coronary angiography is reserved for those cases where there is no ECG gated cardiac CT to exclude coronary artery disease or where the cardiac CT demonstrates flow limiting lesions that must be assessed more precisely for interventional or operative treatment at the time of aneurysm repair. The European and American guidelines recommend no delay in treatment of patients with acute aortic syndromes for coronary imaging [19, 49]. There is no specific provision for symptomatic thoracic aortic aneurysms, but the clinician must balance the risk of waiting for the investigation against the likelihood of positive result that impacts the treatment algorithm.

Guidelines

The American, European and Asian guidelines on thoracic aortic aneurysms recommend that patients with symptoms suggestive of expansion of thoracic aneurysm should have prompt surgical intervention (Class I) [19, 20, 49, 54]. An exception is if comorbidities severely limit patients' life expectancy and quality of life.

Ascending Aorta

Separate aortic valve and ascending replacement is recommended when the root is normal (Class I). Patients with Marfans, Loeys-Dietz and Ehlers-Danlos syndromes and those with aortic root and sinus of Valsalva dilatation should undergo excision of sinuses and a modified valve sparing root replacement or valve graft conduit.

Aortic Arch

Aneurysms involving proximal aortic arch, a hemiarch replacement with ascending aorta replacement using subclavian/ axillary inflow and hypothermic circulatory arrest is reasonable (Class IIa). Total replacement of the aortic arch is warranted for complete arch aneurysms, where the aorta has acute or chronic dissection. For involvement of proximal descending thoracic aorta, an elephant trunk procedure is recommended (Class IIa).

Asymptomatic patients with aneurysms >5.5 cm should be considered for surgery. For isolated arch aneurysms less than 4 cm the patients should undergo annual cross sectional imaging using CT or MRI. For aneurysms greater than 4 cm, 6 monthly imaging is mandated (Class IIa).

Descending Thoracic Aorta

In chronic dissections, specially those in patients with connective tissue disease, aortic diameters >5.5 cm are recommended for open repair (Class I). For degenerative or traumatic aneurysms >5.5 cm, saccular aneurysms or post-operative pseudoaneurysms, endovascular grafting should be considered.

For thoracoabdominal aneurysms where endovascular options are limited and there is high surgical morbidity, elective surgery is recommended if aortic diameter exceeds 6 cm, or if there is a connective tissue disease.

For those with end organ ischaemia or stenosis of branch vessels additional revascularization is recommended.

Connective Tissue Disease

The size criteria cut off for intervention are lower in these patients and more frequent surveillance imaging is of added value when aneurysms are discovered. If maximal cross-sectional area in square centimeters of the ascending aorta or root divided by the patient's height in meters exceeds a ratio of 10, surgical repair is indicated. This is because shorter patients may have dissection at a smaller aortic size. 15% of patients with Marfan syndrome have dissection at a size less than 5.0 cm.

For Loeys-Dietz syndrome or those with mutations in either the transforming growth factor receptor Type I or II (TGFBR1 or TGFBR2 genes) surgical intervention is considered at 4.0 cm. Aortic rupture is reported at diameters below 4.5 cm. For children, once the aortic diameter exceeds the 99th percentile for age and the aortic valve annulus reaches 1.8–2.0 cm, prophylactic root surgery is recommended.

Patients with Type IV Ehlers Danlos syndrome suffer arterial rupture and dissection. The role of prophylactic surgical replacement is not clear.

There are numerous other genetic mutations (for example, FBN1, TGFBR1, TGFBR2, COL3A1, ACTA2, MYH11) associated with risk of thoracic aortic aneurysm. When these are identified, first-degree relatives should be screened for aortic disease.

Bicuspid Aortic Valve

These patients frequently have dilatation of sinuses of Valsalva and/or ascending aortic aneurysms that can extend to the arch. Their aneurysms are more common with right and non-coronary leaflet fusion than those with the most common form, right and left leaflet fusion. Once present, the aortopathy progresses at a mean rate of 0.5 mm per year at the sinuses of Valsalva, and sinotubular junction and 0.9 mm per year at proximal ascending aorta. Operative repair is recommended at a diameter of 5.5 cm for the aortic sinuses and ascending aorta. If there is growth of ≥0.5 cm per year or if there are other risk factors for dissection, a lower threshold of 5 cm is recommended.

Management

Symptomatic aneurysms regardless of size should be treated expediently. This involves admission to an intensive care setting with measurement of heart rate, blood pressure and urine output.

Immediate Medical Treatment and Stabilization

Blood pressure and heart rate reduction are critically important. The goal systolic blood pressure in most patients is 100–120 mmHg and heart rate below 60 whilst maintaining organ perfusion. This is best achieved using beta-blockers and vasodilators, to reduce the force of left ventricular ejection (dP/dt). Commonly used beta-blockers include intravenous labetalol, which has benefit of action on the alpha and beta-receptors, causing reduced arterial pressure and LV contractility. Alternate agents such as esmolol are useful as they have a short half-life, can be titrated and tapered as required. Intravenous nitrates or centrally acting agents such as hydralazine can be added as needed. Monotherapy with nitrates should be avoided as it may raise the dP/dt. In some cases, the venodilatation causes reflex tachycardia, which might worsen the progression of the disease and symptoms. In cases where beta-blockers are contraindicated, alternative therapy with calcium channel blockers may be effective due to their negative inotropic and vasodilator effects.

Surgery

Surgical repair entails resection of the aneurysm and replacement with an appropriately sized prosthetic graft.

Aortic Valve and Aortic Root

Aortic regurgitation due to aortic root dilatation is often treatable by valve sparing root replacement with or without valve repair [55, 56] and valve sparing root replacement [57, 58]. If there is significant intrinsic valve pathology composite root replacement with a mechanical valve conduit (Bentall procedure) or biological valve (Bio-Bentall) and human allografts [59, 60]. In patients with connective tissue diseases (Marfans and Loeys Dietz syndrome) a more aggressive approach is warranted for the management of aortic root disease [61, 62].

Ascending Aorta

Extent of resection depends on the length of aneurysmal segment. For most patients interposition tube graft replacement is the treatment of choice. Patients may require aggressive hemi arch replacement for removal of all aneurysmal disease with an open distal anastomosis under deep hypothermic circulatory arrest with or without cerebral perfusion depending on the surgical and unit expertise, patient variables and technical factors.

Aortic Arch

In cases where there is involvement of the aortic arch, the operative strategy would dependent on:

1. Patient factors such as age, co-morbidities and presence of connective tissue disease
2. Anatomical and technical criteria (such as aortic dimensions, branch vessel involvement, distal embolization or malperfusion)
3. Operative considerations such as site for cannulation, cerebral perfusion strategy and extent of replacement of aorta

In case of aortic arch aneurysm total arch replacement is usually advisable. However, isolated arch arch aneurysms are rare. There is often involvement of the ascending and/or descending thoracic aorta. This mandates an operative strategy to tackle all the diseased segments. The arch vessels may be anastomosed using an island technique or require separate grafts depending on aneurysm morphology and the variables above.

Descending Thoracic Aorta

Patients with symptomatic aneurysms and those with connective tissue disease require a descending thoracic aortic replacement. For patients with traumatic aneurysms, saccular aneurysms and post-operative pseudoaneurysms, TEVAR may be considered. Patients with thoracoabdominal aneurysms and with end-organ ischemia and malperfusion often additional revascularization procedures.

Patients who undergo descending thoracic aorta replacement have a mortality risk of 3–10%, depending on extent of repair. Those undergoing surgery for pain and compressive symptoms have higher mortality between 10–20%. These are still better results than those who undergo emergent surgery for rupture and malperfusion, where mortality of 80% is reported [19, 49, 63].

Extent of repair is described by Crawford type:

1. Type I extends from proximal descending aorta above T6 to renal arteries.
2. Type II extends from proximal descending aorta above T6 to below renal arteries (highest risk)
3. Type III from distal descending aorta below T6 to below diaphragm
4. Type IV from diaphragm to most abdominal aorta.

This classification correlates to risk of paraplegia, stroke, renal failure and death [64–66].

A key consideration of these operations when combined with aortic arch repair is organ protection. This might involve hypothermic circulatory arrest, cerebral and visceral perfusion. Additional technical considerations include protection of the left lung during thoracotomy to prevent lacerations and bleeding from the parenchyma. Identification and protection of the esophagus is important when constructing the anastomoses.

Technical Considerations

Several cannulation and perfusion strategies have been described for aneurysm repair. For arch surgery operative outcomes utilizing right axillary artery, femoral artery or the ascending aorta for cannulation have been reported, with certain advantages and disadvantages described for each [19, 20, 49, 67]. Femoral vessels can be rapidly cannulated, especially in emergency situations using a percutaneous approach, allowing CPB to be established prior to sternotomy/thoracotomy. The main disadvantage is retrograde flow through a diseased aorta, which can cause embolization, alter flow dynamics and worsen organ perfusion in some cases. Central aortic cannulation allows rapid institution of bypass and provides systemic perfusion in an antegrade fashion. However, this technique requires a suitable site for cannulation in a non atheromatous aorta. Right axillary artery cannulation requires extra time and an additional incision to expose the artery. The right axillary artery can either be cannulated directly or via. a graft anastomosed end to side to the artery. The main advantage of using the axillary artery is that it facilitates institution of antegrade cerebral perfusion during circulatory arrest. It is also usually free of atherosclerotic disease. Alternative cannulation sites like the proximal innominate or right subclavian artery have also been described.

Several studies have compared the impact of cannulation site on surgical outcomes. Similar mortality and stroke rates are reported for each technique [68]. Axillary artery cannulation is the predominant cannulation strategy for patients undergoing total arch replacement. A recent large study from the STS database reported lower risk of postoperative stroke when axillary artery was used for cannulation when compared to femoral artery cannulation (OR = 0.6, $P < 0.001$); innominate cannulation was not different from axillary cannulation (OR 0.88; 95% CI 0.57–1.35; $P = 0.5$) [69].

Debate also continues regarding the optimal cerebral protection strategy during circulatory arrest. While safety of both RCP and ACP has been demonstrated for short duration of circulatory arrest (< 30–40 min), most surgeons favor antegrade cerebral perfusion for longer durations of circulatory arrest, as may be required for total arch replacement [70]. Selective myocardial perfusion during arch repair—(the "beating heart" concept) has also been described to reduce cardioplegic arrest time [71].

Studies have compared the 'island' technique (where the cephalad portion of the aortic arch that includes the arch vessels is re-implanted as a patch on the aortic graft) versus individual branch reimplantation; most have reported similar results [72]. There is some concern that the island patch may degenerate over time and lead to aneurysm. The island technique may not be technically feasible if the aneurysm extends to the arch vessels. Individual branch reimplantation is generally preferred in the setting of aortic arch aneurysms, especially in patients with connective tissue disease. Individual reimplantation of the supra aortic vessels has the advantage of removing the dissected tissue in the aortic arch. Additionally, individual branch reimplantation allows early distal reperfusion after the distal anastomosis is performed as opposed to the island technique where both the distal anastomosis and the island reimplantation must be completed before perfusion can be resumed. Several "off the shelf" branched grafts are available and can be used according to surgeon preference. Proximalization of the distal anastomosis to zone II rather than zone III can simplify the distal aortic anastomosis and reduce visceral ischemia time and risk of recurrent laryngeal nerve injury [72, 73]. The base of the left subclavian artery is ligated, and the distal end of the subclavian artery is anastomosed to a branch of the aortic graft. Alternatively, an extra-anatomic bypass can be performed from the aortic graft to the axillary artery.

Total aortic arch replacement can be combined with antegrade delivery of a stent graft into the descending aorta—the "frozen elephant trunk" [73–75]. Since then there have been several new FET devices with various prefabricated grafts, such as the E-vita™ [76], Thoraflex™ [77], Cronus [78] and Frozenix -J graft [79]. These hybrid devices consist of a conventional surgical graft that is mated to a stented endovascular graft, thus eliminating the possibility of a type I endoleak. Presence of a sewing cuff facilitates the distal anastomosis. The endograft helps seal the surgical suture line and reduces the risk of bleeding from fragile aortic tissues. If a distal aortic intervention is required later, shifting the treatment level to the mid thoracic aorta with the use of either a classic or frozen elephant trunk facilitates a technically easier re-operation that avoids hypothermic circulatory arrest and reduces risk of recurrent laryngeal nerve injury. If no pre-mated hybrid FET devices are available, the surgeons can use a commercially available TEVAR graft that is deployed into the descending aorta during circulatory arrest and can be then incorporated into the distal aortic anastomosis [80–82].

Spinal cord ischemia remains a concern with use of FET and in descending aortic replacement. Spinal cord protection strategies might be deployed such as spinal drain, maintain high perfusion pressures, monitoring of spinal cord motor and sensory potentials to alert the surgeon to malperfusion, revascularization of major spinal collaterals and minimal coverage of the aorta [83–85]. Other adjunctive techniques such as, epidural irrigation with hypothermic solutions, high-dose systemic glucocorticoids, osmotic diuresis with mannitol, intrathecal papaverine, and cellular metabolic suppression with anesthetic agents have been described [49].

FET is a useful technique when the aneurysm extends into the descending aorta. The stent graft provides a distal landing zone for later endovascular treatment of the remaining aneurysmal segment. An alternative and more invasive technique to address aneurysm that extends from the arch into the descending thoracic aorta is to perform complete excision and replacement. This can be accomplished by extending the sternotomy transversely into the thirds or fourth interspace, using a bilateral thoraco-sternotomy ("clam shell") incision, or using a left thoracotomy, usually in the fourth intercostal space [86]. When performing a bilateral thoracosternotomy the right pleura is opened widely and the pericardium is not suspended to allow retraction of the heart to the right side. This provides excellent exposure of the descending aorta down to the level of the inferior pulmonary veins or in some patients to the diaphragm.

Thoracic Endovascular Aneurysm Repair (TEVAR)

At present there are no FDA approved endografts for ascending and arch aneurysms. However there are reported cases of arch endografting [87, 88]. For patients who are not operable candidates this treatment might be considered on compassionate use grounds. Data are limited to selected case series [89, 90]. Endograft safety has been demonstrated in other pathological conditions of the aorta including dissection, intramural haematoma, penetrating aortic ulcers, pseudoaneurysms and acute traumatic transections, these though are still considered 'off label' for the devices. There are no published randomized studies comparing open to endovascular treatment. The decision-making is guided by observational retrospective studies and comparisons of patient cohorts.

Aneurysm is excluded from the circulation by implantation of an endograft in a normal diameter aorta above and below the aneurysm. These constitute the proximal and distal landing zones that anchor the graft preventing further aortic enlargement. Pre and post procedure planning is critical for TEVAR. Contrast CT with 1–3 mm slices of the proximal supra aortic vessels down to the femorals are required. Diameter less than 40 mm and length greater than 20 mm of healthy proximal and distal landing zones is needed. The relationship to side branches and the iliofemoral access route assessment is also important. The stent is oversized by 10–15% at the landing zones.

Where there are important aortic side branches (for example the left subclavian), TEVAR is preceded by limited surgical bypass of these branches. Another option is surgical de-branching or the use of fenestrated and branched endografts or 'chimney technique'. In some cases single branched stent grafts might be deployed.

Retrograde open or percutaneous transfemoral access is usually used with devices up to 24Fr carrying the collapsed self-expanding endografts. Contralateral femoral or radial/brachial vessels are used to advance a pigtail catheter for angiography. The endograft is delivered to the aneurysm site over a stiff wire. When the target site is reached, the blood pressure is lowered using rapid right ventricular pacing or using drugs (such as nitroprusside or adenosine) to achieve systolic pressures less than 80 mmHg. The endograft is then deployed and completion angiography performed to detect proximal type I endoleak. In cases where there are branch vessels close to the endograft landing zones or where branched, fenestrated graft deployment needs to be carried out, additional imaging using intravascular ultrasound and TEE might be required. In patients where descending thoracic aorta needs to be treated, spinal protection strategies must be utilized to minimize risk of spinal cord ischemia. Detailed discussion of thoracic endografting is beyond the scope of this chapter; the American and European guidelines are recommended [19, 20, 91].

References

1. Erichsen JE. On the proximate cause of death after the spontaneous introduction of air into the veins, with some remarks on the treatment of that accident. Edinb Med Surg J. 1844;61: 1–24.
2. Swaine, Latham PM. Case of dissecting aneurysm of the aorta. Tr Path Soc London. 1855;7(106):1855–6.
3. Montgomery E. A year-book of medicine, surgery, and their allied sciences, for 1862. London: General Books; 1863.
4. Hirst AE, Johns VJ, Kime SW. Dissecting aneurysm of the aorta: a review of 505 cases. Medicine (Baltimore). 1958;37:217–79.
5. Olsson C, Thelin S, Ståhle E, Ekbom A, Granath F. Thoracic aortic aneurysm and dissection: increasing prevalence and improved outcomes reported in a nationwide population-based study of more than 14,000 cases from 1987 to 2002. Circulation. 2006;114:2611–8.
6. Clouse WD, et al. Acute aortic dissection: population-based incidence compared with degenerative aortic aneurysm rupture. Mayo Clin Proc. 2004;79:176–80.
7. Abdulameer H, Taii ALH, Al-Kindi SG, Milner R. Epidemiology of fatal ruptured aortic aneurysms in the United States (1999–2016). J Vasc Surg. 2019;69:378–384.e2.
8. Hellenthal FAMVI, Buurman WA, Wodzig WKWH, Schurink GWH. Biomarkers of AAA progression. Part 1: extracellular matrix degeneration. Nat Rev Cardiol. 2009;6:464–74.
9. Hellenthal FAMVI, Buurman WA, Wodzig WKWH, Schurink GWH. Biomarkers of abdominal aortic aneurysm progression. Part 2: inflammation. Nat Rev Cardiol. 2009;6:543–52.
10. Ocana E. Characterisation of T and B lymphocytes infiltrating abdominal aortic aneurysms. Atherosclerosis. 2003;170:39–48.
11. De Backer J, Campens L, De Paepe A. Genes in thoracic aortic aneurysms/dissections – do they matter? Ann Cardiothorac Surg. 2013;2:73–82.
12. Hemminki K, Li X, Johansson S-E, Sundquist K, Sundquist J. Familial risks of aortic aneurysms among siblings in a nationwide Swedish study. Genet Med. 2006;8:43–9.
13. Maegdefessel L, et al. Inhibition of microRNA-29b reduces murine abdominal aortic aneurysm development. J Clin Invest. 2012;122:497–506.
14. Boon RA, et al. MicroRNA-29 in aortic dilation: implications for aneurysm formation. Circ Res. 2011;109:1115–9.
15. Jones JA, et al. Selective MicroRNA suppression in human thoracic aneurysms: relationship of miR-29a to aortic size and proteolytic induction. Circ Cardiovasc Genet. 2011;4:605–13.
16. Kim CW, et al. Prevention of abdominal aortic aneurysm by anti-microRNA-712 or anti-microRNA-205 in angiotensin II-infused mice. Arterioscler Thromb Vasc Biol. 2014;34:1412–21.
17. Hellenthal FAMVI, Geenen ILA, Teijink JAW, Heeneman S, Schurink GWH. Histological features of human abdominal aortic aneurysm are not related to clinical characteristics. Cardiovasc Pathol. 2009;18:286–93.
18. Michel J-B, et al. Novel aspects of the pathogenesis of aneurysms of the abdominal aorta in humans. Cardiovasc Res. 2011;90:18–27.

19. Erbel R, Aboyans V, Boileau C, Bossone E. ESC guidelines on the diagnosis and treatment of aortic diseases. Eur Heart J. 2014;35(41):2873–926.
20. Hiratzka LF, Bakris GL, Beckman JA. 2010 ACCF/AHA/AATS/ACR/ASA/SCA/SCAI/SIR/STS/SVM guidelines for the diagnosis and management of patients with thoracic aortic disease. Circulation. 2010;121(13):e266–369.
21. Newman KM, Jean-Claude J, Li H, Ramey WG, Tilson MD. Cytokines that activate proteolysis are increased in abdominal aortic aneurysms. Circulation. 1994;90:II224–7.
22. Wilson NJ, et al. Development, cytokine profile and function of human interleukin 17-producing helper T cells. Nat Immunol. 2007;8:950–7.
23. Abisi S, et al. Cysteine protease activity in the wall of abdominal aortic aneurysms. J Vasc Surg. 2007;46:1260–6.
24. Fiorentino DF, et al. IL-10 acts on the antigen-presenting cell to inhibit cytokine production by Th1 cells. J Immunol. 1991;146:3444–51.
25. Zucker S, Cao J, Chen WT. Critical appraisal of the use of matrix metalloproteinase inhibitors in cancer treatment. Oncogene. 2000;19:6642–50.
26. Brown PM, Zelt DT, Sobolev B. The risk of rupture in untreated aneurysms: the impact of size, gender, and expansion rate. J Vasc Surg. 2003;37:280–4.
27. Elefteriades JA. Natural history of thoracic aortic aneurysms: indications for surgery, and surgical versus nonsurgical risks. Ann Thorac Surg. 2002;74(5):S1877–80.
28. Masuda Y, Takanashi K, Takasu J, Morooka N, Inagaki Y. Expansion rate of thoracic aortic aneurysms and influencing factors. Chest. 1992;102:461–6.
29. Oladokun D, et al. Systematic review of the growth rates and influencing factors in thoracic aortic aneurysms. Eur J Vasc Endovasc Surg. 2016;51:674–81.
30. Cheng SWK, Yiu RS. Natural history and risk factors for rupture of thoracic aortic arch aneurysms. J Vasc Surg. 2015;62:526–7.
31. Gagné-Loranger M, Dumont E, Voisine P, Mohammadi S, Dagenais F. Natural history of 40–50 mm root/ascending aortic aneurysms in the current era of dedicated thoracic aortic clinics. Eur J Cardiothoracic Surg. 2016;50(3):562–6.
32. Francis J, Miller J. Aortic aneurysms. Arterioscler Thromb Vasc Biol. 2002;22:1948–9.
33. Bluth EI, Murphey SM, Hollier LH, Sullivan MA. Color flow Doppler in the evaluation of aortic aneurysms. Int Angiol. 1990;9:8–10.
34. Nakahashi TK, et al. Flow loading induces macrophage antioxidative gene expression in experimental aneurysms. Arterioscler Thromb Vasc Biol. 2002;22:2017–22.
35. Jayarajan SN, Downing BD, Sanchez LA, Jim J. Trends of vascular surgery procedures in Marfan syndrome and Ehlers-Danlos syndrome. Vascular. 2020;13:1708538120925597.
36. Ramirez F, Dietz HC. Marfan syndrome: from molecular pathogenesis to clinical treatment. Curr Opin Genet Dev. 2007;17:252–8.
37. Cury M, Zeidan F, Lobato AC. Aortic disease in the young: genetic aneurysm syndromes, connective tissue disorders, and familial aortic aneurysms and dissections. J Vasc Med. 2013;2013:1–7.
38. Holscher CM, et al. Aortic surgery outcomes of Marfan syndrome and Ehlers-Danlos syndrome patients at teaching and nonteaching hospitals. Ann Vasc Surg. 2019;55:175–181.e3.
39. Coady MA, Rizzo JA, Hammond GL, Kopf GS, Elefteriades JA. Surgical intervention criteria for thoracic aortic aneurysms: a study of growth rates and complications. Ann Thorac Surg. 1999;67:1922–6; discussion 1953–8.
40. Coady MA, et al. What is the appropriate size criterion for resection of thoracic aortic aneurysms? J Thorac Cardiovasc Surg. 1997;113:476–91.
41. Fukui D, et al. Overexpression of transforming growth factor β1 in smooth muscle cells of human abdominal aortic aneurysm. Eur J Vasc Endovasc Surg. 2003;25:540–5.
42. Modarai B, et al. Adenovirus-mediated VEGF gene therapy enhances venous thrombus recanalization and resolution. Arterioscler Thromb Vasc Biol. 2008;28:1753–9.
43. Elefteriades JA, Farkas EA. Thoracic aortic aneurysm: clinically pertinent controversies and uncertainties. J Am Coll Cardiol. 2010;55:841–57.
44. Ruddy JM, Jones JA, Ikonomidis JS. Pathophysiology of thoracic aortic aneurysm (TAA): is it not one uniform aorta? Role of embryologic origin. Prog Cardiovasc Dis. 2013;56:68–73.

45. Collins JS, Evangelista A, Nienaber CA, Bossone E, Fang J, Cooper JV, Smith E, Gara PTO, Myrmel T, Gilon D. Differences in clinical presentation, management, and outcomes of acute type a aortic dissection in patients with and without previous cardiac surgery. Circulation. 2004;110:II237–42.
46. Isselbacher EM. Thoracic and abdominal aortic aneurysms. Circulation. 2005;111:816–28.
47. Laukka D, et al. Prevalence of thoracic aortic aneurysms and dilatations in patients with intracranial aneurysms. J Vasc Surg. 2019;70:1801–8.
48. Lee D, et al. High prevalence of intracranial aneurysms in patients with aortic dissection or aneurysm: feasibility of extended aorta CT angiography with involvement of intracranial arteries. J Neurointerv Surg. 2017;9:1017–21.
49. Hiratzka LF, Bakris GL, Beckman JA. Guidelines for the diagnosis and Management of Patients with Thoracic Aortic Disease: a report of the American Collage of Cardiology Foundation. Circulation. 2010;121(13):e266–369.
50. Grossi EA, et al. High-risk aortic valve replacement: are the outcomes as bad as predicted? Ann Thorac Surg. 2008;85:102–7.
51. Anandaraja S, Mukhopadhyay S, Roy S, Kathuria S, Tyagi S. Left main coronary artery aneurysm in Takayasu arteritis. Echocardiography. 2006;23:430–1.
52. Haddy SM, Bhatt M, Patel JM. Right coronary artery aneurysm in a patient with Takayasu's arteritis. Echocardiography. 2007;24:1108–9.
53. Chun PKC, Jones R, Robinowitz M, Davia JE, Lawrence PJ. Coronary ostial stenosis in Takayasu's arteritis. Chest. 1980;78:330–1.
54. JCS Joint Working Group. Guidelines for diagnosis and treatment of aortic aneurysm and aortic dissection (JCS 2011): digest version. Circulation. 2013;77:789–828.
55. Lansac E, de Kerchove L. Aortic valve repair techniques: state of the art. Eur J Cardiothorac Surg. 2018;53:1101–7.
56. Ehrlich T, et al. State-of-the art bicuspid aortic valve repair in 2020. Prog Cardiovasc Dis. 2020;63(4):457–64. https://doi.org/10.1016/j.pcad.2020.04.010.
57. de Kerchove L, Mosala Nezhad Z, Boodhwani M, Khoury E, G. How to perform valve sparing reimplantation in a tricuspid aortic valve. Ann Cardiothorac Surg. 2013;2:105–12.
58. Ouzounian M, et al. Valve-sparing root replacement compared with composite valve graft procedures in patients with aortic root dilation. J Am Coll Cardiol. 2016;68:1838–47.
59. Cameron DE, et al. Aortic root replacement in 372 Marfan patients: evolution of operative repair over 30 years. Ann Thorac Surg. 2009;87:1344–50.
60. Mookhoek A, et al. Bentall procedure: a systematic review and meta-analysis. Ann Thorac Surg. 2016;101:1684–9.
61. Williams JA, et al. Early surgical experience with Loeys-Dietz: a new syndrome of aggressive thoracic aortic aneurysm disease. Ann Thorac Surg. 2007;83:S757–63. discussion S785–90.
62. Price J, et al. Long-term outcomes of aortic root operations for Marfan syndrome: a comparison of Bentall versus aortic valve-sparing procedures. J Thorac Cardiovasc Surg. 2016;151:330–8.
63. Higgins J, Lee MK, Co C, Janusz MT. Long-term outcomes after thoracic aortic surgery: a population-based study. J Thorac Cardiovasc Surg. 2014;148:47–52.
64. Svensson LG, Crawford ES, Hess KR, Coselli JS, Safi HJ. Experience with 1509 patients undergoing thoracoabdominal aortic operations. J Vasc Surg. 1993;17:357–68., discussion 368–70.
65. Svensson LG, Crawford ES, Hess KR, Coselli JS, Safi HJ. Variables predictive of outcome in 832 patients undergoing repairs of the descending thoracic aorta. Chest. 1993;104:1248–53.
66. LeMaire SA, Miller CC, Conklin LD, Schmittling ZC, Coselli JS. Estimating group mortality and paraplegia rates after thoracoabdominal aortic aneurysm repair. Ann Thorac Surg. 2003;75:508–13.
67. Kreibich M, Desai ND, Interactive JB. Preoperative neurological deficit in acute type A aortic dissection. Interact Cardiovasc Thorac Surg. 2020;30(4):613–9.
68. Kreibich M, et al. Outcome after aortic, axillary, or femoral cannulation for acute type A aortic dissection. J Thorac Cardiovasc Surg. 2019;158:27–34.e9.
69. Ghoreishi M, et al. Factors associated with acute stroke after type A aortic dissection repair: an analysis of the Society of Thoracic Surgeons National Adult Cardiac Surgery Database. J Thorac Cardiovasc Surg. 2019;159(6):2143–2154.e3. https://doi.org/10.1016/j.jtcvs.2019.06.016.

70. Chen E, Gleason T, Yang B, Coselli J, Shrestha M. Discussions in cardiothoracic treatment and care: the contemporary management of acute Type A aortic dissection. Semin Thorac Cardiovasc Surg. 2020;32(2):202–10. https://doi.org/10.1053/j.semtcvs.2020.02.011.
71. Martens A, et al. Do not leave the heart arrested. Non-cardioplegic continuous myocardial perfusion during complex aortic arch repair improves cardiac outcome. Eur J Cardiothorac Surg. 2016;49:141–8.
72. Lin Y, et al. Supra-aortic vessel reconstruction in total arch replacement for acute type A dissection: comparison of en bloc and separate graft techniques. Asian J Surg. 2019;42:482–7.
73. Kato M, et al. New graft-implanting method for thoracic aortic aneurysm or dissection with a stented graft. Circulation. 1996;94:II188–93.
74. Suto Y, et al. Stented elephant trunk procedure for an extensive aneurysm involving distal aortic arch and descending aorta. J Thorac Cardiovasc Surg. 1996;112:1389–90.
75. Fleck T, et al. Combined surgical and endovascular treatment of acute aortic dissection type A: preliminary results. Ann Thorac Surg. 2002;74:761–5; discussion 765–6.
76. Jakob H, Tsagakis K, Leyh R, Buck T, Herold U. Development of an integrated stent graft-dacron prosthesis for intended one-stage repair in complex thoracic aortic disease. Herz. 2005;30:766–8.
77. Shrestha M, Pichlmaier M, Martens A, Hagl C, Khaladj N, Haverich A. Total aortic arch replacement with a novel four-branched frozen elephant trunk graft: first-in-man results. Eur J Cardiothorac Surg. 2013;43(2):406–10.
78. Ma W-G, Zheng J, Sun L-Z, Elefteriades JA. Open stented grafts for frozen elephant trunk technique: technical aspects and current outcomes. Aorta. 2018;03:122–35.
79. Okita Y. Current surgical results of acute type A aortic dissection in Japan. Ann Cardiothorac Surg. 2016;5:368–76.
80. Jassar A, et al. Aortic replacement after TEVAR-diameter correction with modified use of the Siena prosthesis. Ann Thorac Surg. 2018;105:587–91.
81. Eldeiry M, et al. The Buffalo trunk technique for aortic arch reconstruction. Ann Thorac Surg. 2019;108:680–6.
82. Preventza O, et al. The stent is not to blame: lessons learned with a simplified US version of the frozen elephant trunk. Ann Thorac Surg. 2017;104:1456–63.
83. Tanaka A, Safi HJ, Estrera AL. Current strategies of spinal cord protection during thoracoabdominal aortic surgery. Gen Thorac Cardiovasc Surg. 2018;66:307–14.
84. Ghincea CV, Ikeno Y, Aftab M, Reece TB. Spinal cord protection for thoracic aortic surgery: bench to bedside. Semin Thorac Cardiovasc Surg. 2019;31:713–20.
85. Preventza O, et al. Neurologic complications after the frozen elephant trunk procedure: a meta-analysis of more than 3000 patients. J Thorac Cardiovasc Surg. 2019;160(1):20–33.e4. https://doi.org/10.1016/j.jtcvs.2019.10.031.
86. Kim JB, Sundt TM. Best surgical option for arch extension of type B aortic dissection: the open approach. Ann Cardiothorac Surg. 2014;3:406–12.
87. Riambau V. Application of the Bolton relay device for thoracic Endografting in or near the aortic arch. Aorta. 2015;3:16–24.
88. Haverich A. Aortic arch replacement with frozen elephant trunk-when not to use it. Ann Cardiothorac Surg. 2013;2:592–6.
89. Kudo T, Kuratani T, Shimamura K, Sawa Y. Determining the optimal proximal landing zone for TEVAR in the aortic arch: comparing the occurrence of the bird-beak phenomenon in zone 0 vs zones 1 and 2. J Endovasc Ther. 2020;3:1526602820914269.
90. Tsilimparis N, et al. International experience with endovascular therapy of the ascending aorta with a dedicated endograft. J Vasc Surg. 2016;63:1476–82.
91. Grabenwöger M, et al. Thoracic endovascular aortic repair (TEVAR) for the treatment of aortic diseases: a position statement from the European Association for Cardio-Thoracic Surgery (EACTS) and the European Society of Cardiology (ESC), in collaboration with the European Association of Percutaneous Cardiovascular Interventions (EAPCI). Eur Heart J. 2012;33:1558–63.

Future Considerations for Acute Aortic Syndromes

Konstantin von Aspern, Christian D. Etz, and Michael A. Borger

Introduction

Acute aortic syndromes (AAS), including acute aortic dissections (AD), intramural haematomas (IMH) and penetrating aortic ulcers (PAU), remain one of the most unpredictable cardiovascular events and are associated with significant morbidity and mortality. Reports from Europe and Japan analyzing the incidence of aortic diseases—including aneurysms and AAS—reveal slowly increasing numbers over the last two decades [1–5]. For thoracic aortic disease in general, an increase of approximately 28% was noted over the last 20 years [2, 5, 6] with an increase of 36% specifically for AAS [6]. A more recent cohort analysis from the US shows a less pronounced increase in the incidence of AAS from 8.5 to 9.7 cases per 100,000 inhabitants per year [7].

AAS, in particular AD and IMH, are characterised by their sudden onset. When treated conservatively, these pathologies—when originating from the ascending aorta or arch—have a dismal outcome, which is why the number of unknown cases in the population may likely be higher than previously assumed. Contemporary analyses, including data of post-mortem AAS diagnoses, estimate the true incidence at approximately 12 cases per 100,000 inhabitants per year [3, 5]. Regardless of the absolute incidence and regional differences over the last decade, a relatively constant number of open procedures for most thoracic AAS and a relative shift towards endovascular approaches for most descending thoracic, many thoracoabdominal, and the majority of isolated abdominal AAS has been observed [2].

The primary treatment goal of open surgery for AD is to ensure the patient's survival and terminate acute end-organ malperfusion, while prevention of future adverse events from the structurally injured aortic wall is an important secondary

K. von Aspern · C. D. Etz · M. A. Borger (✉)
University Department of Cardiac Surgery, Heart Center Leipzig, Leipzig, Germany
e-mail: Michael.Borger@helios-gesundheit.de

J. S. Coselli et al. (eds.), *Aortic Dissection and Acute Aortic Syndromes*,
https://doi.org/10.1007/978-3-030-66668-2_43

goal. In IMH and PAU, the primary treatment goal is prevention of acute rupture or disease progression to AD. In this regard current guidelines recommend expeditious surgical treatment for all type A AD, IMH (Class I) and PAU (Class IIa). Complicated type B AAS should be managed endovascularly as the first line of treatment (Class I) [8, 9], while management of uncomplicated type B AAS remains a matter of debate. Currently an initial medical approach for type B AAS is recommended (Class I), however, outcome data for endovascularly treated patients (thoracic endovascular aortic repair, TEVAR) suggest a long-term benefit for these patients [10]. TEVAR has therefore been given a IIa recommendation for uncomplicated type B AAS [8, 10].

Diagnostic Considerations and Treatment Outcome

Since AAS share common features with regard to their pathophysiology and diagnostic challenges, a comprehensive approach for early diagnosis and risk stratification is important [2, 11]. Current guidelines for the diagnosis and treatment of AAS recommend pre-test assessments for all suspected cases (Class I) including echocardiography, computed tomography (CT), and magnetic resonance (MR) imaging according to local availability and expertise (Class I) [8, 9]. Developments in CT imaging, in particular, have led to strategies that are very helpful in discerning between AAS and the most common differential diagnoses, i.e. acute myocardial infarction, stroke and pulmonary embolism. The "triple rule-out" strategy using multislice CT imaging with ECG-gated protocols provides high sensitivity and specificity for an early diagnosis of AAS [12]. Advanced imaging devices and protocols, especially CT, also enable detection of additional unrelated, yet relevant and treatable comorbidities [13, 14].

Devastating outcomes have been reported for untreated AAS, particularly for acute type A AD and proximal IMH. Although outcomes of surgical intervention are better than AAS natural history studies, there is still room for improvement, particularly in AD patients with malperfusion syndromes [15]. Current nationwide analyses demonstrate operative mortalities between 17% and 23% [16–19], which have remained relatively stable over the last decade. With the exception of series reported from Japan and South Korea (operative mortality rates 9% and 13%, respectively) [1, 4, 20], registry based outcome data from Europe and the US seem comparable [16, 17].

Although a conclusive explanation as to why Japan and Korea have lower reported operative mortality rates cannot be given, some major differences between these countries and the US and Europe can be highlighted. Japan, for example, has a broader availability of CT imaging throughout the country. While the US and Germany have 44 and 35 CT scanners per one million inhabitants respectively, Japan has over 110 scanners available per one million inhabitants [21] (Fig. 1). The widespread availability and high utilization rates may enable more timely diagnosis and treatment in case of life-threatening AAS. Whether a direct association between

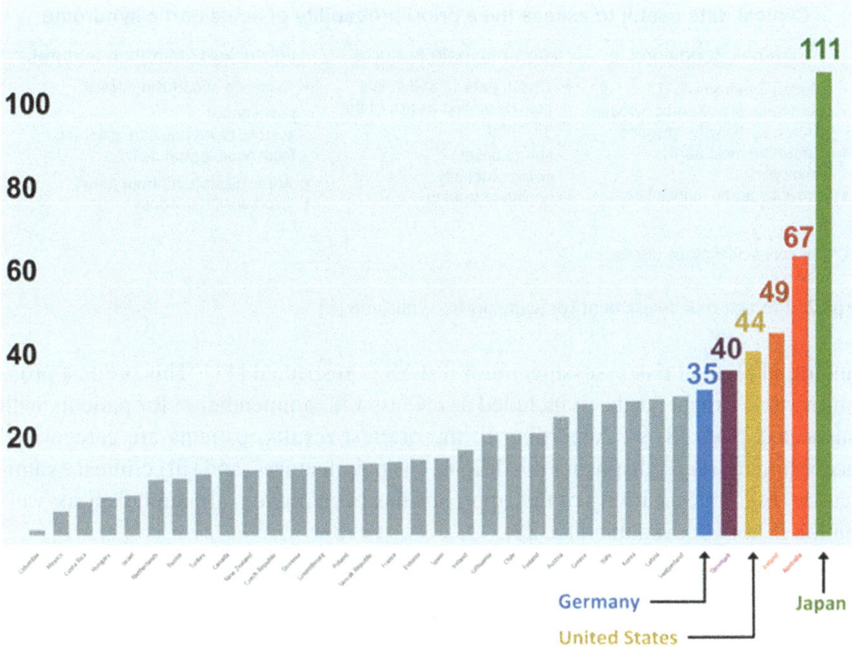

Fig. 1 International comparison of total availability for computed tomography (CT) scanners, shown as CT scanners per one million inhabitants. Top 6 in quantitative order = Japan, Australia, Iceland, United States, Denmark and Germany (figure modified order = from https://data.oecd.org, 2018)

CT availability and treatment outcome exists, however, is questionable given that South Korea has less available CTs and favourable operative mortality rates.

It seems likely that multiple factors influence operative outcome for AAS including the quantity and quality of reported data, disease awareness in the population, and existence of dedicated aortic centres and teams (see The Aortic Team section below). In addition, it is clear that better solutions for AD patients presenting with organ malperfusion need to be developed in order to improve operative mortality rates.

Current Classification Systems, Risk Stratification Tools and Algorithms for Acute Aortic Syndromes

Awareness on the part of all medical professions is pivotal for successful diagnosis and treatment of AAS, which is why several risk stratification models and classification systems were developed.

The American College of Cardiology and the European Society of Cardiology (and other professional societies) suggest a specific diagnostic algorithm as an easy

Clinical data useful to assess the a priori probability of acute aortic syndrome		
High-risk conditions	**High-risk pain features**	**High-risk examination features**
• Marfan Syndrome/CTD • Family history of aortic disease • Known aortic valve disease • Known thoracic aortic aneurysm • Previous aortic manipulation	• Chest, back or abdominal pain described as any of the following: - abrupt onset - severe intensity - ripping or tearing	• Evidence of perfusion deficit: - pulse deficit - systolic blood pressure difference - focal neurological deficit • Aortic diastolic murmur (new) • Hypotension or shock
CTD = connective tissue disease		

Fig. 2 Pre-test risk assessment for acute aortic syndrome [8]

and rapid clinical risk assessment tool if AAS is suspected [11]. This pre-test probability assessment has been included as a Class I recommendation for patients with suspected AAS [8, 9]. According to the pre-test results, patients are categorized according to: (i) predisposing conditions, (ii) pain features, and (iii) clinical examination (Fig. 2). Sensitivity of this approach has been proven, although data for validation is not yet available [17, 22].

Comparable tools, eg. the 'Aortic Dissection Detection Risk Score' (ADDRS) focusing on the clinical features in order to reduce the likelihood of initial misdiagnosis, have been shown to significantly reduce the time to adequate treatment [23]. The most distinct clinical features indicative of AAS were lumbar pain, paresis or sweating [23]. Once AAS is confirmed, additional risk stratification is needed for adequate decision-making with regard to the best-suited type of treatment (surgery vs. endovascular vs. hybrid). Another classification system recognized by the acronym DISSECT has been introduced to further specify the overall clinical and anatomical conditions. It encompasses six features: (i) duration, (ii) intimal tear, (iii) size of aorta, (iv) segmental extent of involvement, (v) clinical complications, and (vi) thrombosis of the false lumen [24]. This system serves as a supplementary to the universally used Stanford and DeBakey classifications.

As mentioned earlier, the primary goal for AAS treatment is to ensure immediate patient survival. Numerous large-scale single centre and registry analyses have shown that malperfusion represents the most potent risk factor for operative mortality in the setting of AAS, particularly for acute type A AD [16, 17, 19]. To address this correlation, the PENN classification system was developed as an easy-to-use clinical assessment tool to predict hospital mortality (Fig. 3) [25, 26].

The established Stanford classification for AD remains the basis for all other classification systems. However, in about 10% of acute aortic pathologies, the binary differentiation between A and B is not appropriate [27]. Therefore a subclassification has been introduced and adopted into clinical practice, categorizing patients with the entry in the descending aorta or arch with proximal extension limited to the arch without involvement of the ascending aorta as 'non-A non-B dissections' [28, 29]. In order to integrate this patient collective, the TEM classification for AAS has been recently developed [27]. According to TEM—which is based on the extended Stanford classification while also incorporating important clinical

PENN Classification in acute (Stanford) type A aortic dissection	
Class A_a	**no ischemia**
Class A_b	**localized ischemia** branch vessel malpersustion (e.g. stroke, renal failure, extremity or mesenteric ishemia)
Class A_c	**generalized ischemia** circulatory collapse with or without cardiac involvement
Class $A_{b\&c}$	**combined ischemia** localized and generalized ischemia together

Fig. 3 PENN classification for acute type A aortic dissection [26]

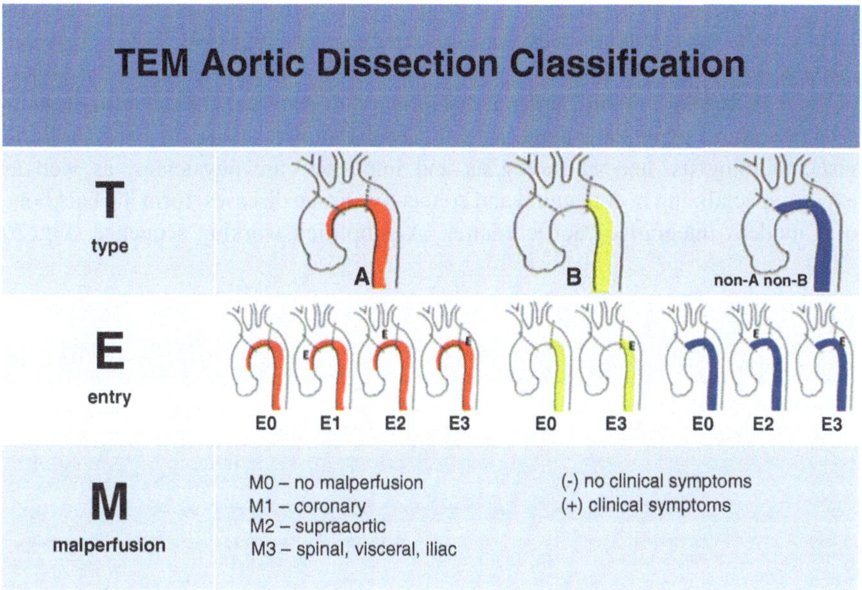

Fig. 4 TEM Aortic dissection classification system (created from [27])

aspects similar to the PENN system—patients are categorized with regard to the: (i) type, (ii) entry/pathology location, and (iii) malperfusion syndrome (Fig. 4). To date only retrospective analyses using the TEM system are available and larger studies are needed for validation.

All the herein described tools (including pre-test assessment and pathology classification systems) have been developed in order to facilitate an unambiguous nomenclature that ensures expeditious diagnosis and treatment. The multidisciplinary character of modern AAS treatment makes a comprehensive team approach to these challenging patients mandatory. The new classification systems will enable stratification of operative and long-term outcomes by crucial clinical risk factors, and enable objective comparisons of outcomes between reported series. Analyses of this data will contribute to future best practice guidelines and improve patient care for this challenging disease.

The Aortic Team: An Interdisciplinary Approach to Acute Aortic Syndromes

AAS patient survival depends on many factors encompassing various specialties within the medical sector. These factors include: (1) expeditious diagnosis, mainly by means of CT (radiology) or echocardiography (cardiology/ intensive care), (2) optimal medical care prior to and during transportation, and (3) a state-of-the-art repair strategy either by open surgery (cardiac/ vascular surgery), endovascular (interventional angiology/ radiology/cardiology), or hybrid procedures [2]. AAS by nature oftentimes involve several aortic segments and traditional borders between medical disciplines are crossed regularly. Treatment should therefore be the subject of joint discussions within an interdisciplinary Aortic Team. Such a multidisciplinary team of experienced cardiac and vascular surgeons, angiologists, cardiologists, radiologists, anaesthesiologists and intensive care physicians, as well as experts specializing in congenital and connective tissue diseases, form the backbone of a modern integrative "aortic centre". A simplified working sequence (Fig. 5)

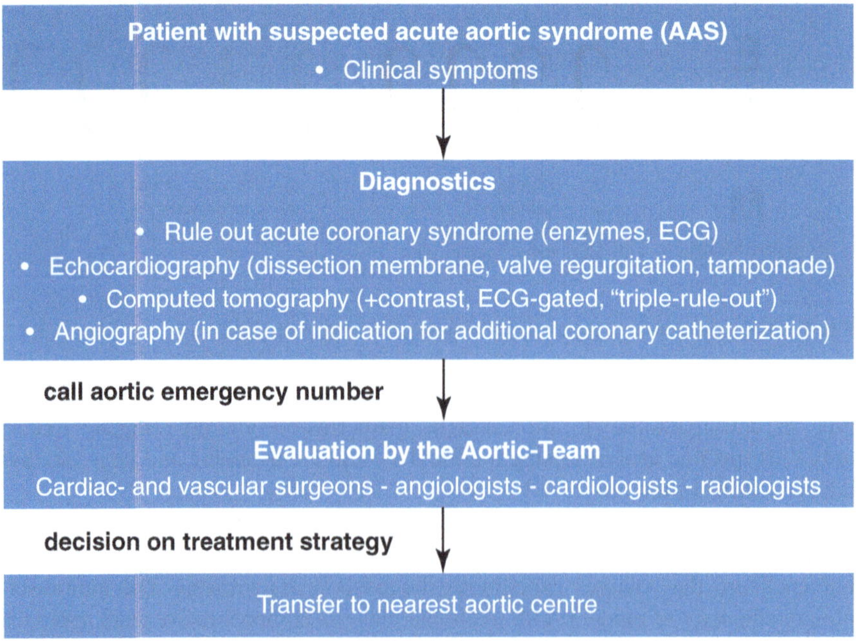

Fig. 5 Working sequence for AAS according to the aortic team principle (created from [2])

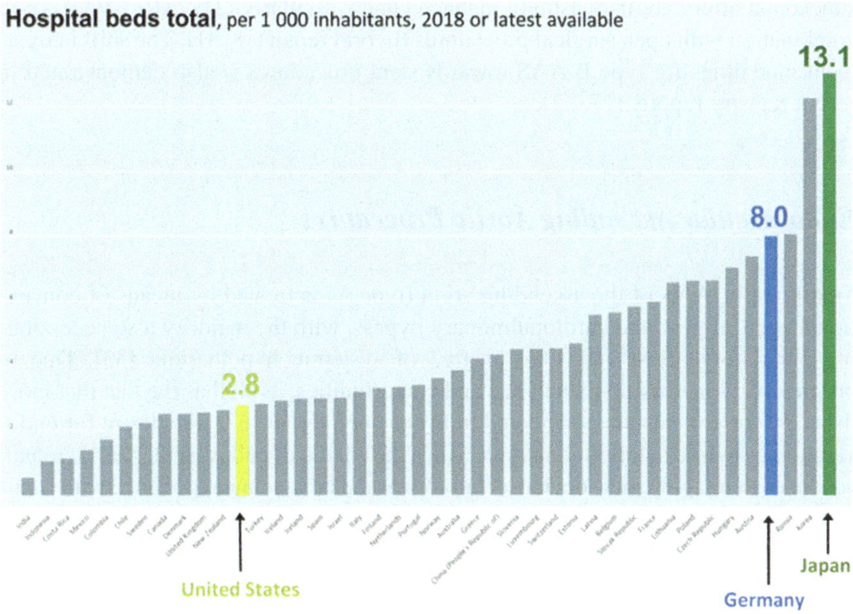

Fig. 6 Number of acute care hospital beds per 1000 inhabitants—international comparison. Highlighted countries: Japan, Germany and United States [21]

incorporating all necessary logistics facilitates smooth and timely patient allocation and treatment as well as subsequent follow-up.

According to recent observational data, implementation of integrative aortic centres and teams is increasing in Europe. In the United States, many specialized and experienced high-volume centres already incorporate infrastructures similar to the herein suggested key elements with great success. However, given the large overall population and differences within regional medical sectors (Fig. 6), a general awareness and optimization of existing structures seems warranted, both in the US and Europe [2].

Initial benefits from an integrative Aortic Team approach may be the decreasing time period from AAS symptom onset to diagnosis and subsequent treatment, which is significantly lower in Europe than in the US (Europe median 6 h, IQR: 3–24 h vs. US median: 15.3 h, IQR: 4.4–48 h; $p < 0.001$) [30].

New Treatment Developments

Open surgical aortic repair remains the mainstay for acute pathologies of the proximal aorta, including the ascending aorta and root as well as the proximal and transverse aortic arch [2, 8, 9]. Acute pathologies of aortic segments distal to the left subclavian artery are increasingly managed endovascularly (TEVAR/ EVAR) or in combination with open surgical procedures (hybrid repair) [8, 31]. The shift in treatment modalities for type B AAS towards stent procedures is also demonstrated in recent registry reports [17, 32].

Endovascular Ascending Aortic Procedures

Traditionally, AAS of the ascending aorta (type A) is treated by means of conventional open surgery and cardiopulmonary bypass, with the majority also necessitating circulatory arrest and some degree of systemic hypothermia [33]. Due to progressively increasing patient age and comorbidities, as well as the fact that more than 25% of patients are considered unfit for open repair [33], the desire for endovascular or hybrid solutions emerged. Since the advent of endovascular aortic repair, advances in imaging, new device technologies and advancing experience with minimally invasive procedures in general have led to a rapid expansion for stent-based treatment indications for aortic pathologies, pushing the boundaries of traditional, anatomical borders between surgeons and interventionists.

To date, few case reports and clinical series regarding endovascular treatment of the ascending aorta for highly selected high-risk AAS patients have been published, with encouraging early results and a technical success rate over 95% [33, 34]. However, patient selection and outcome criteria for proximal aortic TEVAR procedures are controversial [34, 35]. Available data on endovascular ascending aortic repair includes about 60% AAS patients, with the remainder being treated due to aneurysms or pseudoaneurysms [33]. Endovascular repair of the ascending aorta is challenging because of its proximity to the aortic arch and supra-aortic vessels, its curvilinear form, and challenges related to the proximal fixation close to the aortic valve and coronary ostia. Moreover, the ascending aorta is subject to considerable hemodynamic movement and stress during the cardiac cycle and respiration, which further complicates the procedure [33, 34]. In case of acute type A AD, the complexity of the false and true lumen arrangement and potential valve complications oftentimes preclude endovascular repair also in high risk patients unfit for surgery. Challenges with the aortic valve are particularly relevant since the entry tear is frequently located relatively close to the sinotubular junction.

Although a number of different custom-made stent types have been used for endovascular ascending aortic repair, almost all commercially available devices are specifically designed for the descending thoracoabdominal aorta [33], with the exception being the Zenith Ascend TAA Endovascular Graft (Cook Medical, Bloomington, IN; Fig. 7).

The usual device delivery approach—similar to transcatheter aortic valve replacement (TAVR) procedures—is transfemoral (~67%) or transapical (~13%). Alternative approaches are through the left or right carotid or axillary artery (~20%)

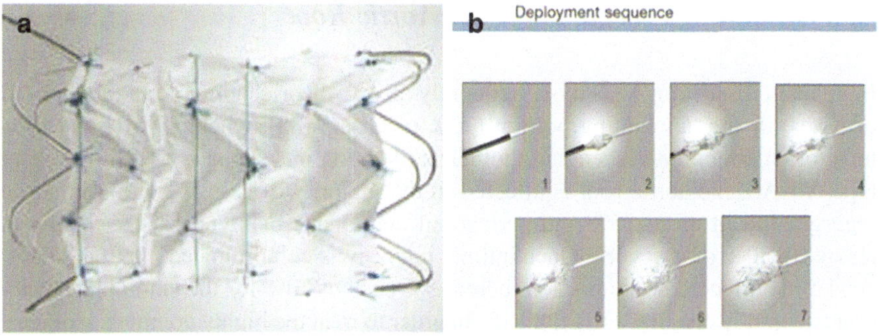

Fig. 7 Zenith Ascend TAA endovascular graft (Cook Medical, Bloomington, IN) (**a**) Stent graft, (**b**) Deployment sequence [36]

[33]. In order to facilitate steady stent placement, rapid ventricular pacing is most commonly used during implantation. Transesophageal echocardiography for adequate procedural guidance has been utilized in the majority of cases.

Perioperative and short-term outcomes for patients treated by TEVAR for the ascending aorta seems encouraging, with a low early conversion rate of less than 1%. Although operative mortality rates have been reported to be approximately 2–4%, early branch vessel occlusion after ascending aortic TEVAR and endoleak (mainly type Ia and Ib) were common in about 12% and 16% of high-risk patients, respectively [33].

To date a major drawback of the procedure remains its applicability, which is limited to highly selected patients with the pathology within a narrow anatomic margin of the ascending aorta. In the case of AD, the intimal tear has to be more than 10 mm above the sinotubular junction and less than 5 mm proximal to the innominate artery. As a result, current experience consists of grafts shorter than 10 cm [33, 34]. Although feasibility for this procedure has been reported in highly selected patients, a multidisciplinary team approach seems mandatory in order to provide adequate patient selection and good procedural outcomes.

In addition to the endovascular treatment of the ascending aorta, few reports and feasibility studies have been conducted using modular, multi-stent approaches for complex treatment of the ascending aorta and arch in AAS [37]. The combination of ascending prostheses with custom made arch prosthesis and side-branches after preliminary carotid-subclavian bypass represents a manageable alternative for high risk patients deemed unfit for emergency surgery [37]. In our opinion, patient selection should be limited strictly to 'high-risk/unfit for surgery' candidates, and performed by an experienced cardiac surgeon within the confines of a multidisciplinary aortic team.

Currently, neither long-term data nor standardized protocols are available for these procedures, warranting larger studies and longer follow up for patients eligible to these novel therapeutic options. Open repair remains the benchmark for these devices.

Endovascular Procedures for the Aortic Root

In general, dissecting AAS most frequently affects the ascending aorta (about 60% of cases) or the descending portion (30% of cases) [38], whereas IMH and PAU most often affect the descending thoracic and abdominal segments [38]. In case of type A AAS, the aortic root is affected in the majority of cases resulting in aortic regurgitation in up to 75% and pericardial tamponade or myocardial ischemia in about 10–20% of cases [8]. Once intimal integrity is compromised, the total diameter of the affected aortic portion increases by about 30% for the sinotubular junction and mid-ascending aorta [39, 40]. In order to treat the highly complex geometry of an acutely injured aortic root—including an altered and frequently regurgitant valve—transcatheter aortic valve procedures in combination with custom-made ascending aortic prostheses have been proposed [41, 42]. However, commercially available self-expandable prostheses are currently only applicable for patients with proximal aortic dimensions smaller than 45 mm [42]. Furthermore, the conundrum of the aortic sinus and the origin of the coronary arteries remain a major obstacle with regard to a fully endovascular treatment of the aortic root.

Initial design and strategy studies have been conducted and delineated several key elements required for a potential complete endovascular solution [42]. Dimensions of both device components need to be defined according to individual imaging studies and the connection between the prosthetic aortic valve and the tubular graft should be coupled in the operating room using clips or single sutures prior to implantation. With regard to achieving unobstructed coronary blood flow, the tubular graft in the proximal portion needs to be uncovered. The endovascular composite valved graft should be implantable from a central or peripheral location (transapical or transfemoral route) in a single-stage procedure, as would be necessary in the setting of AAS [42]. This concept—originally developed for patients with severe aortic stenosis and concomitant ascending aortic aneurysm who are otherwise unfit for open surgery—has been termed the "endo-Bentall", due to its analogy to the surgical root replacement technique [41–43] (Fig. 8).

Conceptualization of the 'endo-Bentall' implies three landing zone regions in order to provide adequate sealing between the covered graft portion and the aortic wall. The first and second landing zone regions are the aortic valve annulus and the sinotubular junction, respectively. The third landing zone region is the distal ascending aorta or proximal aortic arch [41–43]. A recent exploratory study examining the anatomical requirements for an endovascular valve–carrying conduit in the setting of acute type A AD demonstrates that, in theory, up to 68% of all patients could benefit from this novel strategy. However, most patients would require tapered stent-grafts to adequately match aortic root and ascending anatomy [43]. These estimations, however, exclusively focus on the anatomic conditions, not taking into consideration the clinical circumstances and the central issue in AAS, namely the urgency and dynamic nature of the pathology. Without sufficient time to individually design and fabricate an appropriate prosthesis (custom-made), many problems

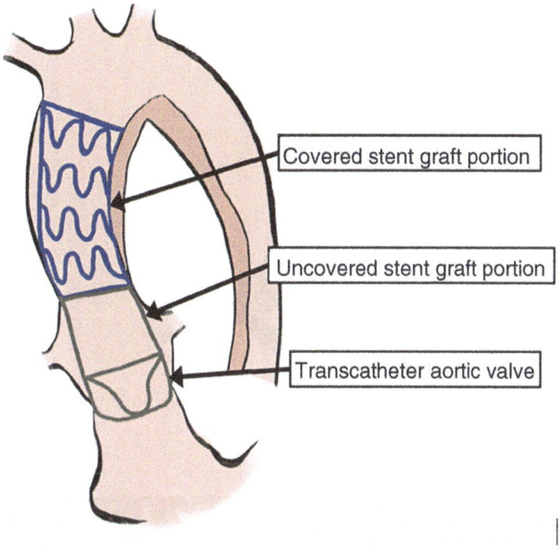

Fig. 8 'Endo-Bentall' conceptualization schematic for aortic root procedures (created from [43]

inherent to this highly variable pathology may not be adequately addressed. Nonetheless—although still in early development—the 'endo-Bentall' may become a promising alternative for otherwise inoperable patients suffering from type A AAS.

Novel Hybrid Approaches to the Aortic Arch

With the introduction of endovascular aortic procedures into the armamentarium of comprehensive aortic repair strategies, hybrid procedures have become a reasonable alternative for various, complex pathologies. Preparatory surgical procedures such as carotid-subclavian bypass or complete debranching have facilitated endovascular aortic repair beyond traditional anatomic borders. Surgical techniques for aortic arch repair using a 'Frozen Elephant Trunk' technique have further simplified subsequent endovascular procedures.

Optimal therapy for acute type A AD ensures patient survival and limits the necessity of secondary procedures. Key elements include resection of the primary entry, elimination of malperfusion, and reinstitution of true lumen perfusion with subsequent positive aortic remodelling/ false lumen thrombosis. Since patency of the false lumen after hemiarch repair of acute DeBakey type I aortic dissection is reported to be up to 70%, patients with untreated false lumen patency develop unfavourable remodelling during the course of follow up [44, 45]. In addition, approximately 50–70% of patients develop distal anastomotic new entry (DANE) sites after hemiarch repair, which are associated with worse downstream aortic remodelling and worse long-term survival [46, 47].

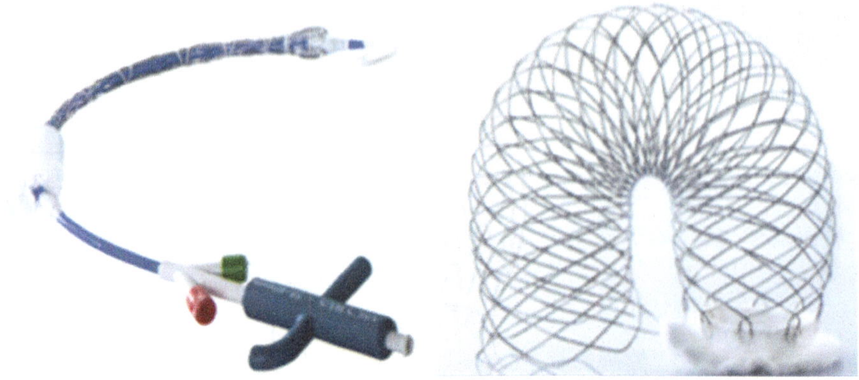

Fig. 9 Ascyrus composite graft. (left) Deployment system and (right) composite prosthesis [44, 45]

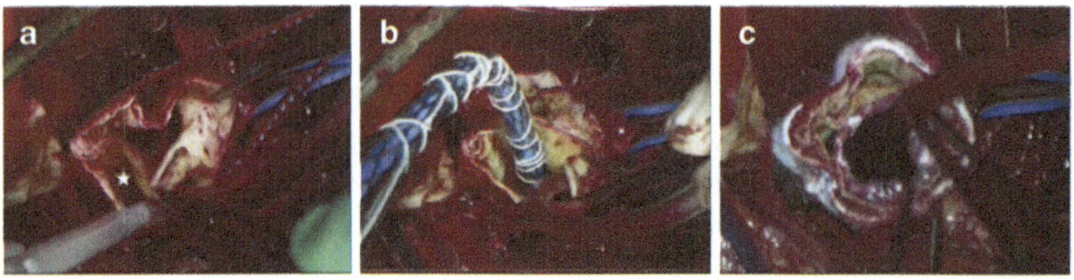

Fig. 10 Ascyrus stent-graft implantation sequence during surgical aortic arch repair [45]. (**a**) dissected aorta (white star indicates the true lumen), (**b**) antegrade insertion of the Ascyrus stent-graft and (**c**) fully deployed Ascyrus stent-graft with the proximal felt sewing cuff visible

To address this problem, a novel composite prosthesis has been designed and recently trialled with regard to its clinical feasibility. The Ascyrus Medical Dissection Stent (AMDS; Ascyrus Medical, Boca Raton, FL) is a partially uncovered aortic arch hybrid graft implanted antegradely during open aortic repair to reduce false lumen perfusion and promote true lumen expansion [44, 45] (Fig. 9).

The device consists of a proximal sewing cuff for the distal aortic anastomosis and an asymmetric helical stent frame for true lumen expansion within the aortic arch and proximal descending aorta [44, 45]. Low outward force of the stent intends to limit iatrogenic damage to the injured and friable aorta (Fig. 10). In addition, the felt sewing ring combined with the radial force of the attached stent results in a strong seal between the dissected aortic layers at the distal suture line, and therefore lower chance of DANE formation.

Initial results in about 50 patients for this new device are promising. Since the AMDS device is primarily intended for type A AD patients presenting with malperfusion syndrome, this cohort seems to benefit most from the stent-based intimal stabilization avoiding complex arch repair and supra-aortic vessel re-implantation. Vessel malperfusion was corrected in over 95% of patients in a small clinical trial,

[45] with an operative mortality of 7.7% in this high-risk malperfusion cohort. Furthermore, all patients with neurologic deficits at presentation recovered completely, while about 8% developed new neurologic deficits postoperatively [44, 45]. -Future studies on larger cohorts, including long-term follow-up and sequential imaging, are required to evaluate device benefits and its clinical significance in comparison to established surgical alternatives.

Summary

Since the first post-mortem description of AAS by Morgagni in 1761, this pathology has challenged the medical and scientific community across many specialties regarding appropriate diagnostic and management strategies [48]. The true incidence of AAS is still uncertain due to the likely substantial number of undiagnosed cases. Recent epidemiologic analyses from Europe have estimated the true incidence for AAS at approximately 12 cases per 100,000 inhabitants per year.

Registry-based, multicentre data reveal an operative mortality of approximately 20% for the surgical treatment of type A AAS, and has remained relatively stable over the last decade. Data from Japan and South Korea, however, have consistently demonstrated lower operative mortalities for this pathology. The reason for these observed differences is likely multifactorial, but a generally heightened awareness for AAS, the implementation of dedicated aortic centres and teams, and the widespread availability of computed tomography likely play a role. Various risk stratification tools and the "triple rule out" strategy may lead to further reductions in mortality in patients with AAS.

With the advent of stent-based aortic repair, a tremendous shift towards endovascular approaches for descending and abdominal AAS has occurred.

As age and comorbidities of patients with AAS are steadily increasing, catheter-based treatment modalities of ascending aorta and arch pathologies have been increasingly developed. A novel device for hybrid stenting of the aortic arch and descending aorta during type A AD repair appears particularly promising. In addition, novel therapeutic options for the treatment of AAS involving the aortic root are being actively investigated. Although several anatomic and technical challenges remain for these procedures, good initial success rates have been reported in highly selected patients. Much more data with longer-term follow will be required, however, before such devices become a standard approach in the management of AAS of the ascending aorta and arch.

References

1. Abe T, Yamamoto H, Miyata H, Motomura N, Tokuda Y, Tanemoto K, Usui A, Takamoto S. Patient trends and outcomes of surgery for type A acute aortic dissection in Japan: an analysis of more than 10 000 patients from the Japan Cardiovascular Surgery Database. Eur J Cardiothorac Surg. 2020 Apr 1;57(4):660–7.

2. Haunschild J, von Aspern K, Scheinert D, Schmidt A, Borger MA, Etz CD. Interdisciplinary treatment of aortic diseases: the A-team. Z Herz- Thorax- Gefäßchir. 2019;33:446–53.
3. Kurz SD, Falk V, Kempfert J, Gieb M, Ruschinski TM, Kukucka M, Tsokos M, Grubitzsch H, Herbst H, Semmler J, Buschmann C Insight into the incidence of acute aortic dissection in the German region of Berlin and Brandenburg. Int J Cardiol [Multicenter Study] 2017 Aug 15;241:326–329.
4. Okita Y. Current surgical results of acute type A aortic dissection in Japan. Ann Cardiothorac Surg. 2016 Jul;5(4):368–76.
5. Olsson C, Thelin S, Stahle E, Ekbom A, Granath F. Thoracic aortic aneurysm and dissection: increasing prevalence and improved outcomes reported in a nationwide population-based study of more than 14,000 cases from 1987 to 2002. Circulation. [Research Support, Non--U.S. Gov't]. 2006 Dec 12;114(24):2611–2618.
6. DeStatis. Federal Office of Statistics (Germany). 2018 (online). Accessed May 2020.
7. DeMartino RR, Sen I, Huang Y, Bower TC, Oderich GS, Pochettino A, Greason K, Kalra M, Johnstone J, Shuja F, Harmsen WS, Macedo T, Mandrekar J, Chamberlain AM, Weiss S, Goodney PP, Roger V Population-based assessment of the incidence of aortic dissection, intramural hematoma, and penetrating ulcer, and its associated mortality from 1995 to 2015. Circ Cardiovasc Qual Outcomes. [Research Support, N.I.H., Extramural Research Support, Non-U.S. Gov't]. 2018 Aug;11(8):e004689.
8. Erbel R, Aboyans V, Boileau C, Bossone E, Bartolomeo RD, Eggebrecht H, Evangelista A, Falk V, Frank H, Gaemperli O, Grabenwoger M, Haverich A, Iung B, Manolis AJ, Meijboom F, Nienaber CA, Roffi M, Rousseau H, Sechtem U, Sirnes PA, Allmen RS, Vrints CJ, Guidelines ESCCfP. 2014 ESC guidelines on the diagnosis and treatment of aortic diseases: document covering acute and chronic aortic diseases of the thoracic and abdominal aorta of the adult. The Task Force for the Diagnosis and Treatment of Aortic Diseases of the European Society of Cardiology (ESC). Eur Heart J. [Practice Guideline]. 2014 Nov 1;35(41):2873–2926.
9. Hiratzka LF, Bakris GL, Beckman JA, Bersin RM, Carr VF, Casey DE, Jr, Eagle KA, Hermann LK, Isselbacher EM, Kazerooni EA, Kouchoukos NT, Lytle BW, Milewicz DM, Reich DL, Sen S, Shinn JA, Svensson LG, Williams DM American College of Cardiology Foundation/American Heart Association Task Force on Practice G, American Association for Thoracic S, American College of R, American Stroke A, Society of Cardiovascular A, Society for Cardiovascular A, Interventions, Society of Interventional R, Society of Thoracic S, Society for Vascular M. 2010 guidelines for the diagnosis and management of patients with thoracic aortic disease. A report of the American College of Cardiology Foundation/American Heart Association Task Force on Practice Guidelines, American Association for Thoracic Surgery, American College of Radiology,American Stroke Association, Society of Cardiovascular Anesthesiologists, Society for Cardiovascular Angiography and Interventions, Society of Interventional Radiology, Society of Thoracic Surgeons,and Society for Vascular Medicine. J Am Coll Cardiol. [Practice Guideline] 2010 Apr 6;55(14):e27–e129.
10. Nienaber CA, Kische S, Rousseau H, Eggebrecht H, Rehders TC, Kundt G, Glass A, Scheinert D, Czerny M, Kleinfeldt T, Zipfel B, Labrousse L, Fattori R, Ince H, Trial I-X Endovascular repair of type B aortic dissection: long-term results of the randomized investigation of stent grafts in aortic dissection trial. Circ Cardiovasc Interv. [Randomized Controlled Trial Research Support, Non-U.S. Gov't]. 2013 Aug;6(4):407–416.
11. Bossone E, LaBounty TM, Eagle KA. Acute aortic syndromes: diagnosis and management, an update. Eur Heart J. [Research Support, Non-U.S. Gov't Review]. 2018 Mar 1;39(9):739–749d.
12. Chae MK, Kim EK, Jung KY, Shin TG, Sim MS, Jo IJ, Song KJ, Chang SA, Song YB, Hahn JY, Choi SH, Gwon HC, Lee SH, Kim SM, Eo H, Choe YH, Choi JH Triple rule-out computed tomography for risk stratification of patients with acute chest pain. J Cardiovasc Comput Tomogr. [Observational Study]. 2016 Jul-Aug;10(4):291–300.
13. Patel A, Mahendran K, Collins M, Abdelaziz M, Khogali S, Luckraz H. Incidental abnormal CT scan findings during transcatheter aortic valve implantation assessment: incidence and implications. Open Heart. 2018;5(2):e000855.

14. Voigt P, Fahnert J, Schramm D, Bach AG, Kahn T, Surov A. Clinically relevant incidental cardiovascular findings in CT examinations. Radiologe. [Review]. 2017 Apr;57(4):296–301.
15. Leontyev S, Legare JF, Borger MA, Buth KJ, Funkat AK, Gerhard J, Mohr FW Creation of a scorecard to predict in-hospital death in patients undergoing operations for acute type A aortic dissection. Ann Thorac Surg. [Multicenter Study]. 2016 May;101(5):1700–1706.
16. Conzelmann LO, Weigang E, Mehlhorn U, Abugameh A, Hoffmann I, Blettner M, Etz CD, Czerny M, Vahl CF Investigators G. Mortality in patients with acute aortic dissection type A: analysis of pre- and intraoperative risk factors from the German Registry for Acute Aortic Dissection Type A (GERAADA). Eur J Cardiothorac Surg. [Multicenter Study Research Support, Non-U.S. Gov't]. 2016 Feb;49(2):e44–e52.
17. Berretta P, Patel HJ, Gleason TG, Sundt TM, Myrmel T, Desai N, Korach A, Panza A, Bavaria J, Khoynezhad A, Woznicki E, Montgomery D, Isselbacher EM, Di Bartolomeo R, Fattori R, Nienaber CA, Eagle KA, Trimarchi S, Di Eusanio M. IRAD experience on surgical type A acute dissection patients: results and predictors of mortality. Ann Cardiothorac Surg. 2016 Jul;5(4):346–51.
18. Etz CD, von Aspern K, Hoyer A, Girrbach FF, Leontyev S, Bakhtiary F, Misfeld M, Mohr FW Acute type A aortic dissection: characteristics and outcomes comparing patients with bicuspid versus tricuspid aortic valve. Eur J Cardiothorac Surg. [Comparative Study]. 2015 Jul;48(1):142–150.
19. Etz CD, von Aspern K, da Rocha ESJ, Girrbach FF, Leontyev S, Luehr M, Misfeld M, Borger MA, Mohr FW. Impact of perfusion strategy on outcome after repair for acute type a aortic dissection. Ann Thorac Surg. 2014 Jan;97(1):78–85.
20. Cho JR, Shin S, Kim JS, Ko YG, Hong MK, Jang Y, Seung KB, Park HS, Tahk SJ, Lim DS, Jeon DW, Chae IH, Kim DK, Yoon J, Jeong MH, Choi D. Clinical characteristics of acute aortic syndrome in korean patients: from the korean multi-center registry of acute aortic syndrome. Korean Circ J. 2012 Aug;42(8):528–37.
21. OECD OECD Health statistics – health care resources. 2018. https://www.oecd.org/health/*
22. Rogers AM, Hermann LK, Booher AM, Nienaber CA, Williams DM, Kazerooni EA, Froehlich JB, O'Gara PT, Montgomery DG, Cooper JV, Harris KM, Hutchison S, Evangelista A, Isselbacher EM, Eagle KA, Investigators I. Sensitivity of the aortic dissection detection risk score, a novel guideline-based tool for identification of acute aortic dissection at initial presentation: results from the international registry of acute aortic dissection. Circulation. [Research Support, Non-U.S. Gov't Validation Study]. 2011 May 24;123(20):2213–2218.
23. Zaschke L, Habazettl H, Thurau J, Matschilles C, Gohlich A, Montagner M, Falk V, Kurz SD. Acute type A aortic dissection: aortic dissection detection risk score in emergency care – surgical delay because of initial misdiagnosis. Eur Heart J Acute Cardiovasc Care. 2020 Mar;30:2048872620914931.
24. Dake MD, Thompson M, van Sambeek M, Vermassen F, Morales JP, Investigators D. DISSECT: a new mnemonic-based approach to the categorization of aortic dissection. Eur J Vasc Endovasc Surg. [Research Support, Non-U.S. Gov't]. 2013 Aug;46(2):175–190.
25. Pisano C, Balistreri CR, Torretta F, Capuccio V, Allegra A, Argano V, Ruvolo G Penn classification in acute aortic dissection patients. Acta Cardiol. [Research Support, Non-U.S. Gov't]. 2016 Apr;71(2):235–240.
26. Augoustides JG, Geirsson A, Szeto WY, Walsh EK, Cornelius B, Pochettino A, Bavaria JE Observational study of mortality risk stratification by ischemic presentation in patients with acute type A aortic dissection: the Penn classification. Nat Clin Pract Cardiovasc Med. [Research Support, Non-U.S. Gov't]. 2009 Feb;6(2):140–146.
27. Sievers HH, Rylski B, Czerny M, Baier ALM, Kreibich M, Siepe M, Beyersdorf F. Aortic dissection reconsidered: type, entry site, malperfusion classification adding clarity and enabling outcome prediction. Interact Cardiovasc Thorac Surg. 2020 Mar 1;30(3):451–7.
28. Rylski B, Perez M, Beyersdorf F, Reser D, Kari FA, Siepe M, Czerny M. Acute non-A non-B aortic dissection: incidence, treatment and outcome. Eur J Cardiothorac Surg. 2017 Dec 1;52(6):1111–7.

29. Pasic M, Knollman F, Hetzer R. Isolated non-A, non-B dissection of the aortic arch. N Engl J Med. [Case Reports Letter]. 1999 Dec 2;341(23):1775.
30. Raghupathy A, Nienaber CA, Harris KM, Myrmel T, Fattori R, Sechtem U, Oh J, Trimarchi S, Cooper JV, Booher A, Eagle K, Isselbacher E, Bossone E International Registry of Acute Aortic Dissection I, Geographic differences in clinical presentation, treatment, and outcomes in type A acute aortic dissection (from the International Registry of Acute Aortic Dissection). Am J Cardiol. [Research Support, Non-U.S. Gov't]. 2008 Dec 1;102(11):1562–1566.
31. Debakey ME, Henly WS, Cooley DA, Morris GC Jr, Crawford ES, Beall AC Jr. Surgical management of dissecting aneurysms of the aorta. J Thorac Cardiovasc Surg. 1965 Jan;49:130–49.
32. Yuan X, Mitsis A, Tang Y, Nienaber CA. The IRAD and beyond: what have we unravelled so far? Gen Thorac Cardiovasc Surg. [Review]. 2019 Jan;67(1):146–153.
33. Baikoussis NG, Antonopoulos CN, Papakonstantinou NA, Argiriou M, Geroulakos G. Endovascular stent grafting for ascending aorta diseases. J Vasc Surg. [Meta-Analysis Review Systematic Review]. 2017 Nov;66(5):1587–1601.
34. Nienaber CA, Sakalihasan N, Clough RE, Aboukoura M, Mancuso E, Yeh JS, Defraigne JO, Cheshire N, Rosendahl UP, Quarto C, Pepper J Thoracic endovascular aortic repair (TEVAR) in proximal (type A) aortic dissection: ready for a broader application? J Thorac Cardiovasc Surg. [Multicenter Study Video-Audio Media]. 2017 Feb;153(2):S3–S11.
35. Plichta RP, Hughes GC. Thoracic endovascular aortic repair for the ascending aorta: experience and pitfalls. Journal of Visualized Surgery. [Review]. 2018;4:92.
36. Ahmad K, Terp K, Andersen G, Hjortdal V. Aortic aneurysms and trans-apical endovascular repair in high risk heart transplant recipient, one year follow up. J Thorac Dis. [Case Reports]. 2015 Nov;7(11):E555–E559.
37. Kolbel T, Detter C, Carpenter SW, Rohlffs F, von Kodolitsch Y, Wipper S, Reichenspurner H, Debus ES, Tsilimparis N Acute type A aortic dissection treated using a tubular stent-graft in the ascending aorta and a multibranched stent-graft in the aortic arch. J Endovasc Ther. [Case Reports] 2017 Feb;24(1):75–80.
38. Tsai TT, Nienaber CA, Eagle KA. Acute aortic syndromes. Circulation. [Review]. 2005 Dec 13;112(24):3802–3813.
39. Rylski B, Munoz C, Beyersdorf F, Siepe M, Reser D, Carrel T, Schoenhoff F, Schlensak C, Lescan M, Eckstein HH, Reutersberg B, Erbel R, Janosi RA, Czerny M. How does descending aorta geometry change when it dissects? Eur J Cardiothorac Surg. 2018 Apr 1;53(4):815–21.
40. Rylski B, Blanke P, Beyersdorf F, Desai ND, Milewski RK, Siepe M, Kari FA, Czerny M, Carrel T, Schlensak C, Kruger T, Mack MJ, Brinkman WT, Mohr FW, Etz CD, Luehr M, Bavaria JE How does the ascending aorta geometry change when it dissects? J Am Coll Cardiol. [Multicenter Study]. 2014 Apr 8;63(13):1311–1319.
41. Kreibich M, Rylski B, Kondov S, Morlock J, Scheumann J, Kari FA, Schrofel H, Siepe M, Beyersdorf F, Czerny M. Endovascular treatment of acute type A aortic dissection-the Endo Bentall approach. Journal of visualized Surgery. 2018;4:69.
42. Rylski B, Szeto WY, Bavaria JE, Branchetti E, Moser W, Milewski RK. Development of a single endovascular device for aortic valve replacement and ascending aortic repair. J Card Surg. 2014 May;29(3):371–6.
43. Kreibich M, Soekeland T, Beyersdorf F, Bavaria JE, Schrofel H, Czerny M, Rylski B Anatomic feasibility of an endovascular valve-carrying conduit for the treatment of type A aortic dissection. J Thorac Cardiovasc Surg. [Research Support, Non-U.S. Gov't]. 2019 Jan;157(1):26–34 e21.
44. Bozso SJ, Nagendran J, MacArthur RGG, Chu MWA, Kiaii B, El-Hamamsy I, Cartier R, Shahriari A, Moon MC Dissected aorta repair through stent implantation trial: Canadian results. J Thorac Cardiovasc Surg. [Clinical Trial Multicenter Study Video-Audio Media]. 2019 May;157(5):1763–1771.
45. Bozso SJ, Nagendran J, Chu MWA, Kiaii B, El-Hamamsy I, Ouzounian M, Kempfert J, Starck C, Shahriari A, Moon MC Single-stage management of dynamic malperfusion using a novel

arch remodeling hybrid graft. Ann Thorac Surg. [Clinical Trial Multicenter Study Research Support, Non-U.S. Gov't]. 2019 Dec;108(6):1768–1775.
46. Evangelista A, Salas A, Ribera A, Ferreira-Gonzalez I, Cuellar H, Pineda V, Gonzalez-Alujas T, Bijnens B, Permanyer-Miralda G, Garcia-Dorado D Long-term outcome of aortic dissection with patent false lumen: predictive role of entry tear size and location. Circulation. [Research Support, Non-U.S. Gov't]. 2012 Jun 26;125(25):3133–3141.
47. Rylski B, Hahn N, Beyersdorf F, Kondov S, Wolkewitz M, Blanke P, Plonek T, Czerny M, Siepe M. Fate of the dissected aortic arch after ascending replacement in type A aortic dissection dagger. Eur J Cardiothorac Surg. 2017 Jun 1;51(6):1127–34.
48. Pretre R, Von Segesser LK. Aortic dissection. Lancet. [Review]. 1997 May 17;349(9063):1461–1464.

The manufacturer's authorised representative in the EU is Springer Nature Customer Service Centre GmbH, Europaplatz 3, 69115 Heidelberg, Germany. If you have any concerns regarding our products, please contact ProductSafety@springernature.com

Printed and bound by CPI Group (UK) Ltd, Croydon, CR0 4YY
30/09/2026
02225238-0018